Review of Surgery for ABSITE and Boards

Review of Surgery for ABSITE and Boards

Christian de Virgilio, MD, FACS

Vice Chair—Education and Director, General Surgery Residency Program,
Department of Surgery, Harbor–UCLA Medical Center, Torrance, California
Professor of Surgery, UCLA School of Medicine, Los Angeles, California

Arezou Tory Yaghoubian, MD

Surgery Resident, Department of Surgery, Harbor–UCLA Medical Center,
Torrance, California

Jennifer Ann Smith, MD

Surgery Resident, Harbor–UCLA Medical Center, Torrance, California

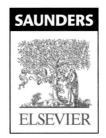

SAUNDERS

ELSEVIER

SAUNDERS
ELSEVIER

1600 John F. Kennedy Boulevard
Suite 1800
Philadelphia, PA 19103-2899

REVIEW OF SURGERY FOR ABSITE AND BOARDS   ISBN: 978-1-4160-4690-5

Library of Congress Cataloging-in-Publication Data

de Virgilio, Christian.
  Review of surgery for ABSITE and boards / Christian de Virgilio, Arezou Yaghoubian and Jennifer Smith. – 1st ed.
    p. ; cm.
  Includes bibliographical references.
  ISBN 978-1-4160-4690-5
1. Surgery–Examinations, questions, etc. 2. Surgeons–Licenses–United States–Examinations–Study guides. I. Yaghoubian, Arezou. II. Smith, Jennifer. III. Title. IV. Title: Review of surgery for American Board of Surgery In-Training Examination and Boards.
  [DNLM: 1. Critical Care–Examination Questions. 2. Surgical Procedures, Operative–Examination Questions. 3. Clinical Medicine–Examination Questions. 4. Specialty Boards. WO 18.2 D495r 2010]
  RD37.2D48 2010
  617.0076–dc22

                    2009034479

Acquisitions Editor: Judy Fletcher
Developmental Editor: Rachel Yard
Project Manager: Bryan Hayward
Design Direction: Lou Forgione

Printed in the United States of America

Last digit is the print number: 9 8 7 6 5 4 3 2

To my wife and fellow surgeon, Kelly, who patiently puts up with my quirks and idiosyncrasies; to my 4.5 kids, Nicholas, Michael, Emma, Sophia, and the highly anticipated but as yet unnamed progeny, who keep me entertained in life; and to the residents at Harbor–UCLA who serve as my academic muse.

—CD

Foreword

This book is a timely addition to learning material for surgical residents at all levels of training. It is in sync with the multitude of changes in surgical education based more on competency and also efficiency within the 80-hour work week. This publication is a product of the training program at Harbor–UCLA Medical Center, which has a disciplined and systematic approach in teaching conferences to include required reading and interactive sessions with the residents on pertinent topics on a weekly basis. This is a key component in their program to prepare trainees in not only clinical care but also preparation for the in-service exams as prepared by the American Board of Surgery. The book includes in 29 chapters the key components of general surgery and asks pertinent questions with answers that are appropriately referenced. This is the product of years of teaching and conferences, which now will be available to all programs preparing residents for eventual board certification. I compliment the authors, Christian de Virgilio, Arezou Yaghoubian, and Jennifer Smith, for their approach to surgical education and believe that this book will assist other program directors and trainees to achieve high levels of competency and success as they prepare the next generation of surgeons.

THOMAS RUSSELL, MD
Former Executive Director
American College of Surgeons

Preface

Eight years ago, I initiated a weekly American Board of Surgery In-Training Examination (ABSITE) and American Board of Surgery (ABS) review for the general surgery residents at Harbor–UCLA Medical Center. The original impetus behind the review was to stimulate the residents to read, to improve performance on the ABSITE, and to enhance the likelihood of passing the ABS examinations on the first try. The review consisted of weekly assigned reading from a major surgical textbook followed by weekly quizzes that I created based on the reading. The plan appeared to have worked, as the following year the mean score on the ABSITE for our residents was at the 75th national percentile.[1] We have continued to conduct the ABSITE/ABS review every year since and are pleased to see that there has been a sustained improvement in ABSITE scores.[2] We were even more delighted when we noticed an uptick in the pass rates of our graduating residents on the ABS Qualifying and Certifying Examinations.[3] In fact, over the past 5 years (2004–2009), the first-time pass rate for our residents is 96% for the qualifying examination and 100% for the certifying examination.

This review book is a compilation of the questions administered to our residents over these years. The intent is to try to cover the major topics in general surgery. Bear in mind, however, that no review book (this one included) can or should replace the importance of regular reading of a major surgical textbook. Many questions have been referenced to a surgical textbook or to the literature. Every effort was made to reference the pertinent papers related to the question or topic. The reference list is by no means comprehensive.

The ideal way to utilize this review book would be to create a reading program for yourself and write down your plan in advance. Read a chapter in a major surgical textbook (such as by Cameron, Sabiston, Schwartz, or Greenfield). After reading the chapter, answer the questions in our review book. Then proceed to read the responses in the back of each section. Go back to each question so that you gain a better understanding of why the incorrect answers are wrong. Then go to the selected references and read further on the topic. Be aware that when you take the ABSITE and ABS qualifying examinations, you will find that there is no textbook or review book that has all the answers. Some answers may be controversial. By approaching the learning process in a multipronged manner, you will maximize your chances of understanding the material and performing well on the examinations. Keep track of how you perform on each section, and if your relative performance in one section is poor, go back to that section again. Finally, add some stress to simulate the examination process. In other words, give yourself a time limit to complete each section. One minute per question is a good rule of thumb. Mild stress seems to facilitate learning.

As residency program director in surgery at Harbor UCLA, I have always advocated to our residents that knowledge provides an invaluable tool to the surgeon. Knowledge gives surgeons the confidence to know that they are providing the best possible care for their patients. Knowledge is also empowering, as it gives surgeons the self-assurance to teach others about the art and science of surgery. Good luck in your pursuit of knowledge. On behalf of my co-editors, I hope you find this review book useful.

References

1. de Virgilio C, Stabile BE, Lewis RJ, Brayack C: Significantly improved American Board of Surgery In-Training Examination scores associated with weekly assigned reading and preparatory examinations, *Arch Surg* 138:1195–1197, 2003.
2. de Virgilio C, Stabile BE: Weekly reading assignments and examinations result in sustained improvement in American Board of Surgery In-Training Examination (ABSITE) scores, *Am Surg* 71:830–832, 2005.
3. de Virgilio C, Chan T, Kaji A, Miller K: Weekly assigned reading and examinations during residency, ABSITE performance, and improved pass rates on the American Board of Surgery Examinations, *J Surg Educ* 65:499–503, 2008.

Acknowledgments

We would like to acknowledge the efforts of Elsevier for the timely preparation and publication of this review book, in particular Judith Fletcher, Publishing Director of Global Medicine, who initiated the development of this book, and supported it throughout production, and the contributions made by Rachel Yard, Editorial Assistant, and Louis Forgione, Senior Book Designer. In addition, we would like to thank the surgery faculty at Harbor–UCLA Medical Center who actively participated in the educational sessions, as well as the surgery residents. Our bright and highly motivated residents were the original inspiration and driving force behind this project.

Contents

Abdominal Wall/ Inguinal Hernias

1

1. Which of the following are true when comparing open mesh with laparoscopic mesh repair of first-time inguinal hernias?
   A. Laparoscopic repair has a lower recurrence rate.
   B. There is no difference in time to return to work.
   C. Open repair is superior.
   D. There is no difference in postoperative pain.
   E. Laparoscopic repair has a lower complication rate.

2. Which of the following is the best option for repair of a unilateral indirect inguinal hernia in a 4-month-old male infant?
   A. High ligation of the sac only
   B. Obliteration of the deep ring
   C. Tension-free repair with mesh
   D. Cooper ligament (McVay) repair
   E. Laparoscopic hernia repair

3. All of the following are good options for repair of a unilateral femoral hernia EXCEPT:
   A. Inguinal approach: Cooper ligament (McVay) repair
   B. Inguinal approach: approximating transverse fascia to inguinal ligament (Bassini operation)
   C. Inguinal approach: standard Lichtenstein tension-free repair with mesh
   D. Infrainguinal approach: polypropylene mesh plug
   E. Open preperitoneal approach

4. The Howship-Romberg sign is associated with which type of hernia?
   A. Spigelian hernia
   B. Richter hernia
   C. Pantaloon hernia
   D. Lumbar hernia
   E. Obturator hernia

5. Which of the following best describes umbilical hernias in children?
   A. They are more common in white children than those of African descent.
   B. Repair is indicated once an umbilical hernia is diagnosed.
   C. Repair should be performed if the hernia persists beyond 6 months of age.
   D. Most close spontaneously.
   E. Repair should be performed only if the child is symptomatic.

6. Which of the following is true regarding umbilical hernias in adults?
   A. Most are congenital.
   B. Repair is contraindicated in patients with cirrhosis.
   C. Strangulation is less common than in children.
   D. Small, asymptomatic hernias can be clinically observed.
   E. Primary closure has recurrence rates similar to those of mesh repair.

7. The hernia bounded by the latissimus dorsi muscle, iliac crest, and external oblique muscle is known as:
   A. Grynfeltt hernia
   B. Richter hernia
   C. Petit hernia
   D. Littre hernia
   E. Obturator hernia

8. Ischemic orchitis after inguinal hernia repair is most often due to:
   A. Too tight a reconstruction of the inguinal ring
   B. Preexisting testicular pathology
   C. Inadvertent ligation of the testicular artery
   D. Completely excising a large scrotal hernia sac
   E. Anomalous blood supply to the testicle

9. The genital branch of the genitofemoral nerve:
    A. Is typically found anteriorly on top of the spermatic cord
    B. Provides sensation to the base of the penis and inner thigh
    C. Typically lies on the anterior surface of the internal oblique muscle
    D. Provides sensation to the side of the scrotum and motor innervations to the cremaster muscle
    E. Often intermingles with the iliohypogastric nerve

10. Four months after inguinal hernia repair, a patient reports moderately severe persistent burning pain at the incision site that radiates to the groin. On examination, there is no evidence of recurrent hernia. Which of the following is true about this condition?
    A. Careful identification of all three sensory nerves will prevent this complication.
    B. Initial management involves wound reexploration.
    C. Local anesthetic nerve blocks are helpful in identifying the nerve involved.
    D. Chronic pain after hernia repair is uncommon.
    E. Reoperation for genitofemoral neuralgia is best approached via the groin.

11. All of the following are true regarding inguinal hernias in children EXCEPT:
    A. They are due to patency of the processus vaginalis.
    B. The incidence is higher in premature infants.
    C. Incarceration risk is higher in children younger than 6 months of age.
    D. Patients with incarcerated hernias should be taken immediately to the operating room.
    E. Right-sided hernias are more common than left-sided ones.

12. All of the following are true regarding hernia anatomy EXCEPT:
    A. The Poupart ligament forms from the inferior edge of the external oblique aponeurosis.
    B. The cremaster muscle arises from the transverse muscle.
    C. The genital branch of the genitofemoral nerve passes through the deep ring.
    D. Cremasteric vessels accompany the genital branch of the genitofemoral nerve.
    E. Indirect hernias arise lateral to the inferior epigastric vessels.

13. A femoral hernia passes:
    A. Anterior to the inguinal ligament
    B. Lateral to the femoral artery
    C. Posterior to the Cooper ligament
    D. Medial to the femoral vein
    E. Anterior to the iliopubic tract

14. Which of the following is true regarding the arcuate line?
    A. It is usually located a few centimeters above the umbilicus.
    B. Below this line, the internal oblique aponeurosis splits.
    C. Below this line, the rectus muscle lies on the transverse fascia.
    D. Below this line, the posterior rectus sheath is thinner.
    E. Below this line, the external oblique muscle does not contribute to the anterior rectus sheath.

15. All of the following statements about hernias in adults are true EXCEPT:
    A. In men, indirect hernias are the most common type.
    B. In women, indirect hernias are the most common type.
    C. Femoral hernias are more common in women.
    D. Umbilical hernias are more common in men.
    E. Aortic aneurysm is a risk factor for inguinal and incisional hernias.

16. A 45-year-old man presents with a small, asymptomatic reducible right inguinal hernia. Which of the following is true about this condition?
    A. The likelihood of incarceration developing is high without surgery.
    B. Without surgery, intractable pain will most likely develop.
    C. Waiting until symptoms develop is a reasonable alternative to surgery.
    D. Laparoscopic repair is the best option.
    E. Without surgery, he is likely to become incapacitated.

17. All of the following are true regarding spigelian hernias EXCEPT:
    A. They occur through the aponeurotic layer between the rectus abdominis muscle and semilunar line.
    B. They tend to be small.
    C. A palpable bulge on examination is uncommon.
    D. The risk of incarceration is low.
    E. A computed tomography scan is useful to establish the diagnosis.

Answers

1. C. In a large, prospective, randomized study comparing open mesh with laparoscopic mesh repair, the following significant findings were noted. Recurrences were more common in the laparoscopic group (10.1% vs. 4.9% in the open group). The rate of complications was higher in the laparoscopic group (39% vs. 33.4%). The laparoscopic group had less pain initially and at 2 weeks and returned to normal activities 1 day earlier. Recurrence rates after repair of recurrent hernias were similar (10.0% for laparoscopic repair and 14.1% for open repair).

Reference: Neumayer L, Giobbie-Harder A, Jonasson O: Open mesh versus laparoscopic mesh repair of inguinal hernia, *N Engl J Med* 350:1819–1827, 2004.

2. A. The etiology of inguinal hernias in infants is a patent processus vaginalis. There is generally no weakness in the floor of the inguinal canal. As such, high ligation of the sac is all that is required. On rare occasions when the hernia is very large, tightening of the internal inguinal ring or even formal repair of the inguinal floor may be necessary.

3. B. It is important to recognize that femoral hernias pass deep (posterior) to the inguinal ligament. As such, repairs to the inguinal ligament (such as a Bassini operation and standard mesh repair) will not obliterate the defect. The femoral hernia can be fixed either through a standard inguinal approach or directly over the bulge using an infrainguinal incision. The essential elements of femoral hernia repair include dissection and removal of the hernia sac and obliteration of the defect in the femoral canal, by either approximation of the iliopubic tract to the Cooper ligament or by placement of prosthetic mesh. Interrupted sutures are placed beginning at the pubic tubercle and continuing laterally along the Cooper ligament, progressively narrowing at the femoral ring. The last stitch to the Cooper ligament is known as a transition stitch and includes the inguinal ligament. Care must be taken not to injure or compress the external iliac vein at this position because it may lead to postoperative venous thrombosis. If the repair is done without mesh, a relaxing incision should always be used given the considerable tension required to span such a large distance. The polypropylene mesh plug (also called a "cigarette plug") technique uses a direct infrainguinal approach. After ligating the sac, a small piece of rolled-up mesh is inserted into the defect. In situations in which there is strangulated bowel in the femoral hernia, the use of mesh should be avoided. Options are either a Cooper ligament repair (without mesh) if using the inguinal approach or simple closure of the aponeurotic defect if using the infrainguinal approach.

4. E. The obturator canal is formed by the union of the pubic bone and ischium. The obturator membrane weakens and predisposes to formation of a hernia sac. It seems to occur more often in elderly, multiparous women with recent weight loss. The hernia is very rare, and the diagnosis is often missed preoperatively. Due to the narrow diameter of the defect, the small bowel is prone to incarceration and strangulation. Patients present with symptoms and signs of small bowel obstruction, but the preoperative diagnosis of obturator hernia is often missed. With the advent of computed tomography, the diagnosis is being made preoperatively with more frequency. Nevertheless, even with newer diagnostic modalities, the mortality rate remains high (11%–25%) due to the frequency of encountering gangrenous bowel and patients' advanced age. Primary closure of the hernia defect is difficult because adjacent tissues are not easily mobilized. For cases in which there is no suspicion of ischemic or dead bowel, the hernia can be repaired using a preperitoneal mesh repair. But in most instances, the hernia is discovered at laparotomy.

References: Bergstein J, Condon R: Obturator hernia: current diagnosis and treatment, *Surgery* 119:133–136, 1996.

Lobo D, Clarke D, Barlow A: Obturator hernia: a new technique for repair, *J R Coll Surg Edinb* 43:33–34, 1998.

5. D. In children, umbilical hernias are congenital. They are formed by a failure of the umbilical ring to close, causing a central defect in the linea alba. Most umbilical hernias in children are small and will close by 2 years of age, particularly if the defect is less than 1 cm in size. If closure does not occur by age 4 or 5 years, elective repair is reasonable. If the hernia defect is large (>2 cm) or the family is bothered by the cosmetic appearance, repair is also indicated. They are eight times more common in children of African descent. Umbilical hernias in children can rarely incarcerate. If the child presents with abdominal pain, bilious emesis, and a tender, hard mass protruding from the umbilicus, immediate exploration and hernia repair are indicated.

6. D. Unlike in children, umbilical hernias in adults are usually acquired. Risk factors are any conditions that increase intra-abdominal pressure, such as pregnancy, obesity, and ascites. Overall strangulation of umbilical hernias is uncommon, but occurs more often than in children. Small barely palpable and asymptomatic hernias can be followed clinically. Larger or symptomatic hernias should be repaired. In patients with cirrhosis and ascites, the markedly increased pressure causes the skin overlying the hernia to become thin and eventually ischemic. One of the most catastrophic complications in this setting is rupture of the hernia through the ischemic skin, leading to peritonitis and death. Thus, patients with cirrhosis and ascites should undergo repair if there is evidence that the skin overlying the hernia is thinning or becoming ischemic. However, repair should be delayed until after medical management of the ascites. If medical management fails and the skin over the hernia is thinned and tense, then a transjugular portosystemic shunt should be considered before repair. Alternatively, if the patient is a transplantation candidate, the hernia can be repaired during the transplantation. Umbilical hernias have historically all been repaired by primary closure. Borrowing from the low recurrence rates using mesh for inguinal hernias, umbilical hernias are now more frequently being repaired using mesh, particularly those with large defects. A recent prospective, randomized study compared primary closure with mesh repair. The early complication rates such as seroma, hematoma, and wound infection were similar in the two groups. However, the hernia recurrence rate was significantly higher after primary suture repair (11%) than after mesh repair (1%). Some authors are now advocating routine use of mesh for all adult umbilical hernias in the absence of bowel strangulation.

References: Arroyo A, García P, Pérez F, et al: Randomized clinical trial comparing suture and mesh repair of umbilical hernia in adults, *Br J Surg* 88:1321–1323, 2001.

Belghiti J, Durand F: Abdominal wall hernias in the setting of cirrhosis, *Semin Liver Dis* 17:219–226, 1997.

7. C. A Petit hernia is bound by the latissimus dorsi muscle, the iliac crest, and the external oblique muscle. A Grynfeltt hernia is a hernia bound by the sacrospinous muscle, the internal oblique muscle, and the 12th rib. A Richter hernia involves one wall of the bowel entering the hernia sac and then becoming incarcerated. It is particularly dangerous because the patient does not exhibit signs of bowel obstruction, yet there is a high risk of ischemia and gangrene of a small knuckle of bowel developing. A hernia containing a Meckel diverticulum is known as a Littre hernia.

8. D. The precise etiology of ischemic orchitis is unclear. The most commonly identified risk factor is extensive dissection of the spermatic cord. This occurs particularly when a patient has a large hernia sac, and the entire distal sac is dissected and excised. As such, it is recommended that the sac instead is divided and the distal sac left in situ. In addition, the cord should never be dissected past the pubic tubercle. Ischemic orchitis is thought to develop as a result of thrombosis of veins of the pampiniform plexus, leading to testicular venous congestion. It has thus been termed *congestive orchitis*. The presentation is that of a swollen, tender testicle, usually 2 to 5 days after surgery. The testicle is often high riding. This may eventually progress to testicular atrophy. Scrotal duplex ultrasonography has been shown to be useful in evaluating the perfusion of the testicle after hernia repair. However, it does not change the management of ischemic orchitis. Management is expectant. In the past, attempts to reexplore the groin were undertaken to try to loosen the internal ring, but this was not successful. The blood supply to the testicle is via the testicular artery, but there are rich collaterals including the external spermatic artery and the artery to the vas. Thus, inadvertent ligation of the testicle does not typically lead to this complication. Ischemic orchitis also occurs more frequently in recurrent inguinal hernia surgery using the anterior approach. Thus, the laparoscopic approach should be considered for recurrent hernias.

References: Holloway B, Belcher H, Letourneau J, et al: Scrotal sonography: a valuable tool in the evaluation of complications following inguinal hernia repair, *J Clin Ultrasound* 26:341–344, 1998.

Wantz G: Testicular atrophy and chronic residual neuralgia as risks of inguinal hernioplasty, *Surg Clin North Am* 73:571–581, 1993.

9. D. The genitofemoral nerve arises from the L1–L2 level. The genital branch innervates the cremaster muscle and sensation to the side of the scrotum and the labia. It is responsible for the cremasteric reflex. In women, it accompanies the round ligament of the uterus. The genital branch of the genitofemoral nerve is part of the cord structures. It lies on the iliopubic tract and accompanies the cremaster vessels. The ilioinguinal nerve lies on top of the spermatic cord. It innervates the internal oblique muscle and is sensory to the upper medial thigh adjacent to the genitalia. The nerve can sometimes splay out over the cord, making dissection difficult. The iliohypogastric and ilioinguinal nerves arise from the T12–L1 level and intermingle. They provide sensation to the skin of the groin, the base of the penis, and the upper medial thigh. The iliohypogastric nerve lies on the internal oblique muscle.

Reference: Wantz G: Testicular atrophy and chronic residual neuralgia as risks of inguinal hernioplasty, *Surg Clin North Am* 73:571–581, 1993.

10. C. Chronic pain after hernia repair is quite common and is present in as many as 10% to 25% of patients at 1 year after surgery. As such, it is imperative that this be discussed in the preoperative consent. The majority of neuralgias are self-limited, resolving within a few weeks of the operation. The etiology is thought to be entrapment of the nerve during surgery or postoperative scarring. Thus, careful identification and preservation of the nerves will not necessarily prevent this complication. In an effort to prevent this complication, some authors have recommended intentional division of the nerves. The results to date on this approach are mixed. Several randomized studies have been conducted. In one study, the risk of developing inguinal pain increased with the number of nerves not detected, and division of nerves was clearly correlated with presence of chronic pain. However, they found that the pain resolved with conservative management. In a second randomized study, pain after open hernia repair with polypropylene mesh was also not affected by elective division of the ilioinguinal nerve, but sensory disturbances in the area of distribution of the transected nerve are significantly increased. Conversely, another randomized study showed that prophylactic ilioinguinal neurectomy significantly decreased the incidence of chronic groin pain after Lichtenstein hernia repair without added morbidity. Initial management of neuralgias after open hernia repair should be conservative. Nerve blocks can help identify which nerve is the source of the problem. If conservative management does not resolve the pain, operative exploration and division of the nerve have met with success. Due to the location of the genitofemoral nerve, however, reopening the groin would not be feasible because the entire repair would need to be taken down. It is probably best managed via a posterior approach.

References: Alfieri S, Rotondi F, Di Giorgio A, et al: Influence of preservation versus division of ilioinguinal, iliohypogastric, and genital nerves during open mesh herniorrhaphy: prospective multicentric study of chronic pain, *Ann Surg* 243:553–558, 2007.

Lik-Man Mui W, Ng C: Prophylactic ilioinguinal neurectomy in open inguinal hernia repair: a double-blind randomized controlled trial, *Ann Surg* 244:27–33, 2006.

Picchio M, Palimento D, Attanasio U, et al: Randomized controlled trial of preservation or elective division of ilioinguinal nerve on open inguinal hernia repair with polypropylene mesh, *Arch Surg* 139:755–758, 2004.

Sherman V, Macho JR, Brunicardi FC: Inguinal hernias. In Brunicardi FC, Andersen DK, Billiar TR, et al, editors: *Schwartz's principles of surgery*, ed 9, New York, 2010, McGraw-Hill, pp 1305–1342.

Wijsmuller A, van Veen R, Bosch J, et al: Nerve management during open hernia repair, *Br J Surg* 94:17–22, 2007.

11. D. The vast majority of inguinal hernias in children are the indirect type due to a persistent patent processus vaginalis. Approximately 1% to 5% of children are born with or develop an inguinal hernia. However, the incidence increases in preterm infants and those with a low birth weight. Right-sided hernias are more common, and 10% of hernias diagnosed at birth are bilateral. Incarceration is a more serious problem in pediatric patients than in adults. Emergent operation on an infant with an incarcerated hernia can be very challenging. Thus, it is preferable to try to reduce the hernia, which is successful in 75% to 80% of cases, allow the inflammation to subside, and then perform the repair semielectively. Methods to achieve reduction include the use of IV sedation, Trendelenburg positioning, ice packs, and gentle direct pressure.

12. B. Poupart ligament is another name for the inguinal ligament. The inguinal ligament is formed from the anteroinferior portion of the external oblique aponeurosis folding back on itself. It extends from the anterosuperior iliac spine to the pubic tubercle, turning posteriorly to form a shelving edge. The cremaster muscle fibers arise from the internal oblique muscle and surround the spermatic cord. The genital branch of the genitofemoral nerve passes through the deep ring, whereas the ilioinguinal nerve passes through the superficial ring. Indirect hernias arise lateral to the inferior epigastric vessels, whereas direct hernias arise medial to the inferior epigastric vessels.

13. D. The boundaries of the femoral canal are the inguinal ligament anteriorly, the Cooper ligament posteriorly, and the femoral vein laterally. The pubic tubercle forms the apex of the femoral canal triangle. A femoral hernia occurs through this space and is medial to the femoral vessels.

14. C. Between the costal margin and the arcuate line, the anterior rectus sheath is made up of a combination of the aponeurosis of the external and internal oblique muscles. The posterior sheath is made up of a combination of the aponeuroses of the internal oblique and transverse abdominal muscles. Below the arcuate line, the anterior sheath is made up of the aponeuroses of all three abdominal muscles. There is no posterior sheath below the arcuate line, and the transverse fascia therefore makes up the posterior aspect of the rectus abdominis muscle.

15. D. Indirect hernias are the most common type of hernias regardless of sex. Femoral hernias are rare in men. In children, congenital umbilical hernias are more common in boys. In adults, acquired umbilical hernias are twice as common in women and are related to pregnancy. Aortic aneurysms are a risk factor for inguinal hernias and for the development of incisional hernias.

16. C. A recent large prospective, randomized study in men demonstrated that watchful waiting for patients with asymptomatic or minimally symptomatic inguinal hernias is an acceptable option to surgery. The patients were followed for as long as 4½ years. Acute hernia incarceration without strangulation developed in only one (0.3%) patient, and acute incarceration with bowel obstruction developed in only one. Approximately one fourth of the watchful waiting group eventually crossed over to receive surgical repair due to increased hernia-related pain.

Reference: Fitzgibbons R, Giobbie-Hurder A, Gibbs J, et al: Watchful waiting vs repair of inguinal hernia in minimally symptomatic men: a randomized clinical trial, *JAMA* 295:285–292, 2006.

17. D. Spigelian hernias are difficult to diagnose because the patient will report abdominal wall pain without an evident bulge on examination because these hernias are interparietal and posterior to the external oblique aponeurosis. They tend to be small with a narrow neck and, as such, are at risk of incarceration and should be repaired. They occur anywhere along the spigelian line, an aponeurotic band at the lateral border of the rectus abdominis muscle. They all occur at or below the arcuate line.

References: Malangoni MA, Rosen MJ: Hernias. In Townsend CM Jr, Beauchamp RD, Evers BM, Mattox KL, editors: *Sabiston textbook of surgery: the biological basis of modern surgical practice*, ed 18, Philadelphia, 2008, WB Saunders, pp 1155–1179.

Seymour NE, Bell RL: Abdominal wall, omentum, mesentery, and retroperitoneum. In Brunicardi FC, Andersen DK, Billiar TR, et al, editors: *Schwartz's principles of surgery*, ed 9, New York, 2010, McGraw-Hill, pp 1267–1281.

Sherman V, Macho JR, Brunicardi FC: Inguinal hernias. In Brunicardi FC, Andersen DK, Billiar TR, et al, editors: *Schwartz's principles of surgery*, ed 9, New York, 2010, McGraw-Hill, pp 1305–1342.

Turnage RH, Richardson KA, Li BD, McDonald JC: Abdominal wall, umbilicus, peritoneum, mesenteries, omentum, and retroperitoneum. In Townsend CM Jr, Beauchamp RD, Evers BM, Mattox KL, editors: *Sabiston textbook of surgery: the biological basis of modern surgical practice*, ed 18, Philadelphia, 2008, WB Saunders, pp 1129–1154.

Aneurysmal Disease and Vascular Trauma

2

1. Hypothenar hammer syndrome is best managed by:
   A. Avoidance of precipitating activity
   B. Aspirin
   C. Coumadin (warfarin)
   D. Resection and reconstruction of ulnar artery
   E. Stenting

2. Dysphagia lusoria is most likely associated with:
   A. Bovine arch
   B. Kommerell diverticulum
   C. Coarctation of the aorta
   D. Ascending aortic aneurysm
   E. Patent ductus arteriosum

3. A 30-year-old woman is found to have an asymptomatic 2-cm splenic artery aneurysm (SAA) within the hilum. Management consists of:
   A. Intervention only if symptoms develop
   B. Intervention only if the aneurysm grows to 3 cm or more
   C. Proximal and distal ligation of splenic artery without arterial reconstruction
   D. Interposition vein graft with excision of aneurysm
   E. Resection of aneurysm with splenectomy

4. Which of the following is true regarding femoral pseudoaneurysms that occur after arteriography?
   A. Ultrasound compression is the procedure of choice.
   B. Ultrasound compression is usually successful even if the patient is receiving anticoagulation therapy.
   C. Surgical repair typically requires interposition vein grafting.
   D. It can be managed with US-guided direct thrombin injection.
   E. A trial of observation is contraindicated because of the high risk of bleeding.

5. All of the following are true regarding human immunodeficiency virus (HIV)–related arterial aneurysms EXCEPT:
   A. They most often involve the aorta.
   B. They have the appearance of pseudoaneurysms on ultrasonography.
   C. They have features of a leukocytoclastic vasculitis.
   D. The inflammation primarily affects the vaso vasorum.
   E. Patients without advanced HIV infection should be managed with interposition grafting.

6. One day after a high-speed motor vehicle accident, a 26-year-old man is noted to have right arm and leg weakness and numbness. He is awake and alert. Findings of a computed tomography (CT) scan of the head are negative. All of the following are true regarding this condition EXCEPT:
   A. CT angiography is indicated.
   B. Systemic anticoagulation may be of benefit.
   C. The neurologic deficit is likely due to a hyperextension injury.
   D. If the carotid artery is occluded, urgent surgical intervention is indicated.
   E. The condition is associated with Horner syndrome.

7. A 40-year-old man sustains a gunshot wound to the right neck just above the clavicle. Initial systolic blood pressure in the emergency department is 70 mm Hg and increases to 90 mm Hg with fluids. The next step in management would be:
   A. Urgent arteriography
   B. Right anterolateral thoracotomy
   C. Median sternotomy
   D. Right supraclavicular and infraclavicular exploration
   E. Insertion of Foley balloon into the bullet wound

8. An 85-year-old woman is brought in by paramedics after a high-speed motor vehicle accident. She has a Glasgow Coma Scale score of 6 with a right blown pupil. A chest radiograph reveals a wide mediastinum, multiple rib fractures, including the first rib, and clear lung fields. A CT scan of the head reveals a right subdural hematoma with midline shift. A CT scan of the chest reveals a mediastinal hematoma and a question of an intimal flap in the thoracic aorta. Management consists of:

   A. Simultaneous craniotomy and left thoracotomy
   B. Craniotomy followed by left thoracotomy
   C. Craniotomy followed by immediate angiography and if positive for aortic injury, then left thoracotomy
   D. Craniotomy only
   E. Craniotomy followed by delayed aortic repair

9. A 25-year-old man presents with a gunshot wound to the left mid cervical region and right hemiparesis. Management would consist of:

   A. Diagnostic arteriography
   B. Carotid duplex scan
   C. Immediate neck exploration with ligation of carotid artery
   D. Immediate neck exploration with repair of carotid artery
   E. Endovascular repair

10. All of the following are true regarding the management of retroperitoneal hematomas EXCEPT:

   A. Zone I hematomas should be explored, regardless of whether they are caused by blunt or penetrating injury.
   B. Penetrating zone III hematomas should be explored.
   C. Blunt zone III hematomas should be observed, even if they are very rapidly expanding.
   D. Blunt nonexpanding zone II hematomas should be observed.
   E. For zone I hematomas, proximal control is best achieved at the aortic hiatus.

11. A 60-year-old man has an asymptomatic 6-cm juxtarenal abdominal aortic aneurysm (AAA). On CT scan, the duodenum is stuck to the anterior aspect of the AAA, the anterior AAA wall is thickened, and there is mild bilateral hydronephrosis. It does not appear to be a candidate for endovascular repair. Which of the following is true?

   A. The duodenum should be carefully peeled off the aorta during surgery.
   B. Ureterolysis should be performed at surgery.
   C. This type of AAA has a higher risk of rupture than other AAAs of the same size.
   D. Patients with this type of AAA often present with back pain, abdominal tenderness, and an elevated erythrocyte sedimentation rate.
   E. The left renal vein and inferior vena cava are not likely to be adherent to the AAA.

12. One day after open AAA repair, watery diarrhea and abdominal distention develop in the patient. On examination, the patient has mild lower left quadrant tenderness without guarding. All of the following are appropriate for this patient EXCEPT:

   A. Proctosigmoidoscopy
   B. Nothing by mouth with nasogastric tube decompression
   C. IV hydration
   D. Broad-spectrum antibiotics
   E. Arteriography

13. A 65-year-old man with a 6-cm AAA is found to have 75% right renal artery stenosis on a preoperative arteriogram. On CT scan, there is a 2-cm proximal neck that measures 20 mm in diameter. He has no history of hypertension. The best management option for this patient would include:

   A. Simultaneous endovascular AAA repair (EVAR) and renal artery stenting
   B. EVAR, leaving the renal artery alone
   C. Open AAA repair and renal artery stenting
   D. Renal artery stenting and then EVAR
   E. Observation of both the AAA and the renal artery

14. A patient with a 7-cm AAA and concomitant iliac occlusive disease undergoes an aortobifemoral bypass. Four hours postoperatively, the nurse notes that his left foot is cold and there is no left femoral pulse. The most appropriate next step would be:
    A. Immediate reexploration via the abdomen
    B. Heparin 10,000 U intravenously
    C. Immediate reexploration via the left groin
    D. Arteriography
    E. Vigorous fluid hydration; then reassess pulse

15. All of the following are known complications of heparin administration EXCEPT:
    A. Skin necrosis
    B. Arterial thrombosis
    C. Osteoporosis
    D. Thrombocytopenia
    E. Cholestatic hepatic injury

16. A 69-year-old man presents to the emergency department with sudden onset of left flank and back pain, abdominal tenderness, a blood pressure of 70/50 mm Hg, and a tender pulsatile midline abdominal mass. Which of the following is true about this condition?
    A. Vigorous intravenous (IV) fluid hydration in the emergency department should be instituted to raise the systolic blood pressure to a target of 110 mm Hg.
    B. A CT scan of the abdomen and pelvis should be promptly performed.
    C. An emergent ultrasound scan should be performed to rule out rupture.
    D. Endovascular repair is the procedure of choice.
    E. Clamping of the aorta at the diaphragm will likely be needed.

17. A 59-year-old man presents with a 4.3-cm asymptomatic AAA. Which of the following is true?
    A. If the patient is at low risk, the aneurysm should be repaired via an open approach.
    B. Endovascular repair should be performed.
    C. There is no benefit to recommending surgery.
    D. Because most aneurysms expand at a rate of 10 to 12 mm per year, the patient should be monitored with an ultrasound scan every 3 months.
    E. Aneurysms this size have approximately an 8% annual risk of rupture.

18. All of the following are indications for inferior mesenteric artery (IMA) reimplantation during AAA surgery EXCEPT:
    A. IMA stump pressure less than 40 mm Hg
    B. Enlarged meandering mesenteric artery visible on preoperative CT angiography
    C. Absent Doppler signals on the serosal surface of the left colon
    D. Brisk back-bleeding from IMA orifice
    E. Intramural colonic pH lower than 6.86

19. During an open AAA repair, before aortic cross-clamping, 7000 U of heparin is administered to a 70-kg man. After completion of the proximal and distal anastomoses, there is no pulse in the graft. On reopening the graft, you notice that there is a red thrombus in it. Activated clotting time is normal. The most appropriate next step would be to:
    A. Administer an additional 5000 U of heparin
    B. Administer IV dextran
    C. Infuse fresh-frozen plasma
    D. Administer lepirudin
    E. Administer argatroban

20. All of the following are true regarding popliteal artery aneurysms EXCEPT:
    A. A 3-cm popliteal aneurysm should be repaired, even if asymptomatic.
    B. Aneurysms with intraluminal thrombus should be repaired regardless of size, even if asymptomatic.
    C. Bypassing the aneurysm with saphenous vein with interval ligation is the standard operative approach.
    D. Patients with acute thrombosis should undergo lytic therapy.
    E. Formal preoperative arteriography is necessary to confirm the presence of an aneurysm.

21. One year after open AAA repair, a patient presents to the emergency department vomiting blood. Vital signs are stable. The results of a routine upper endoscopy are negative. CT scan shows some mild inflammatory changes around the aortic graft. All of the following are true regarding this condition EXCEPT:

    A. Upper endoscopy with a pediatric colonoscope may be helpful.
    B. Arteriography is useful in establishing the diagnosis.
    C. A tagged nuclear white blood cell scan can assist in the diagnosis.
    D. The patient should undergo excision of the aortic graft followed by an axillobifemoral bypass.
    E. In situ placement of an aortic homograft is contraindicated.

22. A 25-year-old man with a history of IV drug abuse presents with fevers, elevated white blood cell count, and a large tender pulsatile mass in his groin at the site of self-injection. The best management of this condition would be:

    A. Ligation of common femoral artery
    B. Axillary to mid–superficial femoral artery bypass followed by ligation of common femoral artery
    C. Obturator bypass, then ligation of common femoral artery
    D. Resection of the infected common femoral artery and in situ reconstruction with panel vein graft
    E. Resection of the infected common femoral artery with polytetrafluoroethylene femoral–femoral crossover

23. A 30-year-old male pedestrian presents with a posterior knee dislocation after being hit by a car. He has no distal pulses. The most appropriate next step in the management would be to:

    A. Take the patient to operating room
    B. Reduce dislocation
    C. Obtain an arteriogram
    D. Check ankle-brachial index
    E. Start heparin

24. The threshold for elective repair of an asymptomatic common iliac aneurysm is greater than:

    A. 2.0 cm
    B. 2.5 cm
    C. 3.5 cm
    D. 4.0 cm
    E. 4.5 cm

25. In which of the following situations would arteriography be LEAST indicated?

    A. Transmediastinal gunshot wound
    B. Zone I neck gunshot wound
    C. Shotgun wound to the groin
    D. Zone III neck gunshot wound
    E. Gunshot wound to the mid thigh with absent pedal pulses

26. The most common symptom of a popliteal aneurysm is:

    A. Rupture
    B. Thrombosis
    C. Distal embolization
    D. Adjacent nerve compression
    E. Adjacent venous compression

27. Which of the following best describes indications for AAA repair?

    A. The appropriate diameter threshold for elective repair for men and women is the same.
    B. The diameter threshold for EVAR in a low-risk patient is lower than that for open repair.
    C. EVAR confers a better long-term survival than open repair.
    D. Careful surveillance of AAA up to 5.5 cm is safe.
    E. In a high–cardiac risk patient with a 5.0-cm AAA, the EVAR approach should be used rather than delay surgery.

28. The most common endoleak after an EVAR is type:

    A. I
    B. II
    C. III
    D. IV
    E. V

29. All of the following are principles of the management of severe frostbite EXCEPT:

    A. Rapid rewarming
    B. Avoidance of débridement
    C. Limb elevation
    D. Early amputation for frank gangrene
    E. Antibiotics

30. All of the following are features of long-standing traumatic arteriovenous fistulas EXCEPT:

    A. Machinery murmur
    B. Dilation of the proximal artery
    C. Decreased diastolic blood pressure
    D. Increased heart rate when the fistula is compressed
    E. Venous hypertension

31. The most common organism cultured from a mycotic aneurysm is:

   A. *Salmonella*
   B. *Streptococcus*
   C. *Staphylococcus*
   D. *Pseudomonas*
   E. *Candida*

32. The best modality for surveillance of an asymptomatic 3.8-cm AAA is:

   A. An annual ultrasound scan
   B. Twice-yearly ultrasound scan
   C. Annual thin-cut (3-mm) CT scan
   D. Twice-yearly thin-cut (3-mm) CT scan
   E. Annual magnetic resonance imaging scan

33. The lower leg compartment most sensitive to compartment syndrome is:

   A. Lateral
   B. Medial
   C. Anterior
   D. Deep posterior
   E. Superficial posterior

Answers

1. D. Hypothenar hammer syndrome is thought to arise from repetitive trauma, such as in carpenters who use the palm of the hand as a hammer. Recent studies suggest that patients with hypothenar hammer syndrome have, in fact, fibromuscular dysplasia in the ulnar artery, which predisposes to aneurysm formation. Aneurysmal degeneration leads to thrombus formation within the aneurysm, with subsequent embolization and digital ischemia. Digital pain, numbness and tingling, weakness of grip, discoloration of the fingers, and digital ulceration may result. Diagnosis is made by arteriography. Surgical management consists of resection of the aneurysmal portion of the vessel with reconstruction using a vein interposition graft.

   Reference: Ferris BL, Taylor LM Jr, Oyama K, et al: Hypothenar hammer syndrome: proposed etiology, *J Vasc Surg* 31:104–113, 2000.

2. B. Dysphagia lusoria (dysphagia by a freak of nature) refers to difficulty in swallowing due to compression of the esophagus by an aberrant right subclavian artery. The aberrant right subclavian artery arises distal to the origin of the left subclavian artery in the descending thoracic aorta, traverses the mediastinum posterior to the esophagus and trachea, and then follows the course of the normal artery into the right upper extremity. It is usually asymptomatic. The most common associated symptom is dysphagia associated with compression of the esophagus between the trachea and the artery. A Kommerell diverticulum occurs as a result of abnormal regression of the fourth aortic arch and persistence of patency of the right eight dorsal aortic segments. An aortic diverticulum is found at the site of origin of the atretic arch. A Kommerell diverticulum can occur in a number of anomalies of the aortic arch system. These abnormalities can, but do not always, cause symptoms of tracheal or esophageal compression. The diverticulum is most frequently present in cases of a right aortic arch with an aberrant left subclavian artery, but can also occur in association with an aberrant right subclavian artery. A "bovine arch" is a normal variant in which the left common carotid artery and the innominate artery share a common origin off the aortic arch. It is important to note that, in a trauma patient, a Kommerell diverticulum can be confused with an aortic transection on angiography.

   Reference: Brown DL, Chapman WC, Edwards WH, et al: Dysphagia lusoria: aberrant right subclavian artery with a Kommerell's diverticulum, *Am Surg* 59:582–586, 1993.

3. E. SAAs seem to form in association with increased splanchnic blood flow, such as in patients with portal hypertension and during pregnancy. They are the most common visceral artery aneurysm. They are four times more common in women. Women of child-bearing age who have SAAs are at significantly increased risk of death from aneurysm rupture. The mortality rate of rupture approaches 70%. Therefore, women of child-bearing age should undergo elective repair. In cases of rupture, bleeding is initially contained in the lesser sac, with subsequent free intraperitoneal rupture resulting in hemodynamic compromise. This pattern is referred to as the double rupture phenomenon. Symptomatic or ruptured SAAs also warrant immediate repair. In men and in asymptomatic women who are not of child-bearing age, observation is recommended for SAAs smaller than 2 cm, and repair is recommended for SAAs larger than 3 cm. For those between 2 and 3 cm, the management is less clear, although newer endovascular approaches make intervention more appealing. For proximal aneurysms, the recommended procedure is exclusion with proximal and distal ligation of the splenic artery. For middle third lesions, excision of the aneurysm is the operation of choice. Distal aneurysms are either treated with splenectomy or aneurysm exclusion and vascular reconstruction. Endovascular therapy with a covered stent represents a new alternative for management of SAAs, but would not be feasible if the aneurysm is in a hilar location.

Reference: Sadat U, Dar O, Walsh S, Varty K: Splenic artery aneurysms in pregnancy: a systematic review, *Int J Surg* 6: 261–265, 2008.

4. D. Pseudoaneurysms can manifest with pain, a pulsatile mass, and/or compression of adjacent structures. Large, expanding, painful pseudoaneurysms are at significant risk of rupture and should be repaired urgently. Smaller, stable pseudoaneurysms may be observed. Duplex ultrasonography has been the diagnostic procedure of choice because it helps define size, morphology, and location. Pseudoaneurysms less than 2 cm in diameter have a higher likelihood of spontaneous thrombosis with compression therapy, whereas larger ones and those in patients receiving anticoagulation therapy are likely to persist. More recent studies, however, have reported high failure rates with this ultrasound compression. Ultrasonography-guided thrombin injection is a newer treatment option, and in many centers is now the treatment of choice. Surgery is reserved for infected or rapidly expanding pseudoaneurysms.

Reference: Wixon CL, Philpott JM, Bogey WM Jr, Powell CS: Duplex-directed thrombin injection as a method to treat femoral artery pseudoaneurysms, *J Am Coll Surg* 187:464–466, 1998.

5. A. The etiology of aneurysms in patients with HIV is unclear. Some authors have theorized that arterial wall weakening occurs from the direct action of HIV itself or from an immune complex mechanism. Patients with HIV-related aneurysms are typically young and lack the usual risk factors associated with vascular disease. The aneurysms are often multiple and occur at unusual sites, particularly in the common carotid and superficial femoral arteries. The abdominal aorta is the third most common site for HIV-related aneurysms. On angiography, they may appear saccular or look like large pseudoaneurysms. On ultrasonography, features are typical of pseudoaneurysms with a blow-out defect and thickening and hyperechoic spotting of the vessel wall. In a seropositive patient without advanced manifestations, the patient should be offered the same treatment as a seronegative patient, via reconstruction using autogenous tissue (such as saphenous vein) for aneurysms of smaller vessels. In patients with advanced HIV and a short life expectancy, the use of endovascular intervention or observation may be a better alternative.

Reference: Nair R: Clinical profile of HIV-related aneurysms, *Eur J Vasc Endovasc Surg* 20:235–240, 2000.

6. D. With the increasing use of diagnostic imaging modalities, recent studies have demonstrated that the incidence of blunt carotid and vertebral artery injury after motor vehicle accidents is higher than previously suspected. Blunt trauma to the neck can cause carotid artery injury either by forceful compression or extension of the artery. After blunt trauma, hemiplegia in the absence of abnormalities on head CT scan should alert the clinician to the possibility of a blunt carotid injury. The injury often

takes the form of a dissection, which can lead to acute occlusion of the internal carotid artery. Patients with blunt carotid trauma often have a paucity of local physical findings in the neck. More generalized findings include a loss of consciousness and lateralizing neurologic deficits. Arteriography (either formal or CT) remains the diagnostic test of choice. Treatment of blunt carotid injuries includes anticoagulation with heparin followed by warfarin for 2 months. Horner syndrome results from the interruption of the sympathetic innervation to the eye and is associated with internal carotid artery dissection. The syndrome includes ptosis, miosis, and anhidrosis.

Reference: Berne J, Norwood S, McAuley C, Villareal D: Helical computed tomographic angiography: an excellent screening test for blunt cerebrovascular injury, *J Trauma* 57:11–17, 2004.

7. C. The patient presented has a zone I penetrating neck injury. In addition, the patient is exhibiting evidence of arterial injury (hypotension). As such, prompt surgical exploration is indicated. Zone I is considered to be the base of the neck and is defined by the thoracic inlet inferiorly and the cricoid cartilage superiorly. Zone II is the mid portion of the neck, from the cricoid cartilage to the angle of the mandible. Zone III includes the area from the angle of the mandible to the base of the skull. Vascular injuries in zone I are often surgically inaccessible from a standard neck incision because one cannot obtain adequate proximal control. For right-sided zone I injuries, proximal control is obtained via a median sternotomy. For left-sided zone I injuries, proximal control is obtained via a left anterolateral thoracotomy because adequate exposure of the left subclavian artery cannot be achieved via a median sternotomy. In situations in which the patient presents to the emergency department with exsanguinating hemorrhage that cannot be controlled by manual compression, rapid insertion of a Foley catheter into the wound and prompt inflation has been performed successfully for temporary tamponade while transporting the patient to the operating room (however, there is no mention of pulsatile hemorrhage in this question).

8. E. The patient presents a surgical dilemma in that there are two injured cavities that need surgical attention. Blunt traumatic rupture of the thoracic aorta is most commonly associated with rapid deceleration injuries, as seen after high-speed motor vehicle accidents. The injury most commonly occurs just distal to the ligamentum arteriosum. Autopsy studies of aviation accidents demonstrate that more than 30% of deaths are due to aortic transection. Overall, immediate mortality is greater than 70%. The majority of patients die instantly of exsanguination. Of those who survive, older literature suggested that as many as 49% died within 24 hours; hence the push for early intervention with thoracotomy and graft replacement of the thoracic aorta. However, in the multiply injured patient, such an approach is associated with a high mortality rate. More recent articles indicate that for patients reaching the hospital alive, the risk of immediate death is overestimated because the injury is contained by the aorta's adventitial layer. The lack of a large hemothorax in the present case further supports contained injury. Thus, attention should focus on treating other major injuries first (in this case, the subdural hematoma with a midline shift). Delayed repair (>48 hours) of blunt aortic thoracic injuries is increasingly being reported, particularly in patients with other life-threatening injuries. Endovascular stent grafting is another new treatment modality and is best used in the elderly who may not withstand a major thoracotomy or in those with multiple other injuries. Patients with delayed repair are treated with beta-blockade, targeting a mean arterial pressure of 70 mm Hg to reduce shear stress on the aorta.

Reference: Buz S, Zipfel B, Mulahasanovic S, et al: Conventional surgical repair and endovascular treatment of acute traumatic aortic rupture, *Eur J Cardiothorac Surg* 33:143–149, 2008.

9. D. The patient has a penetrating zone II injury and a neurologic deficit. First emphasis should focus on airway control because if there is a hematoma, this can lead to airway obstruction. In the presence of a neurologic deficit, expanding hematoma, pulsatile bleeding, or palpable thrill, prompt surgical intervention via neck exploration is indicated. In the past, zone II neck injuries that penetrated the platysma warranted immediate operative exploration, regardless of whether hard signs of injury were present. More recently, however, in the absence of an obvious injury, the trend is to perform diagnostic imaging, such as CT angiography, to detect carotid injuries, as well as injuries to the aerodigestive tract and cervical spine. As a general rule, penetrating injuries to the carotid artery should be repaired when technically feasible, regardless of whether the patient has a neurologic deficit. Ligation of the carotid artery is associated with a poor neurologic outcome in this setting. Repair of the artery by primary repair or interposition grafting would be the procedure of choice. Formal diagnostic arteriography would lead to an inordinate delay, particularly in someone who already has a neurologic deficit. The role of endovascular repair for penetrating arterial injury is still being defined, but is best used in the setting of zone III injuries that are not surgically accessible.

Reference: Feliciano D: Management of penetrating injuries to carotid artery, *World J Surg* 25:1028–1035, 2001.

10. C. The retroperitoneum is divided into three zones: the midline retroperitoneum (zone I), the perinephric space (zone II), and the pelvic retroperitoneum (zone III). As a general rule, any retroperitoneal hematoma from a penetrating injury should be explored because of the concern for a major vascular injury or ureteral injury. Likewise, any hematoma in zone I mandates exploration for both blunt and penetrating trauma because central hematomas have a higher likelihood of a major vascular injury to the aorta or inferior vena cava. Before entering a hematoma, proximal arterial control should be obtained. For zone I or II injuries, proximal control of the aorta should be obtained just below the diaphragm. For penetrating pelvic hematomas, depending on the extent, proximal control can be obtained at the infrarenal aorta. A pelvic retroperitoneal hematoma secondary to penetrating trauma mandates exploration because of the likelihood of iliac vessel injury. However, zone III hematomas resulting from blunt trauma are usually associated with a pelvic fracture and should not be explored because bleeding is due to small vessels

deep in the pelvis. Optimal management involves pelvic stabilization with angiographic embolization. The exception is a rapidly expanding pelvic hematoma because this may indicate a blunt iliac artery injury.

11. D. Inflammatory aneurysms differ from mycotic (infected) aneurysms in that the cause is not an infection. Inflammatory AAA is defined by a constellation consisting of a thickened aneurysmal wall, extensive perianeurysmal and retroperitoneal fibrosis, and dense adhesions of adjacent abdominal structures. Patients with inflammatory aneurysms are more frequently symptomatic at presentation compared with those with noninflammatory AAAs. Patients may present with a combination of low back pain, weight loss, and an increased erythrocyte sedimentation rate. As many as one third of patients may have a tender, pulsatile mass on physical examination. The precise etiology is unclear, but evidence suggests that inflammatory AAA is not a distinct clinicopathologic entity, but rather an inflammatory variant of atherosclerotic AAA. Adjacent structures, such as the fourth part of the duodenum, the inferior vena cava, and the left renal vein may be adherent to the inflammatory AAA, thus making open repair more precarious. The technique of open repair needs to be modified, and any attempts to dissect the duodenum off the aorta should be avoided. Although the ureters are often involved in the inflammatory process, hydronephrosis tends to spontaneously resolve after repair. Because the left renal vein is often densely adherent to the aneurysm neck, this vein may need to be divided close to the inferior vena cava. Division of the retroperitoneal vein can be avoided by using the left retroperitoneal approach, with elevation of the left kidney. Rupture risk does not appear to be greater than noninflammatory aneurysms of the same diameter. Diagnosis is often made by CT scanning, demonstrating the markedly thickened aortic wall. The endovascular approach would be optimal if the patient were a candidate, but the juxtarenal nature currently precludes such an approach.

Reference: Rasmussen T, Hallett J Jr: Inflammatory aortic aneurysms: a clinical review with new perspectives in pathogenesis, *Ann Surg* 225:155–164, 1997.

12. E. Colonic ischemia is a recognized complication after AAA repair, whether open or endovascular. It occurs in approximately 1% to 3% of cases. It is thought to be due to either ligation of the IMA or ligation or exclusion of internal iliac arteries. The most common presentations include an unexpectedly early return of bowel function manifested by diarrhea, left lower quadrant pain, abdominal distention, persistent leukocytosis, elevated white blood cell count, and lactic acidosis. Diagnosis is confirmed by flexible proctosigmoidoscopy, which reveals a friable mucosa. Proctosigmoidoscopy may not be able to accurately distinguish partial ischemia from full-thickness necrosis. Initial management is medical and consists of nasogastric tube decompression, IV hydration, placing the patient on NPO, and broad-spectrum antibiotics. Full-thickness necrosis of the colon should be suspected in patients with evidence of peritonitis or unremitting acidosis. In such cases, laparotomy with colonic resection and colostomy is indicated. The mortality rate after emergent colectomy approaches 50%. Arteriography would not typically be helpful because the usual cause is an intended ligation or exclusion of an internal iliac artery or IMA.

Reference: Becquemin J, Majewski M, Fermani N, et al: Colon ischemia following abdominal aortic aneurysm repair in the era of endovascular abdominal aortic repair, *J Vasc Surg* 47:258–263, 2008.

13. B. Two recent randomized studies comparing observation with open AAA repair for infrarenal AAAs as large as 5.5 cm in maximum diameter demonstrated that the mortality rate for watchful waiting was no different than that for open repair. Thus, the threshold for AAA repair has been raised from 5.0 to 5.5 cm. Other studies comparing open with endovascular repair of infrarenal AAA indicate that in the short term, the endovascular approach is associated with lower perioperative morbidity and mortality rates, but at 2-year follow-up, outcomes for open repair and endovascular repair were the same. Nevertheless, given the appeal of the less invasive endovascular repair, the vast majority of infrarenal AAAs are now being repaired via the endovascular approach. Optimally, a successful endovascular repair requires at least a 15-mm proximal neck, with a maximum diameter of 25 to 30 mm, and less than a 60-degree angulation between the proximal neck and the suprarenal aorta. An adequate diameter of the access vessels (common and external iliac arteries, common femoral arteries) is also important because the outer diameter of the introducer sheaths varies, depending on the device, from 20 to 24 French (3 French is equal to 1 mm). A combination of excessive angulation and severe calcification of the access vessels is a relative contraindication. American Heart Association guidelines for intervention in renal artery stenosis include sudden worsening of preexisting hypertension, resistant hypertension despite at least three antihypertensive drugs, worsening renal function after administration of an angiotensin-converting enzyme inhibitor, unexplained atrophy of one kidney, and hypertension resulting in end-organ damage such as renal insufficiency or recurrent episodes of decompensated congestive heart failure. Thus, in the present case, no renal artery intervention would be recommended with the information given.

References: Blankensteijn J, de Jong S, Prinssen M: Two-year outcomes after conventional or endovascular repair of abdominal aortic aneurysms, *N Engl J Med* 352:2398–2405, 2005.

Lederle F, Johnson G, Wilson S: Rupture rate of large abdominal aortic aneurysms in patients refusing or unfit for elective repair, *JAMA* 287:2968–2972, 2002.

Lederle FA, Wilson SE, Johnson GR, et al: Immediate repair compared with surveillance of small abdominal aortic aneurysms, *N Engl J Med* 346:1437–1444, 2002.

14. C. Immediate postoperative graft occlusion is a known complication of aortobifemoral bypass, emphasizing the importance of a careful neurovascular examination after surgery. Loss of a pulse indicates graft occlusion. Because only one limb is occluded, it suggests that there was a technical error at the femoral anastomosis. Thus, reopening the abdominal incision is not warranted. The operative approach would include a Fogarty embolectomy of the left graft limb proximally and the superficial femoral and profunda femoris arteries distally, followed by intraoperative

arteriography to assess the distal anastomosis. In most instances, the femoral anastomosis would need a revision. If, on the other hand, the patient had a normal femoral pulse and absent distal pulses, this would suggest embolic debris from the aortic aneurysm. A third possibility is the entity known as "trash foot," in which embolic debris from the aortic aneurysm showers both feet. In this situation, they may have normal pulses throughout, but evidence of ischemia of the bilateral toes with mottling and purplish discoloration. In the latter instance, surgical embolectomy would not be of benefit. Because patients are often sedated immediately postoperatively, there is a risk of delay in recognition of the graft occlusion.

15. E. Heparin-induced thrombocytopenia (type I) is typically characterized by a decrease in platelet count (as much as a 50% decrease from baseline) that usually occurs within the first 2 days after heparin initiation and returns to normal despite continued heparin administration. The mechanism of the thrombocytopenia is nonimmune and seems to be due to a direct effect of heparin on platelet activation. A much more serious reaction, known as heparin-induced thrombosis (type II) occurs in 1% to 5% of patients treated with heparin and can lead to both venous and arterial thrombosis. It is an immune-mediated disorder characterized by the formation of antibodies against platelet factor 4, neutrophil-activating peptide 2, and/or interleukin-8. The initial finding in heparin-induced thrombosis is the development of thrombocytopenia. The clot in heparin-induced thrombosis is platelet rich and relatively devoid of fibrin and red cells; thus, the term *white clot syndrome* was coined. Heparin-induced skin necrosis is a well-described complication of either IV or subcutaneous injection of unfractionated heparin. It is also associated with antibody formation against platelet factor 4, creating a local prothrombotic condition. The appearance of erythema is followed by purpura and hemorrhage leading to necrosis. Warfarin can also cause skin necrosis. Another complication of prolonged heparin use is osteopenia, which results from impairment of bone formation and enhancement of bone resorption by heparin. Heparin is a category C drug and can be used in pregnancy, whereas warfarin is teratogenic. Cholestatic hepatic injury is associated with prolonged use of warfarin, not heparin.

16. E. The presentation is consistent with a ruptured AAA. Given the findings and the hemodynamic instability, the patient should be taken directly to the operating room. There would be no role for taking an unstable patient to the CT scanner. The only exception would be centers with a coordinated multidisciplinary ruptured aneurysm team that has immediate endovascular capabilities. In that case, a CT scan might be performed to determine the feasibility of endovascular repair. Although mortality statistics for endovascular repair of ruptured AAAs seem promising compared with open repair, endovascular repair is not readily available emergently at most hospitals, and the improved outcomes compared with open repair may be the result of selection bias. Although ultrasonography is useful for determining the presence of an AAA, it is not accurate for determining the presence of a retroperitoneal rupture. Ultrasonography would be reasonable to perform in this patient if no pulsatile mass could be felt on physical examination to confirm that an aneurysm was present. Once in the operating room, the patient should be prepped and draped before anesthesia induction because the anesthesia may induce a precipitous decrease in blood pressure. Because of the large retroperitoneal hematoma that is typically found, proximal control is best achieved by clamping the aorta at the diaphragm. Most surgeons would recommend a policy of "permissive hypotension" en route to the operating room. Excessive fluid administration and elevation of the blood pressure may further exacerbate bleeding.

Reference: Lee W, Hirneise C, Tayyarah M, et al: Impact of endovascular repair on early outcomes of ruptured abdominal aortic aneurysms, *J Vasc Surg* 40:211–215, 2004.

van der Vliet JA, van Aalst DL, Schultze Kool LJ: Hypotensive hemostatis (permissive hypotension) for ruptured abdominal aortic aneurysm: are we really in control? *Vascular* 15:197–200, 2007.

17. C. For aortic aneurysms less than 5 cm in diameter, there is no benefit of operative intervention because the risk of rupture is low. The risk of rupture is estimated at 1% to 3% per year for aneurysms between 4 and 4.5 cm, which is lower than the operative mortality rate for open repair. With the advent of endovascular techniques and the attendant lower operative mortality, the question is whether the endovascular approach should be offered. This premise has yet to be proven. Surgical intervention is indicated for AAAs larger than 5.5 cm. For aneurysms between 5.0 and 5.5 cm, surgical intervention should be considered on an individual basis, taking into account the patient's age and comorbidities. The average growth rate of AAA is 2 to 3 mm per year, but it accelerates as the aneurysm enlarges. However, not all aneurysms grow. The risk of rupture at 1 year is approximately 9% for AAAs between 5.5 and 5.9 cm, 10% for AAAs between 6.0 and 6.9 cm, and 32% for AAAs larger than 7.0 cm. The threshold for AAA repair in women should be lower than for men because there is a greater tendency for rupture of smaller aneurysms in women. The exact size cutoff, however, is not well defined. The most powerful risk factors for rupture are chronic obstructive pulmonary disease, ongoing cigarette smoking, and poorly controlled hypertension.

References: Blankensteijn J, de Jong S, Prinssen M: Two-year outcomes after conventional or endovascular repair of abdominal aortic aneurysms, *N Engl J Med* 352:2398–2405, 2005.

Lederle F, Johnson G, Wilson S: Rupture rate of large abdominal aortic aneurysms in patients refusing or unfit for elective repair, *JAMA* 287:2968–2972, 2002.

Lederle FA, Wilson SE, Johnson GR, et al: Immediate repair compared with surveillance of small abdominal aortic aneurysms, *N Engl J Med* 346:1437–1444, 2002.

18. D. Numerous authors have attempted to identify guidelines for when to reimplant the IMA to prevent colonic ischemia after open AAA repair. After clamping the aorta and opening the AAA sac, the orifice of the IMA should be examined. If the orifice is occluded, then IMA reimplantation is not needed because the bowel is already receiving blood from other collaterals. If the IMA

is patent and the back-bleeding is poor, this suggests poor collateral flow, and thus the IMA should be reimplanted. If, on the other hand, there is brisk back-bleeding from the IMA, this indicates excellent collateral flow, so that the IMA can be ligated. Because these are subjective observations, some authors have advocated measuring the IMA stump pressure. Pressures greater than 40 mm Hg are indicative of adequate collateral flow and permit safe ligation of the IMA. Collateral blood flow between the superior mesenteric artery and the IMA forms via the Riolan arch, which collateralizes the middle colic artery (a superior mesenteric artery branch) with the left colic artery (an IMA branch). When either the superior mesenteric artery or the IMA is stenosed or occluded, this collateral pathway enlarges, forming the meandering mesenteric artery. Reimplantation of the IMA would be indicated in the presence of a meandering mesenteric artery to maximally preserve mesenteric blood flow. Absent Doppler signals on the bowel surface and a decrease in intramural colonic pH have also been shown to be predictors of colonic ischemia.

Reference: Björck T, Troeng D, Bergqvist M: Risk factors for intestinal ischaemia after aortoiliac surgery: a combined cohort and case-control study of 2824 operations, *Eur J Vasc Endovasc Surg* 13:531–539, 1997.

19. C. The patient is demonstrating evidence of heparin resistance. A relatively high dose of heparin was given, yet the activated clotting time did not change. This scenario is seen more frequently during cardiopulmonary bypass. Heparin binds to antithrombin (AT) III, which becomes activated. Activated AT III inactivates thrombin and factor Xa, inhibiting clot formation. Thus, a deficiency in AT III will lead to a decreased effectiveness of heparin. AT III deficiency can be inherited or acquired. Heparin administration itself lowers AT III levels. Other acquired causes include disseminated intravascular coagulation and liver cirrhosis. Although it may seem counterintuitive, administration of fresh-frozen plasma would provide AT III and should lead to a prolonged activated clotting time. Additional heparin could then be given as needed. Lepuridin and argatroban are direct thrombin inhibitors and are used in the setting of heparin-induced thrombocytopenia. Thrombosis in this setting would produce white clot and is unlikely to occur immediately after heparin administration.

Reference: Spiess B: Treating heparin resistance with antithrombin or fresh frozen plasma, *Ann Thorac Surg* 85:2153–2160, 2008.

20. E. Popliteal aneurysms are the most common peripheral artery aneurysms (overall, aortic and iliac aneurysms are more common). They can be suspected on physical examination. They are bilateral in 50% of patients. Patients who are found to have a popliteal aneurysm should undergo screening for an AAA because 30% will have a concomitant AAA. The most frequent complication of popliteal aneurysms is leg ischemia. Guidelines for repair are controversial. Some authors recommend repair for all popliteal aneurysms. Most would agree that indications for repair are (1) all aneurysms larger than 2 cm, (2) aneurysms with intraluminal thrombus, regardless of size, or (3) those that are symptomatic or have evidence of previous embolization. Diagnosis is made by duplex ultrasonography, which can measure the aneurysm size and detect the presence of thrombus. Arteriography assists in operative planning but should not be used for diagnosis because it does not detect the thrombus nor accurately measure the size. Magnetic resonance imaging and CT angiography can be used as alternatives for operative planning. The standard operative approach involves bypassing the aneurysm with saphenous vein and interval ligation of the popliteal artery. With this approach, the aneurysm sac is not opened, and as such, there is a small risk of continued aneurysm expansion and compression of adjacent structures. Formal endo-aneurysmorrhaphy, as is done with an open AAA repair, is another alternative. In the setting of acute thrombosis, lytic therapy is the initial treatment of choice.

References: Ascher E, Markevich N, Schutzer RW, et al: Small popliteal artery aneurysms: are they clinically significant? *J Vasc Surg* 37:755–760, 2003.

Lowell RC, Glaviczki P, Hallet JW, et al: Popliteal artery aneurysms: the risk of non-operative management, *Ann Vasc Surg* 8:14–23, 1994.

21. B. A patient with an upper gastrointestinal bleed and a history of aortic surgery should be presumed to have an aortoenteric fistula until proven otherwise. The treatment algorithm depends on the hemodynamic stability of the patient. If the patient is unable to be stabilized due to massive hemorrhage, the patient should be taken emergently to the operating room, even if a diagnosis has not yet been established. Oftentimes, the patient will have a so-called herald bleed, after which the bleeding may temporarily stop, allowing a work-up for an aortoenteric fistula. The diagnosis can be difficult to establish. Upper endoscopy has the highest yield, but is surprisingly often negative. Duodenal graft erosion typically occurs at the fourth portion of the duodenum, and findings may be subtle, such as mild mucosal erosion. If the endoscopy findings are negative, repeating the upper endoscopy with a pediatric colonoscope may reveal an abnormality. The next study of choice would be CT. It is unlikely to show blood extravasation, but rather may demonstrate perigraft fluid, air, or inflammation, indicative of a graft infection. Fluid and inflammatory changes around a graft would be abnormal findings beyond 6 weeks after surgery. If the CT scan findings are negative, a nuclear tagged white blood cell scan may be useful for establishing a graft infection. Arteriography is of limited benefit for the diagnosis of vascular graft infections, but can be useful in preoperative planning. In some instances, no source of an upper gastrointestinal bleed is found, and thus one must empirically proceed to graft excision. The operative management consists of obtaining proximal aortic control of the aorta at the diaphragm, graft excision, closure of the aortic stump in two layers, closure of the duodenum, placing omentum in the area of the aortic stump closure, followed by an extra-anatomic axillobifemoral bypass. More recent alternatives are in situ placement of an antibiotic-impregnated graft or a human aortic homograft, and endovascular stent grafting, although the latter approach seems to have a greater risk of recurrent infection.

22. A. The case represents an infected pseudoaneurysm of the common femoral artery from the drug injection. Associated findings at the time of presentation include overlying cellulitis, distal embolization, septic arthritis, endocarditis, and compartment syndrome. Such cases are very difficult to manage. Attempts at revascularization are usually unsuccessful because the artery itself is often friable and does not hold sutures well. The infection is usually multiorganism and includes gram negatives, which have a greater tendency to destroy the native artery. Thus, any autogenous graft placed into the infected field has a high likelihood of becoming itself infected and disrupting the anastomosis. As such, the best option is to ligate the femoral artery proximally and distally. Proximal arterial control needs to be obtained first, and depending on the location of the pseudoaneurysm, this may require a suprainguinal incision first to control the external iliac artery. Ligation in this setting is surprisingly well tolerated, and in one large series, there were no amputations associated with this approach.

Reference: Ganfl J, Leiberman D, Pollock J: Outcome after ligation of infected false femoral aneurysms in intravenous drug abusers, *Eur J Vasc Endovasc Surg* 2:158–161, 2000.

23. B. Posterior knee dislocations are known to have a high risk of associated popliteal artery injury. The popliteal artery is fairly fixed proximally just distal to the adductor hiatus and distally by the soleus muscle. The dislocation stretches the popliteal artery and makes it vulnerable to injury, either an intimal tear, in which case the distal pulse may be intact, or a complete transection. Popliteal artery injury occurs in approximately one third of patients with knee dislocations. The peroneal nerve may also be injured in as many as one fourth of patients. It often also produces compartment syndrome. Popliteal artery injuries result in limb loss more often than any other peripheral vascular injury. This is due in large part to the poor collateralization around the knee. Amputation rates as high as 20% have been reported. The first step in the management of a posterior knee dislocation is to reduce the dislocation and to then reassess the pulse examination. If the pulse is not restored, the patient should be taken to the operating room for revascularization. In the absence of associated injuries, strong consideration should be given to administering IV heparin preoperatively to prevent thrombosis of the distal capillary bed. If the patient will require a major orthopedic intervention and the foot is ischemic, the popliteal artery should be explored and a temporary shunt inserted in the artery while the orthopedic repair is undertaken. A full four-compartment fasciotomy should be performed immediately as well to minimize muscle ischemia from bleeding in the compartments. Arterial repair is completed by interposition reverse saphenous vein grafting from the contralateral leg.

If, on the other hand, a distal pulse is restored in the emergency department with reduction, the patient should undergo arteriography to rule out an intimal injury. If the patient presents with a posterior knee dislocation and has palpable distal pulses, some authors would advocate selective arteriography based on measuring the ankle-brachial index. In those circumstances, arteriography is reserved for situations in which the ankle-brachial index is less than 0.9.

References: Lynch K, Johansen K: Can Doppler pressure measurement replace "exclusion" arteriography in the diagnosis of occult extremity arterial trauma? *Ann Surg* 214:737–741, 1991.

Treiman G, Yellin A, Weaver F, et al: Examination of the patient with a knee dislocation: the case for selective arteriography, *Arch Surg* 127:1056–1062, 1992.

24. C. Common iliac aneurysms are usually diagnosed incidentally. In most cases, they are found in association with an aortic aneurysm. Rare presentation includes the development of a fistula with the adjacent iliac vein or compression of the iliac vein. The natural history of common iliac aneurysms is less well defined. In a recent study, the expansion rate of common iliac aneurysms was 0.29 cm per year, and hypertension predicted faster expansion. Because no rupture of a common iliac aneurysm smaller than 3.8 cm was observed, the recommended threshold for elective repair of asymptomatic patients was larger than 3.5 cm. Treatment options include open surgical replacement with prosthetic graft or endovascular stent grafting. In patients with suitable anatomy, namely, the presence of proximal and distal landing zones, stent grafting has become the treatment of choice. Endovascular repair is associated with fewer complications overall, but poses a higher risk of creating buttock claudication due to occlusion of the internal iliac artery.

Reference: Huang Y, Gloviczki P, Duncan A, et al: Common iliac artery aneurysm: expansion rate and results of open surgical and endovascular repair, *J Vasc Surg* 47:1203–1210, 2008.

25. E. Absent pulses distal to a penetrating injury is considered a hard sign of vascular injury. In this situation, it would be appropriate to proceed directly to the operating room without preoperative arteriography because performing arteriography would lead to an inordinate delay. Because of their relative surgical inaccessibility, zone I and III neck and transmediastinal gunshot wounds are best assessed with preoperative arteriography, provided the patient does not have hard signs of vascular injury (hemodynamic instability, rapidly expanding hematoma, pulsatile hemorrhage). Shotgun wounds have a particularly high rate of arterial injury.

26. B. Popliteal aneurysms rarely rupture. Most commonly, they cause acute or chronic ischemia. In most series, the most common symptom is thrombosis, in as many as 49%, followed by distal embolization. As the aneurysm continues to grow, less commonly, it can compress adjacent structures, such as the popliteal vein. Chronic embolization can lead to occlusions of the infrapopliteal vessels and can complicate revascularization. If they present with acute ischemia, thrombolysis is the intervention of choice, followed by operative repair. Recently, endovascular stent grafting has been used, although long-term patency data are still lacking.

References: Dorigo W, Pulli R, Turini F, et al: Acute leg ischemia from thrombosed popliteal artery aneurysms: role of preoperative thrombolysis, *Eur J Vasc Endovasc Surg* 23:251–254, 2002.

Shortell CK, DeWeese JA, Ouriel K, et al: Popliteal artery aneurysms: a 25-year surgical experience, *J Vasc Surg* 14:771–776, 1991.

27. D. Recent studies have shown that AAAs as large as 5.5 cm in diameter can be safely observed. Another recent randomized study indicated that although the perioperative mortality rate of EVAR is lower than that of open repair, long-term mortality is the same. EVAR should not lower the size threshold for repair in a high–cardiac risk patient if the AAA has not yet reached the 5.5-cm threshold. Guidelines for treatment of AAAs, as reported by a subcommittee of the Joint Council of the American Association for Vascular Surgery and Society for Vascular Surgery, are listed.

1. The arbitrary setting of a single-threshold diameter for elective AAA repair that is applicable to all patients is not appropriate because the decision for repair must be individualized in each case.

2. Randomized trials have shown that the risk of rupture of small AAAs is quite low and that a policy of careful surveillance of those with a diameter of as large as 5.5 cm is safe, unless there is rapid expansion (>1 cm/yr) or symptoms develop. However, early surgery is comparable to surveillance with later surgery, so patient preference is important, especially for AAAs 4.5 to 5.5 cm in diameter.

3. Based on the best available current evidence, a diameter of 5.5 cm appears to be an appropriate threshold for repair in an average patient. However, subsets of younger low-risk patients with a long projected life expectancy may prefer early repair. If the surgeon's personal documented operative mortality rate is low, repair may be indicated at smaller sizes if that is the patient's preference.

4. For women or for AAAs with a greater than average rupture risk, 4.5 to 5 cm is an appropriate threshold for elective repair.

5. For high-risk patients, delay in repair until the diameter is larger is warranted, especially if endovascular aortic repair is not possible.

6. In view of its uncertain long-term durability and effectiveness as well as the increased surveillance burden, EVAR is most appropriate for patients at increased risk of conventional open aneurysm repair. EVAR may be the preferred treatment method if anatomy is appropriate for older high-risk patients, those with a hostile abdomen, or other clinical circumstances likely to increase the risk of conventional open repair.

7. Use of EVAR in patients with unsuitable anatomy markedly increases the risk of adverse outcomes, the need for conversion to open repair, or AAA rupture.

8. At present, there does not seem to be any justification that EVAR should change the accepted size threshold for intervention in most patients.

9. In choosing between open repair and EVAR, patient preference is of great importance. It is essential that the patients be well informed to make such choices.

Reference: Brewster D, Cronenwett J, Hallett J Jr, et al: Guidelines for the treatment of abdominal aortic aneurysms: report of a subcommittee of the Joint Council of the American Association for Vascular Surgery and Society for Vascular Surgery, *J Vasc Surg* 37:1106–1117, 2003.

28. B. Endoleak is a common complication after EVAR that can lead to aneurysm enlargement and even rupture. Endoleaks occur in as many as 40% of patients after EVAR.

Most endoleaks are found in the immediate postoperative period, but late endoleaks also develop. For this reason, routine postoperative surveillance with CT scanning is recommended. New endoleaks have been identified as late as 7 years after EVAR. Endoleaks are classified into four types (types I–IV) based on the source of communication between the circulation and the aneurysm sac. The most common type of leak after endovascular repair is a type II leak, which results from retrograde filling of the aneurysm sac from the lumbar arteries or the IMA. Management of type II leaks is controversial and is based on whether the aneurysm is enlarging or stable. Options include coil embolization of the vessel, laparoscopic ligation, or observation. Type I leaks occur at the stent–graft attachment sites (either at the aorta or at the iliac arteries); type III leaks occur at a stent–stent interface and are also known as modular disassociations; type IV leaks are directly through the graft and are due to graft material porosity. They usually heal spontaneously. The most dangerous type of leak is a proximal type I leak because there is a failure to achieve a proximal seal, leading to continued filling of the aneurysm sac at systemic pressures. Type I leaks require immediate treatment when discovered, typically by deploying another stent or, if unsuccessful, by open surgical conversion. Type III endoleaks represent a true mechanical failure of the endograft, and require repair with an additional endograft to eliminate systemic flow and pressure in the aneurysm.

Reference: Corriere M, Feurer I, Becker S, et al: Endoleak following endovascular abdominal aortic aneurysm repair: implications for duration of screening, *Ann Surg* 239:800–807, 2004.

29. D. Frostbite is defined as local freezing of tissues resulting in ice crystal formation within the extracellular space. This initially causes osmotic transport of water out of the cell and severe cellular dehydration. If prolonged, the process leads to progressive mechanical tissue injury. Eventually this results in the denaturation of protein and inhibition of DNA synthesis. When the tissue is rewarmed, cell swelling ensues, and the limb is at increased risk of developing compartment syndrome. In addition, a procoagulant state is created with increased platelet aggregation and thrombosis of small vessels. This ischemia/reperfusion cycle generates oxygen free radicals, production of prostaglandins, and thromboxane A_2, and the release of proteolytic enzymes. Tissue injury is exacerbated if the area is partially warmed and then reexposed to cold. As such, warming should only be initiated when it can be done rapidly and completely. The currently accepted treatment of frostbite is immersion in a warm water bath until rewarming is complete and sensation returns. The warming should optimally occur in water that is circulating and at a temperature of 40° to 42°C. Circulating water allows the application of a constant temperature. It is recommended to gently remove clear blisters (prevents thromboxane-mediated tissue injury), but to leave hemorrhagic blisters intact (to prevent infection). An important principle is the absolute avoidance of major surgical débridement, even in the face of gangrene. Surgery should be postponed for as long as 3 to 4 months because it may take this long to differentiate between viable and necrotic tissue. This allows the necrotic tissue to autoamputate, thereby maximizing tissue preservation. Antibiotics as well as tetanus prophylaxis should be administered. Local treatment should consist of elevating the affected area to minimize edema, nonabrasive cleaning, air drying, and avoidance of pressure.

30. D. The diagnosis of a traumatic AV fistula can sometimes be delayed. Numerous complications can arise. Venous hypertension distal to the fistula results from high-pressure arterial blood flow into the low-pressure venous system; this situation can lead to significant extremity edema, hyperpigmentation, varicosities, skin induration, and eventual skin ulceration similar to that seen with chronic venous stasis. The diversion of blood flow into the adjacent vein may lead to the steal phenomenon, with distal tissue ischemia. In addition, the marked increase in venous return may lead to high-output cardiac failure. The diagnosis of an arteriovenous fistula can often be established clinically. A history of trauma may be elicited. A "machinery-like" murmur as well as a palpable thrill can be auscultated. The fistula may cause a decrease in both systolic and diastolic blood pressures, an increase in cardiac output, an increase in venous blood pressure, an increase in heart rate, and slight cardiomegaly. On fistula compression, the heart rate decreases (Branham sign). The decrease in heart rate is a result of an arterial baroreceptor reflex triggered by the temporary increase in systolic blood pressure that occurs with closure of the fistula.

31. C. The term *mycotic aneurysm* refers to an infected aneurysm and is a misnomer in that it implies a fungal infection. However, most are bacterial in origin. The most common organisms cultured are *Staphylococcus*, followed by *Salmonella*. The most common location is the aorta. Infected aneurysms most commonly arise from seeding from a remote site, most often the heart, in the setting of endocarditis. Very rarely, infected aneurysms result from direct extension of an adjacent infection. Infected aneurysms require excision and, depending on the location, arterial reconstruction. For the aorta, the options include extra-anatomic reconstruction such as an axillobifemoral bypass and in situ reconstruction with cryopreserved aorta or antibiotic-impregnated grafts. Endovascular techniques, without excision of the infected artery, have been applied, but recurrent infection rates so far have been high.

32. A. Ultrasound scanning is the most cost-effective modality for following an AAA. Given that the AAA presented is small and given that the average annual growth rate of an AAA is 2 to 3 mm, ultrasonography should be performed on a yearly basis. If an AAA is approaching 5 cm in diameter, strong consideration should be given to screening every 3 to 6 months. CT scanning is best used as a preoperative tool to determine suitability for endovascular repair. Thin-cut (3-mm) CT scanning with contrast has become the principal technique for evaluating patients preoperatively for endograft placement. CT permits measurement of the neck diameter, detection of neck thrombus, and measurement of neck length, aneurysm diameter, iliac diameter, and aneurysm length.

33. C. Compartment syndrome can be divided into etiologies that cause external restriction of the compartment and those that lead to an internal increase in compartment volume. External causes include the use of military antishock trousers, splints, casts, or dressings that are placed too tightly, and full-thickness burns, in which the eschar creates a tight restriction. Causes of internal increases in volume include bleeding from trauma or anticoagulation, edema from ischemia/reperfusion, and inadvertent IV fluid infusion. Compartment syndrome can be caused or exacerbated by decreasing the perfusion pressure as well, such as seen with shock. The pathophysiology is thought to be swelling of the injured muscle and soft tissues, which increases the intracompartmental pressure. This leads to closure of lymphatic vessels and small venules. Subsequently, hypertension develops in the capillary bed, and arterioles are compressed. This eventually leads to an ischemia. There are four compartments between the knee and ankle: anterior, lateral, posterior superficial, and posterior deep (there is no medial compartment). The anterior compartment is most commonly involved. This is likely the result of its being a relatively tight compartment with a large muscle mass, combined with limited collateral circulation. It is important to know which nerves run in each compartment. The deep peroneal nerve runs in the anterior compartment, the superficial peroneal nerve in the lateral compartment, the sural nerve in the superficial posterior compartment, and the tibial nerve in the deep posterior compartment. In an awake patient, the earliest symptom is pain, which is often described as out of proportion to the findings. One of the earliest signs is pain on passive dorsiflexion of the foot. Because the anterior compartment is most often affected, one of the earliest sensory deficits is numbness in the web space between the great toe and second toe (deep peroneal nerve). The diagnosis of compartment syndrome is first and foremost a clinical one. In situations in which the diagnosis is in doubt, compartment pressures can be measured via the introduction of a needle connected to a pressure transducer. The most commonly used device is the Stryker intracompartmental pressure monitor system (Stryker Instruments, Kalamazoo, MI). One should measure the pressure in all the compartments in the area of concern. Pressures less than 20 mm Hg are acceptable. Pressures of more than 30 mm Hg are indicative of compartment syndrome, whereas pressures between 20 and 30 mm Hg are in a gray zone. It is important to note, however, that there is no exact threshold of pressure that reliably predicts compartment syndrome.

References: Bullard Dunn KM, Rothenberger DA: Colon, rectum, and anus. In Brunicardi FC, Andersen DK, Billiar TR, et al, editors: *Schwartz's principles of surgery*, ed 9, New York, 2010, McGraw-Hill, pp 1013–1072.

Gloviczki P, Ricotta JJ: Aneurysmal vascular disease. In Townsend CM Jr, Beauchamp RD, Evers BM, Mattox KL, editors: *Sabiston textbook of surgery: the biological basis of modern surgical practice*, ed 18, Philadelphia, 2008, WB Saunders, pp 1907–1940.

Nypaver T: Fasciotomy in vascular trauma and compartment syndrome. In Ernst C, Stanley J, editors: *Current therapy in vascular surgery*, St. Louis, 2001, Mosby, pp 624–628.

Anus and Rectum

3

1. All of the following are true about anorectal anatomy EXCEPT:

   A. The dentate line marks the transition point between columnar and squamous mucosa.
   B. The presacral fascia separates the rectum from the presacral venous plexus and the pelvic nerves.
   C. Waldeyer fascia attaches to the fascia propria at the anorectal junction.
   D. In men, Denonvilliers fascia separates the rectum from the prostate and seminal vesicles.
   E. The surgical anal canal is longer in women than in men.

2. All of the following are true about anorectal lymphatic drainage EXCEPT:

   A. The upper and middle rectum drain to the inferior mesenteric and internal iliac lymph nodes.
   B. The lower rectum drains into the inferior mesenteric and internal iliac lymph nodes.
   C. Proximal to the dentate line, lymph drains into the inferior mesenteric and internal iliac lymph nodes.
   D. Distal to the dentate line, primary drainage is into the inguinal lymph nodes.
   E. Lymphatic drainage of the rectum parallels the vascular supply.

3. The recommended initial treatment of anal canal melanoma is:

   A. Abdominal perineal resection (APR)
   B. Wide local excision
   C. Wide local excision with regional lymph node dissection
   D. Radiation therapy
   E. Radiation therapy and chemotherapy

4. All of the following are true regarding epidermoid cancers of the anal canal EXCEPT:

   A. They include squamous, basaloid, cloacogenic, and transitional carcinomas.
   B. They tend to behave similarly regardless of cell type.
   C. They can generally be excised locally.
   D. They usually present with a mass and rectal bleeding.
   E. They respond to a combination of chemotherapy and radiation therapy.

5. All of the following anal margin lesions are related to human papillomavirus EXCEPT:

   A. Bowen disease
   B. Verrucous carcinoma
   C. Buschke-Löwenstein tumor
   D. Squamous cell carcinoma
   E. Paget disease

6. A 35-year-old man with leukemia and severe neutropenia presents with severe anal pain. Physical examination at the bedside demonstrates induration but no obvious mass in the perianal region. Which of the following is the best management?

   A. Intravenous (IV) antibiotics only
   B. Bedside anoscopy with bedside incision and drainage only if a fluctuant mass is detected
   C. Bedside anoscopy with operative incision and drainage if a fluctuant mass is detected
   D. Examination with patient under anesthesia with wide débridement of perianal area
   E. Examination with patient under anesthesia with biopsy of indurated areas and incision and drainage even if no pus is detected

7. Which of the following is true regarding the blood supply to the rectum?
   A. The superior and middle rectal arteries arise from the inferior mesenteric artery.
   B. The middle rectal veins drain into the internal iliac veins.
   C. The inferior rectal veins drain into the inferior mesenteric vein.
   D. The superior rectal veins drain into the inferior vena cava.
   E. There is poor collateralization between the superior and inferior rectal arteries.

8. A T3 squamous cell cancer of the anal canal is managed by:
   A. Wide local excision
   B. APR
   C. Combined chemotherapy and radiation therapy
   D. Chemotherapy alone
   E. Radiation therapy alone

9. Rectal bleeding due to chronic radiation proctitis that is unresponsive to sucralfate enemas is best managed by:
   A. Argon plasma coagulation
   B. Proximal diverting colostomy
   C. Steroid enemas
   D. APR
   E. Proctectomy

10. Twelve hours after hemorrhoidal banding, a 45-year-old man presents to the emergency department reporting rectal and abdominal pain and an inability to urinate. His temperature is 102°F and heart rate is 110 beats per minute. Management consists of:
    A. Placement of a Foley catheter
    B. Broad-spectrum IV antibiotics
    C. Broad-spectrum antibiotics and rectal examination with the patient under anesthesia
    D. Stool softeners and oral antibiotics
    E. In and out catheterization of bladder and stool softeners

11. The most common cause of a rectovaginal fistula is:
    A. Carcinoma of the rectum
    B. Crohn disease
    C. Obstetric injury
    D. Perianal abscess
    E. Radiation

12. Copious anal bleeding occurring 3 hours after hemorrhoidectomy is best managed by:
    A. Rubber banding the bleeding site
    B. Rectal packing with epinephrine gauze
    C. Suture ligation
    D. Ice packs
    E. Foley catheter balloon compression

13. The prognostic factors of importance in squamous cell cancer of the anus include all of the following EXCEPT:
    A. Positive inguinal versus perirectal nodes
    B. Depth of invasion
    C. Histologic grade
    D. Age
    E. Tumor size

14. The chemotherapeutic agents commonly used and favored for anal canal carcinoma are:
    A. 5-Fluorouracil (5-FU) and mitomycin C
    B. 5-FU and carmustine
    C. Floxuridine and bleomycin
    D. Vincristine and 5-FU
    E. Cyclophosphamide and prednisone

15. A 65-year-old woman presents to the emergency department with severe perianal pain for 12 hours that came on after straining during a bowel movement. Physical examination reveals an exquisitely tender perianal mass with bluish discoloration under the perianal skin. Management consists of:
    A. Stool softeners and sitz baths
    B. Rubber band ligation
    C. Stab incision and drainage with the patient under local anesthesia in the emergency department
    D. Elliptical excision of skin and drainage with the patient under local anesthesia in the emergency department
    E. Rectal examination with the patient under general anesthesia with incision and drainage

16. A 40-year-old man presents with rectal pain and bleeding. He reports a history of prolapsing hemorrhoids with straining for several years that he is simply able to manually reduce. However, he states that this time he is unable to do so. On physical examination, a large mass of edematous hemorrhoidal tissue is evident that you are unable to reduce. Management consists of:

    A. Urgent hemorrhoidectomy
    B. Urgent rubber band ligation
    C. Stab incision and drainage with the patient under local anesthesia in the emergency department
    D. Elliptical excision of skin and drainage with the patient under local anesthesia in the emergency department
    E. Rectal examination with the patient under general anesthesia with incision and drainage

17. Which of the following medical therapies results in the greatest healing rates for chronic anal fissures?

    A. Bulk agents and stool softeners
    B. Topical nitroglycerin
    C. Topical diltiazem
    D. Topical bethanecol
    E. Botulinum toxin injection

18. Which of the following anorectal findings would least likely raise concern for a more serious underlying pathology?

    A. An acute lateral anal fissure
    B. A chronic posterior anal fissure
    C. Recurrent perianal fistula
    D. Multiple perianal fistulas
    E. A perianal fistula with multiple tracts

19. An 80-year-old woman presents with rectal prolapse. She has a history of chronic constipation. Colonoscopy findings are negative. Treatment would be best achieved via:

    A. Fixation of the rectum with prosthetic sling (Ripstein repair)
    B. Anterior resection with rectopexy
    C. Thiersch anal encirclement
    D. Resection of perineal hernia and closure of the cul-de-sac (Moschcowitz procedure)
    E. Perineal rectosigmoidectomy (Altemeier procedure)

20. One week after vaginal delivery of a full-term infant, a 30-year-old woman presents with passage of flatus and small stool particles through her vagina. Endorectal ultrasonography confirms a low rectovaginal fistula. Management consists of:

    A. Two to 3 months of conservative therapy
    B. Endorectal advancement flap
    C. Temporary diverting colostomy
    D. Transabdominal primary repair with simple closure of vagina and rectum
    E. Transabdominal primary repair with interposition of muscle flap between the rectum and vagina

21. The most common bacterial cause of proctitis is:

    A. *Chlamydia trachomatis*
    B. *Neisseria gonorrhoeae*
    C. *Treponema pallidum*
    D. *Haemophilus ducreyi*
    E. *Shigella* species

22. Melanosis coli:

    A. Poses an increased risk of melanoma
    B. Poses an increased risk of colorectal adenocarcinoma
    C. Is related to Peutz-Jeghers syndrome
    D. Is irreversible
    E. Is related to the use of certain laxatives

23. Hirschsprung disease presenting in an adult:

    A. Does not occur
    B. Is not associated with the RET mutation
    C. Is best diagnosed by a barium enema
    D. Requires a pull-through procedure for definitive management
    E. Can be treated with anorectal myomectomy

Answers

1. E. The surgical anal canal is 2 to 4 cm in length and is longer in men. It spans the area from the anorectal junction to the anal verge. The anal transition zone is just proximal to the dentate line and has features of columnar and squamous epithelium as well as cuboidal epithelium. Cancers above this area are usually adenocarcinomas, whereas those distal to this line are squamous or cloacogenic. It is approximately 1 to 2 cm in length. In women, Denovilliers fascia separates the rectum from the vagina. Morgagni columns are found at the dentate line. Anal crypts empty in this area and are the source of abscesses.

2. A. The upper and middle rectum drains into the inferior mesenteric nodes, whereas the lower rectum drains into both the inferior mesenteric nodes and internal iliac nodes. Thus, it parallels the vascular supply. Distal to the dentate line, lymph drains into the inguinal lymph nodes but can also empty into the inferior mesenteric and internal iliac lymph nodes. Thus, an important part of the physical examination in a patient with anal cancer is examining the inguinal region for lymphadenopathy.

3. B. Melanoma of the anal canal is extremely rare, and the overall prognosis is poor. Given its rarity, established management protocols are lacking. A recent meta-analysis showed no stage-specific survival advantage of APR over wide local excision. As such, wide local excision is the recommended management.

   Reference: Droesch JT, Flum DR, Mann GN: Wide local excision or abdominoperineal resection as the initial treatment for anorectal melanoma? *Am J Surg* 189:446–449, 2005.

4. C. Cancers in the anal canal include squamous, basaloid, cloacogenic, and transitional carcinomas, yet despite the variation in cell type, they tend to behave similarly. The currently accepted standard approach is to treat them using a combination of chemotherapy and radiation therapy, which was initially espoused by Nigro. The protocol includes 5-FU and mitomycin C as well as pelvic radiation. Anal canal cancers should be distinguished from anal margin tumors. Anal margin tumors are generally treated by wide local excision.

   Reference: Flam M, John M, Pajak TF, et al: Role of mitomycin in combination with fluorouracil and radiotherapy, and of salvage chemoradiation in the definitive nonsurgical treatment of epidermoid carcinoma of the anal canal: results of a phase III randomized intergroup study, *J Clin Oncol* 14:2527–2539, 1996.

5. E. The human papillomavirus, particularly types 16 and 18, has been linked to anal canal cancers and, in particular, to squamous cell cancers. Bowen disease is a squamous cell carcinoma in situ and is also termed *anal intraepithelial neoplasia*. Verrucous carcinoma is also called a *Buschke-Lowenstein tumor* and is a locally aggressive form of giant condyloma acuminatum. Paget disease of the anus is a form of adenocarcinoma in situ. It does not have the same relationship to human papillomavirus. Both Bowen disease and Paget disease can be confused with an eczematoid rash, thus of persistent perianal rashes is essential. Treatment of both is wide local excision. If an extensive resection is required, closure can be achieved with a V-Y advancement flap. In addition to the previously mentioned lesions, anal margin tumors also include anal margin squamous cell cancer and basal cell carcinoma.

   Reference: Frisch M, Glimelius B, van den Brule AJ, et al: Sexually transmitted infection as a cause of anal cancer, *N Engl J Med* 337:1350–1358, 1997.

6. E. Perianal pain may develop in neutropenic patients, yet the diagnosis of a perianal abscess may be difficult given the lack of inflammatory response to infection. Although broad-spectrum antibiotics may cure some of these patients, an examination with the patient under anesthesia should be performed to rule out an abscess that requires drainage. Although a discrete abscess may not be seen, any areas of induration should be incised and drained and a biopsy specimen obtained to exclude a leukemia infiltrate and cultured to aid in the selection of antimicrobial agents.

   Reference: Cohen J, Paz I, O'Donnell M, Ellenhorn J: Treatment of perianal infection following bone marrow transplantation, *Dis Colon Rectum* 39:981–985, 1996.

7. B. The superior rectal arteries arise from the inferior mesenteric artery, which provides blood to the upper rectum. The middle and inferior rectal arteries arise from the internal iliac arteries, which provide blood to the rest of the rectum and the anal canal. Rich collaterals exist between the rectal arteries such that they are relatively resistant to ischemia. The venous drainage follows the arterial supply. The superior rectal veins drain into the inferior mesenteric vein and then to the portal vein, whereas the middle and inferior rectal veins drain into branches of the internal iliac veins and into the inferior vena cava. The middle rectal arteries are the least consistent and are absent in as many as three fourths of patients.

8. C. As mentioned in question 4, the majority of anal canal cancers behave similarly. At the time of diagnosis, more than 75% are locally invasive, making local excision difficult. If the lesion were confined to the submucosal tissues (T1), wide local excision may be possible. Thus, more invasive lesions are treated according to the Nigro protocol, which consists of chemotherapy with 5-FU and mitomycin C and radiation therapy. APR was the standard treatment before the development of the Nigro protocol. This has since been abandoned because of higher recurrence rates, shorter long-term survival, and increased surgical morbidity. Chemotherapy or radiation therapy alone is not sufficient.

   Reference: Flam M, John M, Pajak TF, et al: Role of mitomycin in combination with fluorouracil and radiotherapy, and of salvage chemoradiation in the definitive nonsurgical treatment of epidermoid carcinoma of the anal canal: results of a phase III randomized intergroup study, *J Clin Oncol* 14:2527–2539, 1996.

9. A. Sucralfate enemas are currently considered to be the first line of treatment for chronic radiation proctitis. Steroid and 5-aminosalicylic acid enemas have not been shown to be effective in the long term for treating radiation proctitis. Thus, if sucralfate enemas have failed, steroid enemas are unlikely to help. For patients with recurrent symptoms, two effective therapies have evolved: endoscopic therapy and topical formulas. Argon plasma coagulation is the currently favored endoscopic technique due to its limited depth of penetration. The success rate of improving bleeding symptoms is 90%, but multiple treatments are necessary. The main drawback is its lack of uniform availability. Formalin therapy has a success rate of 90%; it is inexpensive and effective with a single treatment. Recently, there was a report linking formalin use with anal canal stricturing. Nevertheless, it is an important option when sucralfate enemas fail. The need for surgical therapy is uncommon. For refractory bleeding, a colostomy may be offered, but diversion of the fecal stream is often unsuccessful in stopping the hemorrhage. For incapacitating symptoms from bleeding, strictures, and nonhealing ulcers, proctectomy with a coloanal anastomosis or end colostomy may be offered.

References: de Parades V, Etienney I, Bauer P, et al: Formalin application in the treatment of chronic radiation-induced hemorrhagic proctitis—an effective but not risk-free procedure: a prospective study of 33 patients, *Dis Colon Rectum* 48:1535–1541, 2005.

Gul Y, Prasannan S, Jabar F, et al: Pharmacotherapy for chronic hemorrhagic radiation proctitis, *World J Surg* 26:1499–1502, 2002.

Taïeb S, Rolachon A, Cenni J, et al: Effective use of argon plasma coagulation in the treatment of severe radiation proctitis, *Dis Colon Rectum* 44:1766–1771, 2001.

10. C. Sepsis after the treatment of hemorrhoids has been described after banding, sclerotherapy, and stapled hemorrhoidectomy. Although very rare, it is life threatening. It is most common in immunocompromised patients. The patient usually presents within the first 12 hours after the procedure, but can present in a delayed fashion. The most common symptoms are severe perineal pain, fevers, and urinary retention. Appropriate management of sepsis after hemorrhoidectomy includes hospital admission, fluid resuscitation, and IV antibiotics with coverage of gram-negative rods and anaerobes. Examination with the patient under anesthesia is recommended to rule out a necrotizing infection that may require débridement.

References: Cirocco WC: Life threatening sepsis and mortality following stapled hemorrhoidopexy, *Surgery* 143:824–829, 2008.

McCloud JM, Jameson JS, Scott AN: Life-threatening sepsis following treatment for haemorrhoids: a systematic review, *Colorectal Dis* 8:748–755, 2006.

11. C. A rectovaginal fistula is most often due to an obstetric injury after a vaginal delivery in association with episiotomy typically in primigravidas; to the use of forceps; or due to infection of an episiotomy site. Other causes include inflammatory bowel disease (Crohn disease more than ulcerative colitis), carcinoma of the rectum, radiation therapy for pelvic malignancies, and rarely perianal

abscesses and diverticulitis. It can also be iatrogenic during low anterior resections, particularly in women who have had a hysterectomy. Treatment for low fistulas is with an endorectal advancement flap, and for high fistulas (more likely due to neoplasm, Crohn disease, radiation), management is via a transabdominal approach with resection of the affected rectal segment.

12. C. Bleeding can occur immediately or, in the case of hemorrhoidal banding, after 7 to 10 days, when the necrotic stump sloughs off. Options for the management of bleeding include rectal packing with epinephrine gauze, ice packs, and balloon compression with a Foley catheter. The majority of bleeding is mild and resolves with simple measures. However, if bleeding is copious, the patient should be taken back to the operating/procedure room, where visualization is better, anesthesia is adequate, cautery can be used, and suture ligation can be performed.

References: Jongen J, Bock J, Peleikis H, et al: Complications and reoperations in stapled anopexy: learning by doing, *Int J Colorectal Dis* 21:166–171, 2006.

Ravo B, Amato A, Bianco V, et al: Complications after stapled hemorrhoidectomy: can they be prevented? *Tech Coloproctol* 6:83–88, 2002.

13. D. The size of the tumor, depth of invasion, histologic grade, and nodal status are all important prognostic factors for anal squamous cell cancers. Positive inguinal nodes confer a worse prognosis than positive perirectal nodes. The age of the patient has no prognostic value. Squamous cell cancers can occur at any age, but are typically seen in the sixth and seventh decades. Of note, squamous cell cancers of the anal margin have a better prognosis than do cancers of the anal canal.

14. A. In 1972, the Nigro protocol revolutionized the way in which carcinomas of the anus were managed. This regimen consists of 5-FU and mitomycin C combined with radiation therapy.

15. D. Hemorrhoids should be distinguished as being either internal or external. Internal ones arise above the dentate line and as such are insensate. They may cause painless bleeding during straining to defecate, may prolapse, or may even become strangulated. If they strangulate, they can cause pain due to intense spasm of the anal sphincter. External hemorrhoids originate below the dentate line, are covered with anoderm, and may cause discomfort such as itching, but generally only cause severe pain if they become thrombosed. Treatment of thrombosed external hemorrhoids, as in this case, consists of incision and drainage of the thrombosed hemorrhoid with the patient under local anesthesia. To prevent recurrence or inadequate drainage, it is important to excise an ellipse of skin and not simply perform a stab avulsion. Nonoperative management is acceptable if the patient has had symptoms for many days and the pain is already beginning to subside. Numerous studies have shown that local anesthesia is well tolerated.

Reference: Jongen J, Bach S, Stübinger S, Bock J: Excision of thrombosed external hemorrhoid under local anesthesia: a retrospective evaluation of 340 patients, *Dis Colon Rectum* 46:1226–1231, 2003.

16. A. Internal hemorrhoids are classified into four degrees. First degree, bleeding with no prolapse, is managed with fiber supplements and avoidance of excessive straining. Second degree, prolapse with spontaneous reduction, can be treated with medical management as well as with rubber banding. With third degree, prolapse requiring digital reduction, surgical hemorrhoidectomy should be considered (either standard or stapled), and with fourth degree, nonreducible, strangulated hemorrhoids, urgent hemorroidectomy is often necessary.

17. E. Anal fissures are thought to develop as the result of the passage of hard stools, causing trauma to the anoderm distal to the dentate line. Given their distal location, they cause exquisite pain with each defecation, often accompanied by blood on the toilet paper. To effect healing, softening of the stool is essential, using fiber and stool softeners, as is relaxation of the sphincter. Numerous topical agents have been used with varying degrees of success, including 2% lidocaine jelly, nitroglycerin ointment (0.2%), topical diltiazem, topical arginine (a nitric oxide donor), and topical bethanechol (a muscarinic agonist). However, the best rate of healing with nonoperative treatment is via injection of botulinum toxin, which causes temporary paralysis of the sphincter muscle. Recent studies suggest that healing rates with botulinum toxin approach those of surgery, although surgery remains the gold standard for refractory cases. Surgery is generally reserved for those in whom medical management fails. Surgical treatment is lateral internal sphincterotomy.

References: Giral A, Memisoglu K, Gültekin Y, et al: Botulinum toxin injection versus lateral internal sphincterotomy in the treatment of chronic anal fissure: a non-randomized controlled trial, *BMC Gastroenterol* 4:7, 2004.

Maria G, Cassetta E, Gui D, et al: A comparison of botulinum toxin and saline for the treatment of chronic anal fissure, *N Engl J Med* 338:217–220, 1998.

18. B. Chronic anal fissures are most commonly located in the posterior midline. The next most common site is the anterior midline. Fissures in any other location, such as lateral ones, should raise suspicion for other underlying diseases such as Crohn disease, sexually transmitted diseases, and hidradenitis suppurativa. Likewise, recurrent or complex fistulas should raise concern for Crohn disease.

19. A. Procidentia (rectal prolapse) is much more common in women than men. It is more common in elderly women. In young men, it is more often associated with psychiatric disease. As a general rule, adults with rectal prolapse require surgery, whereas children can often be managed nonoperatively. Procedures are divided into abdominal and perineal procedures. In general, abdominal procedures are associated with a lower recurrence rate but a higher complication rate than are perineal procedures. As such, abdominal procedures are used for younger, lower-risk patients and perineal procedures for older, higher-risk patients. Recent studies have shown favorable results with the perineal rectosigmoidectomy in elderly high-risk patients. The perineal rectosigmoidectomy has a 15% recurrence rate and is a good option for older patients. Another well-accepted

perineal operation is the Delorme procedure, which involves reefing the rectal mucosa. The Thiersch anal encirclement is no longer used.

Reference: Williams J, Rothenberger D, Madoff R, Goldberg S: Treatment of rectal prolapse in the elderly by perineal rectosigmoidectomy, *Dis Colon Rectum* 35:830–834, 1992.

20. A. The treatment of a rectovaginal fistula depends on the size, location, etiology, and condition of surrounding tissues. Most rectovaginal fistulas are due to obstetric injury, and as many as 50% of these fistulas heal spontaneously within 3 months, so initial management should be conservative. If the fistula is caused by an abscess, drainage of the abscess may allow spontaneous closure. Low rectovaginal fistulas are usually best treated via a perineal approach, such as with an endorectal advancement flap (which is the usual case with obstetric fistulas). High fistulas are best treated via a transabdominal approach.

References: Rahman M, Al-Suleiman S, El-Yahia A, Rahman J: Surgical treatment of rectovaginal fistula of obstetric origin: a review of 15 years' experience in a teaching hospital, *J Obstet Gynaecol* 23:607–610, 2003.

Sonoda T, Hull T, Piedmonte M, Fazio V: Outcomes of primary repair of anorectal and rectovaginal fistulas using the endorectal advancement flap, *Dis Colon Rectum* 45:1622–1628, 2002.

21. B. Proctitis typically presents with pain, tenesmus, rectal bleeding, diarrhea, and mucus discharge. It can be due to a bacterial infection, viral infection, trauma, radiation, and inflammatory bowel disease. Bacterial proctitis is often due to sexually transmitted diseases and is associated with anal intercourse. *N. gonorrhoeae* is the most common bacterial cause, followed by *Chlamydia*, which tends to produce fewer symptoms. Bacterial proctitis can also be due to non–sexually transmitted diseases, primarily in association with inflammatory bowel disease. Treatment of bacterial proctitis is with antibiotics, whereas for proctitis in association with inflammatory bowel disease, the treatment includes steroid and 5-aminosalicylic acid enemas.

22. E. Melanosis coli is an accumulation of pigment in the macrophages of the lamina propria of the colon. It is a benign condition noted at colonoscopy that does not seem to increase the risk of malignancy. It has been reported in relation to the use of certain laxatives and cathartics, in particular anthracene cathartics (cascara, senna). It seems to resolve within 6 to 12 months after stopping their use.

Reference: Nascimbeni R, Donato F, Ghirardi M, et al: Constipation, anthranoid laxatives, melanosis coli, and colon cancer: a risk assessment using aberrant crypt foci, *Cancer Epidemiol Biomarkers Prev* 11:753–757, 2002.

23. E. Hirschsprung disease rarely presents in adults. In this setting, the patient typically has a lifelong history of constipation and fecal impaction. A careful history will often reveal symptoms dating back to infancy. In most circumstances, Hirschsprung disease presenting as an adult consists of a short segment of aganglionosis. Although a barium enema can be diagnostic if an extremely dilated proximal colon, transitional zone, and contracted distal colon and rectum are seen, it may miss short-segment Hirschsprung disease if the rectal tube is introduced too far past the anal canal, bypassing the contracted segment. As such, the diagnosis is established by a rectal mucosal biopsy specimen demonstrating aganglionosis. As in children, Hirschsprung disease is associated with the RET mutation in a percentage of patients. Although a pull-through procedure, such as the Soave or Duhamel operation, is performed in children and in those with long segments of aganglionosis, in adults with short-segment aganglionosis, an anorectal myomectomy can be performed.

References: Nelson H, Cima RR: Anus. In Townsend CM, Beauchamp RD, Evers BM, Mattox KL, editors: *Sabiston textbook of surgery: the biological basis of modern surgical practice*, ed 18, Philadelphia, 2008, WB Saunders, pp 1907–1940.

Wu J, Schoetz D Jr, Coller J, Veidenheimer M: Treatment of Hirschsprung's disease in the adult: report of five cases, *Dis Colon Rectum* 38:655–659, 1995.

Appendix

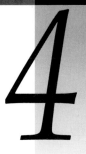

1. Which of the following is true regarding the immune function of the appendix?
   A. It secretes IgA.
   B. It secretes IgE.
   C. It secretes IgM.
   D. It secretes IgG.
   E. It has no immune function.

2. A hernia containing an appendix is known as:
   A. Petit hernia
   B. Amyand hernia
   C. Littre hernia
   D. Spigelian hernia
   E. Grynfeltt hernia

3. Appendiceal rupture occurs most frequently:
   A. At the base
   B. At the tip
   C. At the mesenteric border
   D. At the antimesenteric border
   E. In women

4. The most common cause of acute appendicitis in children is:
   A. Fecalith
   B. Hypertrophied lymphoid tissue
   C. Ascariasis
   D. Pinworms
   E. Vegetable and/or fruit seeds

5. Which of the following is true regarding appendicitis in HIV-infected patients?
   A. It is more frequent than in the general population.
   B. They usually do not manifest abdominal symptoms and signs.
   C. Low CD4 counts are associated with a decreased risk of rupture.
   D. Postoperative morbidity for nonperforated appendicitis is higher than in the general population.
   E. Absolute leukocyte counts are typically elevated.

6. When comparing laparoscopic with open appendectomy, all of the following are true regarding laparoscopic appendectomy EXCEPT:
   A. It is more costly.
   B. It results in shorter length of hospital stay.
   C. It results in a decreased intra-abdominal abscess rate.
   D. It results in a decreased wound infection rate.
   E. It allows a quicker return to work.

7. The most common intestinal parasite causing appendicitis is:
   A. *Enterobius vermicularis*
   B. *Strongyloides stercoralis*
   C. *Ascaris lumbricoides*
   D. *Echinococcus granulosus*
   E. *Clonorchis sinensis*

8. Incidental appendectomy is BEST indicated in which of the following circumstances?
   A. During gastric bypass surgery in a 45-year-old man
   B. During hysterectomy in a 30-year-old woman
   C. During small bowel resection in a 30-year-old woman with Crohn disease
   D. During laparoscopic cholecystectomy in a 25-year-old woman
   E. During a Whipple procedure in a 50-year-old man

9. A 10-year-old boy presents with symptoms and signs of acute appendicitis. At surgery, the appendix appears normal. However, there is diffuse adenopathy within the small bowel mesentery. Which of the following is true about this condition?

  A. The normal appendix should be removed and a biopsy of the mesenteric lymph nodes performed.
  B. This condition usually causes more peritoneal irritation than appendicitis.
  C. The white blood cell count tends to be higher than with appendicitis.
  D. It occurs with equal frequency in adults and children.
  E. It is usually associated with an antecedent upper respiratory tract infection.

10. Which of the following is the most common neoplasm of the appendix?

  A. Adenocarcinoma
  B. Carcinoid
  C. Malignant mucocele
  D. Lymphoma
  E. Lymphosarcoma

11. The most common presentation for appendiceal adenocarcinoma is:

  A. Palpable abdominal mass
  B. Acute appendicitis
  C. Ascites
  D. Incidental finding during unrelated abdominal surgery
  E. Chronic anemia

12. A 40-year-old man undergoes an appendectomy for acute appendicitis. Final pathology reveals a 2.5-cm carcinoid at the tip of the appendix. Lymph nodes are negative. Which of the following is true about this condition?

  A. No further treatment is necessary.
  B. There is a significant chance that carcinoid syndrome will develop in the patient.
  C. The patient should receive chemotherapy.
  D. The patient should undergo reexploration and a right colectomy.
  E. Most appendiceal carcinoids are 2.5 cm or larger when discovered.

13. Five days after appendectomy, liquid stool is noted to be coming out of the right lower quadrant wound. Which of the following is true about this condition?

  A. The patient should have nothing by mouth and be placed on parenteral nutrition.
  B. Octreotide should be started.
  C. The patient should immediately undergo reexploration and a cecostomy.
  D. The patient should immediately undergo reexploration and a right colectomy.
  E. The condition resolves spontaneously in most instances.

14. A 50-year-old woman presents with symptoms and signs of acute appendicitis. At surgery, there is a large amount of gelatinous ascites with peritoneal implants. This most likely represents:

  A. Ovarian cancer
  B. Appendiceal mucinous adenoma
  C. Tuberculous appendicitis
  D. *Salmonella enteritidis*
  E. *Yersinia enterocolitica*

15. A 15-year-old boy presents with a 5-day history of right lower quadrant pain and a fever of 103°F. On examination, he has right lower and right upper quadrant tenderness. Total bilirubin is 3 mg/dL and alkaline phosphatase is 250 IU/L. Computed tomography (CT) with contrast demonstrates multiple densities in the right lobe of the liver, a phlegmon in the right lower quadrant, and stranding around the superior mesenteric vein with air bubbles within the vein. The clinical picture most likely represents:

  A. Amebic liver abscess
  B. Pylephlebitis
  C. Carcinoid syndrome
  D. Metastatic adenocarcinoma
  E. Inflammatory bowel disease

16. A 35-year-old man presents with a 1-day history of anorexia, right lower quadrant pain and tenderness, and low-grade fever. At surgery, the appendix appears normal. However, both the cecum and terminal ileum appear red and inflamed. Management would consist of:

  A. Right hemicolectomy
  B. Appendectomy
  C. Close wound without further intervention
  D. Biopsy of the cecal wall
  E. Biopsy of the terminal ileum

17. Which of the following is true regarding acute appendicitis?
    A. The accompanying nausea and vomiting result from irritation of the parietal peritoneum.
    B. It is a form of closed-loop obstruction.
    C. The male-to-female ratio is 1:1.
    D. The incidence has been increasing over the past 4 decades.
    E. The increasing use of CT has decreased the negative appendectomy rate.

18. All of the following are true regarding acute appendicitis EXCEPT:
    A. The luminal capacity of the appendix is 0.1 mL.
    B. The initial periumbilical pain is due to stimulation of visceral afferent pain fibers.
    C. Hyperperistalsis is a feature of early appendicitis.
    D. Chronic appendicitis does not occur.
    E. Children younger than 5 years have a higher perforation rate.

19. All of the following are signs of acute nonperforated appendicitis EXCEPT:
    A. Voluntary guarding
    B. Psoas sign
    C. Obturator sign
    D. Fever of 103°F
    E. Cutaneous hyperesthesia

20. Which of the following is the most reliable in confirming the diagnosis of acute appendicitis?
    A. Classic history of initial periumbilical pain shifting to the right lower quadrant
    B. Localized tenderness at McBurney point
    C. Rebound tenderness
    D. Presence of obturator sign
    E. Rovsing sign

21. A 30-year-old African American man presents with symptoms and signs of acute appendicitis. At surgery, the appendix appears red and inflamed but without perforation. Approximately 200 mL of purulent fluid is seen in the right paracolic gutter. The patient undergoes appendectomy. Final pathology reveals periappendicitis. This most likely represents:
    A. Acute mesenteric adenitis
    B. Familial Mediterranean fever
    C. Perforated duodenal ulcer
    D. Tuberculosis
    E. Primary peritonitis

22. The most common primary site for carcinoid tumors is:
    A. Rectum
    B. Small intestine
    C. Bronchus
    D. Appendix
    E. Colon

23. A 60-year-old man presents with a 4-day history of right lower quadrant abdominal pain, anorexia, and fever. On physical examination, a mass is palpable in the right lower quadrant. A CT scan shows a small abscess surrounding an inflamed appendix. After fluid resuscitation and intravenous antibiotics, which of the following is the most appropriate management?
    A. CT-guided drainage
    B. Initial nonoperative management followed by interval appendectomy
    C. Laparoscopic appendectomy
    D. Open appendectomy
    E. Ileocecectomy

24. The appendiceal artery is a branch of the:
    A. Right colic artery
    B. Middle colic artery
    C. Left colic artery
    D. Ileocolic artery
    E. Hypogastric artery

25. With appendicitis during pregnancy, the factor most strongly associated with fetal mortality is:
    A. Fetal gestational age
    B. Open appendectomy instead of laparoscopy
    C. Maternal comorbidities
    D. Appendiceal rupture
    E. Delay in antibiotic administration

26. A 55-year-old woman undergoes laparoscopy for presumed appendicitis. At surgery, she is found to have perforated appendicitis with what appears to be peritoneal studding. The patient undergoes appendectomy and biopsy of the peritoneum. Final pathology reveals appendiceal adenocarcinoma. Subsequent work-up reveals no evidence of additional metastatic spread to the liver or lungs. Further treatment would consist of:
    A. No further treatment
    B. Systemic chemotherapy
    C. Intraperitoneal chemotherapy
    D. Cryoreductive surgery and intraperitoneal chemotherapy
    E. Cryoreductive surgery and systemic chemotherapy

Answers

1. A. The appendix is part of the gut-associated lymphoid tissue and primarily secretes IgA. However, removal of the appendix has no known adverse effect on immune function. A recent study from Duke University proposes that the appendix serves as a safe haven or reservoir for healthy bacteria that then repopulate the gut after illnesses have depleted them.

Reference: Bollinger R, Barbas A, Bush E, et al: Biofilms in the large bowel suggest an apparent function of the human vermiform appendix, *J Theoret Biol* (in press).

2. B. The importance of an Amyand hernia is that it can be confused with a standard strangulated hernia. Management should consist of appendectomy without the use of mesh. It is named after Claudius Amyand, who performed the first appendectomy in London in 1746. The patient was an 11-year-old boy with a scrotal hernia that contained the appendix perforated by a pin. Petit hernia is a type of lumbar hernia located in the inferior lumbar triangle. It is bound by the iliac crest inferiorly, the external oblique muscle anteriorly, and the latissimus dorsi muscle posteriorly. Littre hernia is a hernia containing Meckel diverticulum. Spigelian hernia is a hernia through the linea semilunaris. Grynfeltt hernia is another type of lumbar hernia found in the superior lumbar triangle, which is bound by the quadratus lumborum muscle on its floor, the internal oblique muscle anteriorly, and the 12th rib superiorly.

Reference: Logan M, Nottingham J: Amyand's hernia: a case report of an incarcerated and perforated appendix within an inguinal hernia and review of the literature, *Am Surg* 67:628–629, 2001.

3. D. Appendicitis is a form of closed-loop obstruction. The lumen can hold approximately 0.1 mL of fluid. When the base of the appendix becomes obstructed, as by a fecalith, the appendiceal mucosa continues to secrete fluid into the lumen, causing the appendix to distend. Capillary and venule blood flow is obstructed. This leads to infarction, which first occurs at the antimesenteric border because it has the poorest blood supply. Perforation follows at these infarcted areas and typically just beyond the point of obstruction rather than at the tip because, as described by Laplace's law, the wider diameter creates greater intraluminal tension.

4. B. Obstruction of the lumen by hypertrophied lymphoid tissue is the most common cause of acute appendicitis in children. Why the lymphoid tissue hypertrophies is not clear, but some have speculated that it occurs in response to a viral infection. Fecaliths are the usual cause of appendiceal obstruction in adults. Other causes of appendiceal obstruction include inspissated barium from previous x-ray studies, tumors, vegetable and fruit seeds, and intestinal parasites.

5. A. The incidence of acute appendicitis in patients infected with human immunodeficiency virus (HIV) is 0.5%, which is higher than the population as a whole. The overall mode of presentation is similar. However, an absolute leukocyte count is usually not elevated, but rather these patients may have a relative leukocytosis. The rupture risk is higher in HIV-infected patients, which may simply be a manifestation of a delay in presentation, although a low CD4 count seems to increase the risk of appendiceal rupture. Morbidity rates for HIV-infected patients with nonperforated appendicitis are similar to those seen in the general population, but higher with perforation than in patients without HIV.

References: Binderow S, Shaked A: Acute appendicitis in patients with AIDS/HIV infection, *Am J Surg* 162:9–12, 1991.

Bova R, Meagher A: Appendicitis in HIV-positive patients, *ANZ J Surg* 68:337–339, 1998.

6. C. Numerous studies have compared open and laparoscopic appendectomy. Laparoscopic appendectomy seems to be most advantageous in women of child-bearing age, when the diagnosis is in question, or in obese patients. The cost and length of the operation are higher for a laparoscopic appendectomy. Length of hospital stay is slightly shorter, as is the wound infection rate, degree of postoperative pain, and the time to return to work. Interestingly, in one meta-analysis, the rate of intra-abdominal abscess trended toward being higher with a laparoscopic appendectomy, and in another analysis, there was no difference. Wound infections were less likely in a laparoscopic appendectomy.

References: Golub R, Siddiqui F, Pohl D: Laparoscopic versus open appendectomy: a metaanalysis, *J Am Coll Surg* 186:545–553, 1998.

Temple L, Litwin D, McLeod R: A meta-analysis of laparoscopic versus open appendectomy in patients suspected of having acute appendicitis, *Can J Surg* 42:377–383, 1999.

7. C. The association of parasites with appendicitis is somewhat controversial. The debate is whether the parasite is an incidental finding or the actual cause. Ascariasis is the most common parasite worldwide, with an estimated 1.4 billion persons infected. The majority of infections occur in the developing countries of Asia and Latin America. *Enterobius vermicularis* (pinworm) is the second most common parasite. Intestinal parasites can cause appendicitis by obstructing the lumen. Thus, it is always important to check the final pathology because therapy with a helminthicide is necessary postoperatively. Mebendazole, pyrantel pamoate, and albendazole are the drugs of choice.

8. C. When deciding whether to perform an incidental appendectomy during another procedure, one must factor in the lifelong risk of appendicitis versus the risks of appendectomy and the additional costs. Because the lifelong risk of appendicitis is only 8.6% in men and 6.7% in women, incidental appendectomy is rarely recommended. In a large study of patients undergoing cholecystectomy with and without incidental appendectomy, low-risk patients undergoing appendectomy showed a significant increase in nonfatal complications (odds ratio of 1.53). Particular circumstances in which incidental appendectomy (during the course of another operation) would be recommended are for children about to undergo chemotherapy (due to risk of subsequent typhlitis), in the disabled (i.e., para/quadriplegic) who cannot react normally to abdominal pain, Crohn disease patients (because they have a significant risk of subsequent abdominal pain) whose cecum is free of macroscopic disease (to minimize risk of postoperative cecal fistula), and individuals who are about to travel to remote places where there is no access to medical/surgical care.

Reference: Wen S, Hernandez R, Naylor C: Pitfalls in nonrandomized outcomes studies: the case of incidental appendectomy with open cholecystectomy, *JAMA* 274:1687–1691, 1995.

9. E. The presentation and findings are consistent with acute mesenteric adenitis. It is associated with *Yersinia enterocolitica, Helicobacter jejuni, Campylobacter jejuni*, and *Salmonella* or *Shigella* species, as well as streptococcal infections of the pharynx. In children, acute mesenteric adenitis is often preceded by an upper respiratory infection. It is a diagnosis of exclusion. Physical examination typically reveals more vague and diffuse tenderness, without significant guarding, as opposed to the localized tenderness seen in appendicitis. CT may show generalized lymphadenopathy in the small bowel mesentery, but these findings are nonspecific. The diagnosis is often made intraoperatively. There is no need for nodal biopsy.

10. A. Mucinous adenocarcinoma is the most common neoplasm of the appendix, followed by carcinoid. There are three histologic subtypes of appendiceal adenocarcinoma: mucinous, colonic adenocarcinoma, and adenocarcinoid. The overall 5-year survival rate is 55%, but it depends on the histologic type.

Reference: McGory M, Maggard M, Kang H, et al: Malignancies of the appendix: beyond case series reports, *Dis Colon Rectum* 48:2264–2271, 2005.

11. B. Primary adenocarcinoma of the appendix presents most commonly as acute appendicitis. For this reason, it is always important to check the final pathology of the appendiceal specimen. Patients are at increased risk of synchronous neoplasms. Definitive treatment consists of a right colectomy. If the final pathology reveals appendiceal cancer, the patient should be taken back for a right colectomy. In one series, the 5-year survival rate after curative resection was 61% and 31% after palliative surgery.

Reference: Ito H, Osteen R, Bleday R, et al: Appendiceal adenocarcinoma: long-term outcomes after surgical therapy, *Dis Colon Rectum* 47:474–480, 2004.

12. D. Most carcinoids are found at the tip of the appendix. As such, they are not usually the cause of appendicitis, but are rather incidental findings. Tumors less than 1 cm rarely extend outside of the appendix and are treated simply by appendectomy. A right colectomy is indicated for tumors with extension into the mesoappendix or for those greater than 1.5 to 2 cm. Appendiceal carcinoids rarely cause carcinoid syndrome because widespread liver metastases are rare. There is no role for radiation or chemotherapy for

appendiceal carcinoid. In one large series, the overall 5-year survival rate for localized lesions was 94%, 84.6% for regional invasion, and 33.7% for distant metastases. The 5-year survival rate of appendiceal carcinoids was the highest among all types of carcinoid tumors. In approximately 15% of patients, noncarcinoid tumors at other sites were also evident.

References: Jaffe BM, Berger DH: Appendix. In Brunicardi FC, Anderson DK, Billiar TR, et al, editors: *Schwartz's principles of surgery*, ed 9, New York, 2010, McGraw-Hill, pp 1073–1091.

Sandor A, Modlin I: A retrospective analysis of 1570 appendiceal carcinoids, *Am J Gastroenterol* 93:422–428, 1998.

Stinner B, Kisker O, Zielke A, Rothmund M: Surgical management for carcinoid tumors of small bowel, appendix, colon, and rectum, *World J Surg* 20:183–188, 1996.

13. E. The patient has a cecal fistula. The most common causes are slippage of the suture or necrosis of the remaining appendiceal stump. Colocutaneous fistulas, being low-output fistulas, are not associated with losses of large amounts of fluid, electrolytes, and nutrients. Therefore, total parenteral nutrition is not necessary to maintain adequate nutrition. Spontaneous closure is the rule in the majority of patients. Patients can be fed a low-residue diet because absorption is mostly complete by the time the contents reach the cecum. Octreotide does not help in assisting closure of a cecal fistula. If the fistula fails to close, one must suspect the possibility of either a neoplasm in the cecum, inflammatory bowel disease, tuberculosis, or distal obstruction. In a large series of nearly 5000 appendectomies, 4 patients developed cecal fistulas, and 2 closed spontaneously.

Reference: Hale D, Molloy M, Pearl R, et al: Appendectomy: a contemporary appraisal, *Ann Surg* 225:252–261, 1997.

14. B. *Pseudomyxoma peritonei* is a confusing term because it has been applied to several different pathologies. It has been used in reference to any progressive process in which the peritoneal cavity becomes filled with a thick gelatinous substance. This gelatinous substance is thought to arise from mucus-secreting cells from a perforated, mucus-producing tumor, which can be either benign or malignant and can originate from the appendix, small bowel, or ovary. Even if these cells are benign, once it has spread throughout the peritoneum, it is difficult to eradicate, and with time, the patient's small bowel becomes mechanically obstructed. If the source is a malignant tumor, the 5-year survival rate is significantly reduced. The most common source of this condition is a benign mucinous cystadenoma of the appendix. The new terminology has been coined: *disseminated peritoneal adenomucinosis* to define patients with mucinous peritoneal implants that arise from a benign adenoma of the appendix. This is the most common variety. A more aggressive form has been called *peritoneal mucinous carcinomatosis* and features extensive proliferative epithelium, cytologic atypia, and a high mitotic rate. Treatment consists of aggressive removal of all peritoneal implants as well as an appendectomy. Intraperitoneal chemotherapy likewise shows promising results. The 5-year survival rate is approximately 50%, but varies greatly by histology. Tuberculous peritonitis often presents as slowly progressive abdominal distention due to ascites, combined with fever, weight loss, and abdominal pain. Characteristic features at surgery are multiple whitish nodules scattered over the visceral and parietal peritoneum. *Salmonella enteritidis* typically presents with diarrhea, nausea, and vomiting with stool leukocytes. It can rarely lead to intestinal perforation, most commonly through an ulcerated Peyer patch. *Yersinia* infections can lead to mesenteric adenitis, colitis, and ileitis that can present in a similar fashion to acute appendicitis. *Yersinia* infections can also cause appendicitis.

Reference: Wirtzfeld D, Rodriguez-Bigas M, Weber T, et al: Disseminated peritoneal adenomucinosis: a critical review, *Ann Surg Oncol* 6:797–801, 1999.

15. B. Pylephlebitis is essentially an infectious inflammation of the portal venous system. These veins drain the gastrointestinal tract. It typically begins within the small veins draining an area of infection within the abdomen and is most often associated with diverticulitis and appendicitis. Extension of the thrombophlebitis into larger veins can lead to septic thrombophlebitis of the portal vein or its tributaries (superior mesenteric vein, splenic vein) as well as multiple small liver abscesses. Due to laminar flow patterns, the bacteria are more likely to lodge and form abscesses in the right lobe of the liver. Patients are usually not jaundiced but have elevated liver enzymes (particularly alkaline phosphatase). Pylephlebitis was much more common in the preantibiotic era, but it has become very rare due to major advances in antibiotic and surgical treatment. Air bubbles or thrombi of the portal venous system are key findings of pylephlebitis on CT scan. The reported mortality rate is as high as 30% to 50%. Because of the rarity, established management protocols are lacking. The most prudent approach seems to be rapid administration of broad-spectrum antibiotics, removal of the infectious source (in this case by appendectomy), and anticoagulation (for the suspected thrombosed superior mesenteric vein).

References: Chang Y, Min S, Joo S, Lee S: Septic thrombophlebitis of the porto-mesenteric veins as a complication of acute appendicitis, *World J Gastroenterol* 14:4580–4582, 2008.

Vanamo K: Pylephlebitis after appendicitis in a child, *J Pediatr Surg* 36:1574–1576, 2001.

16. C. The condition is consistent with regional enteritis (Crohn disease). The indications for resection would include free perforation, fistula, or stricture. The diagnosis can be confused with appendicitis. Provided the cecum is not inflamed, the appendix should be removed to avoid confusion in the future because recurrent abdominal pain may develop in the patient. However, in the presence of active inflammation of the cecum, appendectomy should not be performed because there is a higher risk of an enterocutaneous fistula formation. Therefore, closure of the wound without further intervention is the correct management for this patient. It is uncommon for acute regional enteritis to progress to chronic ileitis.

17. B. Appendicitis is a form of closed-loop obstruction because the base of the appendix becomes occluded and it is a blind loop. In adults, fecaliths are the most common cause of appendiceal obstruction, but other etiologies

include hypertrophied lymphoid tissue, tumors, foreign bodies, and intestinal parasites. The accompanying nausea and vomiting result from distention of the appendix with stretching of the visceral peritoneum. The male-to-female ratio is approximately 3 to 1. The rate of appendectomy for appendicitis has not changed in the decade from 1987 to 1997. The data on CT scanning for appendicitis, although initially promising, are now conflicting. Although there are some single institutional studies that demonstrate that the use of ultrasound and CT scans has resulted in a decrease in misdiagnosis of appendicitis, the overall rate of misdiagnosis from 1987 to 1997 remained at 15%. In particular, routine use of CT scanning in children should be avoided due to the concerns of radiation exposure. In a young man with a classic history and physical examination, it is unlikely to provide useful additional information and may delay treatment. CT should probably be used selectively in situations in which the diagnosis is unclear or the presentation is atypical or when symptoms are long-standing and a contained abscess is suspected.

References: Lee S, Walsh A, Ho H: Computed tomography and ultrasonography do not improve and may delay the diagnosis and treatment of acute appendicitis, *Arch Surg* 136:556–562, 2001.

Martin A, Vollman D, Adler B, et al: CT scans may not reduce the negative appendectomy rate in children, *J Pediatr Surg* 39:886–890, 2004.

Rao P, Rhea J, Rattner D, et al: Introduction of appendiceal CT: impact on negative appendectomy and appendiceal perforation rates, *Ann Surg* 229:344–349, 1999.

18. D. Because the appendix has a luminal capacity of only 0.1 mL, even small amounts of ongoing intraluminal secretion combined with bacterial overgrowth lead to a rapid increase in intraluminal pressure. Distention of the appendix stretches the surrounding visceral peritoneum and stimulates its afferent fibers, leading to vague and dull pain in the mid-abdomen or lower epigastrium as well as a stimulation of peristalsis and reflex nausea and vomiting. The increasing pressure eventually occludes the blood supply at the capillary and venule levels. Some episodes of acute appendicitis resolve spontaneously. Both recurrent and chronic forms of appendicitis occur and can mislead the clinician because of the longer history. In one study, recurrent episodes were reported in 6.5% of those who ultimately had an inflamed appendix removed. Children have a higher rate of perforation, and the concomitant underdeveloped omentum makes it more difficult to wall off the perforation.

References: Barber M, McLaren J, Rainey J: Recurrent appendicitis, *Br J Surg* 84:110–112, 1997.

Hawes A, Whalen G: Recurrent and chronic appendicitis: the other inflammatory conditions of the appendix, *Am Surg* 60:217–219, 1994.

Rao P, Rhea J, Novelline R, et al: The computed tomography appearance of recurrent and chronic appendicitis, *Am J Emerg Med* 16:26–33, 1998.

19. D. In cases of uncomplicated appendicitis, temperature elevation is rarely greater than 1.8°F. A higher fever would suggest either perforation of the appendix or an alternative diagnosis. Cutaneous hyperesthesia is one of the earliest signs of acute appendicitis and occurs in the distribution of spinal nerves T10–T12. It is elicited by either stroking or mildly pinching the skin in the right lower quadrant.

20. B. All the choices described are associated with acute appendicitis. In fact, Alvarado created a 10-point scoring system for acute appendicitis that included classic migration of pain, anorexia, nausea and vomiting, right lower quadrant tenderness, rebound, fever, leukocytosis, and left shift. Of these, the highest point assignments were given to right lower quadrant tenderness and leukocytosis. However, the most reproducible and reliable finding is localized tenderness at the McBurney point. With early appendicitis, marked leukocytosis with left shift may not be present. The obturator sign is not a constant finding and occurs primarily when the inflamed appendix lies against the obturator internus muscle.

Reference: Alvarado A: A practical score for the early diagnosis of acute appendicitis, *Ann Emerg Med* 15:557–564, 1986.

21. C. Purulent fluid found at appendectomy is indicative of peritonitis. The finding of a large amount of purulent fluid in the absence of a perforation in the appendix should alert the clinician to another diagnosis and should prompt a careful search for another source of perforation. Periappendicitis is a distinct clinical entity that signifies inflammation of the serosa of the appendix, but not a transmural inflammation, as is seen with appendicitis. The serosa becomes inflamed in response to another inciting infection, most often in association with acute salpingitis in women or another gastrointestinal perforation, such as a perforated ulcer. The clinical presentation of a perforated duodenal ulcer can mimic appendicitis, particularly if the perforation seals and the spilled gastroduodenal contents gravitate down the right gutter to the cecal area. Silent 1920s film star Rudolph Valentino reportedly died of a perforated ulcer, although he presented with right lower quadrant pain suggestive of acute appendicitis (since known as Valentino's syndrome). Primary peritonitis occurs most often in patients with nephrotic syndrome or cirrhosis who have ascites that becomes infected, typically by gram-positive cocci. Familial Mediterranean fever occurs primarily in Mediterranean populations and can cause a polyserositis. It would not cause periappendicitis.

References: Fink A, Kosakowski C, Hiatt J, et al: Periappendicitis is a significant clinical finding, *Am J Surg* 159:564–568, 1990.

Hsu CC, Liu YP, Lien WC, et al: A pregnant woman presenting to the ED with Valentino's syndrome, *Am J Emerg Med* 23:217–218, 2005.

Maardh P, Woelner-Hanssen P: Periappendicitis and chlamydial salpingitis, *Surg Gynecol Obstet* 160:304–306, 1985.

22. B. The appendix is listed in most textbooks as the most common site of carcinoids, although some of the large studies on carcinoid tumors are from several decades ago. A recent population-based study using the National Cancer Institute Surveillance, Epidemiology, and End Results program from 1973 to 1997 showed that the incidence rates of carcinoid tumors have increased significantly over the past 25 years. Interestingly, the rates of appendiceal carcinoids have decreased. The gastrointestinal tract accounted for 54.5% of carcinoids. Of those, the small intestine was the most common site (44.7%), followed by the rectum (19.6%), appendix (16.7%), colon (10.6%), and stomach (7.2%). The 5-year survival rates were as follows: stomach (75.1%), small intestine (76.1%), appendix (76.3%), and rectum (87.5%). Another study of more than 15,000 patients also showed that the small intestine was the most common site, with a dramatic decrease in those of appendiceal origin. Associated noncarcinoid tumors were frequent in conjunction with small intestinal (29.0%), gastric (20.5%), colonic (20.0%), and appendiceal (18.2%) carcinoids. The best 5-year survival rates were noted in rectal (88.3%), bronchopulmonary (73.5%), and appendiceal (71.0%) carcinoids.

References: Maggard M, O'Connell J, Ko C: Updated population-based review of carcinoid tumors, *Ann Surg* 240:117–122, 2004.

Modlin I, Lye K, Kidd M: A 5-decade analysis of 13,715 carcinoid tumors, *Cancer* 97:934–959, 2003.

23. B. Patients who present with a protracted history consistent with acute appendicitis and a palpable mass are likely to have a perforated and walled-off abscess. They are best managed by initial nonoperative therapy (IV antibiotics, bowel rest). Taking such a patient to the operating room is acceptable. However, the intense inflammation and scarring will make the operation difficult and significantly increase the chances of having to perform an ileocecectomy. When embarking on nonoperative therapy, whether subsequent interval appendectomy is necessary is controversial. Routine CT-guided drainage of abscesses is not recommended. The timing of interval appendectomy ranges from 6 to 10 weeks after initial presentation. Initial nonoperative management has a failure rate of 9% to 15%. Arguments in favor of interval appendectomy include a significant risk of recurrent appendicitis (as high as 40%), the low morbidity of interval appendectomy, and, in this older patient, the concern that there may be neoplasia within the appendix.

References: Kaminski A, Liu IL, Applebaum H, et al: Routine interval appendectomy is not justified after initial nonoperative treatment of acute appendicitis, *Arch Surg* 140:897–901, 2005.

Oliak D, Yamini D, Udani V, et al: Initial nonoperative management for periappendiceal abscess, *Dis Colon Rectum* 44:936–941, 2001.

Samuel M, Hosie G, Holmes K: Prospective evaluation of nonsurgical versus surgical management of appendiceal mass, *J Pediatr Surg* 37:882–886, 2002.

Yamini D, Vargas H, Bongard F, et al: Perforated appendicitis: is it truly a surgical urgency? *Am Surg* 64:970–975, 1998.

24. D. The appendiceal artery, a branch of the ileocolic artery, supplies the appendix.

25. D. It is important to remember that appendiceal perforation is the most important variable in determining fetal mortality during pregnancy; thus, it is imperative to make the diagnosis early. Conversely, a general anesthetic increases the risk of premature labor. A recent large study was conducted comparing appendicitis in more than 3000 pregnant women with more than 94,000 nonpregnant women. The study found that the rate of negative appendectomy was higher in pregnant compared with nonpregnant women (23% vs. 18%). Rates of fetal loss and early delivery were considerably higher in women with complex appendicitis (6% and 11%, respectively) compared with negative

(4% and 10%, respectively) and simple (2% and 4%, respectively) appendicitis. Complex appendicitis and a negative appendectomy remained risks for fetal loss on multivariate analysis. Interestingly, laparoscopy was associated with a higher rate of fetal loss compared with open appendectomy (odds ratio of 2.31). The study highlights the need for more accurate diagnosis in pregnant women. One must strive to avoid unnecessary appendectomies that place the fetus at risk; however, delays in operative care for appendicitis likewise place the fetus at risk.

Reference: McGory M, Zingmond D, Tillou A, et al: Negative appendectomy in pregnant women is associated with a substantial risk of fetal loss, *J Am Coll Surg* 205:534–540, 2007.

26. D. For patients with peritoneal studding from appendiceal adenocarcinoma, cytoreductive surgery with intraperitoneal chemotherapy has shown promise in patients without evidence of distant organ metastasis. In a large series in which complete cytoreduction was defined as tumor nodules less than 2.5 mm in diameter remaining after surgery, patients with complete cytoreduction and adenomucinosis pathology had a 5-year survival rate of 86%. Incomplete cytoreduction had a 5-year survival rate of only 20%.

References: Jaffe BM, Berger DH: Appendix. In Brunicardi FC, Andersen DK, Billiar TR, et al, editors: *Schwartz's principles of surgery*, ed 9, New York, 2010, McGraw-Hill, pp 1073–1091.

Maa J, Kirkwood KS: The appendix. In Townsend CM Jr, Beauchamp RD, Evers BM, Mattox KL, editors: *Sabiston textbook of surgery: the biological basis of modern surgical practice*, ed 18, Philadelphia, 2008, WB Saunders, pp 1333–1347.

Sugarbaker P, Chang D: Results of treatment of 385 patients with peritoneal surface spread of appendiceal malignancy, *Ann Surg Oncol* 6:727–731, 1999.

Sugarbaker P, Jablonski K: Prognostic features of 51 colorectal and 130 appendiceal cancer patients with peritoneal carcinomatosis treated by cytoreductive surgery and intraperitoneal chemotherapy, *Ann Surg* 221:124–132, 1995.

Breast

5

1. Mondor disease of the breast:

   A. Is a low-grade malignancy
   B. Is a form of thrombophlebitis
   C. Is most often due to a gram-positive organism
   D. Is usually due to autoimmune disease
   E. Occurs exclusively in women

2. Treatment of Mondor disease of the breast consists of:

   A. Local excision
   B. Antibiotics
   C. Systemic anticoagulation
   D. Nonsteroidal anti-inflammatory drugs and warm compresses
   E. Incision and drainage

3. All of the following are true regarding radial scar EXCEPT:

   A. It is an independent risk factor for breast cancer.
   B. It is considered to be a sclerosing disorder.
   C. It demonstrates characteristic spiculation on mammography.
   D. If identified on a mammogram, needle biopsy is necessary.
   E. It has a risk of progressing to malignancy.

4. A 45-year-old woman undergoes excisional biopsy for a mammographic abnormality. Final pathology reveals benign pathology without atypia; however, several foci of lobular carcinoma in situ (LCIS) are detected at the excision margins. Which of the following choices would be the best management option?

   A. Excisional biopsy to achieve negative margin
   B. Mastectomy with sentinel lymph node biopsy
   C. Radiation therapy
   D. Bilateral total mastectomies with immediate reconstruction
   E. Close clinical follow-up

5. All of the following are true regarding patients with the *BRCA1* and *BRCA2* mutations EXCEPT:

   A. Breast cancer in women with the *BRCA2* mutation tends to be more well differentiated than that in women with *BRCA1*.
   B. Both are associated with an increased risk of prostate cancer.
   C. Breast cancer in women with *BRCA1* is more likely to be hormone receptor positive than that in women with *BRCA2*.
   D. The *BRCA2* mutation poses an increased risk of melanoma.
   E. Men with breast cancer and the *BRCA2* mutation present with more advanced cancer than women with breast cancer and the *BRCA2* mutation.

6. Which of the following is true regarding patients with *BRCA1* and *BRCA2* mutations?

   A. In women, both mutations have a similar lifetime risk of breast cancer.
   B. In men, both mutations have a similar lifetime risk of breast cancer.
   C. Both mutations have a similar risk of ovarian cancer.
   D. Both are found on chromosome 13.
   E. For both mutations, the risk of breast cancer can be eliminated by performing bilateral prophylactic simple mastectomy.

7. The guidelines for *BRCA* testing remain controversial. Current guidelines suggest testing in women with an increased-risk family history. Which of the following would best identify a woman as having an increased-risk family history?

   A. Two first-degree relatives with breast cancer at any age
   B. A first-degree relative with breast cancer who is younger than 50 years of age
   C. A first-degree relative with ovarian cancer who is younger than 50 years of age
   D. A woman of Ashkenazi Jewish descent
   E. A male relative with breast cancer

8. A 55-year-old woman presents with a 2.5-cm nodule in the upper outer quadrant of her right breast. In addition to the nodule, mammography reveals two areas of suspicious calcification, one in the upper inner and one in the lower outer quadrant of the same breast. Needle biopsies of the nodule and of the calcifications all reveal high-grade ductal carcinoma in situ (DCIS) with extensive necrosis. Which of the following is the most appropriate recommendation?

   A. Excision of all three lesions to achieve a negative margin followed by radiation therapy to the breast
   B. Excision of all three lesions to achieve a negative margin
   C. Excision of all three lesions to achieve a negative margin followed by radiation therapy to the breast and tamoxifen
   D. Bilateral total mastectomies with immediate reconstruction
   E. Right mastectomy with sentinel lymph node biopsy

9. A 50-year-old woman presents with a palpable mass in her right upper outer quadrant that has been present for 3 months and has not changed in size. She has no family or personal history of breast cancer. On physical examination, the mass feels firm, is nontender, and measures approximately 1.5 cm. Other than the palpable mass, the remainder of the physical examination is unremarkable. Mammography reveals a BI-RADS (Breast Imaging Reporting and Data System) category 2 (benign finding) lesion that corresponds to the mass. Further management consists of:

   A. Observation
   B. Needle biopsy
   C. Magnetic resonance imaging (MRI)
   D. Excision of the mass
   E. Repeat mammogram in 6 months

10. A 45-year-old woman undergoes screening mammography and is found to have a suspicious calcification in the left upper outer quadrant. She undergoes a needle biopsy that confirms DCIS. Needle localized excisional biopsy is performed and reveals DCIS, cribriform type, of a low grade. The deep margin is positive for a focus of DCIS. Management consists of:

    A. Radiation therapy
    B. Close follow-up with repeat mammogram in 6 months
    C. Reexcision of the deep margin
    D. Tamoxifen
    E. Mastectomy

11. Risk factors for male breast cancer include all of the following EXCEPT:

    A. Radiation exposure
    B. Undescended testis
    C. XXY syndrome
    D. Gynecomastia
    E. Obesity

12. Which of the following is true regarding male breast cancer?

    A. Patients present more commonly with DCIS than invasive ductal carcinoma.
    B. It has a worse prognosis than in women at the same stage.
    C. Patients are usually estrogen receptor positive.
    D. It is more common in white men than in African American men.
    E. It occurs at a younger mean age than in women.

13. A 65-year-old woman presents with an eczematoid rash around her right nipple that has not resolved despite numerous applications of steroid creams. Other than the rash, physical examination of the breast is unremarkable. A biopsy of the periareolar skin reveals large, pale vacuolated cells in the epithelium. Immunostaining is positive for carcinoembryonic antigen. Which of the following is true regarding this condition?

    A. The disease process is usually confined to the nipple.
    B. The lesion stains positive for S-100 antigen.
    C. It represents a type of melanoma.
    D. Breast conservation surgery is contraindicated.
    E. Sentinel node sampling is necessary.

14. Which of the following invasive breast cancers has the most favorable prognosis?

    A. Tubular
    B. Papillary
    C. Medullary
    D. Mucinous (colloid)
    E. Lobular

15. Neighborhood calcification is a feature characteristic of:

    A. LCIS
    B. DCIS
    C. Fat necrosis
    D. Radial scar
    E. Fibroadenoma

16. Which of the following is true regarding tamoxifen?

    A. It is not indicated for patients with DCIS.
    B. It is not indicated in men with breast cancer.
    C. It is not effective in preventing invasive cancer in patients with LCIS.
    D. It is equally beneficial in patients with estrogen positive– and estrogen negative–receptor cancers.
    E. It is associated with uterine sarcoma.

17. The primary severe adverse reaction to trastuzumab is:

    A. Liver toxicity
    B. Renal toxicity
    C. Thromboembolic events
    D. Cardiac toxicity
    E. Aplastic anemia

18. Breast lymphoma:

    A. Is usually a T-cell lymphoma
    B. Is much more commonly a secondary than a primary lymphoma
    C. Does not respond well to standard lymphoma chemotherapy
    D. Has a predilection for central nervous system recurrence
    E. Requires mastectomy with node dissection in most instances

19. All of the following are considered risk factors for breast cancer EXCEPT:

    A. Obesity
    B. History of ovarian cancer
    C. Nulliparity
    D. History of endometrial cancer
    E. Women of Japanese descent

20. A 28-year-old lactating woman presents with a 2-day history of right breast pain that is progressively worsening. On examination, a 4-cm area of skin adjacent to the nipple is red and tender with some edema and no detectable fluctuance. Management would consist of:

    A. Fine-needle aspiration
    B. Skin biopsy
    C. Incision and drainage
    D. Oral antibiotics
    E. Mammography

21. After a modified radical mastectomy, a 45-year-old woman reports weakness in her arm. On examination, she has mild weakness when she internally rotates and adducts her arm. This is most likely due to injury to which of the following nerves?

    A. Intercostal brachial
    B. Long thoracic
    C. Thoracodorsal
    D. Supraclavicular
    E. Medial pectoral

22. A 60-year-old woman presents with a large mass that involves the majority of her right breast and has grown rapidly in the past 2 months. The mass causes the breast to take on a "teardrop" configuration. Core needle biopsy findings are consistent with fibroadenoma. A mammogram demonstrates a smooth, rounded mass with well-defined borders. The best management option would be:

    A. Total mastectomy
    B. Modified radical mastectomy
    C. Local excision
    D. Chemotherapy followed by modified radical mastectomy
    E. Lumpectomy plus sentinel node biopsy

23. Eight years ago, a 60-year-old woman underwent lumpectomy and sentinel lymph node biopsy and had radiation therapy to her right breast for invasive ductal cancer. She now presents with what appears to be radiation-induced skin changes diffusely. In addition, the skin over her right breast is edematous and reddened, with multiple bluish nodules. She has no other masses in the breast and no axillary adenopathy. Core needle biopsy of the lesion reveals red blood cells with occasional single cells with pleomorphic nuclei as well as necrosis. Treatment consists of:

    A. Chemotherapy
    B. Observation
    C. Mastectomy with sentinel node biopsy
    D. Wide local excision to negative margins
    E. Radiation therapy

24. Batson plexus provides a potential metastatic route of breast cancer to the:
    A. Diaphragm
    B. Bone
    C. Liver
    D. Adrenal gland
    E. Lung

25. A 30-year-old woman presents with erythema and edema of the skin of most of her right breast. The entire breast feels firm. Despite a course of antibiotics, the erythema persists. The dermatologist performs a skin biopsy that reveals tumor cells in the dermal lymphatics. Initial management consists of:
    A. Chemotherapy
    B. Radiation therapy
    C. Modified radical mastectomy
    D. Chemotherapy and radiation
    E. Simple mastectomy

26. All of the following are true regarding breast cancer staging EXCEPT:
    A. A positive supraclavicular node is at least stage III.
    B. Inflammatory breast cancer is at least stage III.
    C. A positive internal mammary node is at least stage III.
    D. For stage I, the tumor must be 2 cm or less.
    E. The prognosis is no different for 8 versus 11 positive axillary nodes.

27. Comedo-type DCIS is best distinguished from noncomedo-type DCIS by:
    A. Estrogen receptor status
    B. Cytologic grade
    C. Presence of central necrosis
    D. Type of microcalcifications
    E. Aneuploidy

28. The most common cause of bloody nipple discharge is:
    A. Intraductal papilloma
    B. DCIS
    C. Invasive ductal carcinoma
    D. Paget disease
    E. Phyllodes tumor

29. Which of the following is the most important predictor of 10- and 20-year survival for breast cancer?
    A. Tumor size
    B. Tumor pathologic type
    C. The total number of positive lymph nodes
    D. Estrogen receptor status
    E. Age at time of diagnosis

30. All of the following are associated with an increased risk of breast cancer EXCEPT:
    A. Papillomatosis
    B. Sclerosing adenosis
    C. Fat necrosis
    D. Atypical hyperplasia
    E. Florid nonatypical hyperplasia

31. Fifteen years after a modified radical mastectomy for infiltrating ductal carcinoma, reddish blue macules on the skin of her right arm with surrounding satellite lesions and skin blistering develop in a 65-year-old woman. The arm has been chronically swollen since the operation. These lesions most likely represent:
    A. Kaposi sarcoma
    B. Granular cell myoblastoma
    C. Stewart-Treves syndrome
    D. Recurrent breast carcinoma
    E. Hemangioma

32. Relative or absolute contraindications to breast-conserving therapy for invasive breast cancer include all of the following EXCEPT:
    A. Pregnancy
    B. A history of breast irradiation
    C. Clinically palpable abnormal lymph nodes in the axilla
    D. Scleroderma
    E. Two or more primary tumors in separate quadrants of the breast

33. A winged scapula after modified radical mastectomy is most likely due to injury to which nerve?
    A. Intercostal brachial
    B. Long thoracic
    C. Thoracodorsal
    D. Supraclavicular
    E. Medial pectoral

34. Which of the following is true regarding breast cancer during pregnancy?

    A. Stage for stage, breast cancer during pregnancy has a worse prognosis than in nonpregnant women.
    B. If the patient is in the first trimester, chemotherapy should be delayed until after pregnancy.
    C. If the patient is in the first trimester, lumpectomy with sentinel node biopsy is the best alternative.
    D. If breast cancer develops in a patient in the first trimester, therapeutic abortion should be recommended.
    E. Fluorouracil and cyclophosphamide can be safely used in the second and third trimesters.

35. All of the following are true regarding a patient with LCIS EXCEPT:

    A. Patients are at increased risk of the development of invasive lobular cancer.
    B. It is a marker for increased risk of invasive ductal cancer.
    C. The risk of invasive cancer is the same for both breasts.
    D. Tamoxifen alone is an accepted treatment regimen.
    E. It is most commonly detected by its distinctive pattern of calcifications on mammography.

36. Which of the following types of DCIS has the worst prognosis?

    A. Cribriform
    B. Comedo
    C. Solid
    D. Papillary
    E. Focal micropapillary

37. Which of the following is true regarding phyllodes tumor of the breast?

    A. The majority are benign.
    B. They are of epithelial origin.
    C. Benign lesions are managed in a manner similar to that for a fibroadenoma.
    D. Malignant lesions spread via lymphatics more than hematogenously.
    E. Malignancy is determined by cytology.

38. When comparing male and female breast cancers, breast cancer in men:

    A. Is more likely to be DCIS than in women
    B. Is less likely to be HER2 positive
    C. Is less likely to be estrogen receptor positive
    D. Is less likely to require mastectomy
    E. Is less likely to present as stage III or IV

39. The use of MRI as a screening tool for breast cancer is:

    A. Not recommended
    B. Recommended annually in patients with the *BRCA* mutation
    C. Recommended at least every other year in women with very dense breasts
    D. Recommended for women with LCIS
    E. Recommended for all women with a predicted lifetime 10% risk of breast cancer

40. Relative or absolute contraindications to sentinel node biopsy include all of the following EXCEPT:

    A. Previous mastectomy
    B. Inflammatory breast cancer
    C. Breast cancer in multiple quadrants of the breast
    D. Fine-needle aspirate–positive nodes in the axilla
    E. Pregnancy

41. Early-onset breast cancer, sarcomas, leukemia, and brain and adrenocortical tumors would be most consistent with:

    A. Cowden disease
    B. Li-Fraumeni syndrome
    C. Peutz-Jeghers syndrome
    D. Ataxia-telangiectasia
    E. *BRCA2*

Answers

1. B. Mondor disease represents a superficial thrombophlebitis of a vein in the anterior chest wall in the area of the breast. Similar to superficial thrombophlebitis that presents elsewhere, it usually causes an acute onset of pain and tenderness. It typically presents over the lateral aspect of the breast and eventually turns into a palpable cord or hard mass. It is at this point that it becomes of more clinical importance because it can be confused with breast cancer on physical examination. The veins most commonly involved include the lateral thoracic vein, the thoracoepigastric vein, and, less frequently, the superficial epigastric vein. The disorder is benign, self-limited, and not itself a risk factor for breast cancer. It occurs in both men and women.

Reference: Mayor M, Burón I, de Mora J, et al: Mondor's disease, *Int J Dermatol* 39:922–925, 2000.

2. D. The treatment of Mondor disease is the same as for superficial thrombophlebitis in other areas and includes anti-inflammatory drugs and warm compresses. The etiology of Mondor disease is unclear. Whenever one sees a patient with spontaneous superficial venous thrombosis anywhere in the body, one must think of the Virchow triad (injury, stasis, hypercoagulability). Thus, when obtaining a history, one should ask about recent breast surgery, excessive straining, other trauma to the breast, and a history of hypercoagulability. Although the course of Mondor disease itself is benign, mammography is recommended to rule out any other underlying pathology.

Reference: Mayor M, Burón I, de Mora J, et al: Mondor's disease, *Int J Dermatol* 39:922–925, 2000.

3. E. Radial scars are benign lesions that are usually mammographic and histologic findings. They are included in disorders known as complex sclerosing lesions. They are important because they can be confused mammographically with malignant lesions and because they have been shown to be a risk factor for breast cancer. Cancer is not thought to develop within the lesion, but it is rather a marker for cancer in either breast. On mammography, a radial scar classically demonstrates long, thin, radiating spicules with a translucent central area of fat. It has been referred to as a "black star." On physical examination, a palpable mass is rare. Radial scars are characterized microscopically by a fibroelastic core from which ducts and lobules radiate. They may contain microcysts, epithelial hyperplasia, adenosis, and central sclerosis. When a radial scar is identified on mammography, needle biopsy is indicated. Once a radial scar is confirmed histologically and a benign lesion is seen, it is controversial as to whether the entire lesion needs to be excised. Most studies suggest that complete excision of the lesion should be performed to rule out associated malignant or premalignant lesions. Others have stated that the diagnosis of a radial scar based on core needle biopsy is reliable in the absence of associated atypical hyperplasia and when mammographic findings and histologic findings are in accord. Regardless, it is important for the radiologist and pathologist to alert the surgeon to the presence of a radial scar due to its increased risk of associated malignancy and for the need for close surveillance.

References: Alleva D, Smetherman D, Farr G Jr, Cederbom G: Radial scar of the breast: radiologic-pathologic correlation in 22 cases, *Radiographics* 19:S27–S35, 1999.

Cawson J, Malara F, Kavanagh A, et al: Fourteen-gauge needle core biopsy of mammographically evident radial scars: is excision necessary? *Cancer* 97:345–351, 2003.

Fasih T, Jain M, Shrimankar J, et al: All radial scars/complex sclerosing lesions seen on breast screening mammograms should be excised, *Eur J Surg Oncol* 31:1125–1128, 2005.

Jacobs T, Byrne C, Colditz G, et al: Radial scars in benign breast-biopsy specimens and the risk of breast cancer, *N Engl J Med* 340:430–436, 1999.

4. E. LCIS is considered to be a marker for an increased risk of malignancy in either breast. It does not itself progress to invasive cancer. Thus, there is no reason to perform an excision of the area in which the biopsy was performed. Recent studies suggest that most malignancies tend to develop approximately 15 years after the diagnosis of LCIS, that most malignancies are ductal and not lobular (although there is also an increased risk of invasive lobular cancer), and that the cancers are detected early. This latter finding is likely due to the close surveillance of these patients. There are basically three options when LCIS is discovered. One is to have the patient undergo close surveillance to detect new breast cancers. A second option is to administer tamoxifen because it has been shown to reduce the risk of breast cancer. The most aggressive approach is to perform bilateral total mastectomies with immediate reconstruction. This latter option might be considered in a patient with a strong family history of breast cancer. A mastectomy of one breast would not address the risk of malignancy in the contralateral breast.

Reference: Frykberg ER: Lobular carcinoma in situ of the breast, *Breast J* 5:296–303, 1999.

5. C. Breast cancer tends to occur at younger ages than in sporadic cases in those with *BRCA1* and *BRCA2* mutations. It is more likely to be bilateral and associated with other cancers. Breast cancer in women with the *BRCA1* mutation tends to be poorly differentiated and hormone receptor negative, whereas breast cancer in women with the *BRCA2* mutation tends to be well differentiated and hormone receptor positive. Both are associated with an increased risk of prostate cancer. In addition, *BRCA2* is associated with an increased risk of melanoma and cancers of the pancreas, stomach, gallbladder, and bile duct.

Reference: Fossland V, Stroop J, Schwartz R, Kurtzman S: Genetic issues in patients with breast cancer, *Surg Oncol Clin North Am* 18:53–71, 2009.

6. A. Hereditary breast cancer accounts for approximately 5% to 10% of all breast cancers. Carriers of *BRCA1* and *BRCA2* mutations account for the vast majority of hereditary breast cancers. In women with the *BRCA1* and *BRCA2* mutations, the lifetime risk of breast cancer is as high as 80% to 90%. By age 40, breast cancer occurs in approximately 18% of women with *BRCA1* and 15% of those with *BRCA2*. In men, conversely, the lifetime risk of breast cancer is much higher in those with *BRCA2* (approximately 6% vs. 1% in those with *BRCA1*). In fact, the *BRCA2* mutation accounts for nearly 40% of all male breast cancers. The lifetime risk of ovarian cancer is higher with the *BRCA1* mutation (approximately 40%) compared with *BRCA2* (approximately 19%). *BRCA1* maps to chromosome 17p21 and *BRCA2* to chromosome 13. Prophylactic simple mastectomy does not completely eliminate the risk of breast cancer, but leads to a 90% reduction in risk. As such, some have advocated additionally removing the axillary tail, the pectoralis fascia, the subdermal fascia, and the nipple/areolar complex.

References: Fossland V, Stroop J, Schwartz R, Kurtzman S: Genetic issues in patients with breast cancer, *Surg Oncol Clin North Am* 18:53–71, 2009.

Tai Y, Domchek S, Parmigiani G, Chen S: Breast cancer risk among male BRCA1 and BRCA2 mutation carriers, *J Natl Cancer Inst* 99:1811–1814, 2007.

7. E. Increased-risk family history includes three first- or second-degree relatives with breast cancer at any age, two first-degree relatives with breast cancer including one who was younger than age 50 years at diagnosis, a combination of breast and ovarian cancer in first- and second-degree relatives, a male relative with breast cancer, two or more first- or second-degree relatives with ovarian cancer at any age, a woman of Ashkenazi Jewish descent with a first-degree relative with breast or ovarian cancer, or two second-degree relatives.

8. E. Of the choices provided, right mastectomy with sentinel lymph node biopsy is the best option (mastectomy alone would be another). The standard management for DCIS is wide excision with negative margins. However, when DCIS is found to be present in two or more quadrants of the breast (multicentric DCIS), the recommended management is mastectomy. Controversy exists as to whether sentinel lymph node biopsy is necessary when mastectomy is performed for DCIS. Theoretically, there should be no risk of positive axillary lymph nodes. However, in the presence of high-grade DCIS, DCIS with comedonecrosis, or evidence of microinvasion, a growing body of literature indicates that micrometastases are present in the lymph nodes in as many as 10% of patients. In addition, a significant percentage of patients will be found to have a focus of invasive cancer (20% in one study). This would then require a subsequent sentinel lymph node biopsy (which may be technically more difficult and less reliable because the patient had already had a mastectomy). As such, sentinel lymph node biopsy is being recommended in these circumstances. Mastectomy for DCIS is recommended when the DCIS is multicentric (as in this case), when attempts at local excision have yielded persistently positive margins, and for large palpable lesions (>4 cm) because recurrence rates for wide local excision in these settings are significantly increased. Also, recurrences after wide local excision in these cases are more often invasive cancers than simply DCIS.

References: Klauber-DeMore N, Tan LK, Liberman L, et al: Sentinel lymph node biopsy: is it indicated in patients with high-risk ductal carcinoma-in-situ and ductal carcinoma-in-situ with microinvasion? *Ann Surg Oncol* 7:636–642, 2000.

van la Parra RF, Ernst MF, Barneveld PC, et al: The value of sentinel lymph node biopsy in ductal carcinoma in situ (DCIS) and DCIS with microinvasion of the breast, *Eur J Surg Oncol* 34: 631–635, 2008.

9. B. It is important to note that diagnostic mammography should not be used to determine whether to perform a biopsy of a palpable mass. Guidelines issued for mammograms are used for nonpalpable findings. As such, in this patient with a palpable mass, a needle biopsy should be performed. Before performing the needle biopsy, many breast surgeons will first perform a diagnostic ultrasound scan to further characterize the lesion. The Breast Imaging Reporting and Data System (BI-RADS) category classification for mammograms uses a 0 to 6 point scale as follows: 0, assessment incomplete; 1, negative; 2, benign finding; 3, probably benign; 4, suspicious abnormality; 5, highly suspicious of malignancy; 6, known biopsy-proven malignancy. Recommendations by category are as follows: 0, should obtain additional studies (such as ultrasonography); 1 and 2, continue routine screening; 3, short-term follow-up mammogram in 6 months; 4, perform needle biopsy; 5, biopsy and treatment; 6, continue with treatment plan.

References: Eberl M, Fox C, Edge S, et al: BI-RADS classification for management of abnormal mammograms, *J Am Board Fam Med* 19:161–164, 2006.

Kerlikowske K, Smith-Bindman R, Ljung B, Grady D: Evaluation of abnormal mammography results and palpable breast abnormalities, *Ann Intern Med* 139:274–284, 2003.

10. C. DCIS carries a high risk of progression to an invasive cancer (a fivefold increased risk), in the same quadrant of the same breast. Thus, the optimal goal is to completely excise DCIS lesions so as to achieve negative margins. There are three basic treatment strategies for DCIS: wide local excision alone, wide local excision with radiation therapy to the remaining breast, and mastectomy. Long-term survival is the same for each of these approaches, although local recurrences are reduced with mastectomy compared with breast conservation strategies. To date, there are no reliable models or scoring systems that can reliably predict which patients will progress to an invasive malignancy. However, the aggressiveness of DCIS can be classified by using the nuclear grade (high, intermediate, low), the presence of necrosis (extensive, focal, absent), and the DCIS grade (high, intermediate, low). In addition, histology is important, with the comedo type having a worse prognosis. Because DCIS is usually not purely of one type, the histology has been further categorized as comedo, intermediate, and noncomedo. Patients at greatest risk of recurrence and thus most likely to benefit from a more aggressive approach are those with high nuclear and DCIS grades, comedo histology, and extensive necrosis. Compounding the prognostication further, other important features are tumor size and resection margins. In fact, several studies indicate that resection margins are the most important risk for local recurrence. Recurrence risk is greatest if resection margins are less than 1 mm, whereas when resection margins were 10 mm or more, recurrence rates were exceedingly low. When resection margins are positive or very close (<1 mm), the best option is to perform a reexcision, provided that the patient is a good surgical candidate and there is sufficient breast tissue remaining to perform a cosmetically appealing operation.

References: Boyages J, Delaney G, Taylor R: Predictors of local recurrence after treatment of ductal carcinoma in situ: a meta-analysis, *Cancer* 85:616–628, 1999.

Kestin L, Goldstein N, Martinez A, et al: Mammographically detected ductal carcinoma in situ treated with conservative surgery with or without radiation therapy: patterns of failure and 10-year results, *Ann Surg* 231:235–245, 2000.

Neuschatz A, DiPetrillo T, Steinhoff M, et al: The value of breast lumpectomy margin assessment as a predictor of residual tumor burden in ductal carcinoma in situ of the breast, *Cancer* 94:1917–1924, 2002.

Silverstein M, Lagios M, Groshen S, et al: The influence of margin width on local control of ductal carcinoma in situ of the breast, *N Engl J Med* 340:1455–1461, 1999.

11. D. The common denominator that appears to increase the risk of male breast cancer is an increased exposure to estrogen and perhaps androgen deficiency. Thus, any disease that affects testicular function is associated with an increased risk of breast cancer, such as an undescended testis, orchiectomy, orchitis, and testicular injury, as well as with chronic alcohol abuse with cirrhosis and obesity. Other risk factors for male breast cancer include advanced age and radiation exposure. Genetic predisposition includes Klinefelter syndrome, Ashkenazi Jewish ancestry, and the *BRCA2* mutation. Klinefelter syndrome (47,XXY) includes clinical features such as hypothyroidism, infertility, small testicles, and an increased risk of testicular and breast cancer. The *BRCA2* mutation predisposes men to breast cancer (*BRCA1* seems to as well but to a much lesser degree). Gynecomastia has various causes including persistence post-puberty, various drugs, use of anabolic steroids, cirrhosis, testicular tumors, and advanced age. It has not been shown itself be an independent risk factor for breast cancer in men.

References: Olsson H, Bladstrom A, Alm P: Male gynecomastia and risk for malignant tumours—a cohort study, *BMC Cancer* 2:26, 2002.

Thomas D, Jimenez L, McTiernan A, et al: Breast cancer in men: risk factors with hormonal implications, *Am J Epidemiol* 135:734–748, 1992.

12. C. Breast cancer occurring in men is infrequent and accounts for only approximately 1% of breast cancers. The median age at diagnosis is older than in women and averages approximately 68 years. Breast cancer in men tends to develop at a later stage than in women. As such, DCIS is uncommon and more than 90% is invasive, with most being ductal carcinomas. The majority are hormone receptor positive with 80% estrogen receptor positive and 75% progesterone receptor positive. Approximately 35%

express HER2 (epidermal growth factor receptor 2 protein)/neu. Lobular carcinoma is rarely seen (because men do not have terminal lobules). Stage for stage, breast cancer in men has the same prognosis as in women, and prognostic factors such as nodal status, tumor size, histologic grade, and hormone receptor status are the same. The highest rates of breast cancer occur in Jewish and African American men. DCIS makes up less than 15% of male breast cancers, whereas infiltrating no special type makes up more than 85%. Treatment of breast cancer in men is most commonly with modified radical mastectomy.

References: Borgen P, Wong G, Vlamis V, et al: Current management of male breast cancer: a review of 104 cases, *Ann Surg* 215:451–457, 1992.

Guinee V, Olsson H, Moller T, et al: The prognosis of breast cancer in males: a report of 335 cases, *Cancer* 71:154–161, 1993.

13. E. Paget disease of the nipple is a breast cancer that typically starts in the breast ducts near the nipple and then spreads to the nipple itself. It can be confused with eczema and can also have the appearance of a contact dermatitis that can be either moist or dry. As such, any periareolar rash that does not resolve should be evaluated and a biopsy performed and a mammogram obtained to look for underlying associated lesions. Biopsy of the periareolar skin reveals the Paget cell, which is a large, pale vacuolated cell in the rete pegs of the epithelium. Immunostaining is positive for carcinoembryonic antigen. It can be confused with a melanoma (but melanomas stain positive for S-100 antigen). An underlying palpable mass is present in approximately 50% to 60% of patients and is usually centrally located. Paget disease is most commonly treated with mastectomy and sentinel node sampling, particularly if seen in association with a mass. However, if Paget disease is confined clinically and radiologically to the nipple areolar complex, breast-conserving surgery may be performed that must include excision of the nipple areolar complex with at least a 2-cm cone of retroareolar tissue, encompassing all radiographic abnormalities, along with sentinel node sampling and postoperative radiation to the remaining breast.

Reference: Kollmorgen D, Varanasi J, Edge S, Carson W: Paget's disease of the breast: a 33-year experience, *J Am Coll Surg* 187:171–177, 1998.

14. A. Tubular carcinoma of the breast has the most favorable prognosis. It rarely metastasizes. In one large series, 92% of cases were estrogen receptor positive and none had positive lymph nodes. It accounts for only approximately 2% of breast cancers. Long-term survival for tubular carcinoma is nearly 100%. The prognosis for invasive medullary and papillary carcinoma tends to be better than the most common invasive ductal (scirrhous) type and better than lobular.

Reference: Holland D, Boucher L, Mortimer J: Tubular breast cancer experience at Washington University: a review of the literature, *Clin Breast Cancer* 2:210–214, 2001.

15. A. The calcifications seen with LCIS occur in the tissue adjacent to areas of microcalcification on mammography. This feature, which is unique to LCIS, is termed *neighborhood* *calcification.* LCIS has two types, classic and pleomorphic. LCIS is 10 times more common in white than African American women. Invasive breast cancer in either breast eventually develops in as many as one third of women with LCIS and is most often an invasive ductal carcinoma. Thus, a diagnosis of LCIS warrants one of three options: close observation, tamoxifen, or, if at high risk of breast cancer, bilateral prophylactic mastectomies.

16. E. Tamoxifen blocks the uptake of estrogen by breast tissue. Thus, the best response is in patients with estrogen receptor–positive lesions. The indications for tamoxifen include (1) metastatic breast cancer in men and premenopausal women, (2) adjuvant treatment for patients with breast cancer undergoing breast-conserving surgery, (3) DCIS, and (4) breast cancer prevention in high-risk women. Tamoxifen has been demonstrated to improve relapse-free and overall survival in men and women with hormone receptor–positive breast cancer. It has been shown to reduce the risk of invasive breast cancer in either breast in patients with DCIS as well as those with LCIS. It has been shown to reduce the risk of breast cancer in high-risk women. High risk has been defined as women at least 35 years of age with a 5-year predicted risk of breast cancer of 1.67% or greater (as calculated by the Gail model). The decision to give tamoxifen must always be weighed against the potential side effects. It is rarely associated with endometrial adenocarcinoma and even less commonly with uterine sarcoma and with an increased risk of venous thromboembolism. It also increases the risk of cataract formation.

Reference: Wysowski D, Honig S, Beitz J: Uterine sarcoma associated with tamoxifen use, *N Engl J Med* 346:1832–1833, 2002.

17. D. Herceptin (trastuzumab) is a humanized IgG1 kappa monoclonal antibody that selectively binds with high affinity to the epidermal growth factor receptor 2 protein (HER2). Overexpression of HER2/neu (found in approximately 15%–20% of breast cancers) is associated with a worse prognosis and an increased risk of recurrence. Herceptin is indicated for the treatment of HER2-positive node-positive or HER2-positive node-negative breast cancer. It is most often used in conjunction with other agents. It is associated with subclinical and clinical cardiac failure manifesting as congestive heart failure and a decreased left ventricular ejection fraction. Thus, the left ventricular ejection fraction needs to be assessed before instituting the agent and used with caution in conjunction with other agents that are cardiotoxic (such as anthracyclines).

Reference: Seidman A, Hudis C, Pierri M, et al: Cardiac dysfunction in the trastuzumab clinical trials experience, *J Clin Oncol* 20:1215–1221, 2002.

18. D. Breast lymphoma is rare. The majority of cases are B-cell lymphomas, and the most common type is diffuse large B-cell lymphoma (40%–70%). Breast lymphomas are equally divided into primary and secondary. Treatment depends on whether the lesion is localized or diffuse and the grade of lymphoma. With localized and low-grade lymphomas, primary excision may be all that is necessary. With intermediate- or high-grade lymphoma, combination therapy with standard CHOP (cyclophosphamide, hydroxydoxorubicin, vincristine, prednisone) chemotherapy and radiation therapy is recommended. Several studies have noted an unusual predilection for distant dissemination for breast lymphoma to the central nervous system.

References: Brogi E, Harris NL: Lymphomas of the breast: pathology and clinical behavior, *Semin Oncol* 26:357–364, 1999.

Wong W, Schild S, Halyard M, Schomberg P: Primary non-Hodgkin lymphoma of the breast: the Mayo Clinic experience, *J Surg Oncol* 80:19–25, 2002.

19. E. Increased exposure to estrogen is associated with an increased risk of breast cancer, whereas reducing exposure is thought to be protective. Factors that increase estrogen exposure include an increased number of menstrual cycles such as young age at menarche, old age at menopause, and nulliparity. Endometrial cancer is a risk factor due to the fact that endometrial cancer develops secondary to increased estrogen exposure, which leads to endometrial hyperplasia. The terminal differentiation of breast epithelium associated with a full-term pregnancy is protective, so older age at first live birth (older than 30 years) is associated with an increased risk of breast cancer. Obesity is also a risk factor due to the fact that the major source of estrogen in postmenopausal women is the conversion of androstenedione to estrone by adipose tissue. An important nonhormonal risk factor is radiation exposure. Breast cancer is more frequent in white and African American women in the United States and less common in women of Asian descent.

20. D. Erythema, warmth, and tenderness of the breast in a lactating woman is most often mastitis. The majority of patients present without an associated abscess. Mastitis commonly complicates lactation, possibly because of bacteria ascending in the ductal tree of the breast through the nipple. Initial treatment includes the administration of warm compresses and the continuation of breastfeeding. If local measures are not successful, antibiotics are administered. Incision and drainage are not usually needed unless there is a clear area of fluctuance. Because the differential diagnosis of acute mastitis includes inflammatory carcinoma, it is important to follow patients with mastitis and confirm that there has been a complete resolution of symptoms and signs.

21. C. The intercostobrachial nerve is the lateral cutaneous branch of the second intercostal nerve. Resection does not lead to any motor loss, but can cause loss of sensation over the medial aspect of the upper arm. The long thoracic nerve courses along the lateral chest wall in the mid axillary line on the serratus anterior muscle to innervate it. The serratus anterior muscle abducts and laterally rotates the scapula and holds it against the chest wall. Injury to the long thoracic nerve results in a winged scapula. The thoracodorsal nerve courses lateral to the long thoracic nerve on the latissimus dorsi muscle, following the course of the subscapular artery. It innervates the latissimus dorsi muscle. The latissimus dorsi muscle adducts, extends, and medially rotates the arm. Injury to this nerve generally does not cause a major disability, but can lead to difficulty in arm adduction and medial rotation. Furthermore, preservation of this nerve and vessels is important if a subsequent a latissimus dorsi flap is being considered. The medial pectoral nerve runs lateral to or through the pectoral minor muscle, actually lateral to the lateral pectoral nerve, with both innervating the pectoralis minor and major muscles. Injury to the medial pectoral nerve may lead to atrophy of the clavicular portion of the pectoralis muscles. Injury to these nerves would result in atrophy of the pectoralis muscle. The anterior branches of the supraclavicular nerve supply a limited area of skin over the upper aspect of the breast.

22. A. Phyllodes tumors consist of an epithelial component and cellular, spindle cell stroma that forms a leaflike structure (hence the term *phyllodes*). They occur almost exclusively in women and can undergo rapid enlargement, creating a teardrop deformity of the breast and thinning of the skin. On physical examination, they are usually freely mobile. Smaller tumors in particular can be confused clinically, mammographically, and on core biopsy with a fibroadenoma. Phyllodes tumors are usually benign (approximately 65%), but can be of intermediate malignancy (15%) or malignant (25%). However, the distinction between benign and malignant forms can also be difficult to make. Malignant phyllodes tumors have a higher degree of cellular atypia, an increased mitotic count, and an increase in stromal cellularity. The treatment of choice for phyllodes tumors is wide local excision with at least a 1-cm margin. For larger lesions, this may not be possible, and, therefore, mastectomy is required. Wide local excision is acceptable for malignant lesions as well, provided an adequate margin is obtainable. Phyllodes tumors very rarely metastasize to lymph nodes. As such, sentinel node sampling or axillary node dissection is not required. Malignant phyllodes tumors spread hematogenously. Risk factors for distant metastasis include infiltrating tumor margin, severe stromal overgrowth, atypia, and cellularity.

Reference: Chen W, Cheng S, Tzen C, et al: Surgical treatment of phyllodes tumors of the breast: retrospective review of 172 cases, *J Surg Oncol* 91:185–194, 2005.

23. D. The presentation is most consistent with an angiosarcoma (bluish nodules, pleomorphic nuclei, and evidence of necrosis). Radiation-induced skin changes can sometimes be difficult to distinguish from angiosarcomas because the radiation may produce vascular proliferation. As such, biopsy of any new skin changes or new areas of induration is important. Angiosarcomas are rare and may develop after breast cancer surgery (either modified radical mastectomy or breast-conserving surgery with radiation therapy) within the breast or in a lymphedematous extremity after axillary lymph node dissection. The strongest risk for the development of angiosarcoma is lymphedema (not radiation therapy). It may also arise de novo (so-called radiation-naïve angiosarcomas) in the breast. Radiation-naïve angiosarcoma of the breast tends to occur in younger women and typically presents with rapidly enlarging masses with bluish discoloration. It can be confused with a hematoma-filled cyst. Histologically, angiosarcoma consists of an anastomosing tangle of blood vessels in the dermis and superficial subcutaneous fat. Characteristic features include pleomorphic nuclei, frequent mitosis, and stacking up of the endothelial cells lining neoplastic vessels (particularly with high-grade lesions). Another feature that distinguishes it from a hemangioma is the presence of necrosis. The presentation of angiosarcoma includes cutaneous or subcutaneous bluish nodules and red edematous skin. The primary treatment of angiosarcoma is wide excision to a negative margin. This often requires a mastectomy or radical mastectomy. Lymph node metastasis is rare, so sentinel lymph node biopsy is unnecessary. The overall prognosis is poor, particularly with high-grade angiosarcoma.

References: Sher T, Hennessy B, Valero V, et al: Primary angiosarcomas of the breast, *Cancer* 110:173–178, 2007.

Vorburger S, Xing Y, Hunt K, et al: Angiosarcoma of the breast, *Cancer* 104:2682–2688, 2005.

24. B. Batson plexus consists of venules that encircle the vertebrae and course along the spinal column from the sacrum to the cervical vertebrae. Connections exist between these venules and organs located in the thorax, abdomen, or pelvis and are responsible for metastasis to the pelvic bones, spine, skull, or brain. The plexus has been implicated in particular with bony metastasis from prostate and breast cancer. Batson vertebral venous plexus also explains why patients may have bone metastasis without first having pulmonary metastasis because tumor cells enter the plexus and deposit in the vertebrae without first passing through the lungs. The blood flow within the plexus is sluggish, and this is thought to be more conducive to tumor deposition and growth in the spine. Batson plexus may also explain the rare development of metastasis within the spinal cord.

Reference: Mundy G: Mechanisms of bone metastasis, *Cancer* 80(8 Suppl):1546–1556, 1997.

25. A. Inflammatory breast cancer is due to invasion of tumor cells in the subdermal lymphatics, leading to lymphatic obstruction and lymphedema in the breast. It can be confused with an infectious process, particularly in a young patient. In addition, an underlying breast mass may not be palpable, and mammographic abnormalities may not be present. As such, it is important to perform a biopsy in situations in which the skin changes in the breast do not rapidly resolve. Inflammatory breast cancer is by definition at least stage IIIB. At the time of diagnosis, axillary nodal metastases are commonly present. Due to the poor outcome with surgery, the treatment of inflammatory breast cancer has evolved into a multimodality approach with chemotherapy being the first step and the cornerstone of management. Anthracyclines and taxanes are the most effective cytotoxic agents and result in partial or complete response in as many as 75% of cases. Patients who have some response then proceed to surgery for locoregional control, followed by adjuvant radiation and hormone therapy. For those without a response to chemotherapy, radiation therapy to the breast and nodes is given, followed by surgery. The 5-year survival rate is still only 30% to 50%.

Reference: Cristofanilli M, Buzdar A, Hortobágyi G: Update on the management of inflammatory breast cancer, *Oncologist* 8:141–148, 2003.

26. E. The staging system for breast cancer has become increasingly complex. It is based on the TNM system. Factors included in the primary tumor (T) include size, extension into the chest wall or skin, and inflammatory skin changes. Nodal status includes the number of positive nodes and the location of the positive nodes (axillary, internal mammary, infraclavicular/supraclavicular). Nodal prognosis is sequentially determined by the number of nodes: 0, 1 to 3 positive nodes, 4 to 9 positive nodes, and 10 or more positive nodes. A stage I tumor must be 2 cm or less and the nodes negative. Stage II has subcategories A and B. For it to be classified as stage II, there can be no more than three positive nodes and they must be limited to the axilla. Involvement of internal mammary, supraclavicular, or infraclavicular nodes makes it at least a stage III, as does involvement of the chest wall or inflammatory breast cancer. A tumor that extends into the chest wall or skin (including inflammatory breast cancer) makes it a T4 and at least a stage IIIB. Ten or more positive axillary nodes or positive infraclavicular/supraclavicular nodes make it at least a stage IIIC. The 5-year survival rates are 100% for stage I, 86% for stage II, 57% for stage III, and 20% for stage IV.

27. C. DCIS can be classified into papillary, micropapillary, cribriform, solid, and comedo subtypes. Because most lesions do not contain purely one type, classifying the aggressiveness of DCIS is difficult. Factors used in determining aggressiveness include the nuclear and histologic grade (low, intermediate, high), the histologic subtype (comedo, intermediate, and noncomedo), and the presence of necrosis (none, focal, extensive). One must also consider the extent of DCIS and the size of the lesion. The papillary, micropapillary, and cribriform subtypes tend to be thought of as less aggressive and progress to invasive cancer more slowly than the solid and comedo subtypes. The comedo subtype is considered the most aggressive. Because cells are faster growing, the center of the duct may become plugged with dead cellular debris. The rapid growth of these cells may also outstrip the blood supply, leading to the formation of central necrosis, which is the hallmark of comedo DCIS. Comedo DCIS tends to also have a higher cytologic grade and is more likely to produce microcalcifications that deposit around necrotic tissue. They are also more likely to overexpress HER2/neu.

28. A. Intraductal papilloma is a benign intraepithelial tumor of the breast ductal tissues. It can grow as large as a few centimeters in diameter and most commonly presents with unilateral bloody or serosanguineous nipple discharge. It is the most common cause of bloody discharge. Although invasive ductal carcinoma must be ruled out, it accounts for less than 10% of cases of bloody nipple discharge. Treatment for intraductal papilloma is surgical excision. The lesion can sometimes be localized on physical examination by digitally compressing around the areola until bloody discharge is elicited. Ductography can further assist in identifying the affected duct in planning surgical excision.

Reference: Sauter E, Schlatter L, Lininger J, Hewett J: The association of bloody nipple discharge with breast pathology, *Surgery* 136:780–785, 2004.

29. C. The single most important predictor of 10- and 20-year survival rates in breast cancer is the number of axillary lymph nodes involved with metastatic disease. Other prognostic factors include tumor size, estrogen receptor status, ploidy, S phase, cathepsin D, *HER2/neu* oncogene expression, and p53 expression.

30. C. Of the listed lesions, fat necrosis has no known cancer risk. Fat necrosis is usually due to breast trauma. It is of clinical significance only because it can be confused with a malignant process on physical examination and on gross inspection. Microscopically, however, it represents only scarring with associated lipid-containing cystic structures. The risk of breast cancer with benign breast disease is best determined by classifying lesions into proliferative lesions without atypia and proliferative lesions with atypia. Patients with proliferative lesions without atypia (ductal hyperplasia, papillomatosis, radial scar, and sclerosing adenosis) have a 1.88 times increased risk of breast cancer. Papillomatosis is a condition of multiple benign epithelial tumors. Sclerosing adenosis is a fibrosing disease of the glandular tissues of the breast, associated with enlarged, distorted lobular units. Patients with proliferative lesions with atypia have a 4.24 times increased risk of breast cancer. Atypical hyperplasia can be ductal or lobular in origin, has some atypical cellular features, and can be distinguished from DCIS and LCIS. In patients with nonproliferative findings (cysts, fibroadenoma), there is no increased risk of breast cancer if they have no family history of breast cancer.

Reference: Hartmann L, Sellers T, Frost M, et al: Benign breast disease and the risk of breast cancer, *N Engl J Med* 353:229–237, 2005.

31. C. Stewart-Treves syndrome is a deadly malignancy that forms in chronically edematous limbs and is classically described after modified radical mastectomy. It has been described in limbs with chronic lymphedema from other causes. It has been termed *lymphangiosarcoma*, but it seems to actually arise from blood vessels and as such is also called *angiosarcoma*. In addition to chronic lymphedema, some authors have postulated that impaired immunity and radiation therapy may play a role. The diagnosis needs to be established via open biopsy because fine-needle aspiration alone may not be sufficient. The tumor is highly aggressive, with a propensity for early metastasis to the lungs. Treatment consists of early wide surgical débridement, which may require amputation of the limb. Prognosis is poor. Once the lesion develops, the prognosis is poor, with most patients surviving less than 2 years.

Reference: Heitmann C, Ingianni G: Stewart-Treves syndrome: lymphangiosarcoma following mastectomy, *Ann Plast Surg* 44: 72–75, 2000.

32. C. Pregnancy is considered a relative contraindication to breast-conserving therapy because of the concerns of radiation exposure to the fetus. However, if the patient presents in the late second or third trimester, radiation therapy can be given after delivery. A history of radiation therapy to the breast or chest wall will likely preclude being able to administer the full radiation dose. Active connective tissue disorders, and in particular lupus erythematosus and sclero-derma, may be exacerbated by radiation therapy. Two or more primary tumors in separate quadrants of the breast, multicentric disease, or invasive cancer accompanied by diffuse suspicious mammographic abnormalities are considered contraindications to breast-conserving surgery, as is a persistently positive surgical margin after reasonable attempts at local excision. Rheumatoid arthritis is one connective tissue disorder that is not considered a contraindication. The presence of clinically palpable lymph nodes should not influence the decision to proceed with breast-conserving surgery because a lumpectomy with lymph node dissection and subsequent radiation to the breast can still be undertaken.

Reference: Morrow M, Strom E, Bassett L, et al: Standard for breast conservation therapy in the management of invasive breast carcinoma, *CA Cancer J Clin* 52:277–300, 2002.

33. B. Injury to the long thoracic nerve results in a winged scapula secondary to denervation of the serratus anterior muscle. The intercostal brachial nerve is a sensory nerve that supplies the axilla and upper medial arm. Injury does not result in motor deficit, but does cause anesthesia in the medial arm. The thoracodorsal nerve innervates the latissimus dorsi muscle, which adducts and medially rotates the arm. The supraclavicular nerve is also a sensory nerve with anterior and medial branches, supplying a small portion of the upper part of the breast. The medial pectoral nerve innervates the pectoralis major and minor muscles.

34. E. Breast cancer during pregnancy is rare, with a reported rate of 1 in 3000 pregnant women. Stage for stage, the prognosis appears to be the same as for nonpregnant women, although pregnant women tend to present with more advanced disease, and as many as 75% have positive axillary lymph nodes. The diagnosis is made via ultrasonography and core needle biopsy. Mammography is avoided because it may be less sensitive during pregnancy and lactation and because it may expose the fetus to radiation. The surgical treatment for breast cancer during pregnancy in most cases is a modified radical mastectomy. This avoids the issue of fetal exposure to radiation that might occur during breast irradiation and sentinel node biopsy using a radioisotope. Chemotherapy (fluorouracil, doxorubicin, and cyclophosphamide as well as anthracycline based), given during the second or third trimester, has not been shown to be harmful to the fetus. Conversely, chemotherapy given in the first trimester seems to have an increased risk of spontaneous abortion and birth defects. If breast cancer develops during the first trimester, the patient can undergo modified radical mastectomy, but chemotherapy is delayed until the second trimester. If breast cancer develops in the third trimester, the patient could potentially undergo breast-conserving resection with lymph node dissection and undergo radiation therapy after delivery.

References: Berry D, Theriault R, Holmes F, et al: Management of breast cancer during pregnancy using a standardized protocol, *J Clin Oncol* 17:855–861, 1999.

Ring A, Smith I, Jones A, et al: Chemotherapy for breast cancer during pregnancy: an 18-year experience from five London teaching hospitals, *J Clin Oncol* 23:4192–4197, 2005.

35. E. LCIS can lead to calcification, but it does not typically cause a clustering pattern of calcifications that is readily identifiable on mammography. Rather, LCIS is an incidental finding at the time that a biopsy is performed for another mammographic abnormality. Patients with LCIS are at increased risk of the development of both invasive ductal and invasive lobular carcinoma, although invasive ductal carcinoma is more frequent. The cancers develop in both breasts with equal frequency. LCIS occurs 12 times more often in white women than African American women. LCIS has been shown to be present in both breasts as often as 90% of the time. LCIS is a marker for invasive cancer. Tamoxifen as a sole treatment has been shown to decrease the risk of invasive cancer in patients with LCIS.

Reference: Sonnenfeld M, Frenna T, Weidner N, Meyer J: Lobular carcinoma in situ: mammographic-pathologic correlation of results of needle-directed biopsy, *Radiology* 181:363–367, 1991.

36. B. Comedo-type DCIS carries a worse prognosis than all noncomedo types and is used in the classification of DCIS severity. When cancer cells grow rapidly and outstrip their blood supply, necrosis ensues. The presence of necrosis is a prominent feature of comedo-type DCIS. Furthermore, calcium tends to deposit in areas of necrosis.

Reference: Nakhlis F, Morrow M: Ductal carcinoma in situ, *Surg Clin North Am* 83:821–839, 2003.

37. A. A phyllodes tumor is rare, accounting for less than 1% of breast neoplasms. It is the most common neoplasm of nonepithelial origin in the breast. The majority are benign (approximately 65%). It can be confused with a fibroadenoma clinically and pathologically. The distinction is important. Fibroadenomas can be treated with simple enucleation. Benign phyllodes lesions should not be enucleated, but rather excised with a 1-cm margin because recurrence rates are otherwise increased. Malignant phyllodes tumors spread hematogenously and rarely metastasize to the lymph nodes. As such, lymph node dissection is not indicated. Most malignant phyllodes tumors contain liposarcomatous or rhabdosarcomatous elements rather than fibrosarcomatous elements. Cytology is unreliable in differentiating a low-grade phyllodes tumor from a fibroadenoma. Hypercellular stromal fragments can occur in both phyllodes tumors and fibroadenomas, although they are more likely and more prominent in phyllodes tumors. Thus, this feature cannot be used as the sole criterion for distinguishing between the two. Recent studies suggest that the best way to distinguish the two lesions is by the proportion of individual long spindle nuclei (>30% is reliable for phyllodes tumors) amid dispersed stromal cells.

Reference: Krishnamurthy S, Ashfaq R, Shin H, Sneige N: Distinction of phyllodes tumor from fibroadenoma: a reappraisal of an old problem, *Cancer* 90:342–349, 2000.

38. B. In men, more than 95% of cancers are invasive ductal carcinoma, and DCIS is less likely than in women. The majority (95%) of breast cancers in men are estrogen receptor positive compared with 75% in women. Approximately one third of breast cancers in women have overexpression of HER2/neu compared with less than 5% in men. Most men are treated with total mastectomy because there is less tissue for achieving successful margins with breast-conserving surgery. Approximately 40% of men present with stage III or IV cancer, whereas in women, three fourths of breast cancers present as stage I or II. Stage for stage, however, the prognosis is the same.

39. B. MRI in general is not recommended for breast cancer screening due to the cost and a higher likelihood of discovering suspicious lesions that are not malignant, leading to unnecessary biopsies, when compared with mammography. However, MRI has been shown to be a useful adjunct to mammography and, in fact, is better than mammography for detecting breast cancer in certain high-risk patients. As such, MRI is now recommended annually in patients with the *BRCA* mutations, as well as first-degree relatives of *BRCA* carriers who have not been tested. It is also suggested as an adjunct in patients with a more than 20% to 25% lifetime risk of breast cancer, in patients who received chest radiation between the ages of 10 and 30 years, and in other patients and their first-degree relatives with genetic syndromes associated with a high risk of breast cancer (Li-Fraumeni syndrome, Cowden disease, and Bannayan-Riley-Ruvalcaba syndrome). There is as yet insufficient evidence to make a recommendation for or against MRI screening in addition to mammography for patients with LCIS or dense breasts. For patients with a lifetime risk of breast cancer of less than 15%, MRI screening is not recommended.

References: Kriege M, Brekelmans C, Boetes C, et al, Magnetic Resonance Imaging Screening Study Group: Efficacy of MRI and mammography for breast-cancer screening in women with a familial or genetic predisposition, *N Engl J Med* 351:427–437, 2004.

Saslow D, Boetes C, Burke W, et al: American Cancer Society guidelines for breast screening with mri as an adjunct to mammography, *CA Cancer J Clin* 57:75–89, 2007.

40. C. Although the level of evidence is limited or insufficient, relative or absolute contraindications to sentinel lymph node biopsy include locally advanced tumors (such as a T4 lesion) or inflammatory breast cancer; previous mastectomy, previous major breast surgery (such as reduction mammoplasty), or previous major axillary surgery because these will potentially interfere with lymphatic drainage and the ability to accurately identify the sentinel node, in the setting of DCIS when mastectomy is not being performed, when fine-needle aspiration confirms positive nodes in the axilla (because these patients should go directly to lymph node dissection), and pregnancy (because the effects of the radioactive isotope on the fetus are unclear). The finding of clinically suspicious nodes has been included as a relative contraindication, but recent studies indicate that these nodes may often be reactive. As such, it is now recommended to perform a fine-needle biopsy of clinically suspicious nodes, and, if the findings are negative, to proceed with sentinel node biopsy. Breast cancer in multiple quadrants of the breast, although a contraindication to breast-conserving surgery, is not a contraindication to sentinel node biopsy.

References: Schrenk P, Wayand W: Sentinel-node biopsy in axillary lymph-node staging for patients with multicentric breast cancer, *Lancet* 357:122, 2001.

Specht MC, Fey J, Borgen PI, Cody H III: Is the clinically positive axilla in breast cancer really a contraindication to sentinel lymph node biopsy? *J Am Coll Surg* 200:10–14, 2005.

41. B. All are familial cancer syndromes associated with an increased risk of breast cancer. Cowden disease is also associated with multiple hamartomatous lesions and thyroid tumors. Peutz-Jeghers syndrome includes melanocytic macules on the lips and bowel hamartomas, as well as gastrointestinal cancer. Ataxia-telangiectasia is also associated with lymphoma and leukemia.

References: Hunt KK, Newman LA, Copeland EM, Bland KL: Breast. In Brunicardi FC, Andersen DK, Billiar TR, et al, editors: *Schwartz's principles of surgery*, ed 9, New York, 2010, McGraw-Hill, pp 423–474.

Iglehart S, Kaelin C: Breast. In Townsend CM Jr, Beauchamp RD, Evers BM, Mattox KL, editors: *Sabiston textbook of surgery: the biological basis of modern surgical practice*, ed 17, Philadelphia, 2004, WB Saunders, pp 867–928.

Burns

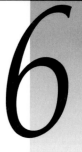

1. The most common type of burn is:
   A. Contact burn
   B. Flame burn
   C. Flash burn
   D. Accidental scald burn
   E. Deliberate scald burn

2. All of the following burn injuries require referral to a burn center EXCEPT:
   A. A 15% total body surface area (TBSA) second-degree burn to the chest in a 30-year-old man
   B. A 5% TBSA second-degree burn of the face in a 40-year-old man
   C. A 3% TBSA second-degree burn of the hand in a 25-year-old woman
   D. An 8% full-thickness burn of the back in a 50-year-old man
   E. A 4% TBSA full-thickness burn of the knee in a 30-year-old woman

3. In a burn patient with suspected smoke inhalation, a useful threshold for endotracheal intubation is a Pa_{O_2}-to-F_{IO_2} ratio less than:
   A. 400
   B. 350
   C. 300
   D. 250
   E. 150

4. The percentage of total burn surface area threshold above which the release of proinflammatory cytokines occurs with a resultant triggering of the systemic inflammatory response is:
   A. 5%
   B. 10%
   C. 20%
   D. 30%
   E. 40%

5. Which of the following is appropriate in the management of burns?
   A. Iced water for a hand burn
   B. Routine central line placement for 20% TBSA burn
   C. Groin intravenous (IV) line in patient with full-thickness arm burns
   D. Antecubital arm lines through eschar in a patient with 40% full-thickness burns of the legs and arms
   E. Intramuscular morphine for pain control

6. Second-degree burns involving the entire head and neck and third-degree burns involving the entire back and half of the chest would be considered:
   A. 12% TBSA
   B. 18% TBSA
   C. 27% TBSA
   D. 36% TBSA
   E. 45% TBSA

7. The percentage of TBSA associated with a 50% mortality rate is:
   A. 40%
   B. 50%
   C. 60%
   D. 70%
   E. 80%

8. Fluid requirements for children with burns is:
   A. 2 mL/kg per % TBSA
   B. 3 mL/kg per % TBSA
   C. 4 mL/kg per % TBSA
   D. 5 mL/kg per % TBSA
   E. 6 mL/kg per % TBSA

9. In patients with major burns, IV infusion of which of the following has been shown to reduce resuscitation volumes and edema?

   A. Vitamin C
   B. Albumin 5%
   C. Vitamin A
   D. Steroids
   E. Vitamin B_6

10. Which of the following is true regarding fluid resuscitation in burn victims?

    A. Normal saline should be avoided.
    B. Hypertonic saline should be used in severe burns to reduce edema.
    C. Dextran is a useful adjunct to prevent protein loss from the burn tissue.
    D. Albumin use is associated with an increased mortality rate
    E. Abdominal compartment syndrome from overresuscitation does not seem to occur.

11. Which of the following is true regarding carbon monoxide (CO) poisoning?

    A. CO shifts the oxygen–hemoglobin dissociation curve to the right.
    B. CO irreversibly binds to the heme molecules of hemoglobin.
    C. Pulse oximetry is an accurate measurement of oxygen saturation after CO poisoning.
    D. CO has 200 times more affinity for hemoglobin than oxygen.
    E. Hyperbaric oxygen therapy should be promptly instituted when CO poisoning is diagnosed in burn victims.

12. According to the Parkland formula, the amount of crystalloid fluids that should be administered in the first 8 hours to a 70-kg man with a 50% TBSA second-degree burn and 20% TBSA third-degree burns should be:

    A. 4900 mL
    B. 5600 mL
    C. 6300 mL
    D. 7350 mL
    E. 9800 mL

13. The main disadvantage of topical mafenide acetate for burn treatment is:

    A. Inability to penetrate eschar
    B. Associated hyponatremia
    C. Associated methemoglobinemia
    D. Associated metabolic acidosis
    E. Ineffectiveness against gram-negative organisms

Answers

1. D. Scalding, typically from hot water, is the most common cause of burns. Water at 140°F (60°C) can quickly (within 3 seconds) create a deep partial-thickness or full-thickness burn.

2. A. The American Burn Association has created guidelines for patients who should be referred to a burn center. These include second- or third-degree burns of more than 10% TBSA in patients younger than 10 or older than 50 years, second- or third-degree burns of more than 20% in other age groups, third-degree burns of more than 5% TBSA in any age group, and any burns to the face, hands, feet, genitalia, perineum, or major joints. In addition, all electrical and chemical burns and those with inhalational injury should be referred.

3. D. Suspected smoke inhalation is not itself an indication for intubation. For example, a coughing patient with a patent airway will be better at clearing secretions than an intubated patient; however, such a patient requires very close monitoring. Smoke inhalation should be suspected in closed-space fires or when the victim was unconscious,

had an acrid smell of smoke on clothing, or had singed nasal hair, hoarseness, wheezing, and facial burns. Hard signs of inhalational injury include the presence of copious sputum production or carbonaceous sputum. Patients with suspected smoke inhalation should have arterial blood gas and CO hemoglobin levels checked. A decreased $Pa_{O_2}{:}F_{I_{O_2}}$ ratio (the ratio of arterial oxygen pressure [Pa_{O_2}] to the percentage of inspired oxygen [$F_{I_{O_2}}$]) is a useful indicator of smoke inhalation. A ratio of 400 to 500 is normal. A ratio of less than 250 is an indication for endotracheal intubation rather than simply increasing the inspired oxygen concentration. Other indications include Pa_{O_2} less than 60, Pco_2 greater than 50, and severe upper airway edema.

Whether routine fiberoptic bronchoscopy should be used in all suspected inhalational injuries is somewhat controversial. In one small study, fiberoptic laryngoscopy allowed differentiation of patients with inhalation injuries who did not require intubation. They recommended observation in a monitored setting with serial fiberoptic examinations. Another study found that fiberoptic bronchoscopy with biopsy was sensitive (79%) and highly specific (94%) for the diagnosis of inhalation injury. In addition, it was more reliable than the circumstances of the injury, clinical findings, and complementary tests. It was also one of the most strongly predictive variables for the onset of acute respiratory distress syndrome and death.

References: Masanès M, Legendre C, Lioret N, et al: Fiberoptic bronchoscopy for the early diagnosis of subglottal inhalation injury: comparative value in the assessment of prognosis, *J Trauma* 36: 59–67, 1994.

Masanès MJ, Legendre C, Lioret N, et al: Using bronchoscopy and biopsy to diagnose early inhalation injury: macroscopic and histologic findings, *Chest* 107:1365–1369, 1995.

Muehlberger T, Kunar D, Munster A, Couch M: Efficacy of fiberoptic laryngoscopy in the diagnosis of inhalation injuries, *Arch Otolaryngol Head Neck Surg* 124:1003–1007, 1998.

4. D. The systemic inflammatory response, triggered by the release of local proinflammatory cytokines, seems to be triggered as burns approach 20% TBSA. This is the basis on which patients with burns of more than 20% TBSA are referred to a major burn center. The inflammatory response triggers a microvascular leak, leading to an immense loss of fluid and protein into the extravascular space from the intravascular compartment. The situation is further exacerbated by a sympathetic response that leads to intense vasoconstriction, resulting in decreased perfusion to the skin and organs.

5. D. Cool water may be appropriate for small burns such as scalds because it may delay edema formation. However, iced water should never be applied. Iced water causes two problems: the ensuing vasoconstriction results in further skin ischemia and if applied to large areas will lead to systemic hypothermia. Central line access is not routinely needed for TBSA burns greater than 20%. They are indicated for patients with burns of more than 50% TBSA or for those with significant other comorbidities. Lower extremity IV lines in burn patients have a high rate of infectious complications and thus should be avoided. It is preferable to use the upper extremities, even if that requires placing the line through burned skin or eschar. Given the variable rate of absorption of medications administered intramuscularly or subcutaneously in burn patients, medications should be given intravenously.

6. D. The TBSA burned can be estimated using the rule of nines. Each upper extremity accounts for 9% of the TBSA, each lower extremity accounts for 18%, the anterior and posterior trunk each accounts for 18%, the head and neck account for 9%, and the perineum accounts for 1%. First-degree burns are not included.

7. E. The total number of burn deaths and the mortality rate both have decreased dramatically in the past 40 years. One way to gauge the improvement in mortality rate is by determining the burn size associated with a 50% mortality rate. The burn size associated with a 50% mortality rate has increased from a 30% TBSA to greater than 80% TBSA in healthy young adults.

8. E. Fluid resuscitation in the pediatric population is particularly challenging and differs from that in adults in several important aspects. Small children (<20 kg) have less energy reserve and thus need supplementation with glucose. Relative to their size, pediatric burn victims need more fluid on a per-kilogram basis than adults. Resuscitation fluid requirements for children are approximately 6 mL/kg per % TBSA of burn. Urine output should be maintained at a higher rate than that of the adult burn victim (1.0–1.5 mL/kg body weight per hour). In addition, the threshold for aggressive resuscitation is lower in children (beginning at 10%–20% TBSA vs. 20% TBSA burns in adults) as is the threshold for burn center referral.

9. A. Recent studies suggest that reactive oxygen species generated by thermal injury are involved in edema formation associated with severe burns. Vitamin C, a free radical scavenge, has been investigated as a potential treatment modality. Tanaka and colleagues reported that the successful use of high-dose (66 mg/kg/hr for 24 hours) IV vitamin C during the first 24 hours after thermal injury significantly reduced resuscitation fluid volume requirements, body weight gain, and wound edema, as well as the severity of respiratory dysfunction. This finding has been observed in an animal model as well.

References: Dubick M, Williams C, Elgjo G, Kramer G: High-dose vitamin C infusion reduces fluid requirements in the resuscitation of burn-injured sheep, *Shock* 24:139–144, 2005.

Matsuda T, Tanaka H, Reyes H, et al: Antioxidant therapy using high dose vitamin C: reduction of postburn resuscitation fluid volume requirements, *World J Surg* 19:287–291, 1995.

Tanaka H, Matsuda T, Miyagantani Y: Reduction of resuscitation fluid volumes in severely burned patients using ascorbic acid administration: a randomized, prospective study, *Arch Surg* 135:326–331, 2000.

10 A. Most burn patients should be resuscitated with crystalloid, specifically lactated Ringer's solution. Some burn specialists recommend the use of colloid, such as albumin, in addition to crystalloid. It has the theoretical advantage of maintaining the plasma oncotic pressure and thus maintaining the intravascular volume without using as large a volume of fluid. One of the few randomized trials comparing crystalloid with colloid in burn patients showed no benefit from albumin in terms of mortality, however. In addition, it is expensive. Albumin is not associated with increased mortality in burn resuscitation. With the aggressive resuscitation approach used currently, compartment syndrome has been reported with increasing frequency in burn patients. One potential benefit of albumin is that it may lead to lower intra-abdominal pressures compared with crystalloid. A recent prospective, randomized trial demonstrated a greater increase in intra-abdominal pressure with crystalloid (26.5 vs. 10.6 mm Hg, $P < 0.0001$) compared with colloid. Thus, albumin may have appeal in patients with massive burns in which large resuscitation volumes are needed. Normal saline should be avoided in burn patients. The large volumes required in burn patients will often lead to hyperchloremia with a metabolic acidosis. A prospective, randomized trial with dextran showed no benefit compared with crystalloid.

References: Monafo W: Initial management of burns, *N Engl J Med* 335:1581–1586, 1996.

O'Mara M, Slater H, Goldfarb I, Caushaj P: **A** prospective, randomized evaluation of intra-abdominal pressures with crystalloid and colloid resuscitation in burn patients, *J Trauma* 58: 1011–1018, 2005.

11. D. CO has 200 times greater affinity for hemoglobin than does oxygen. CO binds to the heme molecules of hemoglobin to form carboxyhemoglobin, although the binding is reversible. It interferes with oxygen delivery in several ways. It prevents oxygen from being displaced on the hemoglobin molecule. It causes the oxygen–hemoglobin dissociation curve to shift to the left. This results in less oxygen being unloaded. CO also inhibits cellular respiration by binding to cytochrome oxidase, a component of the mitochondrial electron transport chain. It is also a direct cardiac and skeletal muscle toxin and causes neurologic symptoms via demyelination. Levels of CO hemoglobin are readily measurable and should be checked in patients with suspected poisoning. Confusion and lethargy typically develop in patients with a CO hemoglobin level of 30%. Levels of 40% to 60% lead to coma, and levels greater than 60% are fatal. To put this in perspective, fatal levels can be reached quickly in smoky fires. Treatment with hyperbaric oxygen is theoretically appealing because it reduces the carboxyhemoglobin dissociation half-life. By inhaling room air, the dissociation half-life is more than 4 hours. By breathing 100% oxygen, it is reduced to 45 minutes. At 2.5 atm with 100% oxygen, the half-life is reduced to approximately 23 minutes. However, there are two randomized trials using hyperbaric oxygen for CO poisoning, one showing worsening neurologic outcome and one showing improvement. Thus, its routine use is not currently recommended. Both studies were conducted in patients without burns. If the patient also has burns, hyperbaric oxygen is not used because it would interfere with the early intense resuscitation efforts that are required. CO gives falsely elevated readings on the pulse oximeter.

References: Ernst A, Zibrak J: Carbon monoxide poisoning, *N Engl J Med* 339:1603–1608, 1998.

Scheinkestel C, Bailey M, Myles P, et al: Hyperbaric or normobaric oxygen for acute carbon monoxide poisoning: a randomised controlled clinical trial, *Med J Aust* 170:203–210, 1999.

12. E. The Parkland formula recommends 4 mL/kg for each percentage of TBSA (second and third degree) burned over the first 24 hours, with one half of that amount administered in the first 8 hours and the remaining half over the next 16 hours. So this patient would require 4 mL × 70 kg × 70% TBSA burn = 19,600 mL, of which half (9800 mL) would be given in the first 8 hours.

13. D. The three agents with proven broad-spectrum antimicrobial activity when applied to the burn wound are silver sulfadiazine (Silvadene), mafenide acetate (Sulfamylon), and silver nitrate. Silver sulfadiazine is the most common agent used in burn centers and has antifungal properties in addition to good bacterial coverage. However, it does not penetrate eschar. Only mafenide acetate is able to penetrate eschar, and it is the only agent capable of suppressing dense subeschar bacterial proliferation. The main disadvantage of mafenide acetate is that it is a carbonic anhydrase inhibitor, which may interfere with renal-buffering mechanisms. Bicarbonate is consumed and therefore chloride is retained, resulting in a hyperchloremic metabolic acidosis. This can lead to mild compensatory respiratory alkalosis. Because silver nitrate does not penetrate the eschar, it should be used before bacteria have penetrated the wound. Two other disadvantages are the associated hyponatremia that occurs, which is common, and methemoglobinemia, which is unusual.

References: Endorf FW, Gibran NS: Burns. In Brunicardi FC, Andersen DK, Billiar TR, et al, editors: *Schwartz's principles of surgery*, ed 9, New York, 2010, McGraw-Hill, pp 197–208.

Wolf SW, Herndon DN: Burns. In Townsend CM Jr, Beauchamp RD, Evers BM, Mattox KL, editors: *Sabiston textbook of surgery: the biological basis of modern surgical practice*, ed 18, Philadelphia, 2008, WB Saunders, pp 559–585.

Cardiac Surgery

7

1. Which of the following are true regarding coronary stenting versus coronary artery bypass for multivessel coronary artery disease?
   A. Stenting is associated with less need for long-term reintervention.
   B. Stenting is associated with a lower rate of long-term myocardial infarction.
   C. Stenting is associated with a higher long-term survival.
   D. Coronary artery bypass results in improved long-term survival, less myocardial infarction, and less need for reintervention.
   E. Stenting and coronary artery bypass have equivalent long-term results.

2. The most common isolated congenital cardiac deformity is:
   A. Atrial septal defect
   B. Ventricular septal defect (VSD)
   C. Atrioventricular defect
   D. Tricuspid atresia
   E. Persistent truncus arteriosus

3. Coarctation of the aorta most commonly occurs in the:
   A. Ascending thoracic aorta
   B. Transverse thoracic aorta
   C. Thoracic aorta just proximal to the left subclavian artery
   D. Thoracic aorta just distal to the left subclavian artery
   E. Descending thoracic aorta just above the diaphragm

4. In patients undergoing coronary artery bypass grafting, all of the following have been identified as being associated with an increased operative risk EXCEPT:
   A. Advanced age
   B. Low ejection fraction
   C. Male sex
   D. Body surface area
   E. Diabetes

5. The most likely cause of a focal neurologic deficit after coronary artery bypass grafting is:
   A. Embolism
   B. Cerebral hypoperfusion
   C. Intracranial thrombosis
   D. Intracranial hemorrhage
   E. Lacunar infarction

6. Five hours after aortic valve replacement, a patient suddenly becomes hypotensive to 80 mm Hg systolic. The cardiac index has decreased from 2.5 L/min to 1.6 L/min. Central venous pressure is 19 mm Hg with a pulmonary artery wedge pressure of 20 mm Hg. Mediastinal drainage, which was approximately 150 mL/hr initially, has been minimal over the past hour. Management consists of:
   A. Echocardiography
   B. Volume resuscitation
   C. Nitroprusside
   D. Nitroglycerin
   E. Mediastinal exploration

7. Which of the following medications would least likely benefit a patient with unstable angina?
   A. Aspirin
   B. Heparin
   C. Statins
   D. Calcium channel blockers
   E. Propranolol

8. Which of the following is not needed in the calculation of systemic vascular resistance?

    A. Systolic blood pressure
    B. Pulmonary capillary wedge pressure
    C. Cardiac output
    D. Diastolic blood pressure
    E. Central venous pressure

9. Which of these veins has the highest venous oxygen saturation?

    A. Superior vena cava
    B. Inferior vena cava
    C. Coronary sinus
    D. Pulmonary artery
    E. Coronary vein

10. Which of the following is NOT an indication for surgical intervention in a patient with aortic stenosis?

    A. Syncope
    B. Angina pectoris
    C. Poor ventricular function
    D. Valve area less than 0.5 cm^2
    E. Calcification of the stenotic valve

11. The intra-aortic balloon pump is associated with all of the following EXCEPT:

    A. Increased coronary blood flow
    B. Increased preload
    C. Improved cardiac index
    D. Improved diastolic perfusion
    E. Decreased afterload

12. Potential indications for the use of an intra-aortic balloon pump include all of the following EXCEPT:

    A. Acute aortic insufficiency
    B. Acute mitral regurgitation after myocardial infarction
    C. Ventricular failure after cardiopulmonary bypass
    D. Postinfarction VSD
    E. Unstable angina

13. Cardiac myxomas most frequently arise in the:

    A. Right atrium
    B. Left atrium
    C. Right ventricle
    D. Left ventricle
    E. Atrial appendage

14. Seventy-five percent of patients have coronary anatomy described as a "right dominant system." Right dominance means that:

    A. The right coronary artery is larger than the left.
    B. The blood flow rate is greater through the right coronary artery than through the left coronary artery.
    C. The posterior aspect of the septum is supplied by the right coronary artery.
    D. The right coronary artery originates from the proximal left anterior descending coronary artery.
    E. The right coronary blood flow occurs during systole.

15. The most common congenital heart defect causing a right-to-left shunt is:

    A. Truncus arteriosus
    B. Total anomalous pulmonary venous return
    C. Tricuspid atresia
    D. Tetralogy of Fallot
    E. Transposition of the great vessels

Answers

1. D. Two recent studies demonstrated that on long-term follow-up, coronary artery bypass for disease of two or more vessels was associated with a higher survival rate, lower rate of myocardial infarction, and less need for reintervention than stenting. The most recent study compared coronary artery bypass with drug-eluting stents.

References: Hannan E, Racz M, Walford G, et al: Long-term outcomes of coronary-artery bypass grafting versus stent implantation, *N Engl J Med* 352:2174–2183, 2005.

Hannan E, Wu C, Walford G, et al: Drug-eluting stents vs. coronary-artery bypass grafting in multivessel coronary disease, *N Engl J Med* 358:331–341, 2008.

2. B. A VSD is a hole between the right and left ventricles. It is the most common isolated congenital cardiac deformity. There are four types. Perimembranous VSDs are the most common. Large VSDs are nonrestrictive in that they allow blood to go freely from the left ventricle to the right ventricle and can lead to early symptoms of congestive heart failure. Small VSDs are considered restrictive in that they limit the shunting of blood. They will not typically cause symptoms early on and therefore may only be detected by auscultation. They carry a long-term risk of causing endocarditis. Small VSDs detected in infancy have a high chance of spontaneous closure and therefore can be monitored. Conversely, large VSDs that are symptomatic will require repair. Traditional repair has been via open cardiac surgery, although more recently VSDs are being repaired using a catheter-directed membranous occluder.

Reference: Hijazi Z, Hakim F, Haweleh A, et al: Catheter closure of perimembranous ventricular septal defects using the new Amplatzer membranous VSD occluder: initial clinical experience, *Catheter Cardiovasc Interv* 56:508–515, 2002.

3. D. Aortic coarctation is a congenital narrowing of the thoracic aorta, usually occurring distal to the left subclavian artery, at the point of insertion of the ductus arteriosus. Coarctation may go undetected until adolescence or young adulthood. Patients may present with severe upper extremity hypertension in association with weak or absent lower extremity pulses. Conventional treatment has been with open thoracic aortic surgery. However, it more recently has been treated successfully with endovascular techniques.

References: Shah L, Hijazi Z, Sandhu S, et al: Use of endovascular stents for the treatment of coarctation of the aorta in children and adults: immediate and midterm results, *J Invasive Cardiol* 17:614–618, 2005.

Thanopoulos B, Hadjinikolaou L, Konstadopoulou G: Stent treatment for coarctation of the aorta: intermediate term follow up and technical considerations, *Heart* 84:65–70, 2000.

4. C. Female sex is associated with increased operative risk with coronary artery bypass. Other factors include renal failure, New York Heart Association functional class IV, peripheral arterial disease, history of stroke, chronic obstructive pulmonary disease, presence of cardiogenic shock, left main disease, recent myocardial infarction, and reoperative cardiac surgery.

5. A. The majority of strokes after coronary artery bypass graft are embolic in etiology. In most instances, the emboli seem to arise during cross-clamping or unclamping of the ascending aorta or during aortic cannulation.

Reference: Likosky D, Marrin D, Caplan L, et al: Determination of etiologic mechanisms of strokes secondary to coronary artery bypass graft surgery, *Stroke* 34:2830–2834, 2003.

6. E. Postoperatively, pericardial tamponade is due to formation of a pericardial clot and compression of the heart. This condition can sometimes be difficult to diagnose. It should be suspected in patients with low cardiac output and hypotension, failure to respond to intravascular volume replacement, increased ionotropic requirements, a sudden decrease in mediastinal tube output, and an increase and equalization of the central venous pressure and pulmonary

capillary wedge pressure. Diagnosis can be assisted by transthoracic and transesophageal echocardiography, although false-negative findings can occur. However, if the patient is clinically decompensating and the presentation is consistent with tamponade, definitive therapy should not be delayed and the patient should be taken back to the operating room.

7. D. There is no benefit from the use of calcium channel blockers. Patients with unstable angina should receive at least aspirin, beta-blockers, and statins. Heparin, clopidogrel, and glycoprotein IIb/IIIa antagonists are also useful.

8. B. Systemic vascular resistance (SVR) is calculated by the following equation:

$$SVR = MAP - CVP/CO \times 80; MAP = DBP + \tfrac{1}{2}(SBP - DBP)$$

where MAP is mean arterial pressure, CVP is central venous pressure, CO is cardiac output, DBP is diastolic blood pressure, and SBP is systolic blood pressure.

9. B. The inferior vena cava has the highest oxygen saturation because it receives venous blood from the kidneys. The kidneys use little oxygen relative to other organs. The kidneys receive a large percentage of the cardiac output but use blood for nonoxidative phosphorylation needs; oxygen extraction is relatively low. The superior vena cava receives blood from the brain, which has a higher oxygen extraction. The pulmonary artery contains a mixture of blood from both the superior vena cava and inferior vena cava, so its oxygen saturation will be somewhere in between.

10. E. Aortic stenosis is caused by acquired calcific disease (most common), congenital bicuspid aortic valve, or rheumatic heart disease. Once a patient becomes symptomatic, surgery is indicated because there is a progressive risk of sudden death. Symptoms include exertional dyspnea, syncope, angina, and heart failure. In the absence of symptoms, surgery is indicated if the valve area is less than 0.5 cm^2. Surgery is still indicated in patients with poor ventricular function.

11. B. The intra-aortic balloon pump inflates at the onset of diastole and deflates just before systole. On inflation, it displaces blood both proximally and distally. It increases myocardial oxygen supply and decreases myocardial oxygen demand. It decreases both preload and afterload. It also improves cardiac output and ejection fraction and increases coronary and systemic perfusion pressure (including renal blood flow). It lowers heart rate, pulmonary capillary wedge pressure, and systemic vascular resistance.

12. A. The most frequent indication for the intra-aortic balloon pump is to provide hemodynamic support during or after cardiac catheterization, in cardiogenic shock, for weaning from cardiac bypass, for preoperative use in high-risk patients, and for those with refractory unstable angina. Because the balloon inflates at the onset of diastole, the intra-aortic balloon pump would increase the regurgitation in an incompetent aortic valve. It is also contraindicated in patients with aortic dissection and those with severe aortoiliac occlusive disease.

13. B. Myxomas are the most common primary tumor of the heart. The majority (60%–75%) arise in the left atrium, with most of the remaining in the right atrium. Very few are found in the right or left ventricle. Myxomas are gelatinous tumors with a propensity for embolization. They can also obstruct or damage the mitral valve, leading to symptoms of heart failure. Diagnosis is made by transthoracic or transesophageal echocardiography. Treatment is surgical excision. They are benign but have a tendency to recur.

14. C. Coronary dominance refers to which coronary artery supplies the posterior descending artery and the posterolateral artery. The right coronary artery is dominant in approximately 70% to 80% of patients. The posterior descending artery supplies blood to the posterior aspect of the septum. A dominant right coronary artery gives off the posterolateral artery, which provides blood to the lower posterolateral part of the left ventricle. If the left coronary artery, via the circumflex artery, provides these branches, it is called a left dominant system (least common). Codominance refers to both right and left coronary arteries providing these branches.

15. D. Tetralogy of Fallot is the most common congenital heart defect presenting as a "blue baby" (cyanosis from a right-to-left shunt). The four features include VSD, dextroposition of the heart (overriding aorta), right ventricular outflow tract obstruction, and right ventricular hypertrophy. Most surgeons recommend repair during infancy, but if the patient is unstable and is younger than 6 months old, Blalock-Taussig shunt placement may be performed.

References: Ferraris VA, Mentzer RM: Acquired heart disease: coronary insufficiency. In Townsend CM Jr, Beauchamp RD, Evers BM, Mattox KL, editors: *Sabiston textbook of surgery: the biological basis of modern surgical practice*, ed 18, Philadelphia, 2008, WB Saunders, pp 1790–1832.

Fraser CD, Carberry KE: Congenital heart disease. In Townsend CM Jr, Beauchamp RD, Evers BM, Mattox KL, editors: *Sabiston textbook of surgery: the biological basis of modern surgical practice*, ed 18, Philadelphia, 2008, WB Saunders, pp 1749–1789.

Karamlou TB, Welke KF, Ungerleider RM: Congenital heart disease. In Brunicardi FC, Andersen DK, Billiar TR, et al, editors: *Schwartz's principles of surgery*, ed 9, New York, 2010, McGraw-Hill, pp 591–626.

LeMaire SA, Sharma K, Coselli JS: Thoracic aortic aneurysms and aortic dissection. In Brunicardi FC, Andersen DK, Billiar TR, et al, editors: *Schwartz's principles of surgery*, ed 9, New York, 2010, McGraw-Hill, pp 665–700.

Schwartz CF, Crooke GA, Grossi EA, et al: Acquired heart disease. In Brunicardi FC, Andersen DK, Billiar TR, et al, editors: *Schwartz's principles of surgery*, ed 9, New York, 2010, McGraw-Hill, pp 627–664.

Cerebrovascular Disease

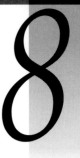

1. Which of the following is true regarding the timing and indication for carotid endarterectomy (CEA) in a patient with a stroke?

   A. The timing of CEA depends on computed tomography (CT) scan findings.
   B. CEA is best performed within 6 to 8 weeks after the stroke.
   C. CEA is best performed 3 months after the stroke.
   D. CEA should be performed urgently.
   E. CEA is indicated if the stroke is completely disabling.

2. All of the following are true regarding CEA for asymptomatic internal carotid artery (ICA) stenosis EXCEPT:

   A. According to the Asymptomatic Carotid Atherosclerosis Study, CEA reduces the 5-year risk of stroke and death from 11% to 5% in patients with high-grade stenosis.
   B. CEA is only beneficial if the perioperative stroke and death rates are less than 3%.
   C. The perioperative stroke rate is surgeon dependent.
   D. The benefit is greatest for women.
   E. CEA is indicated for patients with ICA stenosis ranging from 60% to 99%.

3. Which of the following would provide the greatest benefit from CEA?

Symptom	Percentage of ICA Stenosis
A. Asymptomatic	Right 90%
B. Right eye amaurosis fugax	Right 60%
C. Right arm/leg stroke	Left 60%
D. Left eye amaurosis fugax	Left 80%
E. Right arm/leg stroke	Left 45%

4. Indications for CEA include all of the following EXCEPT:

   A. 55% left ICA stenosis with right arm and leg transient ischemic attack
   B. Asymptomatic 85% right ICA stenosis
   C. 100% right ICA occlusion with right eye amaurosis fugax
   D. 75% left ICA stenosis with transient aphasia
   E. 99% right ICA stenosis with left-sided hemiparesis

5. Thirty minutes after arriving in the recovery room after a right CEA, the patient develops left hemiparesis. The most appropriate next step would be:

   A. Immediate operative re-exploration of the carotid artery
   B. Tissue plasminogen activator infusion
   C. Cerebral angiography
   D. Carotid duplex ultrasound scan
   E. Head CT

6. Accepted guidelines for shunting during CEA include all of the following EXCEPT:

   A. Routine shunting in all cases
   B. Selective shunting in a stroke patient based on intraoperative electroencephalographic changes
   C. Selective shunting based on ICA stump pressure
   D. Selective shunting in an awake patient based on whether hemiplegia on carotid clamping develops
   E. Selective shunting in an asymptomatic patient based on changes on transcranial Doppler ultrasonography

7. All of the following are true regarding the use of patch closure compared with primary closure of the ICA arteriotomy after CEA EXCEPT:

- **A.** Patch closure makes closure of the arteriotomy easier.
- **B.** Patch closure lowers the rate of ICA restenosis at 1 year.
- **C.** Patch closure lowers the risk of postoperative ICA thrombosis.
- **D.** Patch closure lowers the risk of perioperative stroke.
- **E.** Patch closure can be achieved using saphenous vein from the ankle.

8. All of the following are true regarding cerebral hyperperfusion syndrome after CEA EXCEPT:

- **A.** It typically presents within 24 hours after surgery.
- **B.** It can lead to seizures, intracranial hemorrhage, and death.
- **C.** The incidence is higher in patients undergoing CEA for very high grade carotid stenosis.
- **D.** Management includes use of antihypertensive and diuretic agents.
- **E.** The cause is thought to be related to a lack of cerebral autoregulation.

9. Useful and acceptable strategies to gain better exposure of the carotid artery include all of the following EXCEPT:

- **A.** Division of the descendens hypoglossi
- **B.** Division of the posterior belly of the digastric muscle
- **C.** Division of the omohyoid muscle
- **D.** Anterior subluxation of the mandible
- **E.** Division of the superior laryngeal nerve

10. A 45-year-old woman presents with a 2-cm neck mass anterior to the sternocleidomastoid muscle. Duplex ultrasound scan shows a hypervascular solid mass at the carotid bifurcation. Which of the following is NOT true about this lesion?

- **A.** An arteriogram is likely to show splaying of the carotid bifurcation.
- **B.** Surgery carries a significant risk of cranial nerve injury.
- **C.** The lesion is most likely benign.
- **D.** The tumor should be resected in a periadventitial plane.
- **E.** Routine preoperative embolization is recommended to reduce bleeding.

11. Which of the following is NOT true regarding fibromuscular dysplasia (FMD) of the ICA?

- **A.** It primarily affects white women in the fourth and fifth decades of life.
- **B.** It is associated with intracranial aneurysms.
- **C.** It is bilateral in more than 50% of patients.
- **D.** Symptomatic patients can be managed by surgical insertion of dilators into the ICA.
- **E.** The most common type of FMD is intimal fibroplasia.

12. A 65-year-old woman presents with generalized malaise, headache, tenderness over her right temple, and an elevated erythrocyte sedimentation rate. Which of the following is NOT true about this condition?

- **A.** A duplex ultrasound scan may establish the diagnosis.
- **B.** A temporal artery biopsy is indicated.
- **C.** The patient should be immediately started on steroids.
- **D.** It is associated with the development of blindness.
- **E.** Jaw claudication is rare.

13. A 25-year-old woman presents with several episodes of dizziness, syncope, upper extremity claudication, and an elevated erythrocyte sedimentation rate. On examination, she has no radial, brachial, or carotid pulse. Her blood pressure is 70/50 mm Hg in her right arm and 60/40 mm Hg in her left. Magnetic resonance angiography reveals occlusion of both subclavian arteries as well as high-grade stenoses of both common carotid arteries at their origin. Which of the following is true about this condition?

- **A.** Methotrexate is not helpful.
- **B.** Transluminal angioplasty is the treatment of choice.
- **C.** Surgery should be performed urgently.
- **D.** The disease can involve the pulmonary and coronary arteries.
- **E.** Antihypertensive agents are contraindicated.

14. A 40-year-old woman presents to the emergency department after a motor vehicle accident with a seat belt mark across her right neck and weakness and numbness of her left arm and leg. She is otherwise hemodynamically stable, alert, and oriented. A CT scan of the head is negative for an intracranial bleed. Which of the following is true about this injury?

    A. Heparin is contraindicated.
    B. The injury is associated with Horner syndrome.
    C. The injury requires a high degree of force.
    D. If the carotid artery is injured, it is unlikely to heal spontaneously.
    E. Urgent surgical intervention is indicated.

15. A 60-year-old man presents with a right arm and leg hemiparesis that lasted 1 hour. He has a history of a left modified radical neck dissection and neck irradiation for cancer 10 years previously. Magnetic resonance angiography reveals more than 70% stenosis of the left common carotid artery proximal to the bifurcation. Which of the following is recommended as the definitive management?

    A. Aspirin
    B. Aspirin and clopidogrel
    C. Carotid stenting with a cerebral protection device
    D. Resection of the diseased carotid artery with an interposition graft
    E. Standard CEA

16. Which of the following is true regarding penetrating carotid artery injuries?

    A. Associated injuries to the esophagus are uncommon.
    B. Most pseudoaneurysms can be observed.
    C. ICA injury is better tolerated than common carotid injury.
    D. If the patient has a localizing neurologic deficit at presentation, repair should be attempted.
    E. Coma is a contraindication to attempted repair.

17. Indications for CEA include all of the following EXCEPT:

    A. 80% ICA stenosis with contralateral arm and leg hemiparesis
    B. 75% ICA stenosis with ipsilateral amaurosis fugax
    C. 60% ICA stenosis with contralateral arm and leg transient ischemic attack
    D. 80% ICA stenosis with dense contralateral hemiplegia and aphasia
    E. Asymptomatic 80% ICA stenosis

18. Which of the following would be the LEAST likely complication after a right carotid subclavian artery bypass?

    A. Paralysis of the right diaphragm
    B. Chylothorax
    C. Graft infection
    D. Graft occlusion
    E. Hoarseness

19. Four months after CEA, a duplex ultrasound scan reveals recurrent 70% ICA stenosis. The patient reports no symptoms. Optimal management would consist of:

    A. Repeat CEA
    B. Carotid stenting
    C. Observation
    D. Interposition saphenous vein bypass
    E. Interposition polytetrafluoroethylene bypass

20. The most common symptom of nerve injury after CEA is:

    A. Tongue deviation
    B. Hoarseness
    C. Easy voice fatigue
    D. Drooping of nasolabial fold
    E. Swallowing difficulty

21. A 38-year-old woman presents to the emergency department with sudden onset of left arm and leg weakness that lasts 1 hour and then resolves spontaneously. There is no history of trauma. Duplex ultrasound scan of the right carotid artery reveals a complete occlusion of the ICA. Arteriography confirms an occlusion of the ICA approximately 2 to 3 cm distal to the bifurcation. Management consists of:

    A. CEA
    B. Lytic therapy with tissue plasminogen activator
    C. Carotid stenting
    D. Anticoagulation
    E. Fogarty embolectomy

22. Atherosclerosis at the carotid bifurcation tends to occur in all of the following EXCEPT:

    A. Outer (lateral) aspect of the carotid bulb
    B. In areas of low shear stress
    C. In areas of high velocity
    D. In areas of high particle residence time
    E. In areas of flow reversal

23. A patient presents with right eye amaurosis fugax, and magnetic resonance angiography reveals right ICA stenosis of more than 70%. Magnetic resonance angiogram reveals an incidentally discovered 2-mm intracranial berry aneurysm. Management consists of:

A. CEA

B. Surgical clipping of the intracranial aneurysm only

C. Surgical clipping of the intracranial aneurysm, then CEA

D. CEA, then surgical clipping of the intracranial aneurysm

E. Stenting the intracranial aneurysm, then CEA

Answers

1. A. The timing of CEA after a stroke is controversial. A delay in surgery increases the risk of a recurrent stroke. The risk is highest within the first month. Conversely, operating too early creates a potential risk of a reperfusion injury, particularly if a large infarction is present on CT and if hypertension cannot be controlled postoperatively. Intracranial bleeding is thought to occur due to altered autoregulation and hyperperfusion of ischemic tissue. In the North American Symptomatic Carotid Endarterectomy Trial (NASCET), however, postoperative intracranial hemorrhage occurred in only 0.2% of patients. Until recently, CEA was routinely delayed 4 to 6 weeks after a stroke. Subsequent analysis of the NASCET showed that patients with a stable, nondisabling acute stroke, a normal CT scan, and a normal level of consciousness can safely undergo CEA shortly after the diagnosis is made and preoperative evaluation is complete. Current treatment guidelines from the American Academy of Neurology and from the American Stroke Association/American Heart Association recommend that CEA for patients with nondisabling strokes should preferably be performed within 2 weeks of the primary stroke. Patients with a large stroke on CT scan or those with a midline shift may be at higher risk of reperfusion injury, particularly if they have a depressed level of consciousness. Operation should be delayed until these patients improve and plateau in their clinical recovery, in the range of 4 to 6 weeks.

References: Henderson R, Eliasziw M, Fox A, et al: Angiographically defined collateral circulation and risk of stroke in patients with severe carotid artery stenosis. North American Symptomatic Carotid Endarterectomy Trial (NASCET) Group, *Stroke* 31:128–132, 2000.

North American Symptomatic Carotid Endarterectomy Trial Collaborators: Beneficial effect of carotid endarterectomy in symptomatic patients with high-grade carotid stenosis, *N Engl J Med* 325:445–453, 1991.

Sacco R, Adams R, Albers G, et al, American Heart Association; American Stroke Association Council on Stroke; Council on Cardiovascular Radiology and Intervention; American Academy of Neurology: Guidelines for prevention of stroke in patients with ischemic stroke or transient ischemic attack: a statement for healthcare professionals from the American Heart Association/American Stroke Association Council on Stroke: co-sponsored by the Council on Cardiovascular Radiology and Intervention: the American Academy of Neurology affirms the value of this guideline, *Stroke* 37:577–617, 2006.

2. D. The Asymptomatic Carotid Atherosclerosis Study (ACAS) randomized patients with asymptomatic carotid artery stenosis of 60% to 99% to either CEA and aspirin or aspirin alone. The study was interrupted because of a significant benefit identified in patients undergoing CEA. A relative reduction in stroke rate by 50%, from 11% to 5% at 5 years was observed in patients undergoing CEA. The study found that there was no benefit in women. The Asymptomatic Carotid Surgery Trial confirmed the ACAS findings, in that in patients with 60% to 99% stenosis, the net 5-year risk was 6.4% for all strokes or death in patients undergoing CEA versus 11.8% in those not undergoing surgery. This was a net absolute gain of 5.4% (relative risk reduction, 46%). The trial also showed that patients who underwent CEA were much less likely to have a fatal or disabling stroke (3.5% in the surgery group vs. 6.1% in the no-surgery group). The study found that there was less benefit in women. The greatest benefit was in men younger than 75 years of age.

References: Asymptomatic Carotid Surgery Trial (ACST) Collaborative Group: Prevention of disabling and fatal strokes by successful CEA in patients without recent neurological symptoms: randomized controlled trial, *Lancet* 363:1491–1502, 2004.

Executive Committee for the Asymptomatic Carotid Atherosclerosis Study: Endarterectomy for asymptomatic carotid artery stenosis, *JAMA* 273:1421–1428, 1995.

3. D. The first NASCET study found that CEA was of benefit for symptomatic severe ICA stenosis (70%–99%). A symptomatic carotid artery was defined as a nondisabling stroke, a hemispheric transient ischemic attack, or a retinal symptom (amaurosis fugax). Thus, patients with severe neurologic deficits, without meaningful recovery or with marked alteration of consciousness, were not candidates for inclusion in the study. Because the goal of CEA is to prevent further damage to the ipsilateral motor cortex, these latter patients were deemed to have too much injured brain tissue to benefit from a stroke prevention procedure. Life-table estimates of the cumulative risk of any ipsilateral stroke at 2 years were 26% in the aspirin group and 9% in the aspirin and CEA group.

In the second NASCET study, in patients with less than 50% stenosis, the risk of stroke at 5-year follow-up was not different between the CEA plus aspirin group and the aspirin-alone group (14.9% vs. 18.7%, respectively). In patients with stenosis from 50% to 69%, the 5-year risk of ipsilateral stroke was 15.7% in the CEA group and 22.2% in the medical group ($P = 0.04$). Women benefited from surgery only if they met criteria for one or more additional risk factors: age greater than 70 years, severe hypertension, history of myocardial infarction, or a hemispheric (as opposed to a retinal) event. Women also had higher perioperative mortality than men. Patients with only retinal symptoms and 50% to 69% stenosis did not benefit from CEA. Thus, the greatest benefit from CEA is in patients with ICA stenosis between 70% and 99% and recent (within 120 days) ipsilateral symptoms (nondisabling stroke, hemispheric transient ischemic attack, amaurosis fugax). For patients with moderate symptomatic stenosis (50%–69%), CEA is of less benefit, but may be indicated in select cases (hemispheric symptoms, failed medical therapy). ACAS demonstrated the benefit of CEA compared with aspirin for ICA stenosis of 60% to 99%. However, the benefit is much less than for symptomatic high-grade stenosis.

4. C. When deciding whether to perform CEA, it is important to determine whether the patient is symptomatic, whether the ischemic symptoms are compatible with the side of stenosis, and the percentage of stenosis. All options presented represent symptomatic carotid disease. The two NASCET studies demonstrated the benefit of CEA for ICA stenosis ranging from 50% to 69% and from 70% to 99%. However, there is no benefit of CEA with complete (100%) ICA occlusion. The completely occluded ICA has no further prograde flow, and, as such, there is typically no further embolic risk to a completely occluded vessel.

5. A. New neurologic deficits that present within the first 12 hours of operation are almost always the result of thromboembolic phenomena stemming from the CEA site. Possibilities include the development of thrombus on the endarterectomized arterial surface, a residual intimal flap in the ICA leading to occlusion, or a residual flap in the external carotid artery (ECA) leading to ECA thrombosis and retrograde embolization of the clot into the ICA. Immediate heparinization and exploration are indicated without the need for confirmatory arteriography or noninvasive tests. On re-exploring the wound, the ECA and ICA should be palpated for the presence of a pulse. If there is no pulse, this indicates thrombosis, and initial on-table arteriography is not necessary. The artery should be reopened and inspected to look for a cause of the thrombosis. Before closing the arteriotomy, care should be taken to ensure that there is good back-bleeding from the ICA. Fogarty balloon embolectomy of the cephalad ICA should be avoided because this can lead to a carotid-cavernous sinus fistula. The arteriotomy should then be reclosed with a patch. On-table arteriography should then be performed to ensure that the distal ICA is patent and to determine whether there is an embolus in the middle cerebral artery. If an embolus is present in the intracranial carotid or middle cerebral artery, local infusion of a lytic agent should be considered. If on

reopening the wound, an excellent pulse is present in the ICA and ECA, with normal signals on hand-held Doppler ultrasonography, on-table arteriography is performed. If arteriography reveals an intimal flap or irregular mural thrombus at the endarterectomy site, then reopening of the vessel is indicated. Neurologic deficits that develop 12 to 24 hours after the operation are usually due to thromboembolic phenomena stemming from the CEA site, but may also be caused by a postoperative hyperperfusion syndrome. These latter conditions may be worsened by immediate heparinization and re-exploration. Therefore, deficits occurring 12 to 24 hours after the operation should be promptly investigated with CT and arteriography.

6. B. The role of carotid shunting during CEA is controversial. Shunting during CEA decreases the risk of clamp-induced cerebral ischemia. However, overall, only approximately 15% of patients need shunting, as demonstrated by significant electroencephalographic changes with carotid artery clamping. The use of a shunt itself carries risks, including embolization, dissection or intimal injury of the ICA, and hindering the surgeon from visualizing the distal endpoint. Because there is no universal agreement on how to predict who needs shunting, several approaches have been used. One approach is to simply place a shunt in every patient. Others perform CEA under local anesthesia and insert a shunt only if an intraoperative change in neurologic status develops in the patient when the carotid artery is occluded. Intraoperative measurement of ICA back-pressure after clamping the common carotid artery and ECA is another method, with a pressure less than 50 mm Hg indicative of the need to insert a shunt. Other approaches include monitoring intraoperative transcranial Doppler ultrasonography, somatosensory evoked potentials, and electroencephalography. In patients with a history of stroke, all should undergo shunting. Stroke patients have an area surrounding the infarcted brain that is ischemic but not dead, known as the zone of ischemic penumbra. This area is particularly susceptible to alterations in blood flow, and shunting may minimize the risk of further ischemic injury.

Reference: McKinsey J, Gewertz B: Role of shunting in carotid endarterectomy. In Ernst C, Stanley J, editors: *Current therapy in vascular surgery,* St. Louis, 2001, Mosby, pp 55–57.

7. E. The rationale for patch closure after CEA is to reduce technical error and thus lower the risk of perioperative thrombosis and stroke, as well as to lower the risk of long-term restenosis. The majority of randomized studies comparing primary closure with patching were underpowered to demonstrate these differences. However, recent meta-analyses indicate that patching results in a decreased rate of early postoperative ICA occlusion, decreased 30-day perioperative stroke rate, and a decreased incidence of more than 50% restenosis in the first year. When analyzing the type of patch material, the greater saphenous vein seems to be even better than synthetic material, likely the result of the vein endothelium. However, many surgeons use a synthetic Dacron or polytetrafluoroethylene patch to avoid the need for vein harvesting. Vein patching has also been associated with a number of complications, including patch rupture, false aneurysm formation, and thromboembolism arising from the dilated aneurysmal reconstructed bifurcation. If vein is used, it should be harvested from the thigh because the smaller-diameter ankle saphenous vein has been associated with rupture.

Reference: Archie J Jr: Patching with carotid endarterectomy: when to do it and what to use, *Semin Vasc Surg* 11:24–29, 1998.

8. A. The incidence of hyperperfusion syndrome after a CEA is reportedly 0.3% to 1%. It is thought to occur as a result of impaired autoregulation of cerebral blood flow. Severe carotid stenosis leads to hypoperfusion, leading to a compensatory dilation of cerebral vessels distal to the stenosis as part of the normal autoregulatory response to maintain adequate cerebral blood flow. After CEA restores normal pressure, however, autoregulation is impaired and does not immediately adjust to the sudden increase in blood flow. Risk factors associated with cerebral hyperperfusion include recent stroke, surgery for very tight ICA stenosis, concomitant contralateral ICA occlusion, evidence of chronic ipsilateral hypoperfusion, and poorly controlled pre- and postoperative hypertension. Pathologic changes include mild cerebral edema and petechial and intracerebral hemorrhages. The syndrome is heralded by an ipsilateral frontal headache, most commonly on the fifth postoperative day. The headache may be followed by focal motor seizures that are often difficult to control. Management consists of controlling blood pressure, ideally with a beta-blocker, avoidance of vasodilators, and use of antiseizure medications. Sumatriptan, a serotonin receptor agonist, has been shown experimentally to help in the treatment of cerebral hyperperfusion, but this has not been clinically proven.

Reference: Schroeder T, Sillesen H, Sorensen O, Engell H: Cerebral hyperperfusion following carotid endarterectomy, *J Neurosurg* 66:824–829, 1987.

9. E. During CEA or in the trauma setting, difficulty is sometimes encountered in achieving adequate exposure of the carotid artery. This is particularly true for carotid lesions extending beyond the bifurcation into the distal ICA and/or in patients with high carotid bifurcations. The carotid bifurcation is typically at the junction of the third and fourth cervical vertebrae, but it varies. The bifurcation level can be assessed on preoperative imaging such as magnetic resonance imaging or CT angiography. It is also important to determine preoperatively whether the carotid plaque is localized to the bifurcation or whether it extends for some distance distally. If the carotid bifurcation is at the second vertebra or cephalad to it, adjunctive measures to achieve distal exposure may be necessary. Alternatively, a high carotid lesion may need to be treated with stenting.

Useful and acceptable steps to gain better distal exposure include division of the posterior belly of the digastric muscle for better cephalad exposure and division of the omohyoid muscle for better caudad exposure of the common carotid artery. When exposure is required above the second cervical vertebra, anterior subluxation of the mandible is rarely performed, with care not to dislocate the mandible. Division of the superior laryngeal nerve is not indicated because it would result in voice fatigue and difficulty swallowing.

The ansa cervicalis has a superior root and an inferior root. The superior root fibers are formed by branches of the first cervical nerve and accompany the hypoglossal nerve. The ansa cervicalis then branches off and descends in the carotid sheath (where it is called the descendens hypoglossi). It sends off branches to the omohyoid, sternothyroid, and sternohyoid muscles and is then joined by the inferior root. Division of the descendens hypoglossi is sometimes necessary because it allows reflection of the hypoglossal nerve off the ICA. Division of the nerve does not lead to any clinical disability.

10. E. The majority of carotid body tumors are benign. Malignancy occurs in only 6% to 12.5% of cases. Carotid body tumors originate from the chemoreceptor cells located at the carotid bifurcation. They are more prevalent in patients who live at high altitudes. They typically present as a palpable and painless mass over the carotid bifurcation region in the neck. The diagnosis can be established by CT angiography, magnetic resonance imaging, or duplex ultrasound scanning. The classic pathognomonic finding on an arteriogram is widening of the carotid bifurcation by a well-defined tumor blush (lyre sign). Tumors can be bilateral. Biopsy, including fine-needle aspiration, is unnecessary, dangerous, and contraindicated in the evaluation of paragangliomas. The treatment of choice is surgical excision. Preoperative tumor embolization does not lead to a decrease in blood loss or morbidity in most patients and is thus only indicated for large tumors (>4 cm). The tumor should be resected off the carotid artery in a periadventitial plane. If one inadvertently dissects in a subadventitial plane, this can lead to bleeding or postoperative rupture of the carotid artery. Permanent cranial nerve injury has been reported in as many as 20% of cases, with temporary deficits developing in an additional 20%.

Reference: Kafie F, Freischlag J: Carotid body tumors: the role of preoperative embolization, *Ann Vasc Surg* 15:237–242, 2001.

11. E. FMD of the ICA is the most common nonatherosclerotic disease process affecting the ICA. Approximately 25% of patients with carotid FMD have associated intracranial aneurysms and as many as 65% have bilateral carotid FMD. Medial fibrodysplasia is the most common form. It is characterized by stenosis alternating with intervening fusiform dilations that resemble a string of beads. Pathologically, smooth muscle cells in the outer media are replaced by compact fibrous tissue, whereas the inner media contain excess collagen and ground substance in disorganized smooth muscle cells. It is more commonly found in white women. Surgical treatment has been favored for symptomatic patients with angiographically proven disease. Because of the distal location of FMD lesions in the extracranial ICA, resection and repair are not usually feasible. Instead, graduated luminal dilation under direct vision has been used successfully in patients, with antiplatelet therapy continued postoperatively. Open balloon angioplasty of the ICA has been described, which allows precise fluoroscopic guidance, rather than blind dilation with calibrated metal probes, and back-bleeding after dilation to eliminate cerebral embolization. Distal neuroprotective devices may allow this procedure to be performed completely percutaneously, lessening the threat of cerebral emboli.

12. E. The patient most likely has temporal arteritis, also known as giant cell arteritis. It is a vasculitis of medium and large arteries. The cause is unknown. It tends to affect the aortic arch and its branches, including the ICA and ECA. It tends to affect elderly female patients, with a mean age of 69 years. The most devastating complication associated with temporal arteritis is sudden blindness. As such, rapid treatment is indicated with high-dose corticosteroids, even before the diagnosis is established. Because of ECA involvement, jaw claudication, described as a tiring of the jaw with chewing, is one of the most common symptoms. Diagnosis is established via temporal artery biopsy, with at least a 2-cm segment of artery. Duplex ultrasound scanning has been shown to establish the diagnosis, with a clear halo visible around the temporal artery.

Reference: Schmidt W, Kraft H, Vorpahl K, et al: Color duplex ultrasonography in the diagnosis of temporal arteritis, *N Engl J Med* 337:1336–1341, 1997.

13. D. This patient has Takayasu arteritis. Takayasu arteritis is an inflammatory disease of the aorta and its branches as well as the coronary and pulmonary arteries. It occurs most commonly in young women, with a median age of 25 years. The clinical course has been described as beginning with constitutional symptoms such as fever and malaise; however, a National Institutes of Health study showed that only one third of patients recall such symptoms. Characteristic clinical features include hypertension, retinopathy, aortic regurgitation, cerebrovascular symptoms, angina, congestive heart failure, abdominal pain or gastrointestinal bleeding, pulmonary hypertension, and extremity claudication. The gold standard for diagnosis is arterial imaging, with the demonstration of occlusive disease in the subclavian arteries. Unlike atherosclerosis, which tends to affect the origin of these vessels, Takayasu arteritis affects the mid portions of these arteries. Characteristic signs and symptoms include pulselessness or blood pressure differential in the arms, upper or lower extremity claudication, syncope, amaurosis fugax, blurred vision, and palpitations. Treatment consists of steroid therapy initially with cytotoxic agents used in patients who do not achieve remission. Carotidynia, which is pain along inflamed arteries, is pathognomonic for Takayasu arteritis. Surgical treatment with arterial bypass is only performed in advanced states and in situations in which the patient does not respond to medical therapy. It should ideally be performed when the disease is not active. Because the disease causes transmural arterial inflammation with concentric fibrosis, there is no role for endarterectomy, and angioplasty has not met with good results.

14. D. The diagnosis of blunt carotid injury can be difficult, particularly in the multiply injured trauma patient and in those with head injury. As such, the diagnosis has historically been missed or delayed. With the increasingly liberal use of CT angiography of the neck for trauma, the diagnosis is being made with greater frequency. Blunt carotid injury should be suspected if a trauma patient presents with a lateralizing neurologic deficit such as hemiparesis and is not significantly altered mentally, as would be expected with severe head injury. This would be further confirmed by findings of a head CT scan that are not consistent with the neurologic deficit. The most common mechanisms of blunt carotid injury include motor vehicle accidents, fist fights, hanging, and intraoral trauma. However, it has also been reported with relatively minor trauma, such as after chiropractic manipulation of the neck and forceful sneezing. Findings on an initial CT scan of the head and neck may be negative, but the combination of a neurologic deficit with negative head CT findings should prompt further work-up, including angiography. Angiography may reveal an intimal injury or a dissection, which may lead to luminal occlusion. The occlusion has a flame-shaped appearance angiographically, with complete occlusion typically 2 to 3 cm beyond the bifurcation. Autopsy studies have shown a sharply demarcated transition between the normal carotid artery and the dissected segment. Treatment is with anticoagulation and in most cases results in complete resolution within 1 to 2 months. Recently, there has been increased use of stents in severely symptomatic patients.

Reference: Fabian T, Patton J Jr, Croce M, et al: Blunt carotid injury: importance of early diagnosis and anticoagulant therapy, *Ann Surg* 223:513–525, 1996.

15. C. The patient has symptomatic high-grade carotid stenosis, and, as such, an intervention is indicated. With the history of radiation therapy, the stenosis is likely the result of radiation-induced arterial injury. Radiation primarily affects small vessels in the skin, but can also damage medium-sized vessels. Injury to the vasa vasorum leads to ischemic injury to the media, which results in medial fibrosis. Damage to the endothelium also occurs, and in the process of healing, irregular spindle-shaped cells form clumps. The standard approach to radiation-induced carotid stenosis has been to perform CEA. However, the radiation produces local tissue scarring that makes dissection precarious and significantly increases the risk of cranial nerve injury, as well as wound infection and breakdown. The previous neck dissection results in a paucity of tissue coverage between the skin and the carotid artery. This can lead to the catastrophic complication of carotid blow out. The best alternative in this patient would be to perform carotid stenting with a cerebral protection device.

Reference: Harrod-Kim P, Yasha Kadkhodayan Y, Derdeyn C, et al: Outcomes of carotid angioplasty and stenting for radiation-associated stenosis, *AJNR Am J Neuroradiol* 26:1781–1788, 2005.

16. D. Penetrating carotid injuries are highly associated with concomitant esophageal, cervical spine, and laryngeal injuries. For patients with ongoing hemorrhage, prompt operative exploration is indicated. In the hemodynamically stable patient with penetrating neck trauma, imaging of the carotid artery should be performed. This has typically involved formal arteriography, although more recently CT angiography is being used. The decision to operate on an ICA injury is based on whether the ICA is occluded or patent, the patient's neurologic status, the surgical accessibility of the lesion, and whether the ICA injury is minimal or severe. In patients with a neurologic deficit, operative repair should be undertaken, provided the lesion is surgically accessible. For surgically inaccessible lesions near the base of the skull, endovascular approaches should be considered. Coma is not a contraindication to repair, and although coma is predictive of an increased risk of mortality, coma is not a good predictor of neurologic outcome. For very small intimal injuries, observation is indicated. In general, pseudoaneurysms are less likely to resolve nonoperatively than intimal injuries.

17. D. The best indication for CEA is in patients with ICA stenosis between 70% and 99% and recent (within 120 days) ipsilateral symptoms (nondisabling stroke, hemispheric transient ischemic attack, amaurosis fugax). For patients with moderate symptomatic stenosis (50%–69%), CEA is of less benefit, but it is indicated for hemispheric symptoms. The Asymptomatic Carotid Atherosclerosis Study demonstrated the benefit of CEA compared with aspirin for carotid stenosis between 60% and 99%; however, the benefit is much less than for symptomatic patients. Patients with a completely disabling stroke that results in dense hemiplegia with aphasia have been excluded from CEA trials because the goal of CEA is to prevent further damage to the motor cortex from future stroke. In such patients, there is typically no motor cortex left to protect.

18. B. Local complications are related to injury of adjacent structures that may be encountered during the course of the operation and are quite uncommon. Carotid-to-subclavian artery bypasses use polytetrafluoroethylene or Dacron as the conduit. All synthetic grafts are at risk of infection and occlusion. Exposure of the subclavian artery requires division of the anterior scalene muscle, which places the phrenic nerve at risk of injury, with resultant right diaphragm paralysis. Injury to the vagus nerve may also occur during carotid dissection, leading to hoarseness. The thoracic duct is anatomically located on the left side and therefore least likely to be injured because the surgery is being performed on the right side.

Reference: Vitti M, Thompson B, Read R: Carotid subclavian bypass: a twenty-two year experience, *J Vasc Surg* 20:411–418, 1994.

19. C. Recurrent carotid stenosis can occur after CEA. The risk of more than 50% restenosis is 5.8%, 9.9%, 13.9%, and 23.4% at 1, 3, 5, and 10 years, respectively, although severe (>80%) stenosis develops in only 2.1% of patients. Recurrent carotid stenosis occurring within the first 2 years after CEA is usually secondary to myointimal hyperplasia. This type of stenosis tends to have a benign course, with a low risk of recurrent stroke. In addition, reoperative CEA carries a higher risk of cranial nerve injury (7.3% rate if permanent injury in one series). The patient is asymptomatic. If the patient had a symptomatic recurrence, the best option would be carotid stenting. When the recurrent stenosis develops 2 or more years after CEA, recurrent atherosclerosis is the usual cause.

Reference: Mattos M, Van Bemmelen P, Barkmeier J: Routine surveillance after carotid endarterectomy: does it affect clinical management? *J Vasc Surg* 17:819–830, 1993.

20. B. Postoperative cranial nerve dysfunction is reported in approximately 10% of patients after CEA, although the majority of injuries are transient and resolve within a few weeks. Cranial nerve damage may result from nerve transection, excessive nerve traction, or perineural disruption. Common cranial nerve injuries include injury to the vagus or recurrent laryngeal nerve (5%–7%) causing hoarseness, the hypoglossal nerve (4%–6%) causing ipsilateral tongue deviation, and superior laryngeal nerve (1%–3%) causing easy voice fatigability. Less common is injury to the marginal mandibular nerve (1%–3%), which results in drooping of the nasolabial fold ipsilateral to the injury, and the glossopharyngeal nerve, which affects the ability to swallow foods.

Reference: Evans W, Mendelowitz D, Liapis C, et al: Motor speech deficit following carotid endarterectomy, *Ann Surg* 196:461–464, 1982.

21. D. This represents an ICA dissection, which may occur either spontaneously or after trauma. Cervical artery dissection is a significant cause of stroke in patients younger than 40 years. Common presenting symptoms of ICA dissection are headache, transient ischemic attack and/or stroke, and Horner syndrome. Risk factors for dissection include history of infection (syphilis), smoking, Ehlers-Danlos syndrome type IV, cystic medial necrosis, FMD, Marfan syndrome, family history, oral contraceptives, and atherosclerosis. The diagnosis is made by angiography. Angiographic studies suggest that the most likely mechanism of acute dissection is an intimal tear followed by an acute intimal dissection, which produces luminal occlusion due to secondary thrombosis. The occlusion angiographically has a flame-shaped appearance, with complete occlusion typically 2 to 3 cm beyond the bifurcation. Autopsy studies have shown a sharply demarcated transition between the normal carotid artery and the dissected segment. Treatment is with anticoagulation and, in most cases, results in complete resolution within 1 to 2 months. Recently, there has been increasing use of stenting in severely symptomatic patients.

22. C. Atherosclerosis is the most common pathology affecting the carotid artery bifurcation. The tendency for atherosclerotic plaque to occur at the carotid bifurcation is related vessel geometry, velocity profile, and shear stress. It has been demonstrated that plaque formation at the carotid artery bifurcation is increased in areas of low flow velocity and low shear stress and decreased in areas of high flow velocity and elevated shear stress. Atherosclerosis tends to occur along the outer or lateral aspect of the proximal ICA and carotid bulb. This zone corresponds to areas of low velocity and low shear stress. Conversely, the medial or inner aspect of the carotid bulb, which is associated with high blood flow velocity and high shear stress, is generally free of plaque formation.

23. A. Cerebral artery aneurysms (also known as berry or saccular aneurysms) typically develop at vessel bifurcations, where defects in the media are common, and have been postulated to arise from degenerative changes in the wall of the vessel. Berry aneurysms can occur anywhere along the arterial circle of Willis, but they are most common in the anterior circulation: at the junction of the posterior communicating artery and the ICA, at the junction of the anterior communicating artery and anterior cerebral artery, or at the first major branch of the middle cerebral artery. In the posterior circulation, the most common location is at the terminal bifurcation of the basilar artery. The primary concern is rupture, and approximately 10% to 15% of patients in whom rupture occurs die before reaching the hospital. However, rupture is uncommon. Incidentally discovered aneurysms have a very low risk of bleeding, although that depends on the aneurysm size. The yearly risk is approximately 0.05% to 0.5% for aneurysms smaller than 10 mm in diameter. The International Study of Unruptured Intracranial Aneurysms indicated that the risk of morbidity and mortality related to surgery greatly exceeded the 7.5-year risk of rupture among patients with unruptured intracranial aneurysms smaller than 10 mm in diameter. Thus, the recommendation is to observe aneurysms less than 10 mm. For aneurysms greater than 10 mm, the risk of rupture is 1% to 2% per year and is 6% per year for aneurysms greater than 25 mm. For large or symptomatic aneurysms (with evidence of subarachnoid hemorrhage), there are two options for aneurysm exclusion, either craniotomy with clipping or endovascular coiling. Thus, in this case, the aneurysm should be left untreated, and CEA should be performed in the patient.

References: International Study of Unruptured Intracranial Aneurysms Investigators: Unruptured intracranial aneurysms—risk of rupture and risks of surgical intervention, *N Engl J Med* 339: 1725–1733, 1998.

Lin PH, Kougias P, Bechara C, et al: Arterial disease. In Brunicardi FC, Andersen DK, Billiar TR, et al: *Schwartz's principles of surgery*, ed 9, New York, 2010, McGraw-Hill, pp 701–775.

Riles TS, Rockman CB: Cerebrovascular disease. In Townsend CM Jr, Beauchamp RD, Evers BM, Mattox KL, editors: *Sabiston textbook of surgery: the biological basis of modern surgical practice*, ed 18, Philadelphia, 2008, WB Saunders, pp 1882–1906.

Colon 9

1. A 10-year old boy with acute myelogenous leukemia presents with right lower quadrant abdominal pain and tenderness. He recently completed chemotherapy. His temperature is 102°F and white blood cell (WBC) count is 1.9×10^3 cells/μL. A computed tomography (CT) scan reveals inflammation and thickening of the right colon and stranding in the adjacent fat. Management consists of:
   A. IV antibiotics alone
   B. Right hemicolectomy with primary ileotransverse colostomy
   C. Right hemicolectomy with ileostomy and mucus fistula
   D. Cecostomy
   E. Appendectomy

2. A 65-year-old woman presents with a massive lower gastrointestinal (GI) bleed. Her initial blood pressure in the emergency department is 80/60 mm Hg, with a heart rate of 120 beats per minute. After volume resuscitation, the blood pressure increases to 120/80 mm Hg. A nasogastric aspirate is negative for blood. The next step in the management is:
   A. Colonoscopy
   B. Mesenteric arteriography
   C. Tagged red cell scan
   D. Proctoscopy
   E. Exploratory laparotomy

3. A 65-year-old institutionalized patient presents with a 2-day history of abdominal distention, nausea, and obstipation. Physical examination is significant for marked distention with mild diffuse abdominal tenderness, no guarding, and no rebound. The WBC count is 10,000 cells/μL. Plain films reveal a massively dilated, inverted U-shaped (omega sign) loop of bowel. Management should consist of:
   A. Endoscopic detorsion
   B. Endoscopic detorsion followed by elective sigmoid colectomy
   C. Endoscopic detorsion followed by elective sigmoid colectomy if a recurrence
   D. Exploratory laparotomy with sigmoid colectomy, on-table lavage, and primary anastomosis
   E. Exploratory laparotomy with sigmoid colectomy, proximal colostomy, and oversew rectal stump

4. A 75-year-old woman presents with mild diffuse abdominal pain and diarrhea that is guaiac positive. Her medical history is negative. Her WBC count is normal, as is her hematocrit. A CT scan shows mild thickening of the colonic wall at the splenic flexure with some associated pericolic fat stranding. Management consists of:
   A. Diagnostic laparoscopy
   B. Exploratory laparotomy
   C. Intravenous (IV) antibiotics and fluid hydration
   D. Colonoscopy
   E. Mesenteric angiography

5. Which of the following is true about colonic physiology?
   A. The colon absorbs as much as 500 mL/day of water.
   B. Sodium is absorbed actively via Na^+,K^+-ATPase.
   C. Ammonia reabsorption is unaffected by luminal pH.
   D. Chloride is secreted.
   E. It produces no nutrients.

6. A 50-year-old woman presents with rectal pain, incomplete rectal voiding, and bright red blood and mucus per rectum. Colonoscopy reveals a solitary rectal ulcer in the distal rectum on the anterior wall. A biopsy specimen of the ulcer shows chronic inflammation. Management consists of:

   A. Transanal excision of the ulcer
   B. Perineal rectosigmoidectomy
   C. Abdominal rectopexy
   D. High-fiber diet and defecation training
   E. Rectal fixation with prosthetic sling

7. The most common site of involvement by Crohn disease is:

   A. Rectum
   B. Colon
   C. Jejunum
   D. Terminal ileum
   E. Duodenum

8. The most common perianal lesion in Crohn disease is:

   A. Fissures
   B. Skin tags
   C. Perianal abscess
   D. Perianal fistulas
   E. Hemorrhoids

9. A 35-year-old patient with a history of ulcerative colitis (UC) undergoes an ileoanal anastomosis with J-pouch reconstruction. Four months later, he presents with a 3-day history of abdominal pain, diarrhea, hematochezia, and fever. All of the following are true regarding this condition EXCEPT:

   A. The patient should undergo endoscopy with biopsies.
   B. The patient may have undiagnosed Crohn disease.
   C. Use of probiotics is helpful.
   D. Urgent excision of the J pouch is often necessary.
   E. Metronidazole and ciprofloxacin are useful to treat this condition.

10. All of the following are true about familial adenomatous polyposis (FAP) EXCEPT:

    A. The gene mutation is located on chromosome 5q.
    B. The risk of colorectal cancer is nearly 100% by age 50.
    C. Patients with the gene mutation should begin screening with flexible sigmoidoscopy at age 20.
    D. Patients are at risk of periampullary carcinoma.
    E. It is associated with desmoid tumors.

11. A 45-year-old woman with a 15-year history of pancolitis from UC undergoes surveillance colonoscopy. No polyps are detected. Random biopsy samples are taken, and final pathology findings reveal high-grade dysplasia from the sigmoid colon region. Recommended management would be:

    A. Repeat colonoscopy in 6 months with additional random biopsies
    B. Sigmoid colectomy
    C. Total colectomy with ileorectal anastomosis
    D. Total proctocolectomy with ileostomy
    E. Restorative proctocolectomy with ileal pouch–anal anastomosis

12. The earliest manifestation of UC is:

    A. Mucosal ulcerations
    B. Mucosal edema
    C. "Lead pipe" colon
    D. Pseudopolyps
    E. Crypt abscesses

13. All of the following are features more consistent with Crohn colitis rather than UC EXCEPT:

    A. Serosal "fat wrapping"
    B. Segmental disease
    C. Perianal disease
    D. Crypt abscesses
    E. Granulomas

14. A 56-year-old man presents with a 2-day history of fever, nausea, and left lower quadrant pain. His WBC count is 14,000 cells/μL. CT shows a thickened sigmoid colon with fat stranding and a 5-cm pelvic abscess. Optimal management of this patient would be:

    A. Immediate sigmoid colectomy, end colostomy, and drainage of abscess
    B. CT-guided drainage followed in 6 weeks by a sigmoid colectomy
    C. CT-guided drainage alone
    D. IV antibiotics followed in 6 weeks by a sigmoid colectomy
    E. IV antibiotics alone

15. Which of the following are true regarding familial juvenile polyposis?

    A. It is autosomal recessive.
    B. The polyps are hamartomas.
    C. The risk of colon cancer is 100% by age 50.
    D. Once a polyp is detected, total proctocolectomy is recommended.
    E. There is no association with upper GI malignancy.

16. All of the following are true regarding colonic polyps EXCEPT:

A. Tubovillous adenomas have a higher malignancy risk than tubular adenomas.

B. Hyperplastic polyps are not premalignant.

C. The polyps in Peutz-Jeghers syndrome are hamartomas.

D. Inflammatory polyps are pseudopolyps.

E. In an adenomatous polyp, the risk of malignancy is unrelated to size.

17. All of the following are true about hereditary nonpolyposis colon cancer (HNPCC) (Lynch syndrome) EXCEPT:

A. It is associated with a high risk of endometrial cancer.

B. It involves mutations in the mismatch repair genes.

C. Screening colonoscopy should begin at age 25.

D. Colonic malignancy has a worse prognosis than does sporadic cancer.

E. Amsterdam criteria are used for the diagnosis.

18. A 69-year-old woman presents with a 2-day history of abdominal distention, fever to 103°F, mild to moderate diffuse abdominal pain, and diarrhea. The patient is midway through completing a 10-day course of oral Bactrim (sulfamethoxazole/trimethoprim) for pyelonephritis. Plain films reveal a distended colon to 7 cm with no evidence of obstruction. All of the following are true about this condition EXCEPT:

A. Oral metronidazole is the treatment of choice.

B. The bacterium produces two exotoxins.

C. Bactrim (sulfamethoxazole/trimethoprim) should be discontinued and IV cephalosporin given to treat the pyelonephritis.

D. Sigmoidoscopy is useful in establishing the diagnosis.

E. This condition may develop with just one previous antibiotic dose.

19. A 38-year-old woman presents with a 1-day history of nausea, vomiting, abdominal distention, and obstipation. She has no history of surgery and no medical problems. The physical examination is significant for distention with a tympanic mass in the left upper quadrant and mild abdominal tenderness. The WBC count is normal. A plain abdominal radiograph reveals a markedly dilated, kidney-shaped loop of bowel with haustral markings that projects from the right lower quadrant to the left upper quadrant. Which of the following is true about this condition?

A. Cecostomy is the surgical treatment of choice.

B. Operative detorsion with cecopexy is indicated.

C. Right hemicolectomy with an ileostomy and mucus fistula will be required.

D. Endoscopic detorsion with a subsequent right hemicolectomy is indicated.

E. The patient will most likely require a right hemicolectomy with primary anastomosis.

20. All of the following are true regarding diverticular diseases of the lower GI tract EXCEPT:

A. They occur most commonly in the sigmoid colon.

B. The rectum is spared.

C. They are pulsion diverticula.

D. They are true diverticula.

E. They are associated with a low-fiber diet.

21. Which of the following is true regarding UC and colon cancer?

A. The risk of colon cancer is unrelated to the extent of the inflammation.

B. The malignancy typically develops in a polyp.

C. Carcinoembryonic antigen levels are useful in guiding when to perform a colonoscopy.

D. The risk of colon cancer is related to disease duration.

E. Random biopsies are ineffective.

22. After a right colectomy for carcinoma of the cecum, a disruption of the ileocolonic anastomosis occurs. A cutaneous fistula through the midline incision develops in the patient. The major cause of mortality in this patient is:

A. Electrolyte depletion

B. Malnutrition

C. Hypovolemia

D. Sepsis

E. Abdominal wall infection near the fistula

23. A 55-year-old man is undergoing a screening colonoscopy. A benign-appearing 1-cm pedunculated polyp is removed from the sigmoid colon. Four hours later, severe left lower quadrant pain develops in the patient. A CT scan reveals free intraperitoneal air, with minimal fat stranding around the sigmoid colon. The situation is best managed by:

    A. Diverting proximal colostomy
    B. Resection of sigmoid colon with an end colostomy and oversew of the rectum
    C. Resection of the sigmoid colon with primary anastomosis
    D. Primary closure of the perforation
    E. Broad-spectrum antibiotics and nasogastric decompression

24. A 65-year-old man presents with a 2-day history of left lower quadrant abdominal pain, nausea, and low-grade fever. On physical examination, his temperature is 100.5°F and WBC count is 14,000 cells/μL. He has localized, moderate left lower quadrant pain without rebound. Which of the following is indicated as the next step in the patient's management?

    A. Nasogastric tube decompression
    B. IV antibiotics
    C. Flexible sigmoidoscopy
    D. Barium enema
    E. Gastrograffin enema

25. All of the following are true regarding chemotherapy for colon carcinoma EXCEPT:

    A. The combination of 5-fluorouracil and leucovorin prolongs survival in stage IV colon cancer.
    B. Erbitux (cetuximab) prolongs survival in stage IV colon cancer.
    C. Avastin (bevacizumab) prolongs survival in stage IV colon cancer.
    D. 5-Fluorouracil and leucovorin prolong survival in patients with stage III colon cancer.
    E. Avastin (bevacizumab) is a monoclonal antibody against vascular endothelial growth factor.

26. A 40-year-old woman with a 10-year history of Crohn pancolitis undergoes colonoscopy. Biopsy samples of the colonic mucosa at the sigmoid reveal severe dysplasia. Management would consist of:

    A. Restorative proctocolectomy with ileal pouch–anal reconstruction
    B. Total proctocolectomy with ileostomy
    C. Sigmoid colectomy
    D. Repeat colonoscopy with biopsy in 3 months
    E. Course of oral steroids

27. An important source of energy for colonocytes is:

    A. Ketone bodies
    B. Glucose
    C. Amino acids
    D. Butyrate
    E. Glutamine

28. A 15-year-old boy presents to a colorectal clinic with a family history of familial polyposis. *APC* gene testing is performed, and the result is positive. Flexible sigmoidoscopy reveals eight polyps in the sigmoid. Colonoscopy reveals no other polyps. Polyps are consistent with adenomatous polyps without evidence of malignancy. Which of the following is the recommended management?

    A. Repeat sigmoidoscopy in 6 months
    B. Cyclooxygenase-2 inhibitors, repeat sigmoidoscopy in 6 months
    C. Total colectomy with ileorectal anastomosis
    D. Total proctocolectomy with continent ileostomy
    E. Restorative proctocolectomy with ileal pouch–anal anastomosis

29. In female patients with a family history of HNPCC, which of the following is recommended beginning at age 25, in addition to screening colonoscopy?

    A. Annual mammography
    B. Annual CT of the abdomen
    C. Annual endometrial aspiration biopsy
    D. Annual ovarian ultrasound scan
    E. Annual right upper quadrant ultrasound scan

30. A 35-year-old man presents with nausea, two episodes of vomiting, abdominal distention, and obstipation. A plain abdominal radiograph reveals a distended, kidney-shaped segment of bowel in the left upper quadrant. Gastrograffin enema demonstrates abrupt cutoff on contrast in the transverse colon. Management would consist of:

    A. Endoscopic decompression
    B. Endoscopic decompression and, if successful, elective right colectomy
    C. Operative detorsion and cecopexy
    D. Right colectomy with ileostomy and mucus fistula
    E. Right colectomy with primary ileotransverse colostomy

31. A solitary rectal ulcer is most frequently associated with:

    A. A bacterial infection
    B. A viral infection
    C. Malignancy
    D. Internal intussusception
    E. Drug reaction

32. The most common cause of colovesical fistula is:

    A. Colon carcinoma
    B. Diverticulitis
    C. Crohn disease
    D. UC
    E. Bladder carcinoma

33. A 75-year-old woman presents to your clinic for follow-up after three episodes of uncomplicated diverticulitis in the past year, each of which required a 5-day hospitalization for IV antibiotics and bowel rest. The patient is a diabetic. Previous CT scans demonstrated inflammation in the sigmoid colon with fat stranding both times. Subsequent colonoscopy revealed diverticula throughout the entire colon from the ascending colon to the sigmoid, but was negative for other pathology. The recommendation would be:

    A. Continue high-fiber diet
    B. Total colectomy with ileoproctostomy
    C. Sigmoid colectomy with distal margin right at the rectosigmoid junction
    D. Left hemicolectomy with transverse colon-to-rectum anastomosis
    E. Sigmoid colectomy with distal margin at the normal rectum

Answers

1. A. In the neutropenic patient with leukemia who presents with acute abdominal pain, one must suspect neutropenic enterocolitis, which is commonly referred to as typhlitis. The typical patient presents with abdominal pain and tenderness, fever, and diarrhea in association with a neutrophil count less than 1000 cells/μL. A CT scan is helpful in ruling out perforation and in the case of typhlitis will show thickening of the cecal wall with pericolic stranding. Some reports have also shown the utility of ultrasonography in establishing the diagnosis via the demonstration of cecal thickening. The majority of patients respond to bowel rest and IV antibiotics. The mortality rate in children in contemporary series is 8% to 10%. Surgery should be reserved for patients with signs of perforation, although the need for surgical intervention is low.

References: Schlatter M, Snyder K, Freyer D: Successful nonoperative management of typhlitis in pediatric oncology patients, *J Pediatr Surg* 37:1151–1155, 2002.

Sloas M, Flynn P, Kaste S, Patrick C: Typhlitis in children with cancer: a 30-year experience, *Clin Infect Dis* 17:484–490, 1993.

2. D. The most common cause of lower GI bleeding, diverticulosis, accounts for more than one half of cases and is usually from right-sided lesions. Rarely, massive lower GI bleeding can be the result of an upper GI source. As such, placing a nasogastric tube and aspirating for blood is an important first step after the ABCs. Likewise, hemorrhoids can rarely be the cause, particularly in patients with portal hypertension. Thus, the next step is to perform a proctoscopy to rule out hemorrhoids. This will avoid the catastrophic situation of performing a total colectomy only to discover that the patient continues to bleed from a more distal source. After the proctoscopy, the management algorithm depends on the patient's response to resuscitation. If the patient stabilizes, she should undergo colonoscopy after a bowel prep. If the patient continues to bleed, mesenteric arteriography should be performed with possible embolization. If the patient cannot be stabilized and the source is not discovered, the patient should be taken to the operating room for an exploratory laparotomy with intraoperative endoscopy. If the source cannot be localized, a total colectomy should be performed.

Reference: Farner R, Lichliter W, Kuhn J, Fisher T: Total colectomy versus limited colonic resection for acute lower gastrointestinal bleeding, *Am J Surg* 178:587–591, 1999.

3. B. This patient has a sigmoid volvulus. The common denominator in sigmoid volvulus is a large, redundant colon. Individuals with chronic constipation (elderly or institutionalized), a high-fiber diet, or megacolon (Chagas disease) are predisposed. Patients present with symptoms and signs of an acute large bowel obstruction. The important issues are the following:

1. Establishing the correct diagnosis. This can generally be done by classic radiographic findings of a markedly dilated colon with a "bent inner tube" appearance or an omega sign.
2. Determining whether the patient already has an ischemic or dead bowel. This can be achieved via evidence of systemic toxicity (laboratory tests) and physical examination (peritonitis), and if these are present, the patient needs a laparotomy and sigmoid colectomy.
3. The value of endoscopic detorsion. This can be performed with either a rigid proctosigmoidoscope or a flexible endoscope.
4. Awareness that there is a high recurrence rate (as high as 40%). Thus, after detorsion, a recommendation should be made for a subsequent semielective colectomy.
5. Distinguishing it from cecal volvulus, which cannot usually be endoscopically detorsed and requires surgery.

Reference: Chung Y, Eu K, Nyam D, et al: Minimizing recurrence after sigmoid volvulus, *Br J Surg* 86:231–233, 1999.

4. C. Ischemic colitis occurs primarily in elderly patients at an average age of 70 years. Unlike acute small bowel ischemia, which develops in association with mesenteric arterial or venous occlusive disease, colonic ischemia is rarely the result of major vascular occlusion. Rather, it usually occurs as a result of a low-flow state, such as severe dehydration. It tends to develop in watershed areas of blood supply, such as the splenic flexure (most common), known as the Griffith's point, where collaterals are present between the superior mesenteric artery and inferior mesenteric artery (specifically, the ascending left colic artery with the Drummond marginal artery); Sudeck's critical point (rectosigmoid junction), where collaterals are present between the sigmoid artery and superior rectal artery; and the ileocecal area. In addition to advanced age, risk factors for ischemic colitis include underlying cardiovascular disease, diabetes, vasculitis, and hypotension. Most cases are mild and result in painless, bloody diarrhea. More severe cases can result in bacterial translocation with fever and leukocytosis or, rarely, full-thickness necrosis with peritonitis. The diagnosis is via a combination of the history and examination, plain films to rule out an acute abdomen and that sometimes will show signs of mucosal edema (thumb printing), and CT scan (nonspecific colonic wall edema and fat stranding). Because the etiology is not typically major occlusive disease, angiography is not helpful. The surgeon needs to be aware that the differential diagnosis includes colon cancer and inflammatory bowel disease. As such, colonoscopy should eventually be performed, although it is not necessary in the acute phase. The exception is ischemic colitis after aortic surgery, in which case the endoscopy assists in the diagnosis, and CT scan findings may be hard to interpret due to postsurgical changes. Most patients are treated medically with bowel rest and broad-spectrum antibiotics. Surgery is reserved for patients who deteriorate and/or have evidence of diffuse peritonitis.

Reference: Balthazar E, Yen B, Gordon R: Ischemic colitis: CT evaluation of 54 cases, *Radiology* 211:381–388, 1999.

5. B. The colon is responsible for a large amount of water and electrolyte reabsorption. Water absorption averages 1 to 2 L per day, but can be as much as 5 L. Sodium is absorbed actively via Na^+,K^+-ATPase with water following passively. Chloride is actively absorbed, not secreted, through a chloride–bicarbonate exchange. Bacteria fermentation in the colon produces short-chain fatty acids, which are a primary source of energy for colonocytes. Decreasing colonic pH results in a decrease in ammonia reassertion (as occurs with lactulose).

6. D. Solitary rectal ulcer syndrome is an uncommon disorder that can be confused with malignancy because the patient presents with rectal bleeding and pain and evidence of straining during bowel movements. It is a benign process caused by an internal intussusception from chronic straining, leading to repetitive trauma to the mucosa. On proctoscopy, nodules or a mass may be found, in which case the term *colitis cystica profunda* is used. Biopsy should be performed to exclude malignancy. The diagnosis of an internal intussusception can be confirmed with anorectal manometry and defecography. Treatment is nonoperative and includes a high-fiber diet, defecation training to avoid straining, and laxatives or enemas. Either abdominal or perineal repair, as for a patient with rectal prolapse, is recommended for failure of medical management.

Reference: Felt-Bersma R, Cuesta M: Rectal prolapse, rectal intussusception, rectocele, and solitary rectal ulcer syndrome, *Gastroenterol Clin North Am* 30:199–222, 2001.

7. D. The terminal ileum and cecum are the most common sites of involvement in Crohn disease. The next most common site is the small bowel, then the colon and rectum. It can also present with perianal disease (fistulas and abscesses).

8. B. The most common perianal lesion in Crohn disease is a skin tag, followed by fissures. Fissures are tears in the anoderm, and most are superficial and in the posterior midline. A deep fissure or one in an unusual location (lateral) should raise concern for Crohn disease. Most patients with anal manifestations will have Crohn disease elsewhere. Perianal involvement is extremely rare with UC.

9. D. Pouchitis is a nonspecific inflammation of the ileal reservoir that can occur after an ileoanal pouch creation or in a continent ileostomy reservoir. Pouchitis can be acute or can become chronic. Symptoms include increased diarrhea, hematochezia, abdominal pain, fever, and malaise. The diagnosis is established via a combination of the history, endoscopic findings, and histology from biopsy samples. It is the most common long-term complication of this procedure, with an incidence as high as 30% to 55%. Endoscopy with biopsy is important to rule out undiagnosed Crohn disease. The cause is unknown; it may be due to fecal stasis within the pouch, but emptying studies do not confirm this. Antibiotics (metronidazole and ciprofloxacin) are the mainstay of therapy, and most patients will respond rapidly to either oral preparations or enemas. Patients with chronic pouchitis may require ongoing suppressive antibiotic therapy. Salicylate and stool enemas have also been used with some success. Reintroduction of normal flora by probiotics has been shown to be useful in chronic cases. Rarely, the pouch requires excision, but this would not be done urgently.

References: Gionchetti P, Amadini C, Rizzello F, et al: Diagnosis and treatment of pouchitis, *Best Pract Res Clin Gastroenterol* 17:75–87, 2003.

Madiba T, Bartolo D: Pouchitis following restorative proctocolectomy for ulcerative colitis: incidence and therapeutic outcome, *J R Coll Surg Edinb* 46:334–337, 2001.

Shen B, Achkar J, Lashner B, et al: A randomized clinical trial of ciprofloxacin and metronidazole to treat acute pouchitis, *Inflamm Bowel Dis* 7:301–305, 2001.

10. C. Familiar adenomatous polyposis (FAP) is a rare autosomal dominant disease that accounts for approximately 1% of colon cancers. It is due to a mutation in the APC tumor suppressor gene on chromosome 5q. Syndromes that are considered variants include attenuated FAP and Gardner syndrome. If unrecognized or untreated, cancer can develop in all patients by age 35 to 40 years, and, in fact, polyps often begin at puberty. They eventually can develop thousands of polyps. As such, first-degree relatives of FAP patients who are APC positive should begin screening at age 10 to 12 years by flexible sigmoidoscopy. Relatives who are APC mutation negative can wait until age 50 for screening. Adenomas can develop throughout the GI tract in FAP patients, and in particular in the duodenum, and patients are at risk of the development of periampullary carcinoma. Therefore, upper endoscopy for surveillance every 1 to 3 years starting at age 25 to 30 years should be recommended. Once the diagnosis of FAP has been made and polyps are developing, treatment is surgical. FAP may also be associated with extraintestinal manifestations such as congenital hypertrophy of the retinal pigment epithelium, desmoid tumors, epidermoid cysts, mandibular osteomas, and central nervous system tumors.

11. E. The risk of the development of colon cancer in patients with UC increases with time. By 20 years, colon cancer will develop in approximately 10% of patients. Thus, surveillance colonoscopy is recommended. Colon cancer develops in UC in the absence of polyps. In addition, areas of dysplasia may not be readily apparent on standard colonoscopy. As such, once a patient has had UC for 8 years, colonoscopic surveillance is recommended. In addition to biopsies of areas of suspicion, random biopsies are recommended because flat dysplasia develops in the patients. The finding of even high-grade dysplasia is an indication for surgery. Some authors recommend surgery even for low-grade flat dysplasia because the risk of malignancy is also significantly increased. Dysplasia in a flat (nonpolypoid) lesion is concerning because it is more difficult to monitor with follow-up screening. The curative operation is a restorative proctocolectomy with an ileal pouch–anal anastomosis. In addition to dysplasia, the indications for colectomy in patients with UC include toxic megacolon, severe lower GI bleeding, and intractable disease that does not respond to medical management.

Reference: Ullman T, Croog V, Harpaz N, et al: Progression of flat low-grade dysplasia to advanced neoplasia in patients with ulcerative colitis, *Gastroenterology* 125:1311–1319, 2003.

12. B. Mucosal edema is the earliest finding on endoscopy. As the disease advances, friable mucosa and ulcerations develop. A "lead pipe" colon is a feature of long-standing UC seen on barium enema and is the result of a loss of haustral markings and shortening of the colon.

13. D. Findings on gross appearance in Crohn colitis that are not characteristic of UC include a thickened mesentery, thickened bowel wall, segmental disease, and "creeping fat" or "fat wrapping." On microscopic examination, Crohn disease is transmural, whereas UC is limited to the mucosa and submucosa. Noncaseating granulomas are a hallmark feature of Crohn disease, whereas crypt abscesses are characteristic of UC.

14. B. Diverticulitis is divided into simple and complicated diverticulitis. Simple diverticulitis is limited to patients with pericolonic inflammation and/or phlegmon. Once there is fluid/pus beyond the confines of the colon, it is considered complicated. Hinchey devised the following staging system: stage I, pericolonic inflammation with pericolic abscess; stage II, retroperitoneal or pelvic abscess; stage III, purulent peritonitis; and stage IV, fecal peritonitis. Stage I is treated with IV antibiotics. Complicated diverticulitis is treated surgically. Patients with small abscesses (<4 cm) can be treated with antibiotics alone initially, followed in several weeks by elective colectomy after colonoscopy to rule out other etiologies. If the abscess is larger than 4 cm, CT-guided drainage is recommended, followed by elective colectomy. In patients with stage III or IV diverticulitis, urgent colectomy with the Hartmann procedure (proximal colostomy and distal oversew of rectal stump) is recommended. Diverticulitis can also lead to a large bowel obstruction or fistula formation, most commonly to the bladder.

Reference: Siewert B, Tye G, Kruskal J, et al: Impact of CT-guided drainage in the treatment of diverticular abscesses: size matters, *Am J Roentgenol* 186:680–686, 2006.

15. B. Familial juvenile polyposis is an autosomal dominant disorder (just like HNPCC, FAP, and Peutz-Jeghers syndrome). It is a completely different entity from FAP. The polyps are hamartomas (also called *juvenile polyps*), not adenomas. However, the hamartomas can degenerate into adenomas and malignancy. Thus, there is a risk of colon cancer, but not to the same degree as with FAP. The lifetime risk is approximately 10% to 38% (vs. 100% for FAP). Because of this risk and because many polyps occur on the right side, colonoscopic (rather than flexible sigmoidoscopic) surveillance is recommended, beginning at approximately 10 to 12 years of age. Unlike FAP, in which the presence of polyps equates with a need for a restorative proctocolectomy, if a polyp is seen, it should be snared and sent to pathology. In most instances, it will be a hamartoma. If adenomatous changes are seen, then a colectomy should be performed, and if the rectum is spared, an ileorectal anastomosis can be done with close surveillance. Approximately 15% to 20% of FAP patients develop stomach or duodenal cancers, so upper endoscopic surveillance is recommended by age 25.

References: Dunlop M: Guidance on gastrointestinal surveillance for hereditary non-polyposis colorectal cancer, familial adenomatous polyposis, juvenile polyposis, and Peutz-Jeghers syndrome, *Gut* 51(Suppl 5):v21–v27, 2002.

Howe J, Mitros F, Summers R: The risk of gastrointestinal carcinoma in familial juvenile polyposis, *Ann Surg Oncol* 5:751–756, 1998.

16. E. Adenomatous polyps are considered neoplastic and are divided into three types: tubular (<5% risk of malignancy), tubulovillous (20% risk of malignancy), and villous (40% risk of malignancy). Polyp size is also an important determinant, with polyps smaller than 1 cm having an extremely low risk of malignancy versus a nearly 50% risk of malignancy in polyps larger than 2 cm. Most colon cancers develop from adenomatous polyps. Peutz-Jeghers syndrome is characterized by hamartomatous polyps. They present with GI bleeding and intussusception. Although hamartomatous polyps are not considered premalignant, they can degenerate into adenomatous polyps, so there is a risk of malignancy. The polyps in Peutz-Jeghers syndrome occur primarily in the small intestine, but can also occur in the colon and rectum. Patients have melanin spots on the buccal mucosa and lips. Because of the diffuse nature of polyps throughout the GI tract, surgery is only indicated if there is evidence of obstruction or bleeding or evidence that a polyp has undergone adenomatous change. Inflammatory polyps or pseudopolyps are islands of regenerating mucosa seen most often in inflammatory bowel disease. Hyperplastic polyps are not considered premalignant.

17. D. Lynch syndrome or HNPCC arises due to errors in the mismatch repair genes. It is an autosomal dominant syndrome with an increased risk of colorectal carcinoma as well as other malignancies, with a lifetime risk of approximately 80% for colon cancer, 20% for gastric cancer, and a high risk of endometrial cancer. The colon cancers are more commonly right sided (as opposed to left sided in sporadic cancer); as such, screening requires colonoscopy, which is recommended at age 25 or 5 years less than the age at which colon cancer developed in other family members (whichever is earlier). Upper endoscopy screening is also recommended starting at age 50. Interestingly, DNA mismatch repair colon cancers have a better prognosis than sporadic colon cancer regardless of stage. The Amsterdam criteria for clinical diagnosis of HNPCC are three or more family members with colon cancer or two or more family members with colon cancer and one with endometrial cancer. One member must have had colon cancer diagnosed before age 50, and one must be a first-degree relative of the other two.

References: Stigliano V, Assisi D, Cosimelli M, et al: Survival of hereditary non-polyposis colorectal cancer patients compared with sporadic colorectal cancer patients, *J Exp Clin Cancer Res* 27:39, 2008.

Watson P, Lin K, Rodriguez-Bigas M, et al: Colorectal carcinoma survival among hereditary nonpolyposis colorectal carcinoma family members, *Cancer* 83:259–266, 1998.

18. C. Pseudomembranous colitis is predominantly due to *Clostridium difficile*. It is thought to be due to antibiotic administration leading to the elimination of healthy bacteria in the gut and a subsequent overgrowth of *C. difficile*. The antibiotic most commonly implicated is clindamycin, but it can occur with any antibiotic, even after just one dose, and as late as 4 to 5 weeks later. *C. difficile* produces at least two toxins, toxin A and toxin B, which can be detected in the stool. On occasion, the stool toxin test result will be negative. If suspicion for pseudomembranous colitis is high, the patient should undergo sigmoidoscopy to look for the classic yellow plaques called *pseudomembranes*. Pseudomembranous colitis can progress to life-threatening toxic megacolon, which requires emergent total colectomy. Treatment involves immediately discontinuing all antibiotics and instituting oral metronidazole. Oral vancomycin is considered the next drug of choice.

Reference: Hurley B, Nguyen C: The spectrum of pseudomembranous enterocolitis and antibiotic-associated diarrhea, *Arch Intern Med* 162:2177–2184, 2002.

19. E. Cecal or cecocolic volvulus is much less common than sigmoid volvulus. It occurs in younger patients. It is thought to be due to a lack of fixation of the cecum to the retroperitoneum, and as such, the terminal ileum, cecum, and ascending colon twist and can become ischemic. It can sometimes be hard to diagnose radiographically because the patient will often also demonstrate dilated loops of small bowel with air–fluid levels, giving the appearance of a small bowel obstruction. Unlike sigmoid volvulus, endoscopic decompression for cecal volvulus is very difficult. The treatment of choice is to perform a right hemicolectomy with primary anastomosis (despite no bowel preparation). There is a high recurrence rate after operative detorsion and cecopexy. If the right colon is already gangrenous, right hemicolectomy with ileostomy and mucus fistula is the treatment of choice. However, this patient's presentation makes this finding unlikely.

20. D. Diverticular disease is thought to occur due to a low-fiber diet. The diverticula are considered false because they are composed of only mucosa and submucosa. They occur at points of weakness at points between the taeniae coli where blood vessels penetrate the colonic wall. They occur most commonly on the mesenteric side of the antimesenteric taenia. They occur due to increased intraluminal pressure so they are considered pulsion diverticula. Because the taeniae splay out at the rectum, diverticula do not develop in the rectum.

21. D. The association between UC and the development of colon cancer is well known. The risk of colon cancer in these patients has been shown to be related to the extent (pancolitis higher risk) and duration of the inflammation (2% risk at 10 years, 8% risk at 20 years, 18% risk at 30 years), although not related to the intensity of inflammation. The American Society for Gastrointestinal Endoscopy guidelines for cancer screening in patients with UC take into account the extent and duration of the disease. Surveillance at 7 years is recommended for pancolitis and at 10 years if disease is confined to the left colon. Surveillance consists of a full colonoscopy with random segmental biopsies (at least 32 biopsies) because malignancies often develop in flat lesions. If no dysplasia is found, colonoscopy should be performed every 1 to 3 years. If dysplasia is found, the patient should undergo proctocolectomy, particularly if it is high grade, although many surgeons recommend the same management for low-grade flat dysplasia. Carcinoembryonic antigen is a glycoprotein that is not useful in guiding preoperative surveillance. It is not specific and may be elevated in patients with active bowel inflammation without cancer.

Reference: Eaden J, Abrams K, Mayberry J: The risk of colorectal cancer in ulcerative colitis: a meta-analysis, *Gut* 48:526–535, 2001.

22. D. The major source of mortality of fistulas is sepsis. With more distal fistulas such as this one, volume depletion is not as much of a concern.

23. D. In determining management of this case, one must consider the indications for the colonoscopy, the timing of the perforation, and the intraoperative findings. Because the polyp is pedunculated and benign appearing, one can presume that it has been completely removed and that further colon resection is not needed. The vast majority of colonic injuries, whether iatrogenic or from penetrating trauma, can be repaired primarily. Furthermore, this patient has presumably undergone a bowel prep, so the bacterial load is decreased. Resection with colostomy would be reserved for patients with long-standing perforation and diffuse fecal contamination.

24. B. The next step in the management should be institution of broad-spectrum antibiotics. The diagnosis of diverticulitis can be made clinically. Endoscopy in the acute setting is contraindicated because it would risk causing a perforation. Gastrograffin enema is typically not necessary, and barium enema would also be contraindicated due to the risk of causing barium peritonitis. After hydration and the institution of broad-spectrum antibiotics, CT scanning is generally recommended to confirm the diagnosis and rule out an abscess.

25. A. Current guidelines indicate that stage I (node negative, invades submucosa) colon cancer does not need chemotherapy. The role of chemotherapy in stage II (node negative, invades subserosa or direct invasion of adjacent organ) colon cancer remains debatable. The combination of 5-fluorouracil and leucovorin prolongs survival in stage III colon cancer (positive lymph nodes, no distant metastasis). Until recently, there was no effective chemotherapy for stage IV cancers. Two recent drugs have been approved for stage IV colon cancer. They have been shown to prolong life, but not cure this advanced-stage cancer, and are very costly. Erbitux (cetuximab) is a monoclonal antibody that targets epidermal growth factor receptor. Avastin (bevacizumab) is a monoclonal antibody against vascular endothelial growth factor A.

26. B. Both Crohn disease and UC predispose to colon cancer, particularly in the presence of pancolitis. Thus, surveillance colonoscopy with random biopsies is recommended for both. The finding of severe dysplasia would warrant surgery. However, in patients with Crohn disease, the creation of an ileal pouch–anal reconstruction is not recommended because of the risk of the development of Crohn disease within the pouch and the high risk of perianal complications, including fistula, abscess, stricture, pouch dysfunction, and pouch failure.

27. D. Short-chain fatty acids (acetate, butyrate, and propionate) are produced by bacterial fermentation of dietary carbohydrates. Short-chain fatty acids are an important source of energy for the colonic mucosa. The energy is used by colonocytes for processes such as active transport of sodium. The lack of a dietary source for production of short-chain fatty acids or the diversion of the fecal stream by an ileostomy or colostomy may result in mucosal atrophy, which is referred to as diversion colitis.

28. E. In a patient who tests positive for the APC gene, screening via sigmoidoscopy is recommended starting at age 10 to 12 years. Once polyps are detected, the recommendation is to remove the entire colon and rectum. Cyclooxygenase-2 inhibitors were shown to slow the growth of polyps in patients with FAP in a randomized study, but recent studies indicated that these drugs increased the risk of death from cardiovascular events. The best option is a restorative proctocolectomy with an ileal pouch–anal anastomosis. Total abdominal colectomy with ileorectal anastomosis is another option but requires careful lifelong surveillance of the rectal mucosa for polyps.

29. C. Patients with a family history of HNPCC should be screened for colon cancer, upper GI tract cancer, and endometrial cancer. Screening colonoscopy is recommended annually for at-risk patients beginning either at age 20 to 25 years or 10 years younger than the youngest age at diagnosis in the family, whichever comes first. Screening with upper endoscopy in families with a history of gastric cancer should begin at age 50. Transvaginal ultrasound scanning or endometrial aspiration biopsy is also recommended annually after age 25 to 35 years. Prophylactic hysterectomy and bilateral salpingo-oophorectomy should be considered in women who have completed child-bearing.

30. D. Cecal volvulus results from nonfixation of the right colon. Rotation occurs around the ileocolic blood vessels, and vascular impairment occurs early. Plain radiographs of the abdomen show a characteristic kidney-shaped, air-filled structure in the left upper quadrant (opposite the site of obstruction), and a gastrograffin enema confirms obstruction at the level of the volvulus. Unlike sigmoid volvulus, cecal volvulus can almost never be detorsed endoscopically. Moreover, because vascular compromise occurs early in the course of cecal volvulus, surgical exploration is necessary when the diagnosis is made. Right hemicolectomy with a primary ileocolic anastomosis can usually be performed safely and prevents recurrence. Simple detorsion or detorsion with cecopexy is associated with a high rate of recurrence.

31. D. Solitary rectal ulcer syndrome is thought to be due to an internal intussusception of the rectum brought on by chronic straining during bowel movements. On gross endoscopic inspection, it can be confused with malignancy, and biopsy is essential. Treatment is a high-fiber diet and defecation training to avoid straining.

32. B. The most common cause of colovesical fistulas is diverticulitis. Other causes include Crohn disease, radiation therapy, and colon and bladder cancer. The key elements include establishing the diagnosis and ruling out other causes. CT scanning is the best initial study because it will confirm the presence of a fistula by demonstrating air in the bladder and any associated masses. Sigmoidoscopy is useful to rule out any other mucosal abnormalities. A contrast enema may help to define the course of the fistula, but small fistulas may be missed. Surgical management depends on whether the fistula is due to benign or malignant disease. If it is secondary to diverticulitis, management consists of sigmoid colectomy with repair of the bladder. If it is due to a malignancy, en bloc resection of part of the bladder wall should be performed.

Reference: Walker KG, Anderson JH, Iskander N, et al: Colonic resection for colovesical fistula: 5-year follow-up, *Colorectal Dis* 4:270–274, 2002.

33. E. After one episode of uncomplicated diverticulitis, the recommendation is to treat the patient conservatively with a high-fiber diet because the risk of recurrence is less than 25%; after the second attack, the risk increases to 50%, so the standard of care that most surgeons recommend is elective colon resection after two episodes. More recently, studies indicate that the risk of recurrent diverticulitis is much lower, and surgery for uncomplicated diverticulitis

can be safely delayed until the third or fourth episode, provided the patient is not immunocompromised. However, a lower threshold for surgery is recommended for diabetic patients and in immunocompromised (taking steroids) patients. In a patient who is diabetic and with three episodes of diverticulitis in a relatively short time span, surgery would be recommended. One of the principles of surgery for diverticulitis is that one only needs to resect inflamed, thickened colon, despite the presence of diffuse diverticula. Recurrence is primarily the result of an inadequate distal resection, which inadvertently may leave behind sigmoid diverticula. Because diverticula do not occur in the rectum, the distal resection margin should be taken at normal-appearing rectum. The rectum can be identified by the fact that the taenia splay out.

References: Bullard Dunn KM, Rothenberger DA: Colon, rectum and anus. In Brunicardi FC, Andersen DK, Billiar TR, et al: *Schwartz's principles of surgery*, ed 9, New York, 2010, McGraw-Hill, pp 1013–1072.

Chapman J, Davies M, Wolff B, et al: Complicated diverticulitis: is it time to rethink the rules? *Ann Surg* 242:576–581, 2005.

Fry RD, Mahmoud N, Maron DJ, et al: Colon and rectum. In Townsend CM Jr, Beauchamp RD, Evers BM, Mattox KL, editors: *Sabiston textbook of surgery: the biological basis of modern surgical practice*, ed 18, Philadelphia, 2008, WB Saunders, pp 1348–1432.

Janes S, Meagher A, Frizelle F: Elective surgery after acute diverticulitis, *Br J Surg* 92:133–142, 2005.

Salem L, Veenstra D, Sullivan S, Flum DR: The timing of elective colectomy in diverticulitis: a decision analysis, *J Am Coll Surg* 199:904–912, 2004.

Critical Care 10

1. Which of the following is an appropriate definition of shock?

    A. Low blood pressure
    B. Low cardiac output
    C. Low circulating volumes
    D. Inadequate tissue perfusion
    E. Abnormal vascular resistance

2. Mean pulmonary occlusion (wedge) pressure is an indicator of:

    A. Cardiac output
    B. Pulmonary arterial pressure
    C. Left atrial pressure
    D. Pulmonary compliance
    E. Systemic vascular resistance (SVR)

3. After application of positive end-expiratory pressure (PEEP) to 8 cm H_2O, which of the following parameters is likely to increase?

    A. Arterial partial pressure of carbon dioxide (Pa_{CO_2})
    B. Cardiac output
    C. Functional residual capacity
    D. Left ventricular end-systolic volume
    E. Pulmonary edema

4. After surgical drainage of a leaking anastomosis from an esophagogastrectomy, an intubated 60-year-old man was returned to the intensive care unit. Hemodynamic data showed:

Blood pressure	90/60 mm Hg
Heart rate	120/min
Central venous pressure	10 mm Hg
Pulmonary artery pressure	40/14 mm Hg
Pulmonary wedge pressure	8 mm Hg
Cardiac output	10.0 L/min

    His SVR is:

    A. 200 dynes/sec $\times$ cm^{-5}
    B. 360 dynes/sec $\times$ cm^{-5}
    C. 480 dynes/sec $\times$ cm^{-5}
    D. 960 dynes/sec $\times$ cm^{-5}
    E. 1200 dynes/sec $\times$ cm^{-5}

5. Oxygen delivery can be increased by increasing all of the following EXCEPT:

    A. Hemoglobin
    B. Atmospheric pressure
    C. Cardiac output
    D. Inspired oxygen concentration
    E. Oxygen extraction

6. Blood samples for the determination of mixed venous oxygen saturation (Sv_{O_2}) are obtained from:

    A. Right atrium
    B. Pulmonary artery
    C. Pulmonary vein
    D. Two peripheral veins mixed together
    E. Central venous pressure line

7. Which of the following is not a characteristic of acute pulmonary embolism?

A. Heart rate	110/min
B. Blood pressure	90/60 mm Hg
C. Pa_{O_2}	50 mm Hg
D. Pulmonary artery pressure	50/30 mm Hg
E. PCWP	25 mm Hg

8. A 75-year-old man becomes hypotensive (systolic blood pressure of 80 mm Hg) after repair of an inguinal hernia. Urine output is low, and he is unresponsive to fluid administration, although the systolic blood pressure increases to 100 mm Hg. A pulmonary artery catheter is inserted. Cardiac output is 3 L/min; SVR is 2140 dynes/sec $\times$ cm^{-5}; Svo$_2$ is 55%; pulmonary capillary wedge pressure (PCWP) is 24 mm Hg. The next step in treating this patient is:

   A. 500 mL of Ringer's lactate to improve preload
   B. Lasix (furosemide) 20 mg intravenously to improve urine output
   C. Nitroprusside at 0.5 μg/kg/L/min to decrease the SVR
   D. Dobutamine at 5 μg/kg/L/min for inotropic support
   E. Neo-Synephrine (phenylephrine) at 1 μg/L/min to increase blood pressure

9. Each of the following is characteristic of the adult respiratory distress syndrome EXCEPT:

   A. Bilateral pleural infiltrates
   B. Decreased functional residual capacity
   C. Increased plasma thromboxane
   D. Increased pulmonary vascular resistance
   E. PCWP < 20 mm Hg

10. Nosocomial pneumonia among intensive care unit patients:

   A. Has the same mortality rate as does community-acquired pneumonia
   B. Is the most common nosocomial infection
   C. Can be avoided by early tracheostomy
   D. Is directly related to the duration of intubation
   E. Can be prevented by early institution of prophylactic antibiotics

11. In the management of hemorrhagic shock, the best clinical sign of successful fluid resuscitation is:

   A. An increase in blood pressure
   B. An increase in urine output
   C. An increase in arterial oxygenation
   D. A decrease in thirst
   E. A decrease in tachycardia

12. A 50-year-old woman who is septic from cholangitis is transferred to the surgical intensive care unit. She undergoes cholecystectomy and common bile duct exploration after a failed endoscopic sphincterotomy. Because of hypotension and marginal urine output, a Swan-Ganz catheter is placed. Which of the following readings is least consistent with the patient's clinical course?

   A. Central venous pressure 5 cm H$_2$O
   B. SVR 300 dynes/sec $\times$ cm^{-5}
   C. Cardiac index 2.0 L/min/cm^2
   D. Pulmonary capillary wedge pressure 10 cm H$_2$O
   E. Svo$_2$ 86%

13. A 21-year-old man who was the driver in a head-on collision has a pulse of 140 beats per minute, respiratory rate of 36 breaths per minute, and blood pressure of 70 mm Hg palpable. His trachea is deviated to the left, with palpable subcutaneous emphysema and poor breath sounds in the right hemithorax. The most appropriate initial treatment would be:

   A. Immediate thoracotomy
   B. Catheter insertion in the subclavian vein for fluid resuscitation
   C. Intubation and ventilation
   D. Tube thoracostomy
   E. Immediate tracheostomy

14. A 68-year-old (70-kg) male nursing home resident is admitted with cellulitis and dry gangrene of his great toe. His mental status is altered. His vital signs demonstrate orthostatic hypotension. Laboratory studies reveal a serum sodium level of 168 mEq/L, a serum potassium level of 4.0 mEq/L, a serum chloride level of 118 mEq/L, an HCO$_3$ level of 28 mEq/L, a blood urea nitrogen (BUN) of 30 mg/dL, and a serum creatinine level of 1.6 mg/dL. His free water deficit is:

   A. 3 L and all of it should be replaced over the next 12 hours
   B. 4 L and all of it should be replaced over the next 24 hours
   C. 5 L and 2.2 L should be replaced over the next 24 hours
   D. 6 L and 3.0 L should be replaced over the next 24 hours
   E. 7 L and 3.7 L should be replaced over the next 24 hours

15. Which of the following electrocardiographic changes is least likely to occur with hypokalemia?

    A. ST-T segment depression
    B. T-wave inversion
    C. Second- or third-degree atrioventricular block
    D. Premature ventricular complexes
    E. U waves

16. A 42-year-old woman with metastatic breast cancer is lethargic and has mental status changes. Her serum calcium is 20 mg/dL, serum alkaline phosphatase is 2000 IU/L, BUN is 42 mg/dL, and serum creatinine is 1.1 mg/dL. Immediate treatment of her acute hypercalcemia should include intravenous (IV) saline, calcitonin, and:

    A. Mithramycin
    B. Bisphosphonates
    C. Loop diuretics
    D. Gallium nitrate
    E. Glucocorticoids

17. Worsening mental status develops in a 65-year-old man. The patient is postoperative day 2 after an elective transurethral resection of the prostate. He was otherwise in good health and taking no medications. On admission, laboratory data, including a complete blood count, electrolytes, BUN, and creatinine, were within normal ranges. On the first postoperative day, the patient reported headache and nausea. Symptoms progressed, and the patient is now lethargic. On examination, the patient is afebrile, his blood pressure is 150/90 mm Hg, his heart rate is 90 beats per minute, and his respiratory rate is 15 breaths per minute. He is stuporous and unable to follow commands, and he withdraws all four extremities to pain. The patient subsequently experiences a generalized tonic-clonic seizure. Laboratory examination shows a normal complete blood count, a serum sodium level of 114 mEq/L, a serum potassium level of 3.8 mEq/L, a serum chloride level of 78 mEq/L, an HCO_3 level of 20 mEq/L, a BUN of 18 mg/dL, and a serum creatinine level of 1.2 mg/L/dL. Which treatment is most appropriate at this time?

    A. Free water restriction
    B. Isotonic saline
    C. Hypertonic saline
    D. Furosemide
    E. Ringer's lactate

18. Hypophosphatemia increases the risk of the development of each of the following EXCEPT:

    A. Respiratory failure
    B. Tissue anoxia due to decreased hemoglobin
    C. Encephalopathy
    D. Hypothyroidism
    E. Hemolysis

19. After being resuscitated from cardiopulmonary arrest, a 63-year-old man is restless and ataxic and has tonic spasms. Serum osmolality is 330 mOsm/kg. The most likely diagnosis is:

    A. Hyponatremia
    B. Hypercalcemia
    C. Hyperkalemia
    D. Hypernatremia
    E. Hypokalemia

20. Seizures and coma developed in a patient several days postoperatively after removal of a brain tumor and placement of a ventriculostomy for decompression of hydrocephalus. Laboratory values include a serum sodium level of 112 mmol/L, a serum potassium level of 4.1 mmol/L, a serum chloride level of 80 mmol/L, an HCO_3 level of 26 mmol/L, a BUN of 28 mg/dL, and a serum creatinine level of 1.0 mg/dL. Ventilator settings are FIO_2 (fraction of inspired oxygen) of 0.6, PEEP of 12 cm H_2O, and pressure control of 35 cm H_2O. The patient lost 10% of his body weight postoperatively. Urine output is 3 to 4 mL/kg/hr and urine sodium is measured at 170 mmol/L. Results of a urinalysis are normal. Vital signs reveal a heart rate of 112 beats per minute, blood pressure of 110/170 mm Hg, respiration rate of 14 breaths per minute (on ventilator), and temperature of 98°F. Which one of the following is the most likely diagnosis?

    A. Diabetes insipidus
    B. Syndrome of inappropriate antidiuretic hormone (SIADH)
    C. Iatrogenic intoxication
    D. Cerebral salt-wasting syndrome
    E. High-output renal failure

21. A 25-year-old man with insulin-dependent diabetes mellitus is admitted to the intensive care unit with severe hyperglycemia. He has a 1-day history of nausea, vomiting, and diarrhea, and he withheld insulin because of poor oral intake. His blood pressure is 100/60 mm Hg, his heart rate is 104 beats per minute, his respiratory rate is 28 breaths per minute, and his temperature is 99°F. Physical examination reveals dry mucous membranes and mild diffuse abdominal tenderness. Laboratory testing reveals a serum sodium level of 135 mmol/L, a serum potassium level of 3.5 mmol/L, a serum chloride level of 110 mmol/L, a CO_2 of 8 mmol/L, a BUN of 22 mg/dL, a serum creatinine level of 1.2 mg/dL, a serum albumin level of 4.1 g/dL, and a serum glucose level of 350 mg/dL. Arterial blood gas shows FIO_2 of 0.21, pH of 7.25, $PaCO_2$ of 20 Torr, and PaO_2 of 95 Torr. Serum ketones are present at a 1:8 dilution. Which one of the following is the best explanation for the acid-base abnormality in this patient?

    A. Diabetic ketoacidosis
    B. Diabetic ketoacidosis with hyperventilation
    C. Diabetic ketoacidosis and diarrhea
    D. Diabetic ketoacidosis and nausea/vomiting
    E. Laboratory error

22. Which one of the following findings is most likely to be present in a patient with severe magnesium deficiency?

    A. Respiratory depression
    B. Bradycardia
    C. Tetany
    D. Hypotension
    E. Loss of patellar reflex

23. A 54-year-old man who weighs 100 lb comes to the emergency department after vomiting for 3 days and losing 10 lb. His serum electrolytes are as follows: sodium 136 mEq/L, potassium 3.1 mEq/L, chloride 88 mEq/L, and carbon dioxide 37 mEq/L. Which one of the following would be most helpful in determining the cause of his acid-base disorder?

    A. Urine sodium
    B. Urine creatinine
    C. Urine chloride
    D. Urine pH
    E. Urine potassium

24. Which of the following is often associated with early sepsis?

    A. Normal acid-base balance
    B. Metabolic alkalosis
    C. Metabolic acidosis
    D. Respiratory alkalosis
    E. Respiratory acidosis

25. All of the following are true regarding tumor lysis syndrome EXCEPT:

    A. It is associated with renal failure.
    B. Associated hypocalcemia should be aggressively treated.
    C. It is typically seen with poorly differentiated lymphomas.
    D. It usually follows chemotherapy.
    E. It may develop after radiation therapy.

26. Prolonged QT intervals are seen in association with:

    A. Hypomagnesemia
    B. Hypercalcemia
    C. Hyperphosphatemia
    D. Hyperkalemia
    E. Hypokalemia

27. Acute symptoms of hypermagnesemia are treated by:

    A. Fluid hydration with normal saline
    B. IV insulin
    C. Calcium chloride
    D. Dextrose
    E. Dialysis

28. The definitive management of hyperkalemia is by:

    A. Fluid hydration with normal saline
    B. IV insulin
    C. Calcium chloride
    D. Dextrose
    E. Dialysis

29. A complication of the use of hetastarch, which limits its use in trauma patients, is the increased risk of:

    A. Bleeding
    B. Hypochloremic alkalosis
    C. Liver failure
    D. Hyponatremia
    E. Impaired pulmonary function

30. Which of the following bacteria is most commonly associated with transfusion-associated sepsis?

    A. *Staphylococcus aureus*
    B. *Staphylococcus epidermidis*
    C. β-Hemolytic *Streptococcus*
    D. *Bacillus fragilis*
    E. *Pseudomonas* species

Answers

1. D. Shock is defined as tissue perfusion that is insufficient to maintain normal aerobic tissue metabolism. Signs of shock are low blood pressure, tachycardia, and cool or clammy skin. There are four types of shock: hypovolemic, vasogenic, neurogenic, and cardiogenic.

2. C. PCWP provides an indirect estimate of left atrial pressure. Left atrial pressure can be measured by advancing a Swan-Ganz catheter into a branch of the pulmonary artery via the superior vena cava and right atrium, and out the right ventricle into the pulmonary artery. Based on the observed waveform, the balloon is inflated, and thus a branch of the pulmonary artery is temporarily occluded. This measured value is an indirect measurement of left atrial pressure. Normal left atrial pressure is 8 to 10 mm Hg. Mitral valve disease can give a falsely elevated estimate of left atrial pressure.

3. C. PEEP increases intrathoracic pressure, which causes decreased cardiac output by means of decreased preload. PEEP does not decrease lung water, reduce vascular permeability, or hasten the resolution of pulmonary edema. PEEP may shift some edema fluid from the alveolar to the extra-alveolar interstitial space, but PEEP does not reduce the overall degree of pulmonary edema. PEEP is often an effective way of increasing arterial oxygen content by increasing functional residual capacity by recruitment of alveoli in patients who have decreased lung compliance. PEEP does not affect P_{CO_2}. PEEP does not alter cardiac contractility.

4. The formula for SVR is SVR $=$ MAP $-$ CVP/CO $\times$ 80, MAP $=$ DBP $+$ ½ (SBP $-$ DBP), where MAP is the mean arterial pressure, CVP is the central venous pressure, CO is the cardiac output, DBP is the diastolic blood pressure, and SBP is the systolic blood pressure.

5. B. Oxygen delivery (milliliters of oxygen per minute) $=$ cardiac output (liters per minute) $\times$ hemoglobin concentration (grams per liter) $\times$ 1.31 (milliliters of oxygen per grams of hemoglobin) $\times$ percentage of saturation. Cardiac output can be increased by increasing stroke volume, heart rate, or both. In addition, oxygen delivery can be increased by increasing the concentration of hemoglobin, Sa_{O_2} (arterial oxygen saturation), or both.

6. B. Sv_{O_2} is an indirect measurement of tissue oxygenation. It is measured from a blood sample obtained from the pulmonary artery. A true Sv_{O_2} includes blood from the vena cava and the coronary sinus. Sv_{O_2} is a marker for adequacy of resuscitation and reversal of hypoxemia.

7. E. Patients with pulmonary embolism are usually tachycardic, tachypneic, and hypotensive, with elevated pulmonary artery pressures and central venous pressures. In the PIOPED (Prospective Investigation of Pulmonary Embolism Diagnosis) study the most common physical signs of pulmonary embolism were tachypnea (70%), rales (51%), tachycardia (30%), a fourth heart sound (24%), and an accentuated pulmonary component of the second heart sound (23%). Acute respiratory consequences of pulmonary embolism include increased alveolar dead space, pneumoconstriction, hypoxemia, and hyperventilation. This is reflected by decreases in Pa_{O_2} and P_{CO_2}. As time passes, two additional consequences may occur: regional loss of surfactant and pulmonary infarction. Arterial hypoxemia is a frequent but not universal finding in patients with acute embolism. The mechanisms of hypoxemia include ventilation–perfusion mismatch, intrapulmonary shunts, reduced cardiac output, and intracardiac shunt via a patent foramen ovale. Pulmonary infarction is an uncommon consequence because of the bronchial arterial collateral circulation. Pulmonary embolism reduces the cross-sectional area of the pulmonary vascular bed, resulting in increased pulmonary vascular resistance, which, in turn, increases the right ventricular afterload. If the afterload is greatly increased, right ventricular failure may ensue.

8. D. The patient is in cardiogenic shock with a low cardiac output, elevated SVR, and elevated PCWP. Inotropic support such as dobutamine is indicated to improve cardiac contractility and output. His PCWP is already elevated, so he does not need further fluid to increase preload. Lasix (furosemide) is not a good option because his low urine output is a reflection of low cardiac output. Nitroprusside is a vasodilator and could potentially improve cardiac output. It should not be used as the next step in treating this patient. Neo-Synephrine (phenylephrine) is an α_1-agonist that will increase SVR (afterload) and result in decreased cardiac output and low blood pressure.

9. D. The definition of adult respiratory distress syndrome includes (1) a known etiology or disease that would predispose to this syndrome, (2) pulmonary artery pressures less than 18 mm Hg, (3) no clinical evidence of right heart failure subsequent to left heart failure, (4) diffuse bilateral pulmonary infiltrates, and (5) a Pa_{O_2}:Fi_{O_2} ratio less than 200.

10. D. Nosocomial pneumonia is the second most common nosocomial infection and the most common nosocomial infection among ventilated patients. The risk of ventilator-associated pneumonia increases 5% per day and is as high as 70% at 30 days. The 30-day mortality rate from nosocomial pneumonia can be as high as 40%. Nosocomial pneumonias are frequently polymicrobial, and gram-negative rods are the predominant organisms. The criteria for diagnosis include fever, cough, development of purulent sputum in conjunction with radiologic evidence of an infiltrate, suggestive Gram stain findings, and positive sputum, tracheal aspirate, pleural fluid, or blood cultures.

11. B. Hemorrhagic shock is a form of hypovolemic shock. In response to hypovolemia, the cardiovascular system increases the heart rate, myocardial contractility, and SVR to maintain blood pressure. This response occurs secondary to an increase in norepinephrine secretion and a decrease in vagal tone. The cardiovascular system also redistributes blood flow to the brain, heart, and kidneys and shunts it away from the skin, muscle, and gastrointestinal tract. The kidneys respond to hemorrhagic shock by increasing reabsorption of sodium and water, which results in a small volume of concentrated urine. When a patient is adequately resuscitated, the first sign is an improvement in urine output.

12. C. Sepsis produces high-output cardiac failure (elevated cardiac index). SVR is decreased due to toxins that produce vasodilation. This is reflected in a low systemic blood pressure. Central venous pressures are low from the loss of intravascular volume due to third spacing. Wedge pressures are generally unaffected. SvO_2 will be high because the tissues are unable to extract oxygen from the blood for consumption.

13. D. The patient is exhibiting signs of a tension pneumothorax with evidence of hypotension, tracheal deviation, subcutaneous emphysema, and decreased breath sounds over the right hemithorax. The treatment is chest tube insertion. Intubation and mechanical ventilation should not occur before tension decompression because this will do nothing to address the impending cardiovascular collapse.

14. E. Free water deficit = (serum sodium − 140)/(140) × total body water. Total body water is 50% of lean body mass in men and 40% in women. The free water deficit calculates to be 7 L, half of which should be replaced over the next 24 hours. The correction must be made slowly to avoid neurologic complications such as central pontine myelinosis.

15. C. Electrocardiographic changes associated with hypokalemia include U waves, T-wave flattening, ST-segment changes, and arrhythmias. Atrioventricular block is more common with hypercalcemia and hyperkalemia. Hypokalemia is a common electrolyte abnormality in surgical patients, occurring because of inadequate supplementation with total parenteral nutrition and excessive IV fluids.

16. B. The treatment of hypercalcemia of malignancy should begin with saline volume expansion. This alone will decrease renal reabsorption of calcium as the associated volume deficit is corrected. Also calcitonin lowers serum calcium levels within hours by inhibiting bone resorption that is occurring from metastatic disease. Calcitonin is indicated in hypercalcemic crisis. Mithramycin acts directly on bones, lowering calcium levels, but the effect takes more than 24 hours to produce. Loop diuretics help to improve renal potassium excretion but are not indicated in hypercalcemia. Corticosteroids are most useful in hypercalcemia related to sarcoidosis and multiple myeloma. They may be useful in patients with bony metastasis, but take as long

as 1 week to work. Bisphosphonate drugs are indicated immediately in addition to IV hydration and calcitonin. This class includes pamidronate, which inhibits osteoclast activity, resulting in lower calcium levels in patients with bony metastasis.

17. C. This patient has symptomatic hyponatremia. A short-term complication of a transurethral resection of the prostate procedure is severe hyponatremia due to the absorption of hypotonic irrigation used intraoperatively. As serum sodium levels decrease, central nervous system signs are the most prominent, but tissue edema, oliguria, and watery diarrhea also result. Low serum osmolarity causes free water to move by osmosis into brain tissues, increasing intracranial pressure and causing hypertension, seizures, and eventual loss of reflexes. If neurologic symptoms are present, 3% normal saline should be used to increase sodium by no more than 1 mEq/hr until the serum sodium level reaches 130 mEq/L or neurologic symptoms have improved. Free water restriction and isotonic saline will increase sodium levels in patients with mild hyponatremia, but severe symptomatic disease necessitates rapid correction to at least 130 mEq/dL. Furosemide and the use of hypotonic Ringer's lactate (sodium = 130 mg/L) would worsen hyponatremia and therefore are contraindicated.

18. D. Normal serum concentration of phosphorus is 2.5 to 5.0 mg/dL. Severe hypophosphatemia occurs at levels less than 1 mg/dL. Adverse effects of hypophosphatemia are related to the decrease in high-energy phosphates. This can manifest as cardiac dysfunction or muscle weakness. Decreased cardiac output and respiratory failure secondary to muscle weakness may result. Encephalopathy and hemolysis of red blood cells can also result. There is no direct effect on the thyroid with altered phosphate levels.

19. D. The serum osmolality is 330 mOsm/kg, and therefore hyponatremia is not the likely cause of this patient's symptoms. Hypernatremia explains the hyperosmolality, restlessness, and delirium. After cardiopulmonary arrest, the serum potassium level is typically elevated because of cell death, but potassium abnormalities do not typically affect the central nervous system. The serum calcium level may be elevated if it is given during resuscitation, but hypercalcemia is typically manifested by lethargy, stupor, and coma, not restlessness.

20. D. Cerebral salt wasting is a diagnosis of exclusion that occurs in patients with a cerebral lesion and renal wasting of sodium and chloride with no other identifiable cause. Natriuresis in a patient with a contractible extracellular volume should prompt the possible diagnosis of cerebral salt wasting. Only cerebral salt wasting explains the high sodium excretion in the urine and high urine output, resulting in low serum sodium and dehydration. High urine output (200–300 mL/hr) can be explained by diabetes insipidus, cerebral salt wasting, and high-output renal failure, but not likely iatrogenic intoxication or SIADH. Diabetes insipidus is a disorder of antidiuretic hormone stimulation and is manifested by dilute urine in the presence of hypernatremia. Diabetes insipidus can cause seizures, but is characterized by high serum sodium, high serum osmolality, and low urine specific gravity, none of which correlates with this patient. High-output renal failure also does not correlate with this patient's clinical picture because high-output renal failure is usually accompanied by elevated potassium, BUN, and creatinine. SIADH is characterized by low urine output and abnormal retention of free water secondary to the inappropriate antidiuretic hormone action. SIADH should be considered in patients who are euvolemic and hyponatremic with elevated urine sodium and urine osmolarity. Iatrogenic intoxication, most likely referring to narcotics, can cause coma and be confused with the listed syndromes, but does not alter serum and urine electrolytes or osmolality. Water intoxication provokes disturbances in electrolyte balance, resulting in a rapid decrease in serum sodium concentration and eventual death. The development of acute dilutional hyponatremia causes neurologic symptoms because of the movement of water into the brain cells in response to the decrease in extracellular osmolality. Symptoms can become apparent when the serum sodium level falls below 120 mmol/L, but are usually associated with concentrations less than 110 mmol/L. Severe symptoms occur with very low sodium concentrations of 90 to 105 mmol/L. As the sodium concentration decreases, the symptoms progress from confusion to drowsiness and eventually coma. However, the rate at which the sodium concentration decreases is also an important factor.

21. C. This patient has diabetic ketoacidosis, evidenced by hyperglycemia, acidemia, increased anion gap, and the presence of serum ketones. Hyperventilation would cause respiratory alkalosis. Nausea and vomiting would cause a metabolic alkalosis from loss of hydrogen chloride. Diarrhea causes metabolic acidosis due to gastrointestinal loss of bicarbonate.

22. C. Hypomagnesemia results from starvation, malabsorption, IV fluids or total parenteral nutrition without supplementation, gastrointestinal losses, and chronic alcohol use. Neuromuscular and central nervous system hyperactivity is a primary manifestation of magnesium deficiency. Hypomagnesemia is characterized by neuromuscular and central nervous system hyperactivity, and symptoms are similar to those of calcium deficiency, including hyperactive reflexes, muscle tremors, and tetany with a positive Chvostek sign. Severe deficiency can lead to delirium and seizures. Respiratory arrest and cardiac arrest, with loss of tendon reflexes, are characteristic of hypermagnesemia.

23. C. With a bicarbonate level of 37, this patient has a metabolic alkalosis. The cause of metabolic alkalosis can be determined by whether it is chloride responsive or resistant. Chloride-responsive cases (urine chloride < 15 mEq/L) are much more common in surgical patients and result from vomiting (loss of hydrogen ions), diuretics (loss of chloride in the urine), and volume depletion (aldosterone-stimulated hydrogen ion loss in urine). Conversely, chloride-resistant types (urine chloride > 25 mEq/L) result from mineralocorticoid excess or potassium depletion.

24. D. Early sepsis is characterized by tachycardia, increased respiratory rate, and increased catabolic activity. Tachypnea leads to respiratory alkalosis early, as carbon dioxide is blown off.

25. B. Tumor lysis syndrome results when the release of intracellular metabolites is greater than the kidneys' excretory capacity. A rapid release of intracellular contents occurs and is associated with marked hyperuricemia, hyperkalemia, hyperphosphatemia, hypocalcemia, and acute renal failure. It is typically seen with poorly differentiated lymphomas and leukemias, but can also be seen with a number of solid tumor malignancies. Tumor lysis syndrome most commonly develops after chemotherapy or radiotherapy. Once it develops, volume expansion should be undertaken, as should correction of electrolyte abnormalities. Associated hypocalcemia should not be treated unless it is symptomatic. Dialysis may be required for impaired renal function or for correction of electrolyte abnormalities.

26. A. Magnesium depletion is a common problem in hospitalized patients, particularly in the intensive care unit. The kidney is primarily responsible for magnesium homeostasis through regulation by calcium/magnesium receptors on renal tubular cells that sense serum magnesium levels. Hypomagnesemia results from a variety of causes ranging from poor intake (starvation, alcoholism, prolonged administration of IV fluids, and total parenteral nutrition with inadequate supplementation of magnesium), increased renal excretion (alcohol, most diuretics, and amphotericin B), gastrointestinal losses (diarrhea), malabsorption, acute pancreatitis, diabetic ketoacidosis, and primary aldosteronism. Magnesium depletion is characterized by neuromuscular and central nervous system hyperactivity, and symptoms are similar to those of calcium deficiency. Signs include hyperactive reflexes, muscle tremors, and tetany with a positive Chvostek sign. Severe deficiencies can lead to delirium and seizures. Electrocardiographic changes including prolonged QT and PR intervals, ST-segment depression, flattening or inversion of P waves, torsade de pointes, and arrhythmias can also be seen. When hypokalemia or hypocalcemia coexist with hypomagnesemia, magnesium should be aggressively replaced to assist in restoring potassium or calcium homeostasis.

27. C. Treatment of hypermagnesemia includes with holding exogenous sources of magnesium, correcting volume deficits, and correcting acidosis if present. To manage acute symptoms, calcium chloride should be administered to antagonize the cardiovascular effects. If elevated levels or symptoms persist, dialysis is indicated. Insulin, dextrose, and dialysis are typically used in the treatment of hyperkalemia.

28. E. All patients should have exogenous sources of potassium discontinued, including potassium supplementation in IV fluids and enteral and parenteral solutions. Potassium can be removed from the body with a cation-exchange resin, such as Kayexalate (sodium polystyrene), which binds potassium in exchange for sodium. It can be administered either orally (preferred) or rectally. Measures should also include attempts to shift potassium intracellularly with glucose and bicarbonate. Nebulized albuterol (10–20 mg) may also be used. Glucose alone will cause an increase in insulin secretion, but in acutely ill patients, this response may be blunted, and therefore both glucose and insulin are recommended. Circulatory overload and hypernatremia may result from the administration of Kayexalate (sodium polystyrene) and bicarbonate, so care should be exercised when administering these agents. When electrocardiographic changes are present, calcium chloride or calcium gluconate should also be administered to counteract the myocardial effects of hyperkalemia. All of these measures are temporary (lasting from 1 to ~4 hours). Dialysis should be considered when conservative measures fail.

29. A. Hydroxyethyl starch solutions are another group of alternative plasma expanders and volume replacement solutions. Hetastarches are produced by the hydrolysis of insoluble amylopectin, followed by a varying number of substitutions of hydroxyl groups for carbon groups on glucose molecules. The molecular weights can range from 1000 to 3,000,000 Da. The high-molecular-weight hydroxyethyl starch, hetastarch (average molecular weight 480,000 Da), which comes as a 6% solution, is the only hydroxyethyl starch approved for use in the United States. Hemostatic derangements have been related to decreases in von Willebrand factor and factor VIIIc, and its use has been associated with postoperative bleeding in cardiac and neurosurgery patients. Hetastarch can also induce renal dysfunction in patients with septic shock and in recipients of kidneys procured from brain-dead donors. Currently, hetastarch has a limited role in massive resuscitation because of its associated coagulopathy and hyperchloremic acidosis (due to its high chloride content).

30. E. Bacterial contamination of infused blood is rare and can be acquired from contaminated collection bags or poor cleaning of the donor's skin. Gram-negative organisms, especially coliform and *Pseudomonas* species, which are capable of growth at 4°C (39.2°F), are the most common cause. Clinical manifestations include fever, chills, abdominal cramps, vomiting, and diarrhea. There may be hemorrhagic manifestations and increased bleeding. If the diagnosis is suspected, the transfusion should be discontinued and the blood cultured. Emergency treatment includes oxygen, adrenergic blocking agents, and antibiotics.

References: Mullins RJ: Shock, electrolytes, and fluid. In Townsend CM Jr, Beauchamp RD, Evers BM, Mattox KL, editors: *Sabiston textbook of surgery: the biological basis of modern surgical practice*, ed 18, Philadelphia, 2008, WB Saunders, pp 69–112.

Shires GT: Fluid and electrolyte management of the surgical patient. In Brunicardi FC, Andersen DK, Billiar TR, et al, editors: *Schwartz's principles of surgery*, ed 9, New York, 2010, McGraw-Hill, pp 51–66.

Zuckerbraun BS, Peitzman AB, Billiar TR: Shock. In Brunicardi FC, Andersen DK, Billiar TR, et al, editors: *Schwartz's principles of surgery*, ed 9, New York, 2010, McGraw-Hill, pp 89–112.

Esophagus and Diaphragm 11

1. Which of the following statements about achalasia is NOT true?
   A. It can be caused by an infection.
   B. In young patients, videoscopic myotomy is the treatment of choice.
   C. Calcium channel blockers exacerbate the condition.
   D. Botulinum toxin injection can provide short-term relief.
   E. It is presumed to be caused by neurogenic degeneration.

2. All of the following are true regarding carcinoma of the esophagus EXCEPT:
   A. Achalasia is a risk factor.
   B. Squamous cell carcinoma is the most common worldwide.
   C. Adenocarcinoma is decreasing in frequency.
   D. The presence of dysphagia usually signifies advanced disease.
   E. Hyperkeratosis of the palms and soles is a risk factor.

3. Which of the following statements about leiomyomas of the esophagus is NOT true?
   A. They are the most common benign esophageal neoplasm.
   B. The majority occur in the middle and lower third of the esophagus.
   C. They have a risk of malignant degeneration.
   D. They have a characteristic appearance on barium swallow.
   E. A preoperative endoscopic biopsy should be performed.

4. Barrett esophagus:
   A. Is a congenital abnormality
   B. Occurs more frequently in individuals of African descent
   C. When diagnosed, should be treated with an antireflux procedure to prevent cancer
   D. Diagnosis requires replacement of a 3-cm long segment of the squamous cells by columnar epithelium
   E. Features the presence of goblet cells

5. Which one of the following is true about Mallory-Weiss syndrome?
   A. The chief pathologic finding is spontaneous perforation of the esophagus.
   B. It typically presents with forceful vomiting or coughing followed by hematemesis.
   C. It is usually associated with air in the mediastinum.
   D. Endoscopy is contraindicated.
   E. Prompt surgical management is the treatment of choice.

6. Which one of the following statements is NOT true about a foramen of Bochdalek hernia?
   A. It usually has a well-defined sac.
   B. It causes respiratory distress.
   C. It is the most common congenital diaphragmatic hernia.
   D. In infants, it is preferably repaired via an abdominal approach.
   E. It is associated with intestinal malrotation and obstruction.

7. Which of the following is true regarding foramen of Morgagni hernias?
   A. They pose a high risk of intestinal obstruction.
   B. The predominant symptom is respiratory distress.
   C. They typically present in childhood.
   D. They are predominantly on the right side.
   E. Observation is recommended.

8. Over the past 2 years, a 50-year-old man repeatedly reported difficulty swallowing, which he described as a lump in his throat. He has noticed expectoration of excess saliva, intermittent hoarseness, and some weight loss. The most likely diagnosis is:

   A. Cricopharyngeal dysfunction
   B. Achalasia
   C. Diffuse spasm of the esophagus
   D. Scleroderma
   E. Carcinoma of the cervical esophagus

9. Esophageal manometry performed in a patient with a true paraesophageal hernia will demonstrate that the lower esophageal sphincter (LES) is:

   A. Above the normal position
   B. At the normal position
   C. Hypertensive
   D. Hypotensive
   E. Short

10. Which of the following statements about a paraesophageal hernia is true?

    A. It is associated with anemia.
    B. It does not pose a risk for incarceration and strangulation.
    C. Diagnosis is not readily made with upper endoscopy.
    D. It is usually caused by a traumatic injury.
    E. It rarely requires operative repair.

11. Which of the following is true regarding Boerhaave syndrome?

    A. It is the most common cause of esophageal perforation.
    B. It is best diagnosed by measuring the amylase level in pleural fluid.
    C. It causes more bleeding than hemophilia A.
    D. It is best managed nonoperatively.
    E. The majority occur in the left lower esophagus.

12. A 65-year-old man in otherwise good health has persistent heartburn despite aggressive medical antireflux therapy. Esophagoscopy reveals a 6-cm segment of columnar-lined distal esophagus, and high-grade dysplasia is found on multiple biopsy specimens. Which of the following management options is the best?

    A. Antireflux operation
    B. Continued medical therapy
    C. Esophagectomy and reconstruction
    D. Surveillance esophagoscopy and biopsy in 3 months
    E. Surveillance esophagoscopy and biopsy in 1 year

13. Which of the following statements is true about Zenker diverticulum?

    A. It is a true diverticulum.
    B. It is best diagnosed with esophagoscopy.
    C. It is unlikely to cause aspiration.
    D. It is a pulsion diverticulum.
    E. Small diverticula (<3 cm) are best managed endoscopically.

14. During the course of an upper endoscopy for suspected achalasia, the endoscopist thinks he may have caused an inadvertent perforation of the lower esophagus. The patient is stable and shows no signs of sepsis. Esophagogram confirms a markedly dilated esophagus with distal free perforations. Management consists of:

    A. Intravenous (IV) antibiotics, placing patient NPO, and close observation
    B. Resection of the injured esophagus with cervical esophagostomy and gastrostomy and feeding jejunostomy
    C. Primary repair of the esophagus with placement of an intercostal muscle flap over repair
    D. Esophagectomy with immediate reconstruction
    E. Esophageal stent placement

15. A 4-year-old boy presents to the emergency department after an accidental ingestion of lye. The child is exhibiting stridor and hoarseness. The child is emergently intubated and resuscitated with IV fluids. An upright chest radiograph shows no evidence of perforation. The patient is admitted to the intensive care unit. The next step in the management is:

    A. Esophagoscopy
    B. Esophagography
    C. Chest computed tomography scan
    D. Close observation
    E. Immediate exploratory laparotomy

Answers

1. C. Achalasia is a primary motility disorder of the esophagus, specifically of the LES. The pathogenesis is presumed to be neurogenic degeneration (of ganglion cells), which is idiopathic, or infection (Chagas disease, *Trypanosoma cruzi*). The degeneration results in a failure of the LES to relax on swallowing, leading to an increase in intraluminal esophageal pressure, marked esophageal dilation (with an air–fluid level on radiograph), and loss of progressive peristalsis in the body of the esophagus. The classic triad of symptoms is dysphagia, regurgitation, and weight loss. Diagnosis should include manometry (showing failure of the LES to relax with swallowing), barium esophagography (showing a "bird's beak" appearance), and endoscopy (to rule out malignancy). There are four basic treatment options. Early on, medical therapy with calcium channel blockers and nitroglycerin can help relax the LES. In high-risk elderly patients, injection of the LES with botulinum toxin can provide short-term relief. The mainstays of treatment are balloon dilation of the LES and surgical myotomy. All interventions are palliative in that there is no cure. Myotomy can now be done videoscopically and is the treatment of choice for younger patients because it seems to have better long-term durability than dilation.

References: Chapman JR, Joehl RJ, Murayama KM, et al: Achalasia treatment: improved outcome of laparoscopic myotomy with operative manometry, *Arch Surg* 139:508–513, 2004.

Csendes A, Braghetto I, Henríquez A, et al: Late results of a prospective randomized study comparing forceful dilatation and esophagomyotomy in patients with achalasia, *Gut* 30:299–304, 1989.

Hoogerwerf W, Pasricha P: Achalasia: treatment options revisited, *Can J Gastroenterol* 14:406–409, 2000.

Vaezi M, Richter J, Wilcox C, et al: Botulinum toxin versus pneumatic dilatation in the treatment of achalasia: a randomized trial, *Gut* 44:231–239, 1999.

2. C. Worldwide, squamous cell carcinoma is the most common cause, although adenocarcinoma is increasing rapidly and is approaching 50% of cases in the Western world. The main risk factors are smoking and alcohol consumption. Other factors associated include ingestion of nitrosamine compounds, mineral deficiencies, betel nut chewing, long-standing achalasia, Barrett esophagus, caustic burns, and tylosis (an autosomal dominant disorder characterized by hyperkeratosis of the palms and soles). Obesity is emerging as an important risk factor. The esophagus lacks a serosa. As such, it is readily able to accommodate the growth of tumor by dilating. Thus, the presence of dysphagia in most instances indicates a large tumor in an advanced stage. For this reason, screening with endoscopy is advocated in high-risk groups (those with reflux and Barrett esophagus).

3. E. Leiomyomas are the most common benign tumor in the esophagus, accounting for more than 50% of benign tumors. However, benign masses constitute only 10% of esophageal tumors. Leiomyomas only become symptomatic when they are very large (>5 cm). Otherwise, they are incidentally discovered during the course of other studies. They have a characteristic appearance on barium swallow of a smooth, crescent-shaped filling defect that encroaches on the lumen. On endoscopy, the mucosa is usually intact, and the tumor moves up and down with swallowing. If it has the characteristic appearance, the tumor should not undergo biopsy, because of an increased risk of mucosal perforation. Treatment is to enucleate the mass, which can be done via a videoscopic approach, combined with intraoperative esophagoscopy. The cell of origin of these tumors is mesenchymal. The average age at presentation is 38 years, and they are twice as common in males and most commonly located in the lower two thirds of the esophagus. Leiomyomas are usually solitary, but multiple tumors are seen in as many as 10% of patients.

Reference: Aurea P, Grazia M, Petrella F, Bazzocchi R: Giant leiomyoma of the esophagus, *Eur J Cardiothorac Surg* 22:1008–1010, 2002.

4. E. Barrett esophagus occurs in 5% to 7% of patients with gastroesophageal reflux disease. It is an acquired pathology. The hallmark feature is the presence of intestinal goblet cells, which signifies intestinal metaplasia, on endoscopic biopsy. It occurs more commonly in males with a 3:1 ratio and is uncommon in African Americans. Once Barrett esophagus develops, the risk of adenocarcinoma is approximately 0.5% per year. In one large study, the prevalence of cancer was 4%. Management of Barrett esophagus initially is medical, provided there is no evidence of severe dysplasia. However, surveillance of patients with Barrett esophagus for dysplasia is recommended. If severe dysplasia is present, esophagectomy is recommended. Another option for high-grade dysplasia is photodynamic therapy using Photofrin (porfimer sodium), a light-sensitizing drug that is administered orally and concentrates in the area of metaplasia. A laser is then focused on the esophagus, activating the drug and destroying the cells. In patients with Barrett esophagus without dysplasia, a randomized study comparing medical management with antireflux surgery showed that there were no differences between the two treatments with regard to preventing progression to dysplasia and adenocarcinoma, although antireflux surgery was more efficient than medical treatment.

References: Drewitz D, Sampliner R, Garewal H: The incidence of adenocarcinoma in Barrett's esophagus: a prospective study of 170 patients followed 4.8 years, *Am J Gastroenterol* 92:212–215, 1997.

Hameeteman W, Tytgat G, Houthoff H, et al: Barrett's esophagus: development of dysplasia and adenocarcinoma, *Gastroenterology* 96:1249–1256, 1989.

Parrilla P, Martínez de Haro LF, Ortiz A, et al: Long-term results of a randomized prospective study comparing medical and surgical treatment of Barrett's esophagus, *Ann Surg* 237:291–298, 2003.

Jobe BA, Hunter JG, Peters JH: Esophagus and diaphragmatic hernia. In Brunicardi FC, Andersen DK, Billiar TR, et al, editors: *Schwartz's principles of surgery*, ed 9, New York, 2010, McGraw-Hill, pp 803–887.

Maish M: Esophagus. In Townsend CM Jr, Beauchamp RD, Evers BM, Mattox KL, editors: *Sabiston textbook of surgery: the biological basis of modern surgical practice*, ed 18, Philadelphia, 2008, WB Saunders, pp 1049–1107.

5. B. The mechanism of a Mallory-Weiss tear is similar to that of an esophageal perforation (Boerhaave syndrome). It is the result of forceful vomiting or coughing in the presence of a hiatal hernia. This situation exposes the gastroesophageal junction to high pressures, resulting in a partial-thickness mucosal tear and bleeding. Boerhaave syndrome results in a full-thickness tear causing esophageal perforation. Severe sepsis develops in such patients, with air in the mediastinum and pleural effusion, and surgical intervention is required. Most bleeding from Mallory-Weiss tears stops spontaneously with nonsurgical management. Patients should undergo endoscopy to confirm the diagnosis. Recent studies suggest that the area of bleeding is best managed by injecting sclerosing agents or epinephrine to prevent rebleeding.

Reference: Llach J, Elizalde J, Guevara M, et al: Endoscopic injection therapy in bleeding Mallory-Weiss syndrome: a randomized controlled trial, *Gastrointest Endosc* 54:679–681, 2001.

6. A. A Bochdalek hernia is posterolateral in location and is the most common congenital diaphragmatic hernia. It can result in compression of the lung, resulting in pulmonary hypoplasia involving both lungs, with the ipsilateral lung affected more. The most frequent presentation is respiratory distress due to hypoxemia at birth. It can be associated with chronic respiratory disease, pneumonia, or intestinal obstruction. Most pediatric surgeons repair a Bochdalek hernia through an abdominal subcostal incision. In most cases (80%–90%), a hernia sac is not present.

7. D. Foramen of Morgagni hernias are rare congenital diaphragmatic hernias that account for only 5% of cases. The foramen of Morgagni is located in the anterior midline, at the sternocostal hiatus of the diaphragm, between the xiphoid process and the costal margin. Unlike Bochdalek hernias, which are primarily on the left, Morgagni hernias occur on the right 90% of the time. Because they are small, they rarely produce symptoms at birth or in childhood. Most often, they are discovered incidentally on chest radiograph that demonstrates a right-sided middle mediastinal mass. In most cases, the hernia is filled with omentum. Very rarely, bowel can enter the hernia and produce symptoms. When questioned, patients may give a history of eructation or indigestion. Because of the potential risk of incarceration, most surgeons recommend repair, which can be done videoscopically or via an upper abdominal incision. They usually have a well-formed sac.

Reference: Hussong R, Landreneau R, Cole F: Diagnosis and repair of a Morgagni hernia with video-assisted thoracic surgery, *Ann Thorac Surg* 63:1474–1475, 1997.

8. A. Cricopharyngeal dysfunction has multiple causes including neurogenic and myogenic etiologies, such as stroke, multiple sclerosis, peripheral neuropathy, Parkinson disease, and dermatomyositis. The exact cause is unknown, but the primary theory is that the cricopharyngeus muscle, which is normally in a state of tonic contraction, fails to relax and allow the passage of food into the cervical esophagus. Patients describe difficulty swallowing food. A key element of the diagnosis is the classic history of an inability to handle saliva secretion, such that the patient describes expectoration of saliva. Patients also report hoarseness. Weight loss results from a decreased caloric intake. Although one should always be suspicious of carcinoma in a patient with difficulty swallowing and weight loss, the long duration of symptoms makes carcinoma unlikely. Achalasia is failure of the LES to relax. It would not likely lead to excessive expectoration of saliva. The classic triad of presenting symptoms includes dysphagia, regurgitation, and weight loss. The predominant symptom of diffuse spasm of the esophagus is chest pain in association with dysphagia. Patients with scleroderma have a weakening of the LES and a decrease in peristalsis, leading to symptoms of reflux. The work-up for cricopharyngeal dysfunction includes a barium swallow with video or cine radiography, manometry, and esophagoscopy. The barium study should be done before esophagoscopy because it may show a concomitant Zenker diverticulum. Performing esophagoscopy first may be hazardous because there is an increased risk of esophageal perforation owing to the fact that the diverticulum may be inadvertently entered. Treatment of cricopharyngeal dysfunction is with pharyngoesophageal myotomy. If a large Zenker diverticulum is also present, it should be excised, which can be done with a stapling device. Newer alternatives that have emerged are similar to that of achalasia treatment, namely, balloon dilation and injection of botulinum toxin.

9. B. Hiatal hernias are divided into three types. Type I, or a sliding hiatal hernia, is the most common. In this hernia, the gastroesophageal junction moves upward into the posterior mediastinum along with part of the stomach, such that the LES is above its normal position. The majority of these hernias are asymptomatic. Those who do have symptoms typically experience heartburn and regurgitation. In type II or paraesophageal hernias, the gastroesophageal junction and therefore the LES are in their normal positions, as is the cardia. However, the gastric fundus is dislocated upward. A type III hernia is a combination of types I and II. A hypertensive LES is characteristic of achalasia. In gastroesophageal reflux disease, the LES pressure is low. Gastroesophageal reflux disease seems to begin from gastric distention. The distention leads to a shortening of the LES. As the sphincter shortens, its resting pressure decreases. The location of the LES (in the normal abdominal position or in the mediastinum) is important in gastroesophageal reflux disease. Loss of abdominal length of the LES causes a decrease in LES pressure because it is no longer subjected to the positive pressure of the abdomen.

10. A. A paraesophageal hernia, or type II hiatal hernia, is also called a *rolling-type hiatal hernia*. The widened hiatus permits the fundus of the stomach to protrude into the chest, anterior and lateral to the body of the esophagus. The gastroesophageal junction remains below the diaphragm.

The herniated gastric fundus rotates in a counterclockwise direction and is prone to becoming incarcerated and strangulated. The herniated and twisted portion of the stomach develops mucosal erosions, leading to chronic blood loss and anemia in approximately one third of patients, along with dysphagia, heartburn, and abdominal pain. Diagnosis can be made by a barium swallow. Upper endoscopy can readily make the diagnosis on a retroflex view. Although herniation is rare, most surgeons recommend elective repair of paraesophageal hernias because of the potential risk of strangulation.

11. E. Boerhaave syndrome is commonly associated with the Mackler triad (vomiting, chest pain, and subcutaneous emphysema). It accounts for approximately 10% of esophageal perforations (most are iatrogenic). There is usually a history of vomiting. Many patients have a history of gastroesophageal reflux disease. The diagnosis is often missed because the patient will report severe chest pain and commonly have a left pleural effusion. The serum amylase level may be elevated, prompting a misdiagnosis of pancreatitis. The misdiagnosis may be compounded further if a sample of the pleural effusion is sent for laboratory analysis because it will have a high amylase level due to saliva. Boerhaave syndrome may also be misdiagnosed as an acute myocardial infarction or an aortic dissection. More than 80% to 90% of spontaneous esophageal ruptures occur in the lower left esophagus and drain into the left pleural cavity. The diagnosis is confirmed by a contrast esophagogram, using gastrograffin, which shows extravasation in 90% of patients. Surgical management is the treatment of choice. If detected within 72 hours of onset and if there is not severe inflammation, primary repair is recommended with an intercostal muscle or pleural flap.

12. C. If there is evidence of high-grade dysplasia on biopsy, esophagectomy with reconstruction is the best surgical option because there is a significant risk of either finding carcinoma in the specimen or of progression to carcinoma. An antireflux procedure such as a Nissen procedure or medical management will not be sufficient. Newer data suggest that photodynamic therapy may be an alternative to surgery for Barrett esophagus with high-grade dysplasia, but this is as yet not the standard of care.

References: Heitmiller R, Redmond M, Hamilton S: Barrett's esophagus with high-grade dysplasia: an indication for prophylactic esophagectomy, *Ann Surg* 224:66–71, 1996.

Overholt B, Panjehpour M, Halberg D: Photodynamic therapy for Barrett's esophagus with dysplasia and/or early stage carcinoma: long-term results, *Gastrointest Endosc* 58:183–188, 2003.

13. D. Zenker diverticulum is a false diverticulum and is a pulsion diverticulum. A pulsion diverticulum forms at a point of weakness and is due to alterations in luminal pressure, whereas a traction diverticulum forms because of external pulling on the bowel wall such as from an inflamed lymph node. Zenker diverticulum is the most common type of esophageal diverticulum. It usually presents in older patients (older than 60 years). It characteristically arises at a point of weakness, most commonly at the Killian triangle, which is formed by the inferior fibers of the inferior

constrictor muscle and the superior border of the cricopharyngeus muscle. Patients typically present with dysphagia, regurgitation of undigested food, halitosis, episodes of aspiration, and salivation. With the characteristic history, the first diagnostic study is a barium swallow. In the absence of other pathology (such as an irregular mucosa), endoscopy is not needed. Treatment is surgical by either open or endoscopic techniques. The open technique involves cervical esophagomyotomy with stapling and amputation of the diverticulum. The endoscopic technique involves division of the common wall between the diverticulum and the esophagus. Studies have shown that results with the endoscopic technique are better with larger diverticula. Diverticula smaller than 3 cm are too short to accommodate one cartridge of staples and to allow complete division of the sphincter, and therefore this size is considered a contraindication to this technique.

References: Bonavina L, Bona D, Abraham M, et al: Long-term results of endosurgical and open surgical approach for Zenker diverticulum, *World J Gastroenterol* 13:2586–2589, 2007.

Collard JM, Otte JB, Kestens PJ: Endoscopic stapling technique of esophagodiverticulostomy for Zenker's diverticulum, *Ann Thorac Surg* 56:573–576, 1993.

Narne S, Cutrone C, Bonavina L, et al: Endoscopic diverticulotomy for the treatment of Zenker's diverticulum: results in 102 patients with staple-assisted endoscopy, *Ann Otol Rhinol Laryngol* 108:810–815, 1999.

14. C. The decision of how to proceed in an iatrogenic esophageal perforation depends on five things: whether it is a free or contained perforation, the duration of time that the perforation has been present, the underlying pathology in the esophagus, whether severe inflammation is present at surgery, and the patient's condition. As a general rule, if the perforation is contained, as shown on an esophagogram, management can be conservative. If it is a free perforation, surgery is indicated. Resection of an injured esophagus with cervical esophagostomy and gastrostomy and feeding jejunostomy is reserved for situations in which there has been a long delay in diagnosis (>72 hours), severe inflammation is present, or the patient is extremely ill or disabled. If there is underlying disease in the esophagus that will contribute to uncorrectable high esophageal pressures (achalasia) or disease that needs esophagectomy (cancer, severe caustic burn), then immediate esophagectomy is recommended with reconstruction, provided that severe inflammation is not present and there has not been a long delay. Stenting is generally reserved for unresectable cancer.

Reference: Fernandez F, Richter A, Freudenberg S: Treatment of endoscopic esophageal perforation, *Surg Endosc* 13:962–966, 1999.

15. A. Caustic injuries can lead to esophageal perforation in the short term and severe esophageal strictures in the long term. Initial management should focus on the ABCs. An upright chest radiograph should be obtained to look for free air under the diaphragm. Emetics should be avoided. In children, esophagoscopy may not be necessary if the patient is completely asymptomatic. In this patient who is having symptoms and in adults, esophagoscopy is recommended within 12 hours of the ingestion to assess the degree of injury (provided there is no evidence of perforation). It is important to advance the endoscope only to the first area of injury, so as not to increase the risk of iatrogenic perforation. Injury is graded as first degree (mucosal hyperemia, edema), second degree (limited hemorrhage, pseudomembrane formation), or third degree (complete obstruction of lumen by edema, charring). First-degree burns can be treated by observation. Second- and third-degree burns (without perforation) are treated by placing the patient NPO and administering IV antibiotics, H_2-receptor antagonists, proton pump inhibitors, and IV fluids. The use of steroids is controversial.

References: Jobe BA, Hunter JG, Peters JH: Esophagus and diaphragmatic hernia. In Brunicardi FC, Andersen DK, Billiar TR, et al: *Schwartz's principles of surgery*, ed 9, New York, 2010, McGraw-Hill, pp 803–887.

Maish M: Esophagus. In Townsend M Jr, Beauchamp RD, Evers BM, Mattox KL, editors: *Sabiston textbook of surgery: the biological basis of modern surgical practice*, ed 18, Philadelphia, 2008, WB Saunders, pp 1049–1107.

Wilsey M, Scheimann A, Gilger M: The role of upper gastrointestinal endoscopy in the diagnosis and treatment of caustic ingestion, esophageal strictures, and achalasia in children, *Gastrointest Endosc Clin North Am* 11:767–787, 2001.

Gallbladder 12

1. Hemobilia is most frequently accompanied by what other finding?
   A. Arterioportal vein fistula
   B. Arteriohepatic vein fistula
   C. Arterial pseudoaneurysm
   D. Portal venous pseudoaneurysm
   E. Cavernous hemangioma

2. Choledochal cyst disease is thought to be caused by an abnormality of the:
   A. Bile duct smooth muscle
   B. Bile composition
   C. Bile duct adventitia
   D. Pancreaticobiliary duct junction
   E. Bile duct mucosa

3. The most important reason to perform routine intraoperative cholangiography (IOC) during laparoscopic cholecystectomy is to:
   A. Prevent incision of the common bile duct (CBD)
   B. Identify unsuspected common duct stones
   C. Identify anatomic anomalies of the hepatic ducts
   D. Ensure complete removal of the gallbladder and cystic duct
   E. Prevent transection of the CBD

4. The best choice for operative repair of an iatrogenic CBD transection is:
   A. End-to-end CBD anastomosis
   B. Choledochoduodenostomy
   C. Choledochojejunostomy
   D. Hepaticoduodenostomy
   E. Hepaticojejunostomy

5. All of the following are true regarding gallbladder function EXCEPT:
   A. It actively absorbs sodium and chloride.
   B. It passively absorbs water.
   C. It secretes hydrogen ions.
   D. It secretes mucus.
   E. Its contraction is inhibited by vagal stimulation.

6. A 65-year-old woman presents with symptoms and signs of acute cholecystitis and undergoes an uneventful laparoscopic cholecystectomy. On postoperative day 7, the pathology report indicates a superficial gallbladder carcinoma that does not invade the perimuscular connective tissue. Which of the following would be the best management?
   A. Radiation therapy
   B. Chemotherapy
   C. Combined radiation and chemotherapy
   D. Observation
   E. Reoperation with wedge resection of the liver around the gallbladder fossa and regional lymph node resection

7. Which of the following is most commonly associated with sclerosing cholangitis?
   A. Crohn disease
   B. Ulcerative colitis
   C. Riedel thyroiditis
   D. Sarcoidosis
   E. Retroperitoneal fibrosis

8. Which of the following is the best management of a localized Klatskin tumor?
   A. Pancreaticoduodenectomy (Whipple procedure)
   B. Resection of the entire extrahepatic biliary tree with hepatic resection if necessary
   C. Resection of the middle third of the biliary tree with hepaticojejunostomy
   D. Chemotherapy
   E. Radiation followed by chemotherapy

9. A 60-year-old patient presents with nausea, fever, and right upper quadrant pain and tenderness. Ultrasonography (US) reveals gallstones as well as air in the wall of the gallbladder. All of the following are true about this condition EXCEPT:

   A. It is associated with diabetes.
   B. Emergent cholecystectomy is indicated.
   C. There is a high risk of gallbladder perforation.
   D. It is more common in females.
   E. *Clostridia welchii* is a common cause.

10. All of the following are true regarding bile and gallstones EXCEPT:

    A. The primary bile acids are cholic and chenodeoxycholic acid.
    B. The primary phospholipid in bile is lecithin.
    C. Cholecystectomy increases bile salt secretion.
    D. Half a gram of bile salts is produced daily to replace fecal losses.
    E. Bile consists of an equal part bile salts, phospholipids, and cholesterol.

11. A 75-year-old woman presents to the emergency department with a 2-day history of nausea, feculent vomiting, and obstipation. Her blood pressure on admission is 80/60 mm Hg, and her heart rate is 120 beats per minute. Plain films reveal distended loops of small bowel with air–fluid levels as well as air in the biliary tree. After resuscitation, which of the following is the best management option?

    A. Small bowel enterotomy with removal of the gallstone plus cholecystectomy and takedown of the fistula
    B. Small bowel enterotomy with removal of the gallstone alone
    C. Cholecystectomy with CBD exploration
    D. Prolonged nasogastric tube decompression and intravenous (IV) antibiotics
    E. Lysis of adhesions plus resection of the small bowel

12. Aschoff-Rokitansky sinuses are seen with:

    A. Acute cholecystitis
    B. Chronic cholecystitis
    C. Oriental cholangiohepatitis
    D. Sclerosing cholangitis
    E. Acalculous cholecystitis

13. All of the following are true regarding acalculous cholecystitis EXCEPT:

    A. The incidence of perforation is higher than with calculous cholecystitis.
    B. It is seen in association with severe burns.
    C. The US findings may be normal.
    D. In severely ill patients, emergency laparoscopic cholecystectomy is the treatment of choice.
    E. It may be caused by cystic artery thrombosis.

14. All of the following are true regarding brown pigment stones EXCEPT:

    A. They are typically found in Asian patients.
    B. They form primarily in the CBD.
    C. Their formation is aided by bacterial enzymes in the bile.
    D. They form in response to hemolysis.
    E. They tend to be friable.

15. The risk of gallbladder cancer is increased with all of the following EXCEPT:

    A. Calcified gallbladder
    B. Obesity
    C. Male sex
    D. Large gallstones compared with smaller ones
    E. Anomalous pancreaticobiliary junction

16. The most common cause of benign bile duct stricture is:

    A. Ischemia from operative injury
    B. Chronic pancreatitis
    C. Common duct stones
    D. Acute cholangitis
    E. Sclerosing cholangitis

17. Management of type I choledochal cysts consists of:

    A. Excision of the cyst and cholecystectomy with Roux-en-Y hepaticojejunostomy
    B. Excision of the cyst, cholecystectomy, segmental liver resection, and hepaticojejunostomy
    C. Observation
    D. Sphincterotomy
    E. Roux-en-Y cyst jejunostomy

18. Strawberry gallbladder is a gross description given to:

    A. Cholesterolosis
    B. Adenomyomatosis
    C. Porcelain gallbladder
    D. Acalculous cholecystitis
    E. Gangrenous cholecystitis

19. Jaundice with absent urine urobilinogen is most consistent with:
    A. Hepatitis
    B. Cirrhosis
    C. Hemolysis
    D. Biliary obstruction
    E. Sepsis

20. Which of the following best describes the role of preoperative biliary drainage before a Whipple procedure in a patient with obstructive jaundice?
    A. It has been shown to decrease the rate of cholangitis.
    B. It has been shown to increase the rate of wound infections.
    C. It should be performed routinely if the bilirubin level is greater than 8 mg/dL.
    D. It has been shown to shorten the hospital stay.
    E. It has been shown to decrease the mortality rate.

21. US of the gallbladder reveals a polypoid lesion. This most likely represents a:
    A. Cholesterol polyp
    B. Adenomyomatosis
    C. Benign adenoma
    D. Adenocarcinoma
    E. Inflammatory polyp

22. A 45-year-old man has a 50% total body surface area third-degree burn. On hospital day 7, fever, marked leukocytosis, and right upper quadrant pain develop. His blood pressure is 130/80 mm Hg and his heart rate is 110 beats per minute. Ultrasonography shows a distended gallbladder but is negative for gallstones. Antibiotics are initiated. The next step in management would consist of:
    A. Laparoscopic cholecystectomy
    B. Computed tomography
    C. Hepatoiminodiacetic acid (HIDA) scan
    D. Close observation
    E. Upper endoscopy

23. Factors associated with a higher conversion rate from laparoscopic to open cholecystectomy include all of the following EXCEPT:
    A. American Society of Anesthesiologists class
    B. Gallbladder wall thicker than 4 mm
    C. Female sex
    D. Previous surgery
    E. Advanced age

24. Which of the following is true regarding biliary anatomy?
    A. The right hepatic duct tends to be longer than the left and more prone to dilation.
    B. Venous return from the gallbladder is most often via a cystic vein to the portal vein.
    C. Heister valves have an important role in the gallbladder's function as a bile reservoir.
    D. The CBD and pancreatic duct typically unite outside the duodenal wall.
    E. The arterial supply to the CBD derives primarily from the left hepatic and right gastric arteries.

25. During laparoscopic cholecystectomy, bile is noted to be emanating from the region of the CBD/cystic duct junction. Upon conversion to open cholecystectomy, the injury is noted to be a 3-mm longitudinal tear in the anterolateral distal common hepatic duct. The duct itself measures 6 mm in diameter. Management consists of:
    A. Primary repair of the injury
    B. Primary repair of the injury over a T tube
    C. Primary repair of the injury with a T tube placed through a separate choledochotomy
    D. Hepaticojejunostomy
    E. Choledochoduodenostomy

26. Hydrops of the gallbladder:
    A. Poses a significantly increased risk of malignancy
    B. Is due to a stone impacted in the cystic duct
    C. Is typically associated with an enteric bacterial infection
    D. Is associated with marked right upper quadrant tenderness
    E. Results in the gallbladder getting filled with bile-stained fluid

27. Which of the following is true regarding gallstone types?
    A. Pure cholesterol stones are common.
    B. Pigment stones are dark because of the presence of calcium bilirubinate.
    C. Brown stones usually form in association with a hemolytic disorder.
    D. Black stones are associated with bacterial infection.
    E. Most cholesterol stones are radiopaque.

28. A 35-year-old Chinese man presents with a fever of 103.5°F, right upper quadrant pain, and jaundice. Laboratory values are significant for a white blood cell count of 15,000, an alkaline phosphatase level of 400 U/L, and a serum bilirubin level of 3.8 mg/dL. Magnetic resonance cholangiopancreatography demonstrates a markedly dilated CBD, markedly dilated intrahepatic ducts with several intrahepatic ductal strictures, and multiple stones throughout the ductal system. All of the following are true about this condition EXCEPT:

A. Initial management should consist of a hepaticojejunostomy.
B. It is associated with bacteria in the bile.
C. It is associated with *Clonorchis sinesis*.
D. It has a high recurrence rate.
E. It can lead to liver failure.

29. Which of the following best describes the role of early (within 24 hours of admission) laparoscopic cholecystectomy for acute cholecystitis?

A. It results in a shortened hospital stay.
B. It increases the rate of conversion to open cholecystectomy.
C. It should not be performed because the patient should be cooled off for 2 to 3 days with antibiotics.
D. It is associated with a higher overall complication rate.
E. It is associated with a higher mortality rate.

Answers

1. C. Hemobilia presents with a classic triad of upper gastrointestinal bleeding (hematemesis), combined with jaundice and right-sided upper abdominal pain. It is a rare condition. It is most often due to trauma (in >50% of cases), which is mostly iatrogenic injury of the right hepatic artery during laparoscopic cholecystectomy as well as blunt and penetrating injuries. The underlying lesion is typically an arterial pseudoaneurysm that has a connection with the biliary tree (hence the jaundice). It can also occur in association with gallstones, tumors, inflammatory disorders, and vascular disorders. Treatment in most instances involves angiographic embolization of the artery.

    References: Bloechle C, Izbicki J, Rashed M, et al: Hemobilia: presentation, diagnosis, and management, *Am J Gastroenterol* 89:1537–1540, 1994.

    Chari RS, Shah SA: Biliary system. In Townsend CM Jr, Beauchamp RD, Evers BM, Mattox KL, editors: *Sabiston textbook of surgery: the biological basis of modern surgical practice*, ed 18, Philadelphia, 2008, WB Saunders, pp 1547–1588.

    Croce M, Fabian T, Spiers J, et al: Traumatic hepatic artery pseudoaneurysm with hemobilia, *Am J Surg* 168:235–238, 1994.

    Nicholson T, Travis S, Ettles D, et al: Hepatic artery angiography and embolization for hemobilia following laparoscopic cholecystectomy, *Cardiovasc Intervent Radiol* 22:20–24, 1999.

2. D. The exact etiology of choledochal cysts is unclear. The most likely explanation is that there is an anomalous pancreaticobiliary duct junction. Specifically, the pancreatic duct joins the CBD more than 1 cm proximal to the ampulla, resulting in a long common channel. The long channel leads to free reflux of pancreatic secretions into the biliary tract, resulting in increased biliary pressures and inflammatory changes in the biliary epithelium, which eventually lead to dilation and cyst formation. Although an abnormal pancreaticobiliary junction is present in the majority of patients with choledochal cysts, it is not uniformly seen in all. Choledochal cysts are more common in females, and the classic presentation is in childhood with jaundice, an abdominal mass, and abdominal pain. However, less than 50% of patients present with all three features, and thus the diagnosis is often delayed. The diagnosis is made by US, which can sometimes detect the cyst antenatally. There are five types. Type I is the most common (90%) and consists of fusiform dilation of the bile duct. Type V, also known as Caroli disease, is characterized by multiple intrahepatic dilations. Because of the risk of malignant degeneration, treatment involves excising the cyst with a biliary enteric bypass. The risk of malignancy increases with the more advanced age at which the cyst is detected.

    References: Oddsdottir M, Pham TH, Hunter JG: Gallbladder and the extrahepatic biliary system. In Brunicardi FC, Andersen DK, Billiar TR, et al, editors: *Schwartz's principles of surgery*, ed 9, New York, 2010, McGraw-Hill, pp 1135–1166.

    Todani T, Watanabe Y, Fujii T, et al: Anomalous arrangement of the pancreatobiliary ductal system in patients with a choledochal cyst, *Am J Surg* 147:672–676, 1984.

3. E. The routine use of IOC to prevent bile duct injury is controversial. Because the overall risk of bile duct injury is so small, to date there are no sufficiently large-scale randomized studies to answer this question. Most likely the use of IOC will not prevent an injury to the CBD. However, IOC seems to allow earlier recognition of the injury and prevent complete transection of the CBD. Although routine IOC will identify unsuspected CBD stones, in most instances, CBD stones are suspected preoperatively by abnormal liver function tests, a dilated CBD, or a history of gallstone pancreatitis. In a nationwide retrospective analysis, CBD injury was found in 0.39% of patients undergoing cholecystectomy with IOC and in 0.58% of patients without IOC (unadjusted relative risk, 1.49). After controlling for patient-level factors and surgeon-level factors, the risk of injury was increased when IOC was not used (adjusted relative risk, 1.71). Some surgeons prefer selective use of IOC and obtain what is known as the "critical view" whereby the cystic duct and artery are carefully identified and not clipped or cut until conclusive identification has been made. This is done by completely dissecting the Calot triangle free of all fat and fibrous tissue and dissecting the lower part of the gallbladder off the liver bed, such that only two skeletonized structures (the cystic duct and artery) are seen to be entering the gallbladder.

References: Chari RS, Shah SA: Biliary system. In Townsend CM Jr, Beauchamp RD, Evers BM, Mattox KL, editors: *Sabiston textbook of surgery: the biological basis of modern surgical practice*, ed 18, Philadelphia, 2008, WB Saunders, pp 1547–1588.

Detry O, De Roover A, Detroz B, et al: The role of intraoperative cholangiography in detecting and preventing bile duct injury during laparoscopic cholecystectomy, *Acta Chir Belg* 103:161–162, 2003.

Flum D, Dellinger E, Cheadle A, et al: Intraoperative cholangiography and risk of common bile duct injury during cholecystectomy, *JAMA* 289:1639–1644, 2003.

Oddsdottir M, Pham TH, Hunter JG: Gallbladder and the extra hepatic biliary system. In Brunicardi FC, Andersen DK, Billiar TR, et al, editors: *Schwartz's principles of surgery*, ed 9, New York, 2010, McGraw-Hill, pp 1135–1166.

4. E. The management of an intraoperative bile duct injury depends on the type of injury and the clinical setting. If a small lateral injury is created in the CBD, this can be repaired by closing the ductotomy over a T tube. Conversely, if the common duct is transected, this results in an interruption in the blood supply to the duct, and attempts at primary repair will inevitably lead to stricture formation and recurrent episodes of cholangitis. Thus, if a transection is recognized intraoperatively, it is best to repair it immediately and to do so with a biliary enteric bypass. Because most of these injuries will be in the common hepatic duct, the best option is to perform a hepaticojejunostomy. This also depends on whether a surgeon is available with experience in treating complex biliary problems. If one is not available, the best option is to drain the area, place transhepatic catheters, and refer the patient. If the injury is discovered postoperatively and there has been a long delay, the best option is to perform transhepatic drainage and delay primary repair for 6 to 8 weeks to allow the inflammation to subside. A critical element of the repair is to perform a tension-free, mucosa-to-mucosa duct enteric anastomosis.

References: Chari RS, Shah SA: Biliary system. In Townsend CM Jr, Beauchamp RD, Evers BM, Mattox KL, editors: *Sabiston textbook of surgery: the biological basis of modern surgical practice*, ed 18, Philadelphia, 2008, WB Saunders, pp 1547–1588.

MacFadyen B, Vecchio R, Ricardo A, et al: Bile duct injury after laparoscopic cholecystectomy: the United States experience, *Surg Endosc* 12:315–321, 1998.

5. E. The gallbladder concentrates and stores bile. It does this by rapidly absorbing sodium and chloride against a concentration gradient by active transport and passive water absorption. The epithelial cells of the gallbladder secrete mucous glycoproteins and hydrogen ions into the gallbladder lumen. The secretion of hydrogen ions acidifies the bile, increasing calcium solubility, and thus preventing its precipitation as calcium salts. Inflammation of the gallbladder mucosa seems to affect the ability to secrete hydrogen ions, making the bile more lithogenic. Vagal innervation stimulates contraction of the gallbladder.

References: Chari RS, Shah SA: Biliary system. In Townsend CM Jr, Beauchamp RD, Evers BM, Mattox KL, editors: *Sabiston textbook of surgery: the biological basis of modern surgical practice*, ed 18, Philadelphia, 2008, WB Saunders, pp 1547–1588.

Oddsdottir M, Pham TH, Hunter JG: Gallbladder and the extra hepatic biliary system. In Brunicardi FC, Andersen DK, Billiar TR, et al, editors: *Schwartz's principles of surgery*, ed 9, New York, 2010, McGraw-Hill, pp 1135–1166.

6. D. Cancer of the gallbladder is predominantly adenocarcinoma. The majority of cases are discovered in an advanced state with distant metastases. Thus, the overall prognosis is very poor, with a 5-year survival rate of only 5%. The best chance of cure is if it is discovered incidentally at the time of cholecystectomy. Given the overall rarity of gallbladder cancer, the management is somewhat controversial. Recent studies indicate that those that are discovered incidentally and are superficial such as carcinoma in situ and T1 lesions (do not extend into perimuscular connective tissue) and have negative margins can be managed by cholecystectomy alone. Those that are more locally advanced such as T2 through T4 lesions (those that invade the perimuscular connective tissue or directly invade the liver) are treated with a radical cholecystectomy, which includes subsegmental resection of segments IVb and V, plus hepatoduodenal ligament lymphadenectomy, which results in prolonged survival. The caveat is that there must be no evidence of distant metastases. In one series of 48 patients, the overall 5-year survival rate was 13%, but it was 60% for patients who underwent radical cholecystectomy. The radical cholecystectomy group had significantly longer survival than the simple cholecystectomy group for all stages except stage I (T1N0). Radiation therapy with fluorouracil radiosensitization is the most commonly used postoperative treatment.

References: Chari RS, Shah SA: Biliary system. In Townsend CM Jr, Beauchamp RD, Evers BM, Mattox KL, editors: *Sabiston textbook of surgery: the biological basis of modern surgical practice*, ed 18, Philadelphia, 2008, WB Saunders, pp 1547–1588.

Ito H, Matros E, Brooks DC, et al: Treatment outcomes associated with surgery for gallbladder cancer: a 20-year experience, *J Gastrointest Surg* 8:183–190, 2004.

Oddsdottir M, Pham TH, Hunter JG: Gallbladder and the extra hepatic biliary system. In Brunicardi FC, Andersen DK, Billiar TR, et al, editors: *Schwartz's principles of surgery*, ed 9, New York, 2010, McGraw-Hill, pp 1135–1166.

Reid KM, Ramos-De la Medina A, Donohue JH: Diagnosis and surgical management of gallbladder cancer: a review, *J Gastrointest Surg* 11:671–681, 2007.

Taner CB, Nagorney DM, Donohue JH: Surgical treatment of gallbladder cancer, *J Gastrointest Surg* 8:83–89, 2004.

7. B. Sclerosing cholangitis is characterized by the presence of multiple inflammatory fibrous thickenings of bile duct walls resulting in biliary strictures. It is progressive and as such leads eventually to biliary obstruction, recurrent biliary infection, cirrhosis, and liver failure, as well as a significantly increased risk of cholangiocarcinoma (in 10%–20% of patients). It is twice as common in men. Risk factors for sclerosing cholangitis include inflammatory bowel disease, pancreatitis, and diabetes. The strongest association is with ulcerative colitis. Approximately two thirds of patients have ulcerative colitis. In fact, it is usually discovered in these patients when an abnormal liver function test result is noted. It is less commonly associated with

Crohn disease. Other diseases associated with sclerosing cholangitis include Riedel thyroiditis and retroperitoneal fibrosis. Removing the colon in patients with ulcerative colitis does not affect the course of the sclerosing cholangitis. In addition, the severity of inflammation does not predict the onset of malignancy. Currently, the best option is liver transplantation in patients who progress to liver failure.

Reference: Oddsdottir M, Pham TH, Hunter JG: Gallbladder and the extrahepatic biliary system. In Brunicardi FC, Andersen DK, Billiar TR, et al, editors: *Schwartz's principles of surgery*, ed 9, New York, 2010, McGraw-Hill, pp 1135–1166.

8. B. Perihilar cholangiocarcinomas are also known as Klatskin tumors. They are classified into four types based on whether they are limited to the common hepatic duct (type I), involve the bifurcation of the right and left hepatic ducts (type II), or enter into the secondary right (type IIIa) or left (type IIIb) intrahepatic ducts. Surgery is the only treatment that has shown potential for long-term survival, provided the tumor has no evidence of distant spread. Type I and II tumors involve resection of the entire extrahepatic biliary tree with portal lymphadenectomy and bilateral Roux-en-Y hepaticojejunostomies. More recently, an even more aggressive approach has been taken for type I and II tumors to include a hemihepatectomy to achieve negative margins. Using this approach, several authors have shown improved survival. For type III lesions, a similar aggressive approach using lobectomy is advocated. Adjuvant radiation therapy has also not been shown to improve either quality of life or survival in resected patients. Patients with unresectable disease are often offered treatment with 5-fluorouracil alone or in combination with mitomycin C and doxorubicin, but the response rates are low. A Whipple procedure would be appropriate for a distal CBD tumor.

References: Capussotti L, Muratore A, Polastri R, et al: Liver resection for hilar cholangiocarcinoma: in-hospital mortality and longterm survival, *J Am Coll Surg* 195:641–647, 2002.

Dinant S, Gerhards M, Rauws E, et al: Improved outcome of resection of hilar cholangiocarcinoma (Klatskin tumor), *Ann Surg Oncol* 13:872–880, 2006.

Lygidakis N, Sgourakis G, Dedemadi G, et al: Long-term results following resectional surgery for Klatskin tumors: a twenty-year personal experience, *Hepatogastroenterology* 48:95–101, 2001.

Oddsdottir M, Pham TH, Hunter JG: Gallbladder and the extrahepatic biliary system. In Brunicardi FC, Andersen DK, Billiar TR, et al, editors: *Schwartz's principles of surgery*, ed 9, New York, 2010, McGraw-Hill, pp 1135–1166.

9. D. Emphysematous cholecystitis occurs in less than 1% of acute cholecystitis cases. It is a disease that occurs predominantly in elderly diabetic men. The hallmark feature is characterized by gas within the gallbladder wall or lumen. This can be seen on plain radiograph or US or CT scan. Gangrene of the gallbladder is present in three fourths of all cases, and perforation of the gallbladder occurs in more than 20% of cases. In one large series, the mortality rate was 25% and the morbidity rate 50% despite aggressive treatment with broad-spectrum antibiotics and emergent surgery. Coverage should include *Clostridia* and other anaerobes and thus include high-dose penicillin. Common biliary pathogens associated with emphysematous cholecystitis include *Clostridia welchii*, *Escherichia coli*, *Enterococcus*, and *Klebsiella*.

References: Chari RS, Shah SA: Biliary system. In Townsend CM Jr, Beauchamp RD, Evers BM, Mattox KL, editors: *Sabiston*

textbook of surgery: the biological basis of modern surgical practice, ed 18, Philadelphia, 2008, WB Saunders, pp 1547–1588.

Garcia-Sancho Tellez L, Rodriguez-Montes J, Fernandez de Lis S, et al: Acute emphysematous cholecystitis: report of twenty cases, *Hepatogastroenterology* 46:2144–2148, 1999.

10. E. Bile consists of bile salts, phospholipids, and cholesterol in the following concentrations: 80%, 15%, and 5%, respectively. Normally, more than 95% of bile salts are reabsorbed by the enterohepatic circulation and negative feedback accounts for replacement of the 0.5-g loss of bile salts in the stool. The major organic solutes in bile are bilirubin, bile salts, phospholipids, and cholesterol. The primary bile acids are cholic acid and chenodeoxycholic acid. The secondary bile acids are lithocholate and deoxycholate acids. Cholecystectomy has minimal effect on bile acid secretion, but does increase enterohepatic circulation of bile salts.

Reference: Oddsdottir M, Pham TH, Hunter JG: Gallbladder and the extrahepatic biliary system. In Brunicardi FC, Andersen DK, Billiar TR, et al, editors: *Schwartz's principles of surgery*, ed 9, New York, 2010, McGraw-Hill, pp 1135–1166.

11. B. The presentation is consistent with gallstone ileus. *Gallstone ileus* is a misnomer because it is actually a type of mechanical small bowel obstruction. It occurs more commonly in elderly females (older than 70 years). It usually results from a large gallstone (>2.5 cm) that has eroded through the gallbladder into the adjacent duodenum (hence, the air in the biliary tree), creating a cholecystoenteric fistula. Less commonly, the fistula can be between the gallbladder and the colon (hepatic flexure) or the stomach. The stone typically lodges in the narrowest portion of the gastrointestinal tract, the distal ileum, near the ileocecal valve. The diagnosis of gallstone ileus is made preoperatively in only approximately half of cases; because a history of biliary disease may be absent, pneumobilia may not be seen, the gallstone may not be visualized, and/or the abdominal radiographic findings may be nonspecific. Because many of these patients are elderly, have other major comorbidities, and are often markedly dehydrated, initial surgical management should focus on relieving the bowel obstruction, which is best accomplished by a transverse enterotomy, proximal to the palpable stone, and stone removal. It is also important to run the small bowel because a significant portion of patients will have a second gallstone. Cholecystectomy with closure of the fistula should be reserved for young, low-risk, stable patients. Interestingly, in one study, leaving the fistula on long-term follow-up did not seem to lead to significant morbidity, although most surgeons would recommend taking the patient back at a later time for fistula takedown. This decision needs to be individualized.

References: Chari RS, Shah SA: Biliary system. In Townsend CM Jr, Beauchamp RD, Evers BM, Mattox KL, editors: *Sabiston textbook of surgery: the biological basis of modern surgical practice*, ed 18, Philadelphia, 2008, WB Saunders, pp 1547–1588.

Rodríguez-Sanjuán J, Casado F, Fernández M, et al: Cholecystectomy and fistula closure versus enterolithotomy alone in gallstone ileus, *Br J Surg* 84:634–637, 1997.

Tan Y, Wong W, Ooi L: A comparison of two surgical strategies for the emergency treatment of gallstone ileus, *Singapore Med J* 45:69–72, 2004.

12. B. Aschoff-Rokitansky sinuses are associated with chronic cholecystitis. Chronic cholecystitis is the histopathologic result of multiple bouts of symptomatic cholelithiasis or biliary colic. Biliary colic is itself a misnomer because the pain associated with gallstones is typically constant and progressive. On pathologic examination, Aschoff-Rokitansky sinuses develop as a result of atrophy of the mucosa. As the mucosa atrophies, the epithelium protrudes into the muscle coat, leading to the formation of these sinuses.

References: Chari RS, Shah SA: Biliary system. In Townsend CM Jr, Beauchamp RD, Evers BM, Mattox KL, editors: *Sabiston textbook of surgery: the biological basis of modern surgical practice*, ed 18, Philadelphia, 2008, WB Saunders, pp 1547–1588.

Oddsdottir M, Pham TH, Hunter JG: Gallbladder and the extrahepatic biliary system. In Brunicardi FC, Andersen DK, Billiar TR, et al, editors: *Schwartz's principles of surgery*, ed 9, New York, 2010, McGraw-Hill, pp 1135–1166.

13. D. Acalculous cholecystitis typically occurs in critically ill, highly stressed patients, such as those who have experienced severe trauma, sepsis, burns, or multisystem organ failure. The etiology is unclear but is likely related to a combination of ischemia to the gallbladder from a low-flow state and marked gallbladder distention, as well as bile stasis due to a lack of gallbladder contraction (many patients are on total parenteral nutrition). The diagnosis can be very difficult to make because (1) patients are often intubated and sedated, thus not allowing a thorough physical examination; (2) US findings are not pathognomonic; and (3) HIDA scanning can have false-positive results due to the fact that the patients are fasting. Thus, the diagnosis of acalculous cholecystitis requires a high index of suspicion and may need to be a diagnosis of exclusion. The classic findings are fever, leukocytosis, right upper quadrant pain and tenderness, elevation of liver function test results (bilirubin and alkaline phosphatase), a thickened gallbladder wall on US without stones, and nonvisualization of the gallbladder on HIDA scanning. US is the initial diagnostic study of choice and can be performed at the bedside in the intensive care unit. In a recent prospective study, US findings were considered positive if three major criteria were present: wall thickness greater than 4 mm, hydrops, and sludge. The sensitivity was only 50% and the specificity 94%. In stable patients in whom the diagnosis is unclear after US, an HIDA scan can be performed with morphine (67% sensitivity and 100% specificity). Failure to visualize the gallbladder is the most sensitive and specific finding. Leakage into the pericholecystic space suggests perforation. An HIDA scan is not recommended in critically ill patients in whom a delay in therapy can be potentially fatal. Acalculous cholecystitis requires urgent intervention, preferably cholecystectomy. However, if the patient is too ill for surgery, percutaneous US or computed tomography–guided cholecystostomy is the treatment option of choice. Gangrene, perforation, and empyema are seen more frequently than with calculous cholecystitis, and thus, most surgeons would recommend an open cholecystectomy for more stable patients.

References: Chari RS, Shah SA: Biliary system. In Townsend CM Jr, Beauchamp RD, Evers BM, Mattox KL, editors: *Sabiston textbook of surgery: the biological basis of modern surgical practice*, ed 18, Philadelphia, 2008, WB Saunders, pp 1547–1588.

Davis C, Landercasper J, Gundersen L, Lambert P: Effective use of percutaneous cholecystostomy in high-risk surgical patients: techniques, tube management, and results, *Arch Surg* 134:727–731, 1999.

Mariat G, Mahul P, Prévot N, et al: Contribution of ultrasonography and cholescintigraphy to the diagnosis of acute acalculous cholecystitis in intensive care unit patients, *Intensive Care Med* 26:1658–1663, 2000.

14. D. Gallstones are either cholesterol or pigment stones. The majority of stones are cholesterol, although they also contain bile pigments and calcium. Pigment stones are either brown or black. Pigment stones get their characteristic color from calcium bilirubinate, although they also have a smaller amount of cholesterol. Black stones are usually seen in association with hemolytic disorders such as hereditary spherocytosis and sickle cell disease. They form within the gallbladder. Brown stones, conversely, are primarily formed within the bile ducts themselves and are friable. They are associated with parasitic infections and bacteria in the bile. Bacteria secrete β-glucuronidase, which cleaves bilirubin glucuronide to produce unconjugated bilirubin, which is insoluble and precipitates with calcium. Brown stones are primarily composed of precipitated calcium bilirubinate and bacterial cell debris. They are most common in Asian populations.

Reference: Oddsdottir M, Pham TH, Hunter JG: Gallbladder and the extrahepatic biliary system. In Brunicardi FC, Andersen DK, Billiar TR, et al, editors: *Schwartz's principles of surgery*, ed 9, New York, 2010, McGraw-Hill, pp 1135–1166.

15. C. Gallbladder cancer is two to three times more common in females. It is also more common in Native Americans in both North and South America. Approximately 90% of patients with carcinoma have gallstones. Other risk factors include choledochal cysts (which may be due to an abnormal pancreaticobiliary junction), sclerosing cholangitis, gallbladder polyps, and exposure to carcinogens (nitrosamines, azotoluene). Large single stones have a much higher risk of cancer than multiple small stones, likely the result of creating more mucosal inflammation (large stones also are more likely to lead to cholecystoenteric fistulas). Obesity has recently been shown to be a risk factor for a wide range of cancers, including the gallbladder. The risk of gallbladder cancer in porcelain or calcified gallbladders has recently been re-examined. Two types of calcified gallbladders were identified: complete intramural calcification and selective mucosal calcification. The incidence of cancer arising in a gallbladder with selective mucosal wall calcification was approximately 7% (less than previous studies showing a 20% risk), whereas there was no cancer risk in diffuse intramural calcification. Because these calcification characteristics may be difficult to determine noninvasively, current recommendations are to remove porcelain gallbladders even if the patient is asymptomatic.

References: Calle E, Kaaks R: Overweight, obesity and cancer: epidemiological evidence and proposed mechanisms, *Nat Rev Cancer* 4:579–591, 2004.

Oddsdottir M, Pham TH, Hunter JG: Gallbladder and the extrahepatic biliary system. In Brunicardi FC, Andersen DK, Billiar TR, et al, editors: *Schwartz's principles of surgery*, ed 9, New York, 2010, McGraw-Hill, pp 1135–1166.

Stephen A, Berger D: Carcinoma in the porcelain gallbladder: a relationship revisited, *Surgery* 129:699–703, 2001.

16. A. Most benign bile duct strictures are iatrogenic and are due to a technical error during cholecystectomy, such as excessive use of cautery, incorrect placement of a surgical clip, and overly aggressive dissection near the CBD, all of which may be the result of unclear anatomy. Regardless of the cause, the eventual response is fibrosis and stricture formation. As many as three fourths of injuries that lead to strictures are not recognized at surgery, and as many as one third occur 5 years or more after the operation. The majority of iatrogenic strictures are short and occur in the common hepatic duct, distal to the confluence of the right and left hepatic ducts. Bile duct strictures most often present with an episode of cholangitis. The work-up consists of US, which will detect dilated ducts proximal to the stricture, a computed tomography scan to look for masses, and endoscopic retrograde cholangiopancreatography with endoscopic ultrasonography, which can be both diagnostic and therapeutic. Endoscopic ultrasonography can be helpful in detecting a tumor within the bile duct. During endoscopic retrograde cholangiopancreatography, a brushing of the bile duct should be taken for cytology to rule out a malignancy. Management of focal benign strictures by a biliary enteric bypass or stenting remains debatable due to the lack of randomized trials and the lack of good long-term follow-up with stenting. The primary concern with stenting is that the strictures may become obstructed and lead to recurrent cholangitis. Given the much less invasive nature of stenting, however, strong consideration should be given to this approach, and if recurrent obstructive symptoms subsequently develop, a biliary enteric bypass should be performed.

References: Chari RS, Shah SA: Biliary system. In Townsend CM Jr, Beauchamp RD, Evers BM, Mattox KL, editors: *Sabiston textbook of surgery: the biological basis of modern surgical practice*, ed 18, Philadelphia, 2008, WB Saunders, pp 1547–1588.

Costamagna G, Shah SK, Tringali A: Current management of postoperative complications and benign biliary strictures, *Gastrointest Endosc Clin North Am* 13:635–648, ix, 2003.

Lopez R, Cosenza C, Lois J, et al: Long-term results of metallic stents for benign biliary strictures, *Arch Surg* 136:664–669, 2001.

Oddsdottir M, Pham TH, Hunter JG: Gallbladder and the extrahepatic biliary system. In Brunicardi FC, Andersen DK, Billiar TR, et al, editors: *Schwartz's principles of surgery*, ed 9, New York, 2010, McGraw-Hill, pp 1135–1166.

Siriwardana HP, Siriwardena AK: Systematic appraisal of the role of metallic endobiliary stents in the treatment of benign bile duct stricture, *Ann Surg* 242:10–19, 2005.

17. A. Type I choledochal cysts, as discussed in the response to question 2, are the most common and are dilations of either the entire common hepatic duct and CBD or a segment of it. Management consists of excision of the entire cyst (because of the risk of malignancy) and a biliary enteric bypass. Dissection of the posterior wall can sometimes be precarious because it may be stuck to the portal vein. Type II choledochal cysts are diverticula that project from the CBD wall. Type III choledochal cysts are found in the intraduodenal portion of the CBD (also called a *choledochocele*). Type IVa cysts are characterized by multiple dilations of the intrahepatic and extrahepatic biliary tree. Most frequently, a large solitary cyst of the extrahepatic duct is accompanied by multiple cysts of the intrahepatic ducts. Type IVb choledochal cysts consist of multiple dilations that involve only the extrahepatic bile duct. Type V choledochal cysts (Caroli disease) consist of dilations of the intrahepatic biliary tree.

References: Chari RS, Shah SA: Biliary system. In Townsend CM Jr, Beauchamp RD, Evers BM, Mattox KL, editors: *Sabiston textbook of surgery: the biological basis of modern surgical practice*, ed 18, Philadelphia, 2008, WB Saunders, pp 1547–1588.

Oddsdottir M, Pham TH, Hunter JG: Gallbladder and the extrahepatic biliary system. In Brunicardi FC, Andersen DK, Billiar TR, et al, editors: *Schwartz's principles of surgery*, ed 9, New York, 2010, McGraw-Hill, pp 1135–1166.

Todani T, Watanabe Y, Fujii T, et al: Anomalous arrangement of the pancreatobiliary ductal system in patients with a choledochal cyst, *Am J Surg* 147:672–676, 1984.

18. A. Cholesterolosis or strawberry gallbladder is caused by the accumulation of cholesterol in macrophages in the gallbladder mucosa. Cholesterol hypersecretion by the liver promotes excessive accumulation of cholesterol esters within the lamina propria of the gallbladder. The mucosal surface becomes studded with cholesterol deposits, producing the characteristic appearance of the strawberry gallbladder. It is a benign condition. Adenomyomatosis results from hypertrophic smooth muscle bundles and by the ingrowth of mucosa glands into the muscle layer. The cause of this overgrowth is unknown, but it is also a benign condition. Cholecystectomy is not indicated for either of these conditions.

References: Chari RS, Shah SA: Biliary system. In Townsend CM Jr, Beauchamp RD, Evers BM, Mattox KL, editors: *Sabiston textbook of surgery: the biological basis of modern surgical practice*, ed 18, Philadelphia, 2008, WB Saunders, pp 1547–1588.

Oddsdottir M, Pham TH, Hunter JG: Gallbladder and the extrahepatic biliary system. In Brunicardi FC, Andersen DK, Billiar TR, et al, editors: *Schwartz's principles of surgery*, ed 9, New York, 2010, McGraw-Hill, pp 1135–1166.

19. D. Bilirubin is the result of the breakdown of old red blood cells into heme. Heme is broken down into biliverdin and then to bilirubin. Bilirubin is bound to albumin in the circulation, but as it reaches the liver, it is conjugated and eventually enters the gastrointestinal tract. In the gastrointestinal tract, it is deconjugated into urobilinogen by bacteria. Some urobilinogen gets reabsorbed in the gut, returns to the liver, and is excreted in the urine, where it is eventually converted to urobilin, giving urine its yellow appearance. The remaining urobilin is oxidized to stercobilin in the intestines, giving stool its brown appearance. In the presence of biliary obstruction, less bilirubin enters the gut, less urobilinogen is made, and therefore less appears in the urine. Less stercobilin is made and therefore the stools turn pale. Hemolysis would generate an increase in bilirubin and a corresponding increase in urobilinogen in the gut and in the urine.

Reference: Chari RS, Shah SA: Biliary system. In Townsend CM Jr, Beauchamp RD, Evers BM, Mattox KL, editors: *Sabiston textbook of surgery: the biological basis of modern surgical practice*, ed 18, Philadelphia, 2008, WB Saunders, pp 1547–1588.

20. B. Several studies have analyzed the role of preoperative biliary drainage via endoscopic retrograde cholangiopancreatography and stenting in patients with malignant obstructive jaundice who are to undergo a Whipple procedure. Theoretically, relief of jaundice might improve the operative risk of the subsequent Whipple procedure. However, a large meta-analysis and single-center studies failed to show improved morbidity and mortality rates with preoperative biliary drainage. In fact, the routine use of preoperative biliary drainage seems to increase the risk of infectious complications including wound infection (10% with drainage vs. 4% without) as well as increase the risk of pancreatic fistula (10% with drainage vs. 4% without). Thus, it should only be used selectively (such as in the presence of cholangitis or severe intractable pruritus).

References: Chari RS, Shah SA: Biliary system. In Townsend CM Jr, Beauchamp RD, Evers BM, Mattox KL, editors: *Sabiston textbook of surgery: the biological basis of modern surgical practice*, ed 18, Philadelphia, 2008, WB Saunders, pp 1547–1588.

Sewnath ME, Karsten TM, Prins MH, et al: A meta-analysis on the efficacy of preoperative biliary drainage for tumors causing obstructive jaundice, *Ann Surg* 236:17–27, 2002.

Sohn T, Yeo C, Cameron J, et al: Do preoperative biliary stents increase postpancreaticoduodenectomy complications? *J Gastrointest Surg* 4:258–267, 2000.

21. A. Most polypoid lesions of the gallbladder are benign, and of these, cholesterol polyps are the most common. They are usually small (<10 mm), pedunculated, and multiple. They are usually seen in association with cholesterolosis. Adenomyomatosic polyps are the second most common. They appear as sessile polyps that cause focal thickening of the wall. Inflammatory polyps are the third most common. All three are benign and are pseudopolyps. Adenomas and adenocarcinomas of the gallbladder are generally larger than 10 mm. Distinguishing between a benign and a malignant polyp on US, however, is generally not reliable. Thus, when a polyp is found on US, the general indications for cholecystectomy are (1) a symptomatic polyp, (2) a polyp in association with gallstones, (3) a polyp larger than 10 mm, and (4) age older than 50.

References: Chari RS, Shah SA: Biliary system. In Townsend CM Jr, Beauchamp RD, Evers BM, Mattox KL, editors: *Sabiston textbook of surgery: the biological basis of modern surgical practice*, ed 18, Philadelphia, 2008, WB Saunders, pp 1547–1588.

Myers R, Shaffer E, Beck P: Gallbladder polyps: epidemiology, natural history and management, *Can J Gastroenterol* 16:187–194, 2002.

Shinkai H, Kimura W, Muto T: Surgical indications for small polypoid lesions of the gallbladder, *Am J Surg* 175:114–117, 1998.

22. C. The presentation is most consistent with acalculous cholecystitis (see response to question 13). The initial study of choice is US, which can be performed at the bedside. Findings that would confirm the diagnosis would include thickening of the gallbladder wall, sludge, and pericholecystic fluid. If the US findings are negative and the patient is not critically ill, the next study would be an HIDA scan with morphine. A positive study finding would demonstrate nonfilling of the gallbladder with visualization of the tracer in the liver and small bowel. Morphine decreases the rate of false-positive HIDA scan results because it leads to sphincter of Oddi contraction and thus increases the likelihood of filling of the gallbladder in the absence of cholecystitis.

Reference: Chari RS, Shah SA: Biliary system. In Townsend CM Jr, Beauchamp RD, Evers BM, Mattox KL, editors: *Sabiston textbook of surgery: the biological basis of modern surgical practice*, ed 18, Philadelphia, 2008, WB Saunders, pp 1547–1588.

23. C. The need for conversion from laparoscopic to open cholecystectomy has steadily decreased over the past decade. All of the factors listed have been associated with a higher conversion rate except for female sex. Several studies have shown that male sex is associated with a higher conversion rate as well as a higher complication rate. Males also tend to present with more complicated gallbladder disease.

References: Brunt L, Quasebarth M, Dunnegan D: Outcomes analysis of laparoscopic cholecystectomy in the extremely elderly, *Surg Endosc* 15:700–705, 2001.

Chari RS, Shah SA: Biliary system. In Townsend CM Jr, Beauchamp RD, Evers BM, Mattox KL, editors: *Sabiston textbook of surgery: the biological basis of modern surgical practice*, ed 18, Philadelphia, 2008, WB Saunders, pp 1547–1588.

Gharaibeh K, Qasaimeh G, Al-Heiss, et al: Effect of timing of surgery, type of inflammation, and sex on outcome of laparoscopic cholecystectomy for acute cholecystitis, *J Laparoendosc Adv Surg Tech A* 12:193–198, 2002.

24. D. The left hepatic duct is longer than the right and is more likely to be dilated in the presence of distal obstruction. The spiral Heister valves within the cystic duct do not have any true valvular function. In approximately three fourths of individuals, the CBD and the main pancreatic duct unite outside the duodenal wall and traverse the duodenal wall as a single duct. The blood supply to the CBD runs along the lateral and medial walls at 3 and 9 o'clock positions and comes from the right hepatic artery and gastroduodenal artery. Thus, a transverse hemitransection of the duct will likely interrupt the blood supply and render a repair prone to ischemia and stricture.

Reference: Oddsdottir M, Pham TH, Hunter JG: Gallbladder and the extrahepatic biliary system. In Brunicardi FC, Andersen DK, Billiar TR, et al, editors: *Schwartz's principles of surgery*, ed 9, New York, 2010, McGraw-Hill, pp 1135–1166.

25. B. All of the above are potential options for repair of a bile duct injury. Sharp, clean, and small injuries in a large CBD or common hepatic duct are more amenable to primary repair. Repair is generally performed over a T tube. If the duct is transected or nearly transected, a Roux-en-Y hepaticojejunostomy is recommended. Injuries to the distal CBD can be treated with a choledochoduodenostomy.

Reference: Oddsdottir M, Pham TH, Hunter JG: Gallbladder and the extrahepatic biliary system. In Brunicardi FC, Andersen DK, Billiar TR, et al, editors: *Schwartz's principles of surgery*, ed 9, New York, 2010, McGraw-Hill, pp 1135–1166.

26. B. When a gallstone becomes impacted in the cystic duct, the typical course is that acute cholecystitis will develop in the patient. Less frequently, an acute infection does not develop in the patient even though the cystic duct remains obstructed. In this situation, bile within the gallbladder becomes absorbed, but the gallbladder epithelium continues to secrete glycoprotein (mucus). The gallbladder becomes distended with mucinous material. This is known as hydrops. The gallbladder may be palpable, but does not create the Murphy sign. Hydrops of the gallbladder may result in edema of the gallbladder wall and perforation. Although hydrops may persist with few consequences, cholecystectomy is generally indicated to avoid complications.

Reference: Oddsdottir M, Pham TH, Hunter JG: Gallbladder and the extrahepatic biliary system. In Brunicardi FC, Andersen DK, Billiar TR, et al, editors: *Schwartz's principles of surgery*, ed 9, New York, 2010, McGraw-Hill, pp 1135–1166.

27. B. Pure cholesterol stones account for less than 10% of gallstones. Most cholesterol stones are composed of a combination of cholesterol, bile pigments, and calcium. Only approximately 15% of cholesterol stones are radiopaque. As discussed in the response to question 14, pigment gallstones are defined as either black or brown. Pigment stones are dark because of the presence of calcium bilirubinate. They form in association with hemolysis, which increases the concentration of unconjugated bilirubin, which is much less soluble. Brown pigment stones are associated with bacterial infection and parasites.

References: Chari RS, Shah SA: Biliary system. In Townsend CM Jr, Beauchamp RD, Evers BM, Mattox KL, editors: *Sabiston textbook of surgery: the biological basis of modern surgical practice*, ed 18, Philadelphia, 2008, WB Saunders, pp 1547–1588.

Oddsdottir M, Pham TH, Hunter JG: Gallbladder and the extrahepatic biliary system. In Brunicardi FC, Andersen DK, Billiar TR, et al, editors: *Schwartz's principles of surgery*, ed 9, New York, 2010, McGraw-Hill, pp 1135–1166.

28. A. This patient presents with a history and findings consistent with cholangiohepatitis, also known as recurrent pyogenic cholangitis. It is endemic in Asia, although the incidence has been decreasing. Cholangiohepatitis affects both sexes equally. The etiology of cholangiohepatitis seems to be a combination of bacterial and parasitic (*Clonorchis sinensis, Opisthorchis viverrini,* and *Ascaris lumbricoides*) infections in the biliary tree. The bacteria deconjugate bilirubin, which has a greater propensity to precipitate as bile sludge. Brown pigment stones form as a consequence of the sludge and dead bacterial cells. In addition, the nucleus of the stone may harbor a parasite egg. The stones lead to recurrent episodes of cholangitis, liver abscesses, stricture formation, liver failure, and an increased risk of cholangiocarcinoma. Recurrence is high. Initial treatment is with endoscopic retrograde cholangiopancreatography and transhepatic cholangiography. Patients often require multiple interventions to clear the biliary tree. The patient may eventually require a biliary enteric bypass, but this would not be the initial procedure of choice.

29. A. Several prospective, randomized trials, although individually underpowered, have shown that early laparoscopic cholecystectomy (within 24 hours of admission) is safe for acute cholecystitis. The overall complication rate, conversion to open cholecystectomy, bile duct injury rate, and mortality rate are the same as those with delayed cholecystectomy. However, early cholecystectomy shortens the hospital stay.

References: Gurusamy KS, Samraj K: Early versus delayed laparoscopic cholecystectomy for acute cholecystitis, *Cochrane Database Syst Rev* (4):CD005440, 2006.

Lai P, Kwong K, Leung K, et al: Randomized trial of early versus delayed laparoscopic cholecystectomy for acute cholecystitis, *Br J Surg* 85:764–767, 1998.

Lo C, Liu C, Lai E, et al: Early versus delayed laparoscopic cholecystectomy for treatment of acute cholecystitis, *Ann Surg* 223:37–42, 1996.

Head and Neck 13

1. A strong correlation exists between nasopharyngeal carcinoma and:

   A. White race
   B. Alcohol use
   C. Epstein-Barr virus
   D. Betel nut chewing
   E. Plummer-Vinson syndrome

2. Management of nasopharyngeal carcinoma consists primarily of:

   A. Radiation
   B. Chemotherapy
   C. Surgical excision
   D. Combined chemotherapy followed by surgery
   E. Combined chemotherapy and radiation therapy

3. Which of the following is true regarding epistaxis?

   A. Ninety percent of bleeds are from the posterior part of the nose.
   B. Posterior bleeds are associated with hypertension and atherosclerosis.
   C. Anterior bleeds have an associated 5% mortality rate.
   D. Posterior bleeds are best managed by applying digital pressure to the nose.
   E. Anterior bleeds often require packing combined with a Foley catheter.

4. Which of the following statements is true regarding parotid gland tumors?

   A. The majority are malignant.
   B. Pleomorphic adenomas are the most common.
   C. Pleomorphic adenomas are managed by total parotidectomy.
   D. Malignant tumors require en bloc removal of the facial nerve.
   E. Ten percent of pleomorphic adenomas are bilateral.

5. Most salivary gland tumors are in the parotid gland, and approximately 80% of parotid gland tumors are benign. All of the following are true regarding a thyroglossal duct cyst EXCEPT:

   A. It may contain functional thyroid tissue.
   B. Infection is a significant risk.
   C. Malignancy may develop within the cyst.
   D. Management consists of simple cystectomy.
   E. The cyst moves when the tongue is protruded.

6. A 12-week-old male infant presents with a large posterolateral neck mass extending into the axilla that transilluminates. Optimal management would consist of:

   A. Radiation therapy
   B. Repeat needle aspirations
   C. Radical wide excision
   D. Observation
   E. Conservative excision

7. A 54-year-old man presents with a tender left neck mass with a draining sinus. Microscopic examination reveals sulfur granules. Optimal management would be:

   A. Penicillin
   B. Radical excision
   C. Fluconazole
   D. Ciprofloxacin
   E. Radiation

8. Management of a carotid body tumor consists of:

   A. Radiographic embolization
   B. Radiation therapy
   C. Chemotherapy
   D. Surgical excision in a periadventitial plane
   E. Wide excision including carotid bifurcation

9. A 35-year-old man presents with a new dark mole on the face anterior to the tragus as well as clinically suspicious palpable neck nodes. Excisional biopsy confirms melanoma. Optimal management is:
   A. Wide reexcision of the primary tumor and modified radical neck dissection
   B. Modified radical neck dissection only
   C. Wide reexcision of the primary tumor, modified radical neck dissection, and superficial parotidectomy
   D. Wide reexcision of the primary tumor and sentinel node biopsy
   E. Interferon

10. The most likely site of origin for a metachronous cancer in a patient with a history of laryngeal cancer is the:
    A. Esophagus
    B. Lung
    C. Floor of mouth
    D. Tongue
    E. Hypopharynx

11. Which of the following is true regarding carcinoma of the lip?
    A. Upper lip carcinoma is more common.
    B. The majority present with nodal metastasis.
    C. Sun exposure is an important risk factor.
    D. Radiation therapy is the treatment of choice for most lip cancers.
    E. Prophylactic neck dissection is usually indicated.

12. Which of the following is true regarding salivary gland tumors?
    A. Parotid tumors are more likely to be malignant than submandibular gland tumors.
    B. Submandibular gland tumors are more likely to be malignant than minor salivary gland tumors.
    C. Pleomorphic adenomas may undergo malignant degeneration.
    D. Warthin tumors are malignant.
    E. Facial nerve palsy is common, even with benign tumors.

13. The most common malignant salivary gland tumor is:
    A. Acinic cell carcinoma
    B. Mucoepidermoid carcinoma
    C. Adenoid cystic carcinoma
    D. Basal cell adenocarcinoma
    E. Papillary cystadenocarcinoma

14. A 65-year-old man presents with a persistent firm lateral neck mass that measures approximately 2.5 cm. Careful history and physical examination of the head and neck are negative. The next step in the management is:
    A. Positron emission tomography
    B. Computed tomography scan of the head and neck
    C. Fine-needle aspiration of the neck mass
    D. Chest radiograph
    E. Excision of the neck mass

15. The cranial nerve most commonly injured by a temporal bone fracture is the:
    A. Fifth nerve
    B. Seventh nerve
    C. Eighth nerve
    D. Ninth nerve
    E. Eleventh nerve

Answers

1. C. Nasopharyngeal carcinoma is associated with Epstein-Barr virus. In fact, Epstein-Barr virus titers can be used to follow the response to treatment. Nasopharyngeal carcinoma is endemic in certain areas of southern China. It often presents with a middle ear effusion and can initially be confused with otitis media.

   Reference: Al-Sarraf M, LeBlanc M, Giri P, et al: Chemoradiotherapy versus radiotherapy in patients with advanced nasopharyngeal cancer: phase III randomized Intergroup study 0099, *J Clin Oncol* 16:1310–1317, 1998.

2. E. Treatment of nasopharyngeal carcinoma previously consisted of radiation therapy, but more recently, studies have shown that it is better managed with a combination of chemotherapy and radiation. The combination therapy produces superior survival rates for nasopharyngeal carcinoma compared with radiation alone. In a randomized study, the 3-year survival rate for patients randomized to radiation therapy was 46% and 76% for the chemotherapy and radiation therapy group. Surgery is generally not indicated.

Reference: Al-Sarraf M, LeBlanc M, Giri P, et al: Chemo-radiotherapy versus radiotherapy in patients with advanced naso-pharyngeal cancer: phase III randomized Intergroup study 0099, *J Clin Oncol* 16:1310–1317, 1998.

3. B. It is important to recognize that epistaxis has the potential of being life threatening. Epistaxis has anterior and posterior sources. Anterior epistaxis is most common and is caused by trauma in most cases, which causes rupture of superficial mucosal vessels (Kiesselbach plexus). For anterior bleeds, most of them stop with simple direct pressure. If this fails, then anterior packing is performed. Posterior bleeds are more dangerous and potentially life threatening. Bleeding is most commonly from a branch of the sphenopalatine artery. It is associated with hypertension and atherosclerosis. Direct pressure cannot tamponade posterior bleeds. Treatment involves posterior packing. Posterior packing has the potential to compromise the airway and cause hypoventilation; therefore, patients need to be admitted to a monitored setting. Because it occurs more commonly in elderly patients with significant underlying diseases, posterior bleeds are associated with risk of mortality.

4. B. Most salivary gland tumors are in the parotid gland, and approximately 80% of parotid gland tumors are benign. Submandibular and sublingual gland tumors are approximately 50% malignant, and minor salivary gland tumors are predominantly malignant. The most common type of parotid gland tumor is a pleomorphic adenoma (also called a *benign mixed tumor*). The treatment of choice for benign parotid tumors is a superficial parotidectomy. For malignant tumors, every effort should be made to preserve the facial nerve if it is not invaded by tumor.

5. D. A thyroglossal duct cyst is a remnant of thyroid gland descent. It presents as an anterior midline cystic mass that moves with swallowing or sticking out the tongue. Cysts have a risk of infection and of malignant degeneration; thus, excision is recommended. The operation, known as the Sistrunk procedure, removes the cyst, tract, and central portion of the hyoid bone as well as a portion of the tongue base up to the foramen cecum.

6. E. The presentation is consistent with a cystic hygroma given the age of the patient, the location of the mass, and the fact that it transilluminates. A cystic hygroma is a lymphatic malformation. Most present in the posterior neck, and the next most common site is the axilla. More than half present at birth, and the remainder become apparent within the first 2 years of life as baby fat recedes. Complete surgical excision is preferred; however, if the mass is adjacent to nerves, it is best managed with a conservative excision.

7. A. *Actinomyces israelii* and other *Actinomyces* species occur in the normal flora of the mouth and tonsillar crypts. They are anaerobic, gram-positive, branching filamentous bacteria. They are not acid fast. The face and neck are the most common sites of infection and usually develop after minor trauma or a tooth extraction. *Actinomyces* infections generally occur in association with other bacteria. The infection tends to form abscesses that then drain. Microscopic examination may reveal the classic appearance of sulfur granules, which are masses of filamentous organisms. Treatment is with penicillin and surgical drainage.

8. D. Treatment of carotid body tumors is surgical. Excision should be done in a periadventitial plane. If a sub-adventitial plane is inadvertently entered, this increases the risk of hemorrhage and arterial injury. Because of their vascular nature, biopsy is contraindicated. Routine preoperative embolization is not necessary, but should be considered in large tumors (>4 cm).

9. C. For lesions on the face, anterior scalp, and ear, sentinel lymph node biopsy can be performed as in other areas, but is technically more challenging. However, in the situation in which clinically palpable lymph nodes are present, superficial parotidectomy to remove parotid nodes and a modified neck dissection are recommended. The nodes between the lesion and the regional nodes are removed in continuity. If no nodes were palpable, choice D would be appropriate.

References: Barr L, Skene A, Fish S, et al: Superficial parotidectomy in the treatment of cutaneous melanoma of the head and neck, *Br J Surg* 81:64–65, 1994.

Ollila D, Foshag L, Essner R, et al: Parotid region lymphatic mapping and sentinel lymphadenectomy for cutaneous melanoma, *Ann Surg Oncol* 6:150–154, 1999.

10. B. Patients with head and neck cancers have approximately a 14% risk of the development of a second primary tumor. Most of these are metachronous (beyond 6 months). For laryngeal cancer patients, the most common metachronous malignancy is lung cancer. For patients with oral cavity and pharyngeal cancers, the most common metachronous cancer is esophageal.

11. C. Ninety percent to 95% of lip cancers occur in the lower lip. Sun exposure and tobacco use are the most important risk factors. Lip cancers occur most often in elderly white men. They are most often due to squamous cell carcinoma. Upper lip cancers are usually basal cell carcinomas. The most common presentation is an ulcerative lesion on the vermilion or skin surface. Early-stage lesions can be treated with surgery or radiation therapy, but surgical resection is preferred and is the treatment of choice for larger lesions.

12. C. Salivary gland neoplasms are rare. Most arise in the parotid gland. The ratio of malignant to benign tumors varies by site. Parotid gland tumors are 80% benign and 20% malignant, submandibular gland and sublingual gland tumors are 50% benign and 50% malignant, and minor salivary gland tumors are 25% benign and 75% malignant. Warthin tumors are the second most common benign salivary tumor and are strongly related to smoking. The facial nerve involvement is highly suggestive of a malignant tumor. Although benign, pleomorphic adenomas have a known risk of malignant transformation that becomes as high as 10% to 25% when present beyond 15 years. Fine-needle aspiration is useful in the diagnosis.

13. B. Mucoepidermoid carcinoma is the most common malignant salivary gland tumor. It ranges from low to high grade. Treatment depends on the location. Superficial parotidectomy is indicated for superficial tumors, whereas total parotidectomy is indicated for those that extend into the deep lobe. All efforts should be made to preserve the seventh cranial nerve, provided the tumor does not encase the nerve. The second most common malignancy is adenoid cystic carcinoma.

14. C. In adults, the most likely etiology of a persistent neck mass larger than 2 cm is cancer. Most often the cancer is from the head and neck and is squamous cell carcinoma. Careful physical examination is essential. If the physical examination is unremarkable, the next step is to establish whether the mass is malignant. This is best achieved by fine-needle aspiration. Once metastatic cancer is confirmed, a work-up to locate the primary mass is necessary. This includes a chest radiograph, computed tomography scan of the head and neck, and upper endoscopy of the pharynx, hypopharynx, and larynx with guided biopsies. If the primary mass is still not localized, the role of positron emission tomography is debatable. Several studies have shown that it has a low sensitivity and does not alter outcome.

References: Grau C, Johansen L, Jakobsen J, et al: Cervical lymph node metastases from unknown primary tumours: results from a national survey by the Danish Society for Head and Neck Oncology, *Radiother Oncol* 55:121–129, 2000.

Kole A, Nieweg O, Pruim J, et al: Detection of unknown occult primary tumors using positron emission tomography, *Cancer* 82:1160–1166, 1998.

McGuirt W: The neck mass, *Med Clin North Am* 83:219–234, 1999.

15. B. The facial nerve is the nerve most commonly injured by a temporal bone fracture. This fracture is also the most common cause of traumatic facial nerve injury. Partial or delayed paralysis of the face generally resolves spontaneously, whereas immediate paralysis may benefit from nerve decompression.

References: Darrouzet V, Duclos J, Liguoro D, et al: Management of facial paralysis resulting from temporal bone fractures: our experience in 115 cases, *Otolaryngol Head Neck Surg* 125:77–84, 2001.

Lorenz RR, Netterville KL, Burkey BB: Head and neck. In Townsend CM Jr, Beauchamp RD, Evers BM, Mattox KL, editors, *Sabiston textbook of surgery: the biological basis of modern surgical practice*, ed 18, Philadelphia, 2008, WB Saunders, pp 813–847.

Wein RO, Chandra RK, Weber RS: Disorders of the head and neck. In Brunicardi FC, Andersen DK, Billiar TR, et al, editors: *Schwartz's principles of surgery*, ed 9, New York, 2010, McGraw-Hill, pp 475–512.

Hemostasis 14

1. The first step in the process of hemostasis after vessel injury is:
   A. Platelet adherence
   B. Platelet aggregation
   C. Vasoconstriction
   D. Release of thromboxane
   E. Release of adenosine diphosphate

2. The most important preoperative test to assess the risk of abnormal intraoperative bleeding is:
   A. Bleeding time
   B. Activated partial thromboplastin time (aPTT)
   C. International normalized ratio (INR)
   D. History and physical examination
   E. Platelet count

3. Von Willebrand disease is characterized by:
   A. Normal bleeding time
   B. Lack of treatment response to DDAVP (desmopressin) infusion
   C. Types 1 and 2, which demonstrate autosomal recessive inheritance
   D. Defect in platelet adhesion
   E. Prolonged INR

4. Glanzmann thrombasthenia is characterized by:
   A. Normal bleeding time
   B. Treatment response to DDAVP (desmopressin) infusion
   C. Autosomal dominant inheritance
   D. Defect in platelet aggregation
   E. Prolonged INR

5. The most useful laboratory test to assess both risk of bleeding and response to therapy in patients with uremia is:
   A. Bleeding time
   B. Platelet count
   C. INR
   D. aPTT
   E. Thrombin time

6. Which of the following is least likely to be useful in the treatment of bleeding in the uremic patient?
   A. Desmopressin
   B. Cryoprecipitate
   C. Fresh-frozen plasma
   D. Recombinant human erythropoietin
   E. Estrogens

7. Vitamin K–dependent factors include all of the following EXCEPT factor:
   A. II
   B. V
   C. VII
   D. IX
   E. X

8. In a patient with abnormal bleeding, which of the following findings would make primary fibrinolysis more likely the cause of the bleed than disseminated intravascular coagulation (DIC)?
   A. Normal platelet count
   B. Prolonged thrombin time
   C. Prolonged aPTT
   D. Low fibrinogen level
   E. Increase in fibrin degradation products

9. A 55-year-old patient undergoes surgery, during which a blood transfusion is given. One week later, purpura develops. The platelet count decreases from 250,000/μL to 10,000/μL; and an upper gastrointestinal bleed develops. Laboratory studies establish a diagnosis of posttransfusion purpura. All of the following are true about this condition EXCEPT:
   A. It is more common in middle-aged women.
   B. Severe bleeding is best managed by platelet transfusions.
   C. It can occur after transfusion of packed red blood cells.
   D. It is an antibody-mediated reaction.
   E. Platelet counts typically decrease more than with heparin-induced thrombocytopenia.

10. A 10-year-old boy with a history of hemophilia A presents to the emergency department reporting crampy abdominal pain, nausea, and vomiting. Computed tomography demonstrates mucosal fold thickening and what appears to be a large duodenal hematoma. Definitive management is best achieved by:

    A. Exploratory laparotomy
    B. Laparoscopic drainage
    C. Factor VIII replacement
    D. DDAVP (desmopressin)
    E. Recombinant factor VIIa

11. Which of the following is NOT true about patients with hemophilia B (Christmas disease)?

    A. It is X-linked recessive.
    B. It prolongs the aPTT.
    C. It causes less bleeding than hemophilia A.
    D. DDAVP (desmopressin) is not useful.
    E. It is due to a factor IX deficiency.

12. All of the following statements are true regarding hypocalcemia after massive blood transfusion EXCEPT:

    A. It usually does not correct spontaneously.
    B. It is more common in children.
    C. It is more common in patients with liver disease.
    D. It results from citrate toxicity.
    E. It is more common in patients with severe hypotension.

13. A 35-year-old man has been in the intensive care unit with severe pancreatitis, ventilator dependence, and pneumonia for 2 weeks. He is receiving nutrition parenterally. The INR is 2.0. The aPTT is normal. The total bilirubin level is normal. The platelet count is normal. Which of the following is the most likely etiology?

    A. Factor VII deficiency
    B. DIC
    C. Vitamin K deficiency
    D. Primary fibrinolysis
    E. Chronic liver disease

14. A normal INR and a prolonged aPTT would suggest all of the following EXCEPT:

    A. Factor II deficiency
    B. Factor VIII deficiency
    C. Factor IX deficiency
    D. Factor XI deficiency
    E. Exogenous heparin

15. A 60-year-old man with diabetes presents with right upper quadrant pain and leukocytosis. The patient has a prolonged INR of 2.5 and an aPTT of 60 seconds, a low fibrinogen level, and a platelet count of 70,000/μL. An ultrasound scan reveals gas in the wall of the gallbladder. The most important part of management in this patient would be:

    A. Administration of fresh-frozen plasma
    B. Administration of cryoprecipitate
    C. Checking the D-dimer assay
    D. Emergent cholecystectomy
    E. Administration of platelets

16. Cryoprecipitate contains high concentrations of all of the following EXCEPT:

    A. Fibrinogen
    B. Factor VIII
    C. Von Willebrand factor
    D. Fibronectin
    E. Factor XI

17. The most common cause of transfusion-related death is:

    A. Infection
    B. ABO incompatibility
    C. Acute lung injury
    D. Delayed transfusion reaction
    E. Graft-versus-host reaction

18. Death from a transfusion-related infectious disease is most likely due to:

    A. Human immunodeficiency virus
    B. Hepatitis B
    C. Hepatitis C
    D. Cytomegalovirus
    E. Bacterial contamination of blood

19. Persistent life-threatening bleeding in a factor VIII–deficient hemophiliac with high titers of inhibitors (factor VIII alloantibodies) is best treated with:

    A. A higher dose of factor VIII
    B. Fresh-frozen plasma
    C. Cryoprecipitate
    D. Recombinant factor VIIa
    E. DDAVP (desmopressin)

20. Levels of factor VIII/IX should be increased to what level before major surgery in a hemophiliac?

    A. 10%
    B. 30%
    C. 50%
    D. 75%
    E. 100%

21. Indications for red blood cell transfusion include all of the following EXCEPT:

    A. Availability of predonated autologous blood

    B. Hemoglobin < 10 g/dL, heart rate 110 beats per minute, patient with history of myocardial infarction

    C. Hemoglobin < 8 g/dL in a patient with shortness of breath and oliguria

    D. Hemoglobin < 8 g/dL, diastolic blood pressure 55 mm Hg, heart rate 110 beats per minute

    E. Hemoglobin < 10 g/dL in a patient with chronic obstructive pulmonary disease and confusion

22. After a transurethral prostate resection in a 50-year-old man, persistent bloody urine develops. The patient has no history of bleeding disorders, has had previous surgery without incident, and had a normal preoperative coagulation profile and platelet count. Which of the following is most likely to be of benefit?

    A. Fresh-frozen plasma

    B. Platelets

    C. Cryoprecipitate

    D. Amicar (aminocaproic acid)

    E. DDAVP (desmopressin)

23. Bleeding time is prolonged by all of the following EXCEPT:

    A. Aspirin

    B. Von Willebrand disease

    C. Hemophilia A

    D. Severe thrombocytopenia

    E. Qualitative platelet disorders

24. Which factor deficiency does the INR detect that is not detected by the aPTT?

    A. II

    B. V

    C. VII

    D. IX

    E. X

25. All of the following are true regarding Plavix (clopidogrel) EXCEPT:

    A. It inhibits the binding of adenosine diphosphate to its platelet receptor.

    B. It inhibits activation of the glycoprotein IIb/IIIa complex.

    C. The risk of bleeding complications is increased if it is used with aspirin.

    D. When discontinued, bleeding time normalizes in approximately 2 to 3 days.

    E. It inhibits platelet aggregation within 2 hours of oral administration.

26. Plavix (clopidogrel) has been linked to fatal episodes of:

    A. Aplastic anemia

    B. Thrombotic thrombocytopenic purpura

    C. Idiosyncratic liver failure

    D. Pulmonary hypertension

    E. Pulmonary fibrosis

27. Severe life-threatening hemorrhage is a potential indication for the use of recombinant factor VIIa for all of the following indications EXCEPT:

    A. In association with DIC

    B. In a patient with hemophilia A

    C. In a patient with hemophilia B

    D. In a patient with intracranial hemorrhage

    E. In congenital factor VII deficiency

Answers

1. C. Hemostasis involves four steps in the following sequence: vascular constriction, platelet plug formation, fibrin formation, and fibrinolysis. Hemostasis is also divided into primary and secondary hemostasis. Vasoconstriction is the first response and relies on a reflexive smooth muscle contraction. Vasoconstriction is subsequently maintained by the release of thromboxane A_2, serotonin, and bradykinin. The exposure of subendothelial collagen leads to platelet adhesion, which is mediated by von Willebrand factor. Platelets then release granules and factors into the bloodstream, and form pseudopods. The released substances attract more platelets, which leads to an initial aggregation of platelets. This initial process is termed *primary hemostasis*, is reversible, and is not inhibited by heparin. It is followed by a second wave of platelet aggregation, mediated by serotonin, adenosine diphosphate, calcium, and fibrinogen, which results in an irreversible plug. Aspirin and nonsteroidal anti-inflammatory drugs inhibit this second wave. Fibrin is then formed by activation of the coagulation cascade by either the intrinsic or extrinsic pathway, leading to cleavage of prothrombin to thrombin, which then cleaves fibrinogen into fibrin.

Extensive cross-linking of fibrin leads to formation of a stabilized clot. To prevent excessive thrombosis, fibrinolysis via plasmin follows, which degrades the fibrin clot, thus preventing blood vessel occlusion.

2. D. The most important element in detecting an increased risk of abnormal bleeding before surgery is a detailed history and physical examination. One study showed that in low-risk patients, the aPTT result does not predict the risk of bleeding. Other studies have likewise shown that routine use of laboratory testing is neither sensitive nor specific for determining the increased risk of bleeding. One needs to inquire about a history of prolonged bleeding after minor trauma, tooth extraction, menstruation, and in association with major and minor surgery. In addition, one must make inquiries into medications and over-the-counter supplements that might affect hemostasis. If a careful history is negative and the planned surgical procedure is minor, then further testing is not necessary. A potential pitfall in relying solely on the history is that the history obtained might not be sufficiently thorough or the patients might not recall or recognize that they had previous abnormal bleeding after an operation. If a major operation is planned that is not a high bleeding risk, then a platelet count, a blood smear, and an aPTT are recommended. If the history suggests abnormal bleeding or the operation is either a high bleeding–risk operation or one in which even minor bleeding may have dire consequences (neurosurgery), then a bleeding time and INR should be added and a fibrin clot to detect abnormal fibrinolysis. If there is high suspicion for a history of abnormal bleeding, a hematology consult should be obtained.

References: Chee Y, Greaves M: Role of coagulation testing in predicting bleeding risk, *Hematol J* 4:373–378, 2003.

Klopfenstein C: Preoperative clinical assessment of hemostatic function in patients scheduled for a cardiac operation, *Ann Thorac Surg* 62:1918–1920, 1996.

Suchman A, Mushlin A: How well does the activated partial thromboplastin time predict postoperative hemorrhage? *JAMA* 256:750–753, 1986.

3. D. There are three different types of von Willebrand disease: types 1,2, and 3. Types 1 and 2 are inherited in an autosomal dominant fashion. Type 3 is inherited in an autosomal recessive fashion. Patients have a low level of von Willebrand factor and consequently of factor VIII (because it is a factor VIII carrier). Von Willebrand factor is important in platelet adhesion and platelet aggregation. Patients with von Willebrand disease do not typically present with early spontaneous bleeding in childhood. Rather, they may report easy bruising, mucosal bleeding, or a history of excessive bleeding with a tooth extraction. Treatment is with either intermediate purity factor VIII concentrate (Humate-P) or with DDAVP (desmopressin). Pure factor VIII concentrates do not have sufficient von Willebrand factor. Not every patient responds to DDAVP (desmopressin), so they should be pretested. Von Willebrand disease causes a prolonged bleeding time and a prolonged aPTT. Bleeding time tests platelet function and will also be prolonged with marked thrombocytopenia.

4. D. Glanzmann thrombasthenia is an autosomal recessive disorder resulting from an absence of functional glycoprotein IIb/IIIa. Glycoprotein IIb/IIIa is a receptor for fibrinogen and von Willebrand factor. It results in a defect in platelet aggregation. As such, bleeding time is prolonged. Understanding the pathophysiology of Glanzmann thrombasthenia led to the development of glycoprotein IIb/IIIa inhibitors such as ReoPro (abciximab) and Integrilin (eptifibatide). Treatment is with platelets. Repeated use of platelet transfusions can induce antiglycoprotein IIb/IIIa alloimmunization, rendering the treatment ineffective. In this circumstance, recombinant factor VIIa may be useful.

Reference: d'Oiron R, Ménart C, Trzeciak M, et al: Use of recombinant factor VIIa in 3 patients with inherited type I Glanzmann's thrombasthenia undergoing invasive procedures, *Thromb Haemost* 83:644–647, 2000.

5. A. In uremic patients, the bleeding time is the most useful clinical laboratory test to assess both bleeding risk and response to therapy. The etiology of abnormal bleeding in uremic patients is multifactorial, but one of the most important aspects is impairment of platelet function due to a functional defect in von Willebrand factor, which leads to impaired platelet aggregation. Uremic patients may also have a decreased platelet count, but the absolute count does not accurately reflect their risk of bleeding. The most common bleeding manifestation in uremic patients is excessive bleeding from puncture sites, followed by nasal, gastrointestinal, and genitourinary bleeding. Thrombin time will be prolonged with a low fibrinogen level, which can be congenital or acquired. Acquired causes of low fibrinogen include DIC, liver disease, elevated fibrin degradation products, and primary fibrinolysis, and it may develop during institution of thrombolytic therapy. Warfarin does not prolong thrombin time, whereas heparin does.

References: Hedges S, Dehoney S, Hooper J, et al: Evidence-based treatment recommendations for uremic bleeding, *Nat Clin Pract Nephrol* 3:138–153, 2007.

Weigert A, Schafer A: Uremic bleeding: pathogenesis and therapy, *Am J Med Sci* 316:94–104, 1998.

6. C. DDAVP (desmopressin) seems to enhance the release of von Willebrand factor by endothelial cells. A single dose of 0.3 to 0.4 μg/kg is given intravenously or subcutaneously. It has a rapid onset and relatively short duration. Cryoprecipitate has high concentrations of von Willebrand factor as well as factor VIII and fibrinogen. Recombinant human erythropoietin (Epogen [epoetin alfa]) has been shown to help uremic bleeding in several studies. In addition to stimulating erythropoiesis, Epogen (epoetin alfa) enhances platelet aggregation. The increased red cell mass also seems to displace platelets from the center of the blood vessel and place them closer to the endothelium. Estrogens have been shown to improve bleeding in men and women. The exact mechanism is unknown, but it is theorized that they decrease arginine levels, which decreases nitric oxide. This may lead to increases in thromboxane A_2 and adenosine diphosphate. Dialysis is also effective in the treatment of uremic bleeding. It removes uremic toxins that are associated with bleeding and may improve platelet function. Fresh-frozen plasma does not have high concentrations of von Willebrand factor and thus is not effective for uremic bleeding.

Reference: Hedges S, Dehoney S, Hooper J, et al: Evidence-based treatment recommendations for uremic bleeding, *Nat Clin Pract Nephrol* 3:138–153, 2007.

7. B. Vitamin K–dependent factors include factors II, VII, IX, and X and proteins C and S.

8. A. Primary fibrinolysis is rare and can be very difficult to distinguish from DIC. This is because DIC itself leads to a secondary fibrinolysis. Thus, the coagulation profile can be very similar. Primary fibrinolysis can be triggered by several conditions, including malignancies, shock, sepsis, cirrhosis, and the use of cardiopulmonary bypass. It seems to be induced by the release into the circulation of excess plasminogen activator. Tumor cells contain plasminogen activators. Plasminogen is then converted to plasmin, which degrades fibrin, fibrinogen, and factors V and VIII. The primary treatment for both DIC and primary fibrinolysis is to correct the underlying trigger. However, with primary fibrinolysis, the use of inhibitors of fibrinolysis can be helpful, such as aminocaproic acid, which acts by inhibiting plasminogen activation. Both DIC and primary fibrinolysis result in decreased fibrinogen levels and a prolonged thrombin time. DIC results in the consumption of coagulation factors, so both the INR and PTT will be prolonged. Because plasmin can degrade factors V and VIII, both the INR and aPTT may be prolonged in primary fibrinolysis (depending on the severity, these can be normal). Fibrin degradation products will be increased in both. In pure primary fibrinolysis, the platelet count is normal (as opposed to decreased in DIC). Another distinguishing feature is a normal D-dimer in primary fibrinolysis (as opposed to increased in DIC). Amicar (aminocaproic acid) and antifibrinolytic agents Cyklokapron and Transamin (tranexamic acid) have been used in orthopedic surgery to reduce bleeding. Another antifibrinolytic, aprotinin, was frequently used in cardiac surgery for bleeding but was withdrawn because recent studies showed an increased long-term mortality rate. There is no evidence of an increased mortality rate with the use of Amicar (aminocaproic acid) and Cyklokapron or Transamin (tranexamic acid).

Reference: Ray M, Hatcher S, Whitehouse SL, et al: Aprotinin and epsilon aminocaproic acid are effective in reducing blood loss after primary total hip arthroplasty—a prospective randomized double-blind placebo-controlled study, *J Thromb Haemost* 3: 1421–1427, 2005.

9. B. Transfusion purpura is an uncommon cause of thrombocytopenia and is associated with bleeding after transfusion. It is caused by platelet alloantibodies formed from a previous exposure (pregnancy, previous blood transfusion). The platelet is antigenic, and most people have human platelet alloantigen 1a, but a small minority have human platelet alloantigen 1b. These latter patients, when exposed to human platelet alloantigen 1a platelets, form antibodies against them. The exposure may come from a transfusion of red blood cells or fresh-frozen plasma that was contaminated with a few platelets. Transfusion purpura is most common in women with previous multiple pregnancies. It is much less common in men. It can occur after red blood cell transfusion but has become less common with leukocyte-reduced red cells. The mortality rate is as high as 10% to 20% due to hemorrhage. Diagnosis is made by demonstrating platelet alloantibodies with an absence of the corresponding antigen on the patient's platelets. Treatment is with IV IgG. The resultant thrombocytopenia and bleeding may continue for several weeks. Corticosteroids may also be helpful. The presentation can easily be confused with heparin-induced thrombocytopenia without appropriate testing. A platelet count of less than 15,000/μL is more highly suggestive of transfusion purpura.

Reference: Lubenow N, Eichler P, Albrecht D, et al: Very low platelet counts in post-transfusion purpura falsely diagnosed as heparin-induced thrombocytopenia: report of four cases and review of literature, *Thromb Res* 100:115–125, 2000.

10. C. Spontaneous duodenal hematomas occur primarily in patients with bleeding tendencies. They occur most often in patients who are inadvertently excessively anticoagulated as well as in patients with hemostatic defects. They are well described in hemophilia. Management of duodenal hematomas is conservative, with correction of the underlying bleeding disorder. An upper gastrointestinal study would show a "stack of coins" appearance. Hemophilia A is the result of factor VIII deficiency. Patients are prone to spontaneous bleeding in childhood, particularly hemarthrosis. The most appropriate management would be recombinant factor VIII replacement. DDAVP (desmopressin) can increase factor VIII activity and is most useful in situations of minor bleeding. Factor VIIa is useful but should be reserved for patients who have developed inhibitors.

References: Abbes MA, Collins JM, Olden KW, Kelly KA: Spontaneous intramural small-bowel hematoma: clinical presentation and long-term outcome, *Arch Surg* 137:306–310, 2002.

Gonzalez EA, Jastrow KM, Holcomb JB, et al: Hemostasis, surgical bleeding, and transfusion. In Brunicardi FC, Andersen DK, Billiar TR, et al, editors: *Schwartz's principles of surgery*, ed 9, New York, 2010, McGraw-Hill, pp 67–87.

Jewett TC Jr, Caldarola V, Karp MP, et al: Intramural hematoma of the duodenum, *Arch Surg* 123:54–58, 1988.

Lusher JM, Arkin S, Abildgaard CF, Schwartz RS: Recombinant factor VIII for the treatment of previously untreated patients with hemophilia A: safety, efficacy, and development of inhibitors. Kogenate Previously Untreated Patient Study Group, *N Engl J Med* 328:453–459, 1993.

Rutherford EJ, Brecher ME, Fakhry SM, Sheldon GF: Hematologic principles in surgery. In Townsend CM Jr, Beauchamp RD, Evers BM, Mattox KL, editors: *Sabiston textbook of surgery: the biological basis of modern surgical practice*, ed 18, Philadelphia, 2008, WB Saunders, pp 113–142.

11. C. Both hemophilia A (factor VIII deficiency) and hemophilia B (factor IX deficiency) are X-linked recessive. They are clinically indistinguishable. The severity of symptoms and timing of presentation depend on the percentage of normal factor present, so that patients with less than 1% of normal factor levels present with spontaneous hemarthroses, retroperitoneal bleeds, or intramuscular hematomas. Laboratory features for both hemophilias include a prolonged aPTT and a normal INR and bleeding time. Treatment of hemophilia B is with factor IX concentrate. DDAVP (desmopressin) increases factor VIII levels and is ineffective for hemophilia B. For patients undergoing surgery, factor replacement should begin pre-operatively, be increased to 100% initially, continued to keep blood levels at 50% to 70% of normal until wound healing begins (at approximately postoperative day 2), and then reduced to 30% for a total of 7 to 10 days.

References: Biggs R, Douglas AS, Macfarlane RG, et al: Christmas disease: a condition previously mistaken for haemophilia, *Br Med J* 2:1378–1382, 1952.

Nilsson I, Berntorp E, Löfqvist T, et al: Twenty-five years' experience of prophylactic treatment in severe haemophilia A and B, *J Intern Med* 232:25–32, 1992.

12. A. Severe hypocalcemia with massive blood transfusion is uncommon and does not typically manifest unless the patient is receiving more than one unit of packed red blood cells every 5 minutes. The hypocalcemia is the result of citrate toxicity because the citrate in the transfused blood binds to circulating calcium in the patient. Because citrate is metabolized in the liver, hypocalcemia can be more severe in patients with hepatic dysfunction. It occurs more commonly in children and in patients with severe hypotension. It resolves spontaneously in most patients and does not require aggressive treatment unless the patient is demonstrating abnormalities such as a prolonged QT interval and refractory hypotension.

13. C. Several studies have demonstrated that patients in the ICU have a high incidence of coagulopathy and that vitamin K deficiency is the most common cause. The differential diagnosis for an elevated INR with a normal aPTT would include a factor VII deficiency, warfarin administration, the acute phase of liver disease, and vitamin K deficiency. Vitamin K is not stable in patients receiving total parenteral nutrition, and therefore, in this case, the prolonged prothrombin time correlates with vitamin K deficiency. Factors II, VII, IX, and X as well as proteins C and S all require vitamin K. Vitamin K should be given by parenteral injection at least 6 to 12 hours before a procedure in patients with adequate liver function. In patients with hepatocellular disease, fresh-frozen plasma or whole blood is required. Platelets and cryoprecipitate are unrelated to prolonged prothrombin time.

References: Chakraverty R, Davidson S, Peggs K, et al: The incidence and cause of coagulopathies in an intensive care population, *Br J Haematol* 93:460–463, 1996.

Crowther M, McDonald E, Johnston M, et al: Vitamin K deficiency and D-dimer levels in the intensive care unit: a prospective cohort study, *Blood Coagul Fibrinolysis* 13:49–52, 2002.

14. A. A normal INR and prolonged aPTT indicate an abnormality of the intrinsic system and an intact extrinsic system. Deficiency of factors VIII, IX, XI, and XII would cause this problem. Heparin also prolongs the aPTT without prolonging the INR. Factor II (prothrombin) is common to both pathways, and a deficiency would cause both the INR and aPTT to be prolonged.

15. D. This is a classic presentation of emphysematous cholecystitis complicated by DIC. Elderly male diabetic

patients are at higher risk of emphysematous cholecystitis, and gas in the gallbladder confirms the primary diagnosis. The initial event in DIC is introduction into the circulation of thromboplastic material. This creates a generalized, or disseminated, coagulation, which consumes fibrinogen, platelets, and coagulation factors, resulting ultimately in diffuse bleeding. There is no specific test for DIC, but thrombocytopenia, hypofibrinogenemia, prolonged prothrombin time and PTT, and the presence of fibrin degradation products are sufficient indications to warrant treatment of DIC. Fresh-frozen plasma, platelets, and cryoprecipitate are all important components of the treatment, especially for an actively bleeding patient, but the most important part of the management of DIC is to identify and correct the underlying cause, which in this case is by broad-spectrum intravenous (IV) antibiotics and emergent cholecystectomy. Without removal of the source, DIC will continue to consume transfused products.

16. E. Cryoprecipitate contains all items listed as well as factor XIII. It does not have high concentrations of factor XI. Factor XI deficiency is also known as hemophilia C, occurs more often in the Ashkenazi Jewish population, and is treated with fresh-frozen plasma.

17. B. In a large series of transfusion-associated deaths, just more than half were due to ABO incompatibility, followed by acute lung injury. Graft-versus-host reaction can occur if competent lymphocytes are transfused into an immunocompromised patient, leading to the lymphocytes attacking the recipient's bone marrow and subsequent aplasia.

Reference: Sazama K: Reports of 355 transfusion-associated deaths: 1976 through 1985, *Transfusion* 30:583–590, 1990.

18. E. Bacterial contamination of blood is the most frequent cause of death from transfusion-transmitted infectious disease and was the third most common cause of death overall in a large series (after ABO incompatibility and acute lung injury). The highest risk of bacterial infection is from pooled platelet transfusions. Gram-negative sepsis is the most lethal. Cytomegalovirus is the most common infectious agent transmitted, but because it is so ubiquitous, it is generally not a threat to most patients. One exception is the transplant recipient.

Reference: Kuehnert M, Roth V, Haley N, et al: Transfusion-transmitted bacterial infection in the United States, 1998 through 2000, *Transfusion* 41:1493–1499, 2001.

19. D. With time, as many as 20% to 30% of patients with factor VIII–deficient hemophilia develop inhibitors (alloantibodies) against factor VIII. In situations in which life-threatening hemorrhage develops, recombinant factor VIIa is the best option. Another option is porcine factor VIII, but there is approximately a 25% cross-reactivity with inhibitors. Factor VIIa complexes with tissue factor at the site of injury, resulting in an activation of factor X, which then results in clot formation. The primary concern with recombinant factor VIIa is the potential for inducing thrombosis (stroke, deep venous thrombosis) as well as the cost.

Reference: Kenet G, Lubetsky A, Luboshitz J, Martinowitz UA: New approach to treatment of bleeding episodes in young hemophilia patients: a single bolus megadose of recombinant activated factor VII (NovoSeven), *J Thromb Haemost* 1:450–455, 2003.

20. E. The levels of factors VIII and IX should be increased to 30% of normal to prevent bleeding after dental extraction. Levels should be increased to 50% of normal if major joint or intramuscular bleeding is already present and to 100% in cases of life-threatening bleeding or before a major operation.

21. A. In patients with cardiopulmonary disease, transfusion may be considered because a decrease in cardiac output may cause myocardial ischemia. Stable asymptomatic patients should not receive red blood cells solely because their hematocrit is less than 30%. Indications for transfusion include hemoglobin less than 8 g/dL or acute blood loss in an otherwise healthy patient with signs and symptoms of decreased oxygen delivery. Patients at increased risk of cardiopulmonary disease should be transfused when hemoglobin is less than 10 g/dL.

References: Gonzalez EA, Jastrow KM, Holcomb JB, et al: Hemostasis, surgical bleeding, and transfusion. In Brunicardi FC, Andersen DK, Billiar, et al, editors: *Schwartz's principles of surgery*, ed 9, New York, 2010, McGraw-Hill, pp 67–87.

Rutherford EJ, Brecher ME, Fakhry SM, Sheldon GF: Hematologic principles in surgery. In Townsend CM Jr, Beauchamp RD, Evers BM, Mattox KL, editors: *Sabiston textbook of surgery: the biological basis of modern surgical practice*, ed 18, Philadelphia, 2008, WB Saunders, pp 113–142.

22. D. Patients undergoing a transurethral prostate resection are at increased risk of bleeding from primary fibrinolysis. The fibrinolytic agent urokinase was originally made from urine. Transurethral prostate resection leads to the release of urokinase and tissue plasminogen activator from the prostate. The urine bathes the resected area, potentially leading to bleeding. Bleeding after any operation should always be considered a surgical bleed until proven otherwise. However, several studies have demonstrated efficacy of antifibrinolytic agents such as Amicar (aminocaproic acid) and Transamin (tranexamic acid) in the treatment of bleeding during transurethral prostate resection.

References: Nielsen J, Gram J, Holm-Nielsen A, et al: Postoperative blood loss after transurethral prostatectomy is dependent on in situ fibrinolysis, *Br J Urol* 80:889–893, 1997.

Rannikko A, Pétas A, Taari K: Tranexamic acid in control of primary hemorrhage during transurethral prostatectomy, *Urology* 64:955–958, 2004.

23. C. Bleeding time tests platelet adhesion to an injured blood vessel wall (endothelium). Hemophilia A is associated with a factor VIII deficiency, which manifests as a prolonged aPTT, but does not manifest abnormalities in bleeding time. Drugs that inhibit platelet function, such as aspirin (which works by inhibiting cyclooxygenase), will increase bleeding time. Von Willebrand disease is due to low von Willebrand factor, which serves as a carrier for factor VIII and is necessary for normal platelet adhesion to exposed subendothelium and for normal platelet aggregation. Severe thrombocytopenia (quantitative) and platelet dysfunction (qualitative) both prolong bleeding time. Fibrinogen deficiency also prolongs bleeding time because fibrinogen is required for platelet aggregation.

24. C. The INR detects abnormalities in the extrinsic and common pathways. The extrinsic pathway is triggered by exposure of the injured vessel to tissue factor and starts with factor VII. It then merges with the intrinsic pathway at factor X and is followed by activation of factors V and II and fibrinogen (factor I). Thus, both the prothrombin time and the aPTT will detect abnormalities in factors I, II, V, and X.

25. D. Plavix (clopidogrel) irreversibly inhibits platelet aggregation, so its effect lasts 5 to 7 days. It is indicated in the treatment of acute coronary syndromes and in patients with a recent stroke or myocardial infarction. Use with aspirin increases the risk of bleeding. It has been shown to decrease the rate of a combined endpoint of cardiovascular death, myocardial infarction, or stroke in patients with acute coronary syndromes.

26. B. Plavix (clopidogrel) has been associated with the development of thrombotic thrombocytopenic purpura, even with short-term use (<2 weeks). Treatment is with plasma exchange. The mortality rate is as high as 29%.

27. A. Recombinant factor VIIa binds with tissue factor to initiate the activation of factor X, thus initiating the coagulation cascade via the extrinsic pathway. It was originally designed for treatment of hemophilia A and B as well as congenital factor VII deficiency, but its use has been expanded to other situations with life-threatening hemorrhage, including abdominal trauma and intracranial hemorrhage. In addition to cost, the primary drawback is an increased risk of thromboembolic events. Thus, it is contraindicated for bleeding due to DIC.

References: Gonzalez EA, Jastrow KM, Holcomb JB, et al: Hemostasis, surgical bleeding and transfusion. In Brunicardi FC, Andersen DK, Billiar TR, et al, editors: *Schwartz's principles of surgery*, ed 9, New York, 2010, McGraw-Hill, pp 67–87.

Mayer S, Brun N, Begtrup K, et al: Recombinant activated factor VII for acute intracerebral hemorrhage, *N Engl J Med* 352:777–785, 2005.

O'Connell K, Wood J, Wise R, et al: Thromboembolic adverse events after use of recombinant human coagulation factor VIIa, *JAMA* 295:293–298, 2006.

Rutherford EJ, Brecher ME, Fakhry SM, Sheldon GF: Hematologic principles in surgery. In Townsend CM Jr, Beauchamp RD, Evers BM, Mattox KL, editors: *Sabiston textbook of surgery: the biological basis of modern surgical practice*, ed 18, Philadelphia, 2008, WB Saunders, pp 113–142.

Liver 15

1. Which of the following is true regarding the portal vein?

   A. It typically has one or two valves.
   B. It supplies approximately one third of the blood to the liver.
   C. The normal pressure is 10 to 12 mm Hg.
   D. It is formed by the confluence of the inferior mesenteric and splenic veins.
   E. In the hepatoduodenal ligament, it is usually posterior to both the bile duct and hepatic artery.

2. Focal nodular hyperplasia:

   A. Is typically symptomatic
   B. Is usually centrally located in the liver
   C. Is best resected via formal lobectomy
   D. Poses a significant risk of rupture
   E. Is thought to be due to an embryonic disturbance in liver blood flow

3. The best screening approach for detecting early hepatocellular carcinoma (HCC) in patients with chronic viral hepatitis is:

   A. Alpha fetoprotein (AFP) level
   B. AFP level and ultrasonography
   C. Computed tomography (CT)
   D. Carcinoembryonic antigen level
   E. Alkaline phosphatase level

4. A 36-year-old woman presents with right upper quadrant pain, jaundice, evidence of ascites, and an enlarged liver on physical examination. CT demonstrates marked hypertrophy of segment I of the liver, free fluid in the peritoneum, and inhomogeneous contrast enhancement of the remainder of the liver. This most likely indicates:

   A. Budd-Chiari syndrome
   B. Ruptured hepatic adenoma
   C. Ruptured hemangioma
   D. Acute hepatitis
   E. Schistosomiasis

5. Which of the following is true regarding hepatic adenomas?

   A. They exhibit a central scar.
   B. They tend to appear "hot" on a sulfur colloid liver scan.
   C. Rapid contrast enhancement on CT distinguishes them from focal nodular hyperplasia (FNH).
   D. Management of an asymptomatic 4-cm lesion is surgical resection.
   E. They contain an abundance of nonparenchymal (Kupffer) cells.

6. Management of a hydatid cyst with free-floating echogenic material (type II) of the liver located in the mid right lobe of the liver is best achieved by:

   A. Long-term oral albendazole
   B. Long-term oral mebendazole
   C. Laparoscopic cyst excision with omentoplasty
   D. Open hepatic lobectomy
   E. Percutaneous aspiration and injection of scolicidal agents is contraindicated

7. Management of ascites due to cirrhosis includes all of the following EXCEPT:

   A. Transjugular intrahepatic portosystemic shunt (TIPS) placement in a patient with advanced liver disease
   B. Six-liter paracentesis followed by intravenous (IV) albumin replacement
   C. Spironolactone
   D. Furosemide
   E. Sodium restriction

8. The most common identifiable source of a pyogenic liver abscess is:

   A. Seeding from the portal vein
   B. The biliary tree
   C. Hematogenous from endocarditis
   D. Direct extension of a nearby focus
   E. Trauma

9. The principal mediators of fibrosis leading to cirrhosis in the liver are:

    A. Kupffer cells
    B. Ito (liver stellate) cells
    C. Endothelial cells
    D. Hepatocytes
    E. Clefts of Mall

10. Which of the following is true with regard to the TNM system for patients with HCC?

    A. It includes tumor grade.
    B. It includes AFP levels.
    C. It does not factor in liver function.
    D. It is considered the best classification system for long-term prognosis.
    E. It does not include the number of tumors.

11. An 8-year-old girl presents with upper gastrointestinal (UGI) bleeding. The physical examination demonstrates splenomegaly. Her medical history is significant for a prolonged stay in the neonatal intensive care unit at birth due to prematurity, complicated by necrotizing enterocolitis. She has no history of travel outside the United States. Laboratory testing reveals a hematocrit of 20% and normal bilirubin, albumin, and international normalized ratio. After fluid resuscitation, an upper endoscopy is performed that reveals esophageal varices. The patient is given octreotide and undergoes sclerotherapy. Which of the following studies will most likely determine the cause of her UGI bleed?

    A. Duplex ultrasonography of the portal vein
    B. Duplex ultrasonography of the splenic vein
    C. CT scan of the abdomen
    D. Magnetic resonance imaging (MRI) of the abdomen
    E. Liver biopsy

12. For the patient in question 11, persistent UGI bleeding refractory to repeated efforts at medical management would be best managed by:

    A. TIPS placement
    B. Superior mesenteric vein–to–left portal vein bypass at the Rex recessus
    C. Mesocaval shunt
    D. Splenectomy
    E. Liver transplantation

13. A 45-year-old man with a history of alcohol abuse presents with recurrent UGI bleeding. His history is significant for alcoholic pancreatitis. On upper endoscopy, he is found to have bleeding from isolated gastric varices. The bleeding is controlled medically. On splenoportography, the portal and superior mesenteric veins are patent, whereas the splenic vein is not visualized. Optimal management for this patient would be:

    A. Side-to-side portacaval shunt
    B. Mesocaval shunt
    C. Distal splenorenal shunt
    D. Long-term beta-blocker therapy
    E. Splenectomy

14. A 30-year-old Hispanic man with a history of alcohol abuse presents with high fevers, right upper quadrant pain, and leukocytosis. Ultrasonography reveals a 5-cm fluid collection in the right lobe of the liver. On the CT scan, the fluid collection shows a peripheral rim of edema. The cause of the fluid collection is most likely to be determined by:

    A. Blood cultures
    B. Stool cultures
    C. Percutaneous aspiration of liver
    D. Serologic tests
    E. Liver function tests

15. Definitive management of the patient in question 14 consists of:

    A. Oral metronidazole
    B. Broad-spectrum antibiotics and open surgical drainage
    C. Broad-spectrum antibiotics and early percutaneous aspiration of the abscess
    D. Broad-spectrum antibiotics and CT-guided catheter insertion to drain the abscess
    E. Broad-spectrum antibiotics and laparoscopic drainage

16. The most common benign tumor of the liver is:

    A. FNH
    B. Hepatic adenoma
    C. Hemangioma
    D. Mesenchymal hamartoma
    E. Inflammatory pseudotumor

17. All of the following are acceptable treatment options for symptomatic liver cysts associated with polycystic liver disease EXCEPT:

    A. Percutaneous aspiration, instillation of alcohol, and reaspiration
    B. Laparoscopic fenestration
    C. Open hepatic resection
    D. Oral estrogen therapy
    E. Liver transplantation

18. Which of the following is the best method to prevent a first bleed in a patient with known esophageal varices?
    A. Beta-blockade
    B. TIPS placement
    C. Sclerotherapy
    D. Endoscopic ligation
    E. Selective portosystemic shunt placement

19. A 45-year-old man with Child-Pugh B cirrhosis presents with recurrent bleeding esophageal varices and refractory ascites. The patient is currently awaiting liver transplantation. Which of the following would be the best option if the bleeding is not controlled with medical management?
    A. TIPS placement
    B. End-to-side portacaval shunt placement
    C. End-to-end portacaval shunt placement
    D. Distal splenorenal shunt placement
    E. H-type portacaval shunt placement

20. Which of the following is considered a selective portacaval shunt?
    A. Large-diameter mesocaval shunt
    B. End-to-side portacaval shunt
    C. Small-diameter portacaval H graft
    D. Central splenorenal shunt
    E. Side-to-side portacaval shunt

21. Fibrolamellar carcinoma (FLC) of the liver:
    A. Is strongly associated with hepatitis B
    B. Most often occurs in elderly men
    C. Causes a marked elevation in AFP levels
    D. Often contains a central scar
    E. Has a worse prognosis than HCC

22. All of the following are risk factors for HCC EXCEPT:
    A. Toxins from *Aspergillus*
    B. Hepatitis B
    C. Smoking
    D. Wilson disease
    E. Hepatitis A

23. The Model for End-stage Liver Disease (MELD) score:
    A. Includes an assessment of the severity of ascites
    B. Includes the presence of encephalopathy
    C. Was originally designed to determine operative mortality for portacaval shunting
    D. Is not as useful as the Child-Pugh classification
    E. Predicts 3-month mortality in patients awaiting liver transplantation

24. Which of the following is true regarding the blood supply to the liver?
    A. The middle hepatic vein joins the right hepatic vein as it enters the inferior vena cava.
    B. Veins from the caudate lobe drain primarily into the right hepatic vein.
    C. The ligamentum venosum marks the location of the intrahepatic portal vein.
    D. A replaced right hepatic artery arises from the superior mesenteric artery and is posterior to the portal vein.
    E. The proper hepatic artery gives rise to the gastroduodenal artery in most instances.

25. A 72-year-old woman presents with a sigmoid colon cancer. Metastatic work-up reveals a 4-cm mass in the right lobe of the liver involving segments V and VIII. Which of the following is most appropriate?
    A. Simultaneous sigmoid colectomy and resection of liver metastasis
    B. Chemotherapy followed by sigmoid colectomy
    C. Sigmoid colectomy and 8 weeks later performance of hepatic resection after reimaging
    D. Sigmoid colectomy followed by chemotherapy
    E. Chemotherapy only

26. Which of the following is not considered a poor predictor of survival after hepatic resection for a metastatic colorectal cancer?
    A. Hepatic metastasis measuring 4 cm
    B. Nodes positive in colon primary
    C. Four small hepatic metastases
    D. Hepatic metastasis developing 6 months after primary resection
    E. Very high carcinoembryonic antigen levels

27. The most common primary liver malignancy in children is:
    A. HCC
    B. FLC
    C. Intrahepatic cholangiocarcinoma
    D. Giant cell carcinoma
    E. Hepatoblastoma

28. All of the following are part of the Child-Pugh scoring system EXCEPT:
    A. Overall nutritional state
    B. Presence of ascites
    C. Presence of encephalopathy
    D. Serum bilirubin
    E. International normalized ratio

29. The most widely used test for assessment of hepatic reserve before major hepatic resection is:

    A. Aminopyrine breath test
    B. Indocyanine green clearance
    C. Bromsulphthalein retention
    D. Sulfur colloid scan
    E. Bile acid tolerance

30. Which of the following is true regarding Budd-Chiari syndrome?

    A. Immediate heparinization is indicated.
    B. Diagnosis is best made by portal venography.
    C. The jaundice is caused by presinusoidal liver failure.
    D. TIPS placement is contraindicated.
    E. A nonselective portosystemic shunt is contraindicated.

31. In patients with fulminant hepatic failure, the complication that most frequently leads to death is:

    A. Renal failure
    B. Hypoglycemia
    C. Pneumonia
    D. Intracranial hypertension
    E. Coagulopathy

32. A 30-year-old woman is found to have an incidental 3-cm mass in the liver on CT scan that intensely enhances in the arterial vascular phase. The lesion is "hot" on a technetium-99m–macroaggregated albumin liver scan. Which of the following is true about this lesion?

    A. It is usually centrally located.
    B. It poses a significant risk of rupture.
    C. It poses a significant risk of malignancy.
    D. It is thought to be caused by an embryologic vascular injury.
    E. It is composed of sheets of hepatocytes with no Kupffer cells.

33. Which of the following is true regarding preoperative portal vein embolization before hepatic resection?

    A. If liver function is normal, the threshold for portal vein embolization is a calculated future liver remnant of less than 50%.
    B. It is contraindicated in patients with cirrhosis.
    C. It should not be used in conjunction with hepatic artery chemoembolization.
    D. The preferred approach is the percutaneous transhepatic route.
    E. For a planned extended right lobectomy, embolization of segment IV branches should be avoided.

34. Which of the following factors has the shortest half-life?

    A. I
    B. II
    C. VII
    D. IX
    E. X

35. All of the following are true regarding comparisons of amebic and pyogenic liver abscesses EXCEPT:

    A. Amebic abscesses have a much higher male preponderance.
    B. Mortality rates are similar.
    C. Both are more likely to occur in the right lobe.
    D. Percutaneous aspiration is more likely to be needed with pyogenic abscesses.
    E. Pyogenic abscesses are more likely to be multiple.

36. A 30-year-old woman who is taking oral contraceptives is discovered to have a 4-cm asymptomatic solid mass in the right lobe of the liver on an ultrasound scan. CT demonstrates a central stellate scar within the mass that enhances on arterial phase. Management consists of:

    A. Observation
    B. Discontinuing oral contraceptives, repeating the CT scan in 6 months, and resection if the mass has not decreased in size
    C. Resection of the mass with a 1-cm margin
    D. Radiofrequency ablation
    E. Formal hepatic lobectomy

37. All of the following are true regarding liver hemangioma EXCEPT:

    A. Radiolabeled red blood cell scans are useful in establishing the diagnosis.
    B. Large lesions can lead to thrombocytopenia.
    C. If surgery is necessary, the procedure of choice is a formal resection.
    D. They are associated with high-output cardiac failure in children.
    E. The majority are asymptomatic.

38. A 30-year-old woman with symptoms and signs of symptomatic cholelithiasis is found to have gallstones and a 4-cm mass in the left lateral lobe of the liver on an ultrasound scan. The patient takes oral contraceptives but no other medications. Contrast-enhanced MRI reveals a lesion of low signal intensity with peripheral nodular enhancement, and T2-weighted images reveal high signal intensity. Management consists of:

A. Laparoscopic cholecystectomy with a needle biopsy of the liver mass
B. Laparoscopic cholecystectomy alone
C. A trial of contraceptive cessation
D. Open cholecystectomy with a wedge liver resection
E. Open cholecystectomy with a left lateral segmentectomy

39. The most common cause of intrahepatic presinusoidal portal hypertension is:

A. Alcohol
B. Budd-Chiari syndrome
C. Schistosomiasis
D. Hemochromatosis
E. Portal vein thrombosis (PVT)

40. Which of the following is true regarding a TIPS?

A. It is contraindicated in patients with poorly controlled ascites.
B. It has a significant rate of causing encephalopathy.
C. It is considered to be a selective shunt.
D. It is best used for long-term portal decompression.
E. It has a low 1-year rate of shunt occlusion.

41. A 40-year-old man presents with recurrent bleeding esophageal varices. Medical management and an attempt at TIPS placement also fails. He is still actively bleeding. He is classified as Child-Pugh B. Liver transplantation is a future possibility. Which of the following would be the best shunt option?

A. End-to-side portacaval shunt placement
B. End-to-end portacaval shunt placement
C. Distal splenorenal shunt placement
D. Mesocaval shunt placement
E. Portocaval H graft

42. All of the following are true regarding bile acids EXCEPT:

A. Cholic and chenodeoxycholic acids are primary bile acids.
B. Deoxycholic acid and lithocholic acid are secondary bile acids.
C. Secondary bile acids are formed by intestinal bacteria.
D. After ingestion of food, bile acid concentration in the portal vein increases.
E. Fasting leads to an inhibition of cholesterol 7-hydroxylase.

Answers

1. E. The portal vein has no valves. It supplies approximately 75% of the blood flow to the liver compared with 25% by the hepatic arteries. It is formed by the confluence of the superior mesenteric and splenic veins. The normal pressure in the portal vein is 3 to 5 mm Hg. The portal vein is most commonly located posterior to the common bile duct and hepatic artery in the hepatoduodenal ligament.

2. E. FNH is usually an incidental finding on a CT scan because most patients are asymptomatic, and it is not associated with a risk of rupture or subsequent malignancy. A hallmark feature of FNH is the presence of a central scar on CT or MRI that enhances with contrast. It may on occasion be difficult to distinguish from hepatic adenoma or fibrolamellar HCC. An early embryologic disturbance in liver blood flow is the postulated cause of FNH, which is supported by the findings of regenerative nodules. Resection is indicated when patients are symptomatic or if a definitive diagnosis cannot be made. Lesions are usually located in the periphery of the liver.

Reference: Wanless IR, Mawdsley C, Adams R: On the pathogenesis of focal nodular hyperplasia of the liver, *Hepatology* 5:1194–1200, 1985.

3. B. Screening for HCC is only of potential benefit in patients at high risk of developing HCC. The role and best test for screening for HCC carcinoma in high-risk patients remain controversial. Studies in Asian patients with chronic viral hepatitis showed that a combination of ultrasonography and AFP is an effective screening tool. Recommendations are that AFP alone should not be used and that ultrasonography seems to be more efficient. The benefits of screening high-risk white patients are unclear, as is the cost-effectiveness.

References: Daniele B, Bencivenga A, Megna A, Tinessa V: Alpha-fetoprotein and ultrasonography screening for hepatocellular carcinoma, *Gastroenterology* 127:S108–S112, 2004.

Tong M, Blatt L, Kao V: Surveillance for hepatocellular carcinoma in patients with chronic viral hepatitis in the United States of America, *J Gastroenterol Hepatol* 16:553–559, 2001.

4. A. The patient most likely has Budd-Chiari syndrome, a rare disorder caused by thrombosis of the hepatic inferior vena cava or the hepatic veins themselves that leads to hepatic venous outflow obstruction, postsinusoidal liver failure, and cirrhosis. The classic triad includes abdominal pain, ascites, and hepatomegaly. There are four forms: acute, chronic, asymptomatic, and fulminant. It is often associated with a hypercoagulable state that is either inherited (protein C, protein S, factor V Leiden, or antithrombin III deficiency) or acquired (myeloproliferative disorders, polycythemia vera, thrombocytosis, pregnancy). It is more common in women. The diagnosis can be made by duplex ultrasonography, which will show the thrombosed hepatic veins or inferior vena cava. The most prominent feature on a CT scan is caudate lobe (segment I) hypertrophy and inhomogeneous contrast enhancement. The treatment depends on the acuity of the presentation. Immediate treatment is with anticoagulation. There are rare reports of successful thrombolysis. Subsequent treatment depends on whether the primary indication for an intervention is portal hypertension (TIPS or nonselective shunt) or liver failure (transplantation).

References: Kim T, Chung J, Han J, et al: Hepatic changes in benign obstruction of the hepatic inferior vena cava: CT findings, *AJR Am J Roentgenol* 173:1235–1242, 1999.

Slakey D, Klein A, Venbrux A, Cameron J: Budd-Chiari syndrome: current management options, *Ann Surg* 233:522–527, 2001.

5. D. Distinguishing between FNH and a hepatic adenoma is important because the management of the former is observation, whereas the treatment of hepatic adenomas often requires surgical resection because of their known risk of malignant degeneration and risk of hemorrhage and spontaneous rupture. In a recent study, 70% of hepatic adenomas were symptomatic (abdominal pain), 29% of resected hepatic adenomas had evidence of hemorrhage, and 5% had malignancy present. Thus, current recommendations are that all hepatic adenomas should be resected, provided they are surgically accessible and the patient is at reasonable operative risk. Differentiating FNH and hepatic adenoma is not always straightforward. Both may show contrast enhancement in the arterial phase of a CT scan, so this does not help to differentiate them. FNH characteristically demonstrates a central scar. Hepatic adenomas present in young women and in association with oral contraceptive use. There have been a few scattered reports of the adenomas shrinking with discontinuation of oral contraceptives. Adenomas may demonstrate increased fat signal on MRI compared with FNH. When CT and MRI are unable to distinguish adenoma from FNH, a sulfur colloid scan may be beneficial because adenomas will appear "cold" and FNHs "hot" because of the presence of Kupffer cells. Radiofrequency ablation is another potential option in managing hepatic adenomas, especially when multiple adenomas are present or the patient is not a candidate for a major liver resection.

References: Cho S, Marsh J, Steel J, et al: Surgical management of hepatocellular adenoma: take it or leave it? *Ann Surg Oncol* 15:2795–2803, 2008.

Daniele B, Bencivenga A, Megna A, Tinessa V: Alpha-fetoprotein and ultrasonography screening for hepatocellular carcinoma, *Gastroenterology* 127:S108–S112, 2004.

Herman P, Pugliese V, Machado M, et al: Hepatic adenoma and focal nodular hyperplasia: differential diagnosis and treatment, *World J Surg* 24:372–376, 2000.

Toso C, Majno P, Andres A, et al: Management of hepatocellular adenoma: solitary-uncomplicated, multiple and ruptured tumors, *World J Gastroenterol* 11:5691–5695, 2005.

6. E. Cystic hydatid disease of the liver is due to infection by the tapeworm *Echinoccocus granulosus*. Another species, *Echinoccocus multilocularis*, causes alveolar echinococcosis. Humans (and sheep) are intermediate hosts, whereas dogs are the definitive host. Diagnosis is established by an enzyme-linked immunosorbent assay test for echinococcus antigen, coupled with an ultrasound or CT scan. Characteristic features have led to four types described (Gharabi types): a simple cyst (type I), a cyst with free-floating hyperechogenic material called *hydatid sand* (type II), a cyst with a rosette appearance suggesting daughter cyst (type III), and a cyst with a diffuse hyperechoic solid pattern (type IV). Treatment options for hydatid disease include oral anthelmintic agents (albendazole, mebendazole), laparoscopic or open cyst excision with omentoplasty, formal liver resection, and PAIR (percutaneous aspiration, injection of a solicidal agent, and reaspiration). PAIR has emerged as the preferred definitive treatment for type I and II cysts that are anatomically accessible. It has similar success to surgery with a shorter hospital stay. Drug therapy alone is curative in only a small percentage of patients. For patients whose disease is refractory to PAIR, laparoscopic or open complete cyst removal with instillation of a scolicidal agent generally is curative. If this is not technically feasible, formal liver resection may rarely be performed. During aspiration or surgical treatment of hydatid cysts, extreme caution must be taken to avoid rupture of the cyst. Cyst rupture can result in release of protoscolices into the peritoneal cavity and can lead to anaphylaxis.

References: Etlik O, Arslan H, Bay A, et al: Abdominal hydatid disease: long-term results of percutaneous treatment, *Acta Radiol* 45:383–389, 2004.

Kabaalioglu A, Ceken K, Alimoglu E, Apaydin A: Percutaneous imaging-guided treatment of hydatid liver cysts: do long-term results make it a first choice? *Eur J Radiol* 59:65–73, 2006.

Khuroo M, Wani N, Javid G, et al: Percutaneous drainage compared with surgery for hepatic hydatid cysts, *N Engl J Med* 337:881–887, 1997.

7. A. The initial treatment of ascites in a patient with cirrhosis includes a low sodium diet and the use of the diuretics spironolactone and furosemide. In the majority of patients, this approach is successful. If the ascites is refractory to this management, the next step is large-volume (4–6 L) paracentesis. The paracentesis should be followed by an IV infusion of 25% salt-poor albumin. If the ascites is still not responsive, serial large-volume paracentesis can be used. A TIPS is another option, but should be reserved for patients with reasonably good liver function because those with advanced liver disease will have a high risk of the development of encephalopathy and hepatic decompensation. In the latter patient, the ideal option would be a liver transplantation. Peritoneovenous shunting is now rarely used because it has a high rate of shunt clotting and can induce disseminated intravascular coagulation.

Reference: Choudhury J, Sanyal A: Treatment of ascites, *Curr Treat Options Gastroenterol* 6:481–491, 2003.

8. B. The classic triad associated with pyogenic liver abscess consists of right upper quadrant pain, fever, and jaundice, although only 10% of patients have all three features. Pyogenic liver abscess remains a highly lethal disease, with mortality rates, even in more recent large series, ranging from 10% to 20%. The most common etiology of pyogenic liver abscesses is the biliary tract. In most instances, management consists of IV antibiotics with percutaneous aspiration of the abscess with or without catheter drainage. Other etiologies include seeding of the portal vein from diverticular disease, appendicitis, inflammatory bowel disease, and systemic infections such as bacterial endocarditis. In a high percentage of pyogenic liver abscesses, the source is unclear, however.

Reference: Chu K, Fan S, Lai E, et al: Pyogenic liver abscess: an audit of experience over the past decade, *Arch Surg* 131:148–152, 1996.

9. B. The Ito cells are also known as the hepatic stellate cells. They are located in the Disse space and are characterized by the presence of lipid droplets because they store vitamin A. Ito cells play an important role in the liver's response to acute liver injury as well as in chronic liver injury. In these settings, the Ito cell differentiates into a myofibroblast-like cell that has a high capacity for fibrogenesis.

Reference: Hautekeete ML, Geerts A: The hepatic stellate (Ito) cell: its role in human liver disease, *Virchows Arch* 430:195–207, 1997.

10. C. Numerous classification systems have been developed for HCC. None have been universally accepted as the gold standard. The primary critique of the TNM system is that it does not factor in hepatic reserve, which is an important predictor of long-term survival in these patients. Several classification systems have been devised to try to incorporate tumor characteristics with liver function. These include the Japan Integrated Staging score, Cancer of the Liver Italian Program score, and Barcelona Clinic Liver Cancer Staging score. The Japan Integrated Staging score appears to be the most promising and includes the Child-Pugh grade (based on bilirubin, albumin, prothrombin time, presence of ascites or encephalopathy) and TNM staging. Other factors that have been shown to be important prognosticators in HCC include the AFP level, the alkaline phosphatase level ($<$/$>$400 IU/L), the presence of portal

hypertension, and the presence of PVT. The TNM staging does include the number and size of tumor nodules and whether vascular invasion is present. Tumor grade is not included and does not appear to be an independent predictor of outcome.

References: Cillo U, Vitale A, Grigoletto F, et al: Prospective validation of the Barcelona Clinic Liver Cancer staging system, *J Hepatol* 44:723–731, 2006.

Huang Y, Chen C, Chang T, et al: Evaluation of predictive value of CLIP, Okuda, TNM and JIS staging systems for hepatocellular carcinoma patients undergoing surgery, *J Gastroenterol Hepatol* 20:765–771, 2005.

11. A. Variceal bleeding in children is rare. The combination of esophageal varices and splenomegaly, in the absence of evidence of cirrhosis (normal hepatic function), is highly suggestive of PVT. The diagnostic test of choice is a duplex ultrasound scan of the portal vein. PVT likely occurs due to a combination of factors that contribute to the Virchow triad (injury, stasis, and hypercoagulability). Many children with PVT have a history of neonatal umbilical vein catheterization (leading to portal venous injury), neonatal omphalitis (umbilical sepsis), or neonatal intra-abdominal sepsis (leading to infectious seeding of the portal vein). Some patients may have congenital webs in the portal vein (leading to stasis), and a smaller fraction have inherited hypercoagulable states. In one study of 100 neonates who underwent umbilical vein catheterization, portal vein ultrasonography demonstrated clinically silent portal venous thrombosis in 43%, and only 56% had complete or partial resolution. The etiology of PVT in adults is different. It is more likely associated with malignancy and cirrhosis. In most children, PVT is clinically silent until esophageal varices and UGI bleeding develop. Initial treatment of the bleeding varices is similar to that for adults and includes the use of sclerotherapy or banding as well as octreotide. Because PVT in children is not usually associated with cirrhosis, liver function is intact, and the overall prognosis for these children is reasonably good. Nevertheless, a portosystemic shunt should be considered in patients who are refractory to medical management.

References: Kim JH, Lee YS, Kim SH, et al: Does umbilical vein catheterization lead to portal venous thrombosis? Prospective US evaluation in 100 neonates, *Radiology* 219:645–650, 2001.

Schettino GC, Fagundes ED, Roquete ML, et al: Portal vein thrombosis in children and adolescents, *J Pediatr (Rio J)* 82: 171–178, 2006.

12. B. For children with PVT and recurrent refractory UGI bleeding, the superior mesenteric vein–to–left portal vein bypass at the Rex recessus (known as the Rex shunt) seems to be the most advantageous shunt because it serves the dual function of decompressing the portal system while simultaneously restoring some blood flow to the liver. The bypass is performed most often using the internal jugular vein. This shunt seems to have the best chance to prevent long-term behavioral, growth, and personality disorders noted after the use of other portosystemic shunts in children.

References: Ates O, Hakgüder G, Olguner M, et al: Mesenterico left portal bypass for variceal bleeding owing to extrahepatic portal hypertension caused by portal vein thrombosis, *J Pediatr Surg* 41:1259–1263, 2006.

Fuchs J, Warmann S, Kardorff R, et al: Mesenterico-left portal vein bypass in children with congenital extrahepatic portal vein thrombosis: a unique curative approach, *J Pediatr Gastroenterol Nutr* 36:213–216, 2003.

13. E. The finding of isolated gastric varices, without esophageal varices, is highly suggestive of splenic vein thrombosis. This condition leads to venous outflow obstruction of the spleen, resulting in massively dilated short gastric veins. The most common cause of splenic vein thrombosis is chronic pancreatitis, which leads to perivenous inflammation. It has been reported to occur in 4% to 8% of patients with chronic pancreatitis. Splenic vein thrombosis with gastric variceal formation is referred to as left-sided or sinistral portal hypertension. The mortality rate for gastric variceal bleeding exceeds 20%. Splenectomy is curative. Controversy exists as to whether prophylactic splenectomy is necessary when asymptomatic gastric varices are discovered in association with splenic vein thrombosis. A recent study suggests that gastric variceal bleeding from pancreatitis-induced splenic vein thrombosis occurs in only 4% of patients. Thus, prophylactic splenectomy is not recommended in asymptomatic patients, nor is it recommended concomitant with another planned abdominal operation.

References: Agarwal A, Raj Kumar K, Agarwal S, Singh S: Significance of splenic vein thrombosis in chronic pancreatitis, *Am J Surg* 196:149–154, 2008.

Heider TR, Azeem S, Galanko J, Behrns K: The natural history of pancreatitis-induced splenic vein thrombosis, *Ann Surg* 239: 876–880, 2004.

Weber S, Rikkers L: Splenic vein thrombosis and gastrointestinal bleeding in chronic pancreatitis, *World J Surg* 27:1271–1274, 2003.

14. D. The diagnosis of an amebic liver abscess is made using a combination of the clinical presentation, ultrasound and CT scan features, and serologic testing. The causative organism is *Entamoeba histolytica*. Humans ingest the cysts through a fecal-oral route. The cyst becomes a trophozoite in the colon and invades the colonic mucosa, resulting in a diarrheal illness. The organism then reaches the liver via the portal vein. It leads to a liquefaction necrosis of the liver, leading to the description of an "anchovy paste" appearance of the fluid, which is a combination of blood and liquefied hepatic tissue. The infection is much more common in endemic areas such as Central and South America, India, and Africa or in those individuals who have had recent travel to those locations. Less than one third of patients will have a history of a diarrheal illness. Amebic liver abscesses are much more common in patients with a history of heavy alcohol consumption, suggesting that alcohol increases susceptibility. CT scanning can help distinguish amebic liver abscesses from other entities, such as a pyogenic abscess and echinococcal cysts. The classic finding on CT is that of a single fluid collection in the right lobe with a rim of peripheral edema. Culturing the liver abscess or stool does not usually yield ameba. The best test to establish the diagnosis is serologic testing using enzyme immunoassays. Conservative medical management of amebic liver abscess is safe. Percutaneous ultrasonography-guided aspiration is indicated only in patients who fail to improve clinically after 48 to 72 hours.

References: Blessmann J, Binh H, Hung D, et al: Treatment of amoebic liver abscess with metronidazole alone or in combination with ultrasound-guided needle aspiration: a comparative, prospective and randomized study, *Trop Med Int Health* 8:1030–1034, 2003.

McGarr PL, Madiba TE, Thomson SR, Corr P: Amoebic liver abscess—results of a conservative management policy, *S Afr Med J* 93:132–136, 2003.

15. A. Amebic liver abscesses respond very well to oral metronidazole. Several studies have investigated whether percutaneous drainage is needed. Given the rapid response to oral metronidazole, aspiration or catheter-directed drainage is unnecessary in the majority of cases. Aspiration is only indicated if the diagnosis of amebic liver abscess is uncertain or if the patient does not respond appropriately to antibiotics within a few days. Metronidazole is administered for 7 to 10 days.

References: Akgun Y, Tacyildiz I, Celik Y: Amebic liver abscess: changing trends over 20 years, *World J Surg* 23:102–106, 1999.

Blessmann J, Binh H, Hung D, et al: Treatment of amoebic liver abscess with metronidazole alone or in combination with ultrasound-guided needle aspiration: a comparative, prospective and randomized study, *Trop Med Int Health* 8:1030–1034, 2003.

McGarr PL, Madiba TE, Thomson SR, Corr P: Amoebic liver abscess—results of a conservative management policy, *S Afr Med J* 93:132–136, 2003.

16. C. Hemangiomas are the most common benign tumors of the liver. They are usually discovered incidentally and are usually asymptomatic. Diagnosis is generally made by characteristic features of CT and MRI. The main issues to be aware of are that they can sometimes be difficult to distinguish from malignancy and that in children, in particular, giant hemangiomas can lead to arteriovenous shunting with congestive heart failure and thrombocytopenia.

17. D. Polycystic liver disease is an autosomal dominant disorder that is seen in patients with polycystic kidney disease or can be seen with liver cysts alone. The majority of patients are asymptomatic from their liver, but on rare occasion, large cysts can produce severe abdominal pain requiring intervention. Given the rarity of polycystic liver disease, a uniform therapeutic approach has not been established. Various strategies have been used with varying degrees of success in symptomatic patients. Percutaneous aspiration, instillation of alcohol, and reaspiration (PAIR) is optimally suited for patients with single cysts, but has been used in polycystic liver patients with a dominant cyst. In patients who are not candidates for PAIR or in whom PAIR failed, fenestration or resection of the cyst can be undertaken, either via an open or a laparoscopic approach. Formal lobectomy is another option. When all other options have been exhausted, liver transplantation has been successful. To date, there is no successful medical management. However, patients are instructed to avoid factors that have been associated with increased cyst growth. Hormone replacement therapy with estrogens in particular has been linked to cyst growth and should therefore be avoided. Recently, octreotide has shown some preliminary promise in retarding cyst growth.

References: Que F, Nagorney D, Gross J Jr, Torres V: Liver resection and cyst fenestration in the treatment of severe polycystic liver disease, *Gastroenterology* 108:487–494, 1995.

Sherstha R, McKinley C, Russ P, et al: Postmenopausal estrogen therapy selectively stimulates hepatic enlargement in women with autosomal dominant polycystic kidney disease, *Hepatology* 26:1282–1286, 1997.

18. D. Because of the high risk associated with esophageal varices, numerous studies have been undertaken to try to prevent first-time bleeds. The objective is to reduce portal venous pressure to less than 12 mm Hg without adding morbidity. Prophylaxis is important as the 1-year mortality rate is as high as 70% in cirrhotic patients. Prophylactic sclerotherapy, TIPS placement, and portosystemic shunting have not been shown to be effective. Conversely, both prophylactic β-adrenergic blockade and endoscopic ligation have been shown to be effective. Two large randomized studies demonstrated that endoscopic ligation is even more effective than beta-blockade in bleed prevention.

References: Psilopoulos D, Galanis P, Goulas S, et al: Endoscopic variceal ligation vs. propranolol for prevention of first variceal bleeding: a randomized controlled trial, *Eur J Gastroenterol Hepatol* 17:1111–1117, 2005.

Sarin SK, Lamba GS, Kumar M, et al: Comparison of endoscopic ligation and propranolol for the primary prevention of variceal bleeding, *N Engl J Med* 340:988–993, 1999.

19. A. In patients who are candidates for liver transplantation and have esophageal bleeding that is not controlled by medical management, a TIPS is the best bridge while awaiting transplantation. Emergent portacaval shunting is associated with a prohibitive mortality in most series. In addition, the dissection around the portal vein makes subsequent transplantation much more challenging. Distal splenorenal shunt is a technically demanding, long operation that is not well suited for emergent indications. In addition, it tends to exacerbate ascites, so refractory ascites is a relative contraindication. It is best indicated in the semielective situation in patients who need long-term decompression, who are not candidates for transplantation, and who have recurrent variceal bleeding (once the bleeding has been medically controlled). A recent prospective, randomized study comparing TIPS placement with distal splenorenal shunting demonstrated equal effectiveness of both procedures for refractory bleeding, but with more of a need for reintervention with TIPS.

References: Colombato L: The role of transjugular intrahepatic portosystemic shunt (TIPS) in the management of portal hypertension, *J Clin Gastroenterol* 41(Suppl 3):S344–S351, 2007.

Henderson J, Boyer T, Kutner M, et al, DIVERT Study Group: Distal splenorenal shunt versus transjugular intrahepatic portal systematic shunt for variceal bleeding: a randomized trial, *Gastroenterology* 130:1643–1651, 2006.

20. C. Portal vein–to–systemic vein shunts are classified as either being selective or nonselective. Nonselective shunts are much more effective at decompressing portal hypertension and stopping variceal hemorrhage at the expense of diverting all the portal venous blood flow. Thus, there is a high risk of encephalopathy, especially if the patient already has poor function. Examples of nonselective

shunts include the end-to-side portocaval shunt, side-to-side portacaval shunt, mesocaval shunt, large-diameter interposition shunts, and a central splenorenal shunt. Selective shunts include the distal splenorenal shunts, and a small-diameter portocaval H graft shunt. Selective shunts selectively decompress the portal venous system, theoretically leading to less encephalopathy and less diversion of portal venous flow to the liver.

21. D. FLC has been considered to be a variant of HCC, but recent studies suggest that it is a distinct pathologic entity. FLC generally occurs in younger patients (median age, 25 years) and HCC in older patients (median age, 55 years). Unlike HCC, the majority of patients with FLC do not have cirrhosis, are not hepatitis B positive, and do not have elevated AFP levels. The tumor is usually well demarcated and may have a central fibrotic area. This can make it hard to distinguish from FNH. In the arterial phase of CT scan, the central scar in FNH enhances because it actually represents a vascular entity, whereas the central scar in FLC does not enhance. Likewise, the central scar in FNH is hyperintense on gadolinium MRI. The prognosis overall tends to be better than that of HCC, mostly due to the absence of cirrhosis, but it still only carries a 5-year survival rate of 45%. It is associated with elevated neurotensin levels. Treatment is surgical resection.

References: Ichikawa T, Federle MP, Grazioli L, et al: Fibrolamellar hepatocellular carcinoma: imaging and pathologic findings in 31 recent cases, *Radiology* 213:352–361, 1999.

Kakar S, Burgart LJ, Batts KP, et al: Clinicopathologic features and survival in fibrolamellar carcinoma: comparison with conventional hepatocellular carcinoma with and without cirrhosis, *Mod Pathol* 18:1417–1423, 2005.

22. A. Both hepatitis B and C virus infections are factors for the development of HCC, whereas hepatitis A is not. Cirrhosis is not required for the development of HCC, and HCC is not an inevitable result of cirrhosis. Chronic alcohol abuse and smoking are also associated with an increased risk of HCC. Aflatoxin is linked to HCC. It is produced by *Aspergillus* species and can be found on contaminated peanuts and other grains. Other hepatic carcinogens include nitrites, hydrocarbons, solvents, pesticides, vinyl chloride, and Thorotrast (a contrast agent no longer used). HCC has also been linked to metabolic liver diseases such as hereditary hemochromatosis, α-antitrypsin deficiency, and Wilson disease.

23. E. The MELD score was originally designed to prioritize patients awaiting liver transplantation and includes the serum bilirubin and serum creatinine levels and the international normalized ratio. The score ranges from 6 to 40. It has since been modified to add the serum sodium level because low serum sodium (<126 mEq/L) has been shown to be an independent risk of mortality in liver transplant recipients. The MELD score, in combination with American Society of Anesthesiologists class and patient age, has been shown to be predictive of perioperative mortality in patients with cirrhosis undergoing a wide variety of surgical procedures. The MELD score removes the subjectivity associated with other classification systems. In patients with end-stage liver disease awaiting transplantation, the 3-month mortality rate was 1.9% for those with a MELD score less than 9, whereas patients with a MELD score of 40 or more had a mortality rate of 71.3%.

Reference: Wiesner R, Edwards E, Freeman R, et al: Model for end-stage liver disease (MELD) and allocation of donor livers, *Gastroenterology* 124:91–96, 2003.

24. D. The right hepatic vein drains segments V, VI, VII, and VIII and enters the vena cava. The middle hepatic vein drains segments IVA, IVB, V, and VIII. The middle hepatic vein enters the inferior vena cava jointly with the left hepatic vein via a common orifice. The left hepatic vein drains segments II and III. The round ligament is a remnant of the umbilical vein and marks the location of the intrahepatic location of the left portal vein. The ligamentum venosum is a remnant of the ductus venosus and marks the border between the caudate lobe and the left lateral sector. In most instances, the common hepatic artery gives rise to the gastroduodenal artery and right gastric artery, after which the name changes to the proper hepatic artery. The proper hepatic artery becomes the right and left hepatic arteries. A replaced right hepatic artery arises from the superior mesenteric artery and is posterior to the portal vein.

25. C. The role of simultaneous colon and hepatic resection remains controversial. In highly experienced hands and well-selected patients, the outcomes are favorable. However, simultaneous resection is best conducted in young patients (younger than 70 years old) with favorable operative risk who do not need a major hepatic resection but rather a segmentectomy. Given the patient's age and the size and location of the hepatic tumor, the safest answer would be to perform the colonic resection first.

References: Reddy SK, Pawlik TM, Zorzi D, et al: Simultaneous resections of colorectal cancer and synchronous liver metastases: a multi-institutional analysis, *Ann Surg Oncol* 14:3481–3491, 2007.

Thelen A, Jonas S, Benckert C, et al: Simultaneous versus staged liver resection of synchronous liver metastases from colorectal cancer, *Int J Colorectal Dis* 22:1269–1276, 2007.

26. A. Several studies have analyzed predictors of poor long-term outcome after resection of hepatic metastasis from colorectal cancer. In one study, the factors were positive tumor margin, presence of extrahepatic disease, node-positive primary tumor, disease-free interval from primary tumor to metastases less than 12 months, more than one hepatic tumor, the largest hepatic tumor more than 5 cm, and carcinoembryonic antigen level greater than 200 ng/mL. Using the last five factors, the authors recommended against hepatic resection for those with 3 or more points because the long-term outcome was poor. In another large study, the factors for adverse outcome were similar and included the number of hepatic metastases greater than three node-positive primary tumor, poorly differentiated primary tumor, extrahepatic disease, tumor diameter 5 cm or larger, carcinoembryonic antigen level greater than 60 ng/mL, and positive resection margin.

References: Fong Y, Fortner J, Sun R, et al: Clinical score for predicting recurrence after hepatic resection for metastatic colorectal cancer: analysis of 1001 consecutive cases, *Ann Surg* 230:309–318, 1999.

Rees M, Tekkis P, Welsh F, et al: Evaluation of long-term survival after hepatic resection for metastatic colorectal cancer: a multifactorial model of 929 patients, *Ann Surg* 247: 125–135, 2008.

27. E. Hepatoblastoma is the most common primary liver malignancy in children. It has been associated with familial polyposis syndrome. It presents typically with an asymptomatic abdominal mass, anemia, thrombocytosis, and elevated AFP levels. Treatment is with chemotherapy first and then resection. Chemotherapy enables the subsequent hepatic resection to be less and may make tumors resectable that appear initially to be unresectable.

Reference: Seo T, Ando H, Watanabe Y, et al: Treatment of hepatoblastoma: less extensive hepatectomy after effective preoperative chemotherapy with cisplatin and adriamycin, *Surgery* 123:407–414, 1998.

28. A. The Child-Pugh modification is thought to be a better predictor of hepatic reserve than the original Child scoring system. It includes ascites (none, mild, tense), encephalopathy (none, stage I–II, stage III–IV), international normalized ratio (<1.7, 1.7–2.3, >2.3), bilirubin (<2, 2–3, >3), and albumin (>3.5, 2.8–3.5, <2.8) levels. For each of the five criteria, a point (1–3) is assigned. Child-Pugh A includes 5 to 6 points (no mortality risk at 1 year), Child-Pugh B includes 7 to 9 points (20% 1-year mortality rate), and Child-Pugh C includes 10–15 points (55% 1-year mortality rate).

Reference: Schneider P: Preoperative assessment of liver function, *Surg Clin North Am* 84:355–373, 2004.

29. B. In general, the Child-Pugh scoring system is useful in predicting hepatic reserve after hepatic resection. However, it loses its predictive value in Child-Pugh A patients. The indocyanine green clearance test is the most widely used study for measuring hepatic reserve before hepatic resection in combination with the Child-Pugh score. Indocyanine green binds to albumin and α_1-lipoproteins in liver parenchymal cells and thus rapidly clears from the plasma. It is then secreted in the bile. Hepatic reserve is measured by the amount of indocyanine green retained in the plasma after 15 minutes. If more than 15% remains in the plasma at 15 minutes, this is considered abnormal.

Reference: Schneider P: Preoperative assessment of liver function, *Surg Clin North Am* 84:355–373, 2004.

30. A. Budd-Chiari syndrome is due to thrombosis of the hepatic veins or intrahepatic vena cava. It is often due to an underlying hypercoagulable state. It leads to postsinusoidal portal hypertension, and jaundice develops from hepatic venous congestion. Diagnosis is made by CT scan and duplex ultrasound scan of the hepatic veins. Initial management is with heparinization. Rare reports exist of successful thrombolysis. However, the majority will require some type of surgical nonselective portosystemic shunt. A TIPS has also been used successfully. Those with decompensated liver function may require liver transplantation.

Reference: Slakey D, Klein A, Venbrux A, Cameron J: Budd-Chiari syndrome: current management options, *Ann Surg* 233: 522–527, 2001.

31. D. Cerebral edema and intracranial hypertension are the complications of fulminant hepatic failure, most likely to result in adverse outcome and death. Thus, it is essential to monitor intracranial hypertension as hepatic coma develops with intracranial pressure monitoring. This technology has been shown to be critical to the ongoing determination of a patient's candidacy for liver transplantation. Patients whose intracranial pressure increases to more than 20 mm Hg or whose cerebral perfusion pressure decreases to less than 60 mm Hg will have a high risk of irreversible brain injury. If the intracranial pressure is more than 50 mm Hg or the cerebral perfusion pressure is less than 40 mm Hg, transplantation is contraindicated.

Reference: Sass DA, Shakil A: Fulminant hepatic failure, *Liver Transpl* 11:594–605, 2005.

32. D. The patient has FNH. In contrast to hepatic adenomas, FNH typically is not associated with symptoms and does not pose any risks of rupture or malignant degeneration. These lesions intensely enhance in the arterial vascular phase of axial imaging studies. Characteristically, as many as two thirds of lesions will demonstrate a central scar that enhances in the arterial phase (versus FLC, which remains hypodense). The lesions are often peripherally located. On a technetium-99m–macroaggregated albumin liver scan, FNH appears "hot" because of the presence of Kupffer cells. The etiology is thought to be the result of an early embryologic vascular injury. FNH is rarely symptomatic. In patients with symptoms related to FNH, resection is indicated. Because the lesions are often peripheral, minimally invasive (laparoscopic) approaches to resection should be advocated. Resection of the lesion with a thin margin of normal liver parenchyma is curative, but formal segmental resection should be considered because such procedures are associated with lower morbidity.

33. D. The primary cause of mortality after major hepatic resection in patients with underlying cirrhosis is liver failure. The premise behind preoperative portal vein embolization is to increase the safety margin of a planned hepatic resection. By embolizing and inducing atrophy of the planned area of resection, compensatory hypertrophy of the remaining liver ensues, reducing the likelihood that liver failure will develop. There are two approaches: a transileocolic one that requires general anesthesia and a laparotomy and a percutaneous one. The percutaneous transhepatic approach is generally preferred. In addition to the advantage of requiring only local anesthesia, the transhepatic approach permits direct access to the portal venous branches of the lobe and segments to be embolized via an ipsilateral approach, thereby reducing the risk of thrombosis of the main trunk of the portal vein and vascular injury to the portal venous branches supplying the future liver remnant. Interestingly, hepatocytes in the embolized lobe undergo apoptosis, not necrosis. Main side effects are pain from the transhepatic access site and low-grade fever. If an extended right lobectomy is to be performed, it is important to embolize not only the main right portal vein but also the portal venous branches to segment IV. This approach is important to prevent accelerated growth of tumor, and it also ensures adequate hypertrophy of segments I, II, and III. Transarterial hepatic artery chemoembolization can be used before portal vein embolization. This approach is particularly appealing in patients with HCC because it further helps to prevent tumor growth during the waiting period after portal vein embolization. Portal vein embolization is indicated when the remnant liver volume is expected to be less than 40% with normal liver function and less than 50% when liver function is abnormal, as measured by the presence or absence of obstructive jaundice or an abnormal indocyanine green test result (normal study result is <10% retention of indocyanine green at 15 minutes).

Reference: Kokudo N, Makuuchi M: Current role of portal vein embolization/hepatic artery chemoembolization, *Surg Clin North Am* 84:643–657, 2004.

34. C. Warfarin acts in the liver by blocking the vitamin K–dependent factors (II, VII, IX, and X). Of these, factor VII has the shortest half-life. A deficiency in factor VII manifests by a prolongation of the prothrombin time and the international normalized ratio. Vitamin K is critical in the γ-carboxylation of these factors that are synthesized in the liver. Patients with hepatic dysfunction would similarly display prolongation of the prothrombin time.

35. B. The male-to-female ratio for amebic liver abscesses is approximately 10:1 versus 1.5:1 for pyogenic abscesses. Three fourths of liver abscesses involve the right lobe of the liver. Pyogenic abscesses are more likely to be multiple. Amebic abscesses tend to occur in younger patients and in endemic areas. Heavy alcohol consumption is commonly reported for amebic infection and is also a risk factor for pyogenic abscesses. The majority of amebic abscesses are managed with antibiotics alone, whereas pyogenic abscesses often require aspiration or catheter-based drainage. The mortality for patients with amebic liver abscesses is 2% to 4%; however, the mortality for patients with pyogenic abscesses ranges from 10% to 20%.

36. A. The presence of a central stellate scar is considered diagnostic of FNH when the scar enhances in the arterial phase. FNH is thought to be the result of a response to an in utero disturbance in liver blood supply with a subsequent liver regeneration. There does not seem to be any link to oral contraceptive use and no risk of rupture or malignancy, so the management is observation. The size of the FNH lesion does not seem to be influenced by oral contraceptive use. The only indications for surgery would be if the diagnosis cannot be made preoperatively (particularly to distinguish FNH from FLC) with certainty or if the patient has symptoms (although the presence of symptoms suggests another pathology). Change in the size of FNH on follow-up is rare.

Reference: Mathieu D, Kobeiter H, Maison P, et al: Oral contraceptive use and focal nodular hyperplasia of the liver, *Gastroenterology* 118:560–564, 2000.

37. C. Hemangiomas are the most common benign tumor of the liver and are more common in women. Most are asymptomatic and are incidental findings. Giant cavernous hemangiomas (>5 cm) can occasionally be symptomatic, causing vague upper abdominal pain, and have rarely been associated with the Kasabach-Merritt syndrome, which consists of intravascular coagulation with platelet trapping and activation and the consumption of coagulation factors. It can also lead to symptoms of congestive heart failure. CT and MRI usually establish the diagnosis. Radiolabeled red blood cell scans are accurate but reserved for situations in which CT and MRI are not diagnostic. If surgical resection is indicated and the diagnosis of hemangioma is established, the recommended approach is enucleation, not formal hepatic resection.

References: Hochwald S, Blumgart L: Giant hepatic hemangioma with Kasabach-Merritt syndrome: is the appropriate treatment enucleation or liver transplantation? *HPB Surg* 11:413–419, 2000.

Yoon S, Charny C, Fong Y, et al: Diagnosis, management, and outcomes of 115 patients with hepatic hemangioma, *J Am Coll Surg* 197:392–402, 2003.

38. B. The MRI findings are characteristic of a hemangioma, given the peripheral nodular enhancement and the brightness on T2-weighted images. They have low signal intensity on T1-weighted imaging. Hemangiomas are common benign liver lesions generally discovered incidentally on imaging studies. They may on occasion be difficult to distinguish from other lesions. MRI findings tend to be more specific than CT scan for hemangiomas. Rarely, hemangiomas are difficult to differentiate on MRI or CT scan. Hemangiomas can be definitively diagnosed by a technetium-99–labeled red cell scan with single-photon emission CT. Diagnostic findings include decreased activity on early images and subsequent delayed filling from the periphery. CT criteria that are specific for hemangioma include diminished attenuation on precontrast scan, peripheral contrast enhancement during the dynamic bolus phase of scanning, and complete isodense fill-in on delayed imaging. Given the vascular nature of hemangiomas, needle biopsy is contraindicated. Resection is also unnecessary. Hemangiomas are not associated with oral contraceptive use.

References: Freeny P, Marks W: Hepatic hemangioma: dynamic bolus CT, *AJR Am J Roentgenol* 147:711–719, 1986.

Reimer P, Rummeny E, Daldrup H, et al: Enhancement characteristics of liver metastases, hepatocellular carcinomas, and hemangiomas with Gd-EOB-DTPA: preliminary results with dynamic MR imaging, *Eur Radiol* 7:275–280, 1997.

39. C. Portal hypertension is classified into three types: presinusoidal, sinusoidal, and postsinusoidal. Distinguishing between these causes is important because treatment may differ. Also, unlike the sinusoidal and postsinusoidal types, presinusoidal portal hypertension is more likely to be associated with a preserved liver function. Presinusoidal hypertension is further divided into intrahepatic and extrahepatic causes. Extrahepatic causes include portal and splenic vein thromboses. The most common intrahepatic etiology is schistosomiasis (*Schistosoma japonicum* and *Schistosoma mansoni*). The infection by a fluke leads to fibrosis and granulomatous reactions. In children, congenital hepatic fibrosis is another cause.

Sinusoidal causes include alcoholism and other causes of cirrhosis. Other etiologies include hemachromatosis and Wilson disease. Postsinusoidal portal hypertension includes Budd-Chiari syndrome and congenital webs in the intrahepatic inferior vena cava.

40. B. A TIPS has been shown to be useful in patients who do not respond to medical management of variceal bleeding. It is considered to be a nonselective shunt and is highly effective in the short term in preventing rebleeding. However, because it is nonselective, it has a significant risk of encephalopathy. Thus, it should be used with caution in patients who already have marginal hepatic reserve. A TIPS is also useful in patients with refractory ascites. Recent studies suggest that it is also useful as a bridge to liver transplantation in patients with hepatorenal syndrome. It is not a good alternative to long-term portal decompression because the 1-year patency rate is only approximately 50%. Absolute contraindications to TIPS placement are polycystic liver disease and right heart failure.

References: Colombato L: The role of transjugular intrahepatic portosystemic shunt (TIPS) in the management of portal hypertension, *J Clin Gastroenterol* 41(Suppl 3):S344–S351, 2007.

Testino G, Ferro C, Sumberaz A, et al: Type-2 hepatorenal syndrome and refractory ascites: role of transjugular intrahepatic portosystemic stent-shunt in eighteen patients with advanced cirrhosis awaiting orthotopic liver transplantation, *Hepatogastroenterology* 50:1753–1755, 2003.

41. D. Portal vein–to–systemic vein bypasses are rarely used given the success rates of medical management, TIPS placement, and liver transplantation. The few indications for shunting are when medical management and a TIPS have failed. It can then be a bridge to transplantation. However, if the patient is Child-Pugh C, the quoted operative mortality rate is exceedingly high due to further hepatic decompensation. Thus, it is ideal in patients with better hepatic reserve. The distal splenorenal shunt is too time-consuming to be used in the emergent setting. The mesocaval shunt is the best option of those given. It avoids dissection of the portal vein, thus avoiding the complication of a difficult reoperation for future liver transplantation.

Reference: Ezzat FA, Abu-Elmagd KM, Aly MA, et al: Selective shunt versus nonshunt surgery for management of both schistosomal and nonschistosomal variceal bleeders, *Ann Surg* 212:97–108, 1990.

42. D. Bile salts are made in the liver and then secreted to be used in the biliary tree and the intestine. Bile is composed of bile acids, pigments, phospholipids, cholesterol, proteins, and electrolytes. Bile salts are important for small intestinal absorption of fats and vitamins. Cholic acid and chenodeoxycholic acid are primary bile acids. They are made in the liver from cholesterol and then conjugated with glycine and taurine in the hepatocytes. The secondary bile acids are deoxycholic and lithocholic acids and are formed by intestinal bacterial modification of the primary bile acids. As a result of enterohepatic circulation, 95% of bile acids are returned to the liver via the portal circulation. They are reabsorbed passively in the jejunum and actively in the ileum. Bile salts are important in the absorption of dietary fats and fat-soluble vitamins. Major resection of the distal ileum results in fat malabsorption and deficiency in fat-soluble vitamins because it impairs the circulation of bile acids. It also lowers cholesterol levels because more cholesterol is used to make new bile salts. After ingestion of food, bile acid concentration in the liver decreases and the inhibition of cholesterol 7-hydroxylase decreases, resulting in an increase of bile acid secretion in the liver.

References: D'Angelica M, Fong Y: The liver. In Townsend CM Jr, Beauchamp RD, Evers BM, Mattox KL, editors: *Sabiston textbook of surgery: the biological basis of modern surgical practice*, ed 18, Philadelphia, 2008, WB Saunders, pp 1463–1523.

Geller DA, Gross JA, Tsung A: Liver. In Brunicardi FC, Andersen DK, Billiar TR, et al, editors: *Schwartz's principles of surgery*, ed 9, New York, 2010, McGraw-Hill, pp 1093–1133.

Pancreas 16

1. All of the following are true about tropical pancreatitis EXCEPT:

   A. It is common in adolescents.
   B. It is associated with protein-caloric malnutrition.
   C. It has a familial pattern.
   D. It frequently leads to chronic pancreatitis.
   E. It is not associated with diabetes.

2. Which of the following is the least favorable management option for a chronic large pancreatic pseudocyst?

   A. Endoscopic transpapillary drainage using a stent
   B. Laparoscopic cystogastrostomy
   C. Computed tomography (CT)–guided drainage with a pigtail catheter
   D. Open Roux-en-Y cystojejunostomy
   E. Endoscopic transgastric cystogastrostomy

3. A 65-year-old man presents with a persistent skin rash of the lower abdomen and perineum, accompanied by intermittent vague left upper quadrant pain. A chemistry panel reveals a serum glucose of 160 mg/dL but results are otherwise unremarkable. CT reveals a large mass in the tail of the pancreas. This most likely represents:

   A. VIPoma
   B. Glucagonoma
   C. Somatostatinoma
   D. Gastrinoma
   E. Insulinoma

4. A 45-year-old woman presents with intermittent vague right upper quadrant pain and jaundice. In addition, she notes having greasy, floating stools. A right upper quadrant ultrasound scan reveals gallstones as well as a mass in the pancreatic head. This most likely represents:

   A. VIPoma
   B. Glucagonoma
   C. Somatostatinoma
   D. Gastrinoma
   E. Insulinoma

5. A 35-year-old cachectic woman presents with episodic severe watery diarrhea that has led to multiple hospital admissions for replacement of fluids and electrolytes over the course of several months. Stool cultures are repeatedly negative, and she has no history of travel abroad. On examination, a mass is palpated in the epigastrium/right upper quadrant. CT reveals a large, bulky pancreatic mass with extension into the superior mesenteric vein and adjacent organs. The best palliative management option for this patient's symptoms is:

   A. Octreotide
   B. Streptozotocin
   C. Embolization
   D. Chemotherapy
   E. Radiation therapy

6. Known risk factors for the development of pancreatic cancer include all of the following EXCEPT:

   A. Chronic pancreatitis
   B. Diabetes
   C. Smoking
   D. *BRCA2*
   E. Coffee consumption

7. The most common functional pancreatic endocrine neoplasm is:

   A. VIPoma
   B. Glucagonoma
   C. Somatostatinoma
   D. Gastrinoma
   E. Insulinoma

8. Octreotide scanning is most useful for localization of which of the following tumors?

   A. VIPoma
   B. Glucagonoma
   C. Pancreatic polypeptide-secreting tumor
   D. Gastrinoma
   E. Insulinoma

9. Admission data that have prognostic value for mortality in patients with alcoholic pancreatitis include all of the following EXCEPT:

   A. Age
   B. White blood cell count
   C. Amylase
   D. Glucose
   E. Lactate dehydrogenase

10. Which of the following is true regarding the role of endoscopic retrograde cholangiopancreatography (ERCP) and timing of surgery for acute biliary pancreatitis?

   A. In mild pancreatitis, laparoscopic cholecystectomy can be safely performed within 48 hours of admission.
   B. ERCP with sphincterotomy should be used routinely before surgery.
   C. If a common duct stone is suspected, ERCP with sphincterotomy should always be performed preoperatively.
   D. In severe pancreatitis, early cholecystectomy reduces morbidity and mortality.
   E. There is minimal risk of worsening the pancreatitis with the performance of ERCP.

11. A 60-year-old woman presents with gallstone pancreatitis. Which of the following is the best predictor of a residual gallstone persisting in the common bile duct?

   A. Persistent elevation of the total bilirubin level
   B. A dilated common bile duct on admission
   C. Persistent elevation of the alkaline phosphatase level
   D. Persistent elevation of the serum amylase level
   E. Persistent abdominal pain

12. A 55-year-old man presents with a 12-hour history of epigastric pain, nausea, and vomiting. He has diffuse mild abdominal tenderness to palpation. Laboratory values are significant for a serum amylase of 800 U/L, serum glucose of 130 mg/dL, white blood cell count of 12,000 cells/μL, serum sodium of 125 mEq/L, and triglyceride levels of 1800 mg/dL. The most likely explanation for the hyponatremia is:

   A. Excessive fluid loss
   B. Inappropriate antidiuretic hormone response
   C. Excessive free water replacement
   D. Pseudohyponatremia
   E. Adrenal insufficiency

13. All of the following are true regarding hereditary pancreatitis EXCEPT:

   A. It increases the risk of pancreatic cancer.
   B. It has an autosomal dominant pattern of inheritance.
   C. Patients typically present with abdominal pain in childhood.
   D. Progressive pancreatic dysfunction is common.
   E. It is due to a defect in the steapsin gene.

14. Which of the following are true regarding pancreas divisum?

   A. The duct of Santorini ends in a blind pouch.
   B. The inferior portion of the pancreas drains through the duct of Santorini.
   C. The majority of the pancreas drains through the duct of Wirsung.
   D. The duct of Santorini drains through the major papilla.
   E. The ducts of Wirsung and Santorini fail to fuse.

15. The preferred definitive treatment for recurrent acute pancreatitis due to pancreas divisum is:

   A. Lateral pancreaticojejunostomy (Puestow procedure)
   B. Pancreaticoduodenectomy (Whipple procedure)
   C. Minor papilla sphincterotomy
   D. Major papilla sphincterotomy and pancreatic ductal septotomy
   E. Distal pancreatectomy

16. A 50-year-old man with chronic pancreatitis presents with chronic pain. A CT scan demonstrates no inflammatory masses in the pancreas but does show a markedly dilated pancreatic duct with evidence of strictures, calcifications, and distal obstruction. The best management option is:

   A. Pancreaticoduodenectomy (Whipple procedure)
   B. Total pancreatectomy
   C. Endoscopic stent placement
   D. Extracorporeal lithotripsy
   E. Lateral pancreaticojejunostomy (Puestow procedure)

17. Adenocarcinoma of the pancreas arises most often from which anatomic site?

   A. Main pancreatic duct
   B. Branch pancreatic duct
   C. Pancreatic acinus
   D. Ampulla of Vater
   E. Pancreatic islet

18. A 60-year-old man presents with obstructive jaundice, acholic stools, and weight loss. An ultrasound scan demonstrates a dilated biliary tree and no gallstones. A dynamic contrast-enhanced CT scan demonstrates a mass localized to the head of the pancreas without evidence of distant metastasis, adenopathy, or vascular invasion. The patient is otherwise in good health. Which of the following best describes the role of preoperative percutaneous biopsy of the mass in this setting?

    A. It is highly sensitive.
    B. It is nonspecific.
    C. It is associated with a high complication rate.
    D. It should be routinely performed.
    E. It is unnecessary.

19. All of the following are true regarding alcohol and its relation to the pancreas EXCEPT:

    A. It relaxes the sphincter of Oddi.
    B. It is a metabolic toxin to the pancreatic acinar cells.
    C. It increases pancreatic duct permeability.
    D. It transiently decreases pancreatic blood flow.
    E. It inappropriately activates trypsin.

20. Which of the following is true regarding alcohol and pancreatitis?

    A. It commonly occurs after a single binge of alcohol.
    B. The type of alcohol consumed is an important risk determinant.
    C. Patients consuming a high protein and fat diet are at greater risk.
    D. There is a threshold amount of alcohol consumption below which pancreatitis does not occur.
    E. It typically develops after a mean of 5 years of heavy drinking.

21. Which of the following is true regarding pancreatogenic (type 3) diabetes?

    A. Ketoacidosis is common.
    B. The diabetes is easily controlled.
    C. Peripheral insulin sensitivity is decreased.
    D. Glucagon and pancreatic polypeptide (PP) levels are low.
    E. Hyperglycemia is usually severe.

22. All of the following are true regarding PP EXCEPT:

    A. Proximal pancreatectomy is associated with a greater PP deficiency than distal pancreatectomy.
    B. Patients with PP producing pancreatic tumors present with severe hypoglycemia.
    C. PP regulates expression of the hepatic insulin receptor gene.
    D. PP deficiency correlates with severity of chronic pancreatitis.
    E. It is secreted by F cells.

23. A 60-year-old alcoholic man presents with chronic abdominal pain. He denies a history of pancreatitis and is otherwise in good health. CT reveals a 6-cm multiloculated, septated cyst at the tail of the pancreas. Management consists of:

    A. Distal pancreatectomy and splenectomy
    B. CT-guided drainage of the cyst
    C. Endoscopic cystogastrostomy
    D. Roux-en-Y cystojejunostomy
    E. ERCP with stent placement

24. After a motor vehicle accident, persistent ascites develops in a 55-year-old man. Other than the ascites, CT findings are unremarkable. Paracentesis reveals clear fluid with an amylase level of 5000 U/L and a protein level of 40 g/L. Which of the following is true regarding this condition?

    A. He will likely need surgical intervention.
    B. ERCP is unnecessary.
    C. He will likely need a pancreatic resection.
    D. Paracentesis to completely drain the fluid should be performed.
    E. Somatostatin is unlikely to be of benefit.

25. A 60-year-old man presents with chronic epigastric abdominal pain and jaundice. CT reveals diffuse swelling of the pancreas with compression of the intrapancreatic common duct. Needle biopsy of the pancreas reveals diffuse fibrosis and a plasma and lymphocytic infiltrate. Serum IgG levels are increased. Primary management consists of:

    A. Whipple procedure
    B. Steroids
    C. Chemotherapy
    D. Hepaticojejunostomy
    E. ERCP with stenting

26. A 30-year-old nurse presents with intermittent diaphoresis, trembling, and palpitations. Her fasting blood sugar is 50 mg/dL. C peptide levels are low, and the insulin level is high. Which of the following is the next step in management?

A. CT scan of the abdomen
B. Endoscopic ultrasound
C. Psychiatric counseling
D. Octreotide scan
E. Magnetic resonance imaging

27. Management of pancreatic lymphoma is by:

A. Pancreaticoduodenectomy
B. Chemotherapy
C. Pancreaticoduodenectomy with postoperative chemotherapy
D. Radiation therapy
E. Preoperative chemoradiation followed by pancreaticoduodenectomy

28. The most common cause of chronic pancreatitis worldwide is:

A. Gallstones
B. Alcohol abuse
C. Hereditary
D. Hypertriglyceridemia
E. Infectious

Answers

1. E. Tropical pancreatitis is a form of chronic pancreatitis that occurs in young patients in tropical regions of the world. It is associated with a genetic mutation of the pancreatic secretory trypsinogen inhibitor or *SPINK1* gene. It is also associated with ingestion of the cassava root, which contains toxic glycosides that may lead to free radical injury to the pancreas. There is a familial pattern, and as such, some have theorized that it is simply a variant of hereditary pancreatitis. Patients present with abdominal pain, and diabetes commonly develops as the pancreatitis often becomes chronic. It is also associated with pancreatic duct stone formation. Treatment is with pain medication and digestive enzyme supplementation. Progression may require endoscopic decompression or rarely surgical decompression, although the latter has unsatisfactory results. It is associated with an increased risk of pancreatic cancer.

Reference: Tandon R, Garg P: Tropical pancreatitis, *Dig Dis* 22:258–266, 2004.

2. C. Internal drainage is usually preferred to external drainage for a symptomatic pancreatic pseudocyst that has failed to resolve with conservative therapy. External drainage is associated with a higher rate of complications, including infection and pancreaticocutaneous fistula. Pseudocysts communicate with the pancreatic ductal system in 80% of cases. Internal drainage can be achieved endoscopically via a transmural approach or a transpapillary approach. Surgical options include a cystogastrostomy, a Roux-en-Y cystojejunostomy, and a cyst duodenostomy. Cystogastrostomy can be performed endoscopically, laparoscopically, or with a combined approach. Failure of the endoscopic approach can be predicted by the finding of major ductal disruption or stenosis on ERCP or magnetic resonance cholangiopancreatography.

References: Nealon W, Walser E: Surgical management of complications associated with percutaneous and/or endoscopic management of pseudocyst of the pancreas, *Ann Surg* 241:948–957, 2005.

Yusuf T, Baron T: Endoscopic transmural drainage of pancreatic pseudocysts: results of a national and an international survey of ASGE members, *Gastrointest Endosc* 63:223–227, 2006.

3. B. New-onset diabetes in association with a skin rash and a pancreatic mass in the tail is highly suggestive of a glucagonoma. The rash is termed *necrolytic migratory erythema* and tends to manifest on the lower abdomen or perineum. The diagnosis is confirmed by measuring glucagon levels. Because the tumors are in the distal pancreas, the patient does not usually present with jaundice; as such, the diagnosis is often made late when the tumor is large.

4. C. Most pancreatic head tumors represent adenocarcinoma. However, in the setting of pancreatic exocrine insufficiency, as manifested by steatorrhea and gallstones, the most likely endocrine tumor would be somatostatinoma because it inhibits pancreatic and biliary secretions. They are most common in the proximal pancreas and are usually metastatic at the time of presentation. The diagnosis is confirmed by an elevated somatostatin level.

5. A. The patient most likely has a VIPoma (vasoactive intestinal polypeptide). It has also been termed *WDHA* (watery diarrhea, hypokalemia, and achlorhydria) and Verner-Morrison syndrome. Patients have large-volume secretory diarrhea and can lose enormous amounts of fluids and electrolytes. Diagnosis is by CT scan, and most tumors are in the tail of the pancreas and have metastasized at the time of diagnosis. Another useful imaging tool is endoscopic ultrasonography. Even with distant metastasis, however, tumor debulking, hepatic artery embolization, and radiofrequency ablation of liver metastasis are useful in controlling symptoms. The best medical treatment of symptoms is achieved with octreotide, a somatostatin analogue.

Reference: Nguyen H, Backes B, Lammert F, et al.: Long-term survival after diagnosis of hepatic metastatic VIPoma: report of two cases with disparate courses and review of therapeutic options, *Dig Dis Sci* 44:1148–1155, 1999.

6. E. Coffee drinking has not been shown to be a risk factor for pancreatic cancer. Factors that are associated with a risk for pancreatic cancer include obesity, atypical multiple mole melanoma, hereditary pancreatitis, familial adenomatous polyposis, hereditary nonpolyposis colon cancer, and Peutz-Jeghers syndrome. The role of alcohol in pancreatic cancer is debatable.

7. E. Insulinoma is the most common functional pancreatic endocrine neoplasm. The classic feature is the Whipple triad, which includes symptomatic fasting hypoglycemia, a documented serum glucose level of less than 50 mg/dL, and relief of symptoms with the administration of glucose. Patients will often present with recurrent episodes of syncope. They may also report palpitations, trembling, diaphoresis, confusion or disorientation, and seizures. The diagnosis is confirmed by demonstrating a low fasting blood sugar and an elevated C peptide level. Localization is achieved by CT scan and endoscopic ultrasonography. They are evenly distributed throughout the head, body, and tail of the pancreas. The majority are benign (90%). On occasion, they cannot be localized preoperatively, in which case, intraoperative ultrasonography is useful. They can be treated with enucleation.

Reference: Halfdanarson T, Rubin J, Farnell M, et al: Pancreatic endocrine neoplasms: epidemiology and prognosis of pancreatic endocrine tumors, *Endocr Relat Cancer* 15:409–427, 2008.

8. D. Many pancreatic endocrine tumors have high concentrations of somatostatin receptors and can therefore be imaged with a radiolabeled form of the somatostatin analogue octreotide (indium-111 pentetreotide). Octreotide scanning has the advantage of whole-body scanning, which is useful in gastrinomas because they can present in a wide area. Used in combination with endoscopic ultrasonography, it detects more than 90% of gastrinomas. It is also useful for localizing carcinoid tumors. As many as 90% of gastrinomas are found in the Passaro triangle, an area defined by the junction of the cystic duct and common bile duct, the second and third portions of the duodenum, and the neck and body of the pancreas. Although a CT scan is also useful, the octreotide scan is particularly helpful in localizing gastrinomas smaller than 1 cm. Somatostatinomas and VIPomas tend to be large bulky tumors and are thus readily seen by CT. Octreotide scanning will miss as many as 40% of insulinomas because they may not express sufficient somatostatin receptors.

Reference: de Herder W, Kwekkeboom D, Valkema R, et al: Neuroendocrine tumors and somatostatin: imaging techniques, *J Endocrinol Invest* 28(11 Suppl Int):132–136, 2005.

9. C. The amylase level does not correlate with severity of pancreatitis. Admission Ranson criteria for acute pancreatitis

not due to gallstones include age older than 55 years, white blood cell count more than 16,000 cells/μL, blood glucose level greater than 200 mg/dL, serum lactate dehydrogenase greater than 350 IU/L, and aspartate aminotransferase level greater than 250 IU/L. Additional criteria at 48 hours include hematocrit decrease more than 10%, blood urea nitrogen elevation more than 5%, serum calcium level less than 8 mg/dL, arterial P_{O_2} less than 60 mm Hg, base deficit more than 4 mg/dL, and fluid sequestration more than 6 L.

10. A. Gallstones are the most common cause of acute pancreatitis worldwide and thought to be due to a gallstone-causing transient obstruction at the ampulla of Vater. It most cases, the inflammation is mild to moderate, and the stone passes into the intestine spontaneously. In patients with severe pancreatitis, early cholecystectomy is associated with an increased morbidity and mortality, so that cholecystectomy should be delayed until the pancreatitis is resolved. In mild to moderate pancreatitis, the timing of surgery is not critical, and early cholecystectomy (within 48 hours) can be performed safely. However, long delays result in as much as a 30% recurrence of pancreatitis. Routine ERCP to detect the presence of common duct stones is unnecessary because the probability of finding residual stones is low and the risk of ERCP-induced pancreatitis is significant. Preoperative ERCP should be reserved for patients with concomitant cholangitis or clear evidence of biliary obstruction (jaundice, persistent elevation of total bilirubin > 4 mg/dL). Otherwise, an intraoperative cholangiogram should be performed, and if a common bile duct stone is detected, either a laparoscopic common duct exploration or a postoperative ERCP should be performed.

References: Chang L, Lo S, Stabile B, et al: Preoperative versus postoperative endoscopic retrograde cholangiopancreatography in mild to moderate gallstone pancreatitis: a prospective randomized trial intervention, *Ann Surg* 231:82–87, 2000.

Kelly T, Wagner D: Gallstone pancreatitis: a prospective randomized trial of the timing of surgery, *Surgery* 104:600–605, 1988.

Rosing D, de Virgilio C, Yaghoubian A, et al: Early cholecystectomy for mild to moderate gallstone pancreatitis shortens hospital stay, *J Am Coll Surg* 205:762–766, 2007.

11. A. Persistent elevation of the total bilirubin is the best predictor of a residual common bile duct stone. Because the pathophysiology of gallstone pancreatitis is transient obstruction of the ampulla of Vater by a gallstone, a significant number of patients will have some degree of common bile duct dilation on admission; as such, common bile duct dilation is not a specific finding. This differs from patients with symptomatic cholelithiasis in which ductal dilation is frequently associated with common duct stones.

References: Chan T, Yaghoubian A, Rosing D, et al: Total bilirubin is a useful predictor of persisting common bile duct stone in gallstone pancreatitis, *Am Surg* 74:977–980, 2008.

Chang L, Lo S, Stabile B, et al: Gallstone pancreatitis: a prospective study on the incidence of cholangitis and clinical predictors of retained common bile duct stones, *Am J Gastroenterol* 93:527–531, 1998.

12. D. Severe hypertriglyceridemia leads to a falsely low sodium level. Water is displaced in the serum by lipids, resulting in an error in measurement. The danger is that the clinician who is unaware may try to correct the hyponatremia with hypertonic saline, leading to severe hypernatremia.

   Reference: Howard J, Reed J: Pseudohyponatremia in acute hyperlipemic pancreatitis: a potential pitfall in therapy, *Arch Surg* 120:1053–1055, 1985.

13. E. Hereditary pancreatitis is thought to be due to a defect in trypsin inactivation in the pancreas. It is an autosomal dominant condition with equal distribution in both sexes. The genetic defect is localized to chromosome 7q35 and is caused by a missense mutation resulting in Arg to His substitution at position 117 of the trypsinogen gene or *PRSS1*. This mutation prevents trypsin from being inactivated and results in uncontrolled proteolytic activity and autodestruction of the pancreas. Typically, patients present in childhood or adolescence with abdominal pain and are found to have calcifications within the pancreas on imaging studies. Progressive pancreatic dysfunction is common, and many patients present with symptoms caused by pancreatic duct obstruction. The risk of subsequent carcinoma has been reported to be as high as 40%. Patients typically present within the first two decades of life. Steapsin degrades triglycerides into fatty acids and glycerol, but is not defective in this condition.

   Reference: Whitcomb D, Preston R, Aston C, et al.: A gene for hereditary pancreatitis maps to chromosome 7q35, *Gastroenterology* 110:1975–1980, 1996.

14. E. In pancreatic divisum, the ducts of Wirsung and Santorini fail to fuse. The result is that the majority of the pancreas drains through the duct of Santorini and through the lesser papilla. The inferior portion of the pancreatic head and uncinate process drains through the duct of Wirsung and the major papilla. It is considered a normal anatomic variant and is seen in 10% of individuals. It is thought to lead to an increased risk of pancreatitis because the minor papilla sometimes cannot handle the higher flow of pancreatic juices. In another more common variant, the duct of Santorini ends in a blind pouch but still fuses with the Wirsung duct.

15. C. Pancreas divisum can lead to recurrent episodes of acute pancreatitis as well as chronic pancreatitis with intractable pain. Unlike other forms of chronic pancreatitis, however, marked dilation of the dorsal duct is unusual. As such, surgical decompressive procedures are not successful. For patients with recurrent attacks of acute pancreatitis, the best option is sphincterotomy of the minor papilla because the duct of Santorini is providing the primary drainage to the pancreas. A recent study from Marseille found a decreased rate of acute pancreatitis in 24 patients after minor papilla sphincterotomy and dorsal duct stenting. The complication rate was lower with sphincterotomy than with stent insertion. Major papilla sphincterotomy would not likely be helpful because it drains a minority of the pancreas in pancreatic divisum.

   Reference: Heyries L, Barthet M, Delvasto C, et al: Long-term results of endoscopic management of pancreas divisum with recurrent acute pancreatitis, *Gastrointest Endosc* 55:376–381, 2002.

16. E. Surgical drainage of a dilated pancreatic duct with distal obstruction is more effective than endoscopic approaches in patients with chronic pancreatitis. The Puestow procedure involves cutting open the length of the main pancreatic duct and anastomosing a Roux limb of jejunum to the duct.

   Reference: Cahen D, Gouma D, Nio Y, et al: Endoscopic versus surgical drainage of the pancreatic duct in chronic pancreatitis, *N Engl J Med* 356:676–684, 2007.

17. A. The majority of adenocarcinomas of the pancreas arise from the main pancreatic duct. Approximately 66% of pancreatic adenocarcinomas develop within the head or uncinate process of the pancreas.

18. E. In a patient with obstructive jaundice, the first study to perform is an ultrasound scan. In the absence of abdominal pain and in the presence of weight loss, it is highly likely that the diagnosis is malignancy. A dynamic, contrast-enhanced CT scan is highly effective in determining the resectability of the mass. More recently, the addition of endoscopic ultrasonography has aided in determining resectability. In particular, it is useful in determining invasion of the superior mesenteric vein or portal vein, which most surgeons would consider a contraindication to surgery. In the situation in which the mass appears to be resectable, percutaneous or endoscopic ultrasonography–guided biopsy is not considered necessary. Needle biopsy is prone to sampling error; therefore, a negative biopsy finding would not alter the plan to perform a Whipple procedure. Likewise a positive biopsy finding would not alter the operative decision. Operative morbidity and mortality after the Whipple procedure are sufficiently low that one would accept the low likelihood (~5%) that the lesion is benign. Biopsy should be reserved for situations in which the lesion appears to be unresectable because it may guide chemotherapy. It is also indicated in situations in which the appearance of the mass suggests other less common pathologies such as pancreatic lymphoma.

19. A. The exact mechanism by which alcohol induces pancreatitis is unclear; however, all the listed effects have been shown to be adverse effects of alcohol. Ethanol actually induces spasm of the sphincter of Oddi, and this may lead to an increase in ductal pressure with a simultaneous brief stimulation of pancreatic secretion.

20. C. Most patients with alcohol-related pancreatitis have a long-standing history of heavy drinking. The mean number of years of drinking at the time of presentation with pancreatitis is 18 years in men and 11 years in women. The type of alcohol consumed is not important, but rather the quantity and duration. The mean amount consumed in patients in whom pancreatitis develops is 100 to 175 g/day, although it can rarely develop after just one binge. In alcoholics, the first attack of pancreatitis may represent an acute exacerbation of chronic pancreatitis, and the patient may have had repeat subclinical bouts of acute pancreatitis previously. The risk of pancreatitis seems to be higher in patients who have a diet high in protein and fat.

21. D. For diabetes to develop as a result of pancreatitis, extensive destruction of the pancreas must occur. Diabetes in the setting of chronic pancreatitis or after pancreatic resection is termed *type 3 diabetes*. It differs from type 1 and 2 diabetes in that it is associated with decreased glucagon and PP levels as well as insulin due to pancreatic loss or destruction. Because all three of these hormones regulate glucose levels, the diabetes that ensues is considered to be difficult to control. Furthermore, peripheral insulin sensitivity is increased, whereas hepatic insulin sensitivity is decreased. The result is that patients are prone to the development of hypoglycemia, but ketoacidosis and marked hyperglycemia are rare.

22. B. PP seems to have an important role in glucose metabolism. PP regulates the expression of the hepatic insulin receptor gene. PP cells are primarily located in the proximal pancreas, in the uncinate process and posterior head. Thus, proximal pancreatic resections are more likely to result in PP deficiency than distal pancreatectomy. Therefore, in patients who have undergone proximal pancreatectomy or have severe chronic pancreatitis, diminished hepatic insulin sensitivity develops. A few rare cases of PPomas have been reported. However, they do not seem to cause any specific symptoms. PP cells are also called *F cells*.

References: Brunicardi F, Chaiken R, Ryan A: Pancreatic polypeptide administration improves abnormal glucose metabolism in patients with chronic pancreatitis, *J Clin Endocrinol Metab* 81:3566–3572, 1996.

Slezak L, Andersen D: Pancreatic resection: effects on glucose metabolism, *World J Surg* 25:452–460, 2001.

23. A. It is important to be aware that not all fluid-filled pancreatic abnormalities in a patient with a history of drinking represent pseudocysts. Some of these lesions may represent cystic neoplasms of the pancreas. Suspicion of a cystic neoplasm should be particularly increased in the absence of a history of pancreatitis, as in this patient. A cystic neoplasm should also be suspected when the CT scan demonstrates a solid component in the cystic lesion or septations within the cyst. The differential diagnosis includes serous cystadenoma, mucinous cystic neoplasm, intraductal papillary-mucinous adenoma, and solid pseudopapillary neoplasm. On a CT scan, a central scar is characteristic of a serous cystadenoma (although present in only 20%), whereas the finding of peripheral eggshell calcifications, although rare, is diagnostic of mucinous cystic neoplasm and highly suggestive of cancer. In the patient presented, the procedure of choice is surgical resection with distal pancreatectomy and splenectomy. This is based on several factors: The patient is having symptoms; he is a good candidate for surgery; the lesion is readily amenable to resection; and the lesion's size, its septations, and its multiple loculations. If, conversely, a patient has an incidentally discovered pancreatic cyst without symptoms, surgery is generally recommended if the risk of surgery is low. Before surgery, further studies are recommended to attempt to determine the malignant potential. The work-up may include magnetic resonance imaging, endoscopic ultrasonography to better delineate the mass, and CT-guided aspiration of the fluid for amylase level and tumor markers (carcinoembryonic antigen, CA 19-9, CA 125, CA 72-4, CA 15-3).

24. D. After surgery, trauma, or bouts of pancreatitis, persistent ascites or pleural effusions can develop. These are generally caused by a disruption of the pancreatic duct, with free extravasation of pancreatic fluid, leading to the development of an internal pancreatic fistula, which is rare. More commonly, the extravasated fluid leads to the formation of a contained fluid collection known as a pseudocyst. Management of pancreatic ascites or effusion first requires establishing the diagnosis by obtaining a sample of the fluid and demonstrating a markedly elevated amylase level and a protein level greater than 25 g/L. Serum amylase may be elevated from reassertion across the peritoneal membrane. The recommended management is a stepwise progression, first with conservative management with bowel rest, parenteral nutrition, and placing the patient NPO. If this fails to resolve the internal fistula, ERCP with pancreatic stenting is recommended. If this fails, surgery is indicated and should be tailored to the location of the ductal injury. For distal duct disruptions, a distal pancreatectomy is recommended, whereas for disruption of the body, a Roux-en-Y pancreaticojejunostomy is performed. Conservative therapy is successful in only approximately 50%, so that nearly one half will require an invasive procedure.

References: Gómez-Cerezo J, Barbado Cano A, Suárez I, et al: Pancreatic ascites: study of therapeutic options by analysis of case reports and case series between the years 1975 and 2000, *Am J Gastroenterol* 98:568–577, 2003.

O'Toole D, Vullierme M, Ponsot P, et al: Diagnosis and management of pancreatic fistulae resulting in pancreatic ascites or pleural effusions in the era of helical CT and magnetic resonance imaging, *Gastroenterol Clin Biol* 31:686–693, 2007.

25. B. Autoimmune pancreatitis is a form of chronic pancreatitis that is increasingly being recognized and can be confused with pancreatic lymphoma or pancreatic cancer. It presents most often as a diffusely enlarged hypoechoic pancreas. A CT scan often shows diffuse narrowing of the main pancreatic duct without the typical calcifications seen with chronic alcoholic pancreatitis. Pathology reveals a plasma cell and lymphocytic infiltrate. Laboratory values reveal increased levels of IgG and often diabetes. Antibodies against lactoferrin and carbonic anhydrase have been reported, but they are not a specific finding. The treatment of choice is steroid therapy, and the disease responds well to this management.

References: Ketikoglou I, Moulakakis A: Autoimmune pancreatitis, *Dig Liver Dis* 37:211–215, 2005.

Okazaki K: Autoimmune-related pancreatitis, *Curr Treat Options Gastroenterol* 4:369–375, 2001.

26. C. Although the patient has symptomatic hypoglycemia, seemingly consistent with an insulinoma, her C peptide levels are low and the insulin-to-C peptide ratio is greater than 1. This combination is highly suggestive of factitious hypoglycemia (self-administration of insulin). The precursor to insulin is proinsulin. Proinsulin is packaged in the pancreatic B cell where it is cleaved to insulin and C peptide, which are then released into the circulation at an equal ratio. Endogenous insulin is cleared by the liver, whereas C peptide is cleared by the kidney and is cleared more slowly than insulin, such that the normal insulin-to-C peptide ratio is less than 1 during fasting. With a true insulinoma, both insulin and C peptide levels would be elevated and the ratio would be less than 1. Factitious hypoglycemia has been reported more frequently in health care workers and is associated with a higher incidence of suicide, depression, and personality disorders. Thus, the patient should be referred for psychiatric counseling.

References: Lebowitz M, Blumenthal S: The molar ratio of insulin to C-peptide: an aid to the diagnosis of hypoglycemia due to surreptitious (or inadvertent) insulin administration, *Arch Intern Med* 153:650–655, 1993.

Waickus C, de Bustros A, Shakil A: Recognizing factitious hypoglycemia in the family practice setting, *J Am Board Fam Pract* 12:133–136, 1999.

27. B. Primary pancreatic lymphoma is extremely rare. Thus, the management approach is based on case series and experience with lymphoma at other sites. Patients with pancreatic lymphoma may present with symptoms and CT findings suggestive of pancreatic adenocarcinoma, and as such, it may be difficult to diagnose preoperatively. However, suspicion of lymphoma should be raised in the presence of a large bulky pancreatic tumor or with more diffuse pancreatic involvement. This is one situation in which CT-guided needle biopsy of the mass is indicated because the majority of studies indicate that pancreatic lymphoma responds to chemotherapy as the primary modality.

References: Arcari A, Anselmi E, Bernuzzi P, et al: Primary pancreatic lymphoma: report of five cases, *Haematologica* 90: ECR09, 2005.

Bouvet M, Staerkel G, Spitz F, et al: Primary pancreatic lymphoma, *Surgery* 123:382–390, 1998.

Grimison P, Chin M, Harrison M, Goldstein D: Primary pancreatic lymphoma—pancreatic tumors that are potentially curable without resection: a retrospective review of four cases, *BMC Cancer* 6:117, 2006.

28. B. For acute pancreatitis, gallstones and alcohol abuse are by far the two most common etiologies, with a slightly higher incidence of biliary pancreatitis. Biliary pancreatitis, however, leads to chronic pancreatitis far less often. Alcohol abuse is by far the most common cause of chronic pancreatitis.

References: Fisher WE, Andersen DK, Bell RH, et al: Pancreas. In Brunicardi FC, Andersen DK, Billiar TR, et al, editors: *Schwartz's principles of surgery*, ed 9, New York, 2010, McGraw-Hill, pp 1167–1243.

Steer ML: Exocrine pancreas. In Townsend CM Jr, Beauchamp RD, Evers BM, Mattox KL, editors: *Sabiston textbook of surgery: the biological basis of modern surgical practice*, ed 18, Philadelphia, 2008, WB Saunders, pp 1589–1623.

Pediatric Surgery 17

1. A 4-year-old boy presents with a midline anterior neck cystic mass that moves up and down when he sticks his tongue out. Which of the following is true about this condition?

   A. Most of these masses are symptomatic.
   B. The most common complication is fistula formation.
   C. It presents no risk of future malignancy.
   D. Surgical resection requires removal of part of the hyoid bone.
   E. It is most commonly detected at birth.

2. Which of the following is true regarding congenital diaphragmatic hernia (CDH) (Bochdalek hernia)?

   A. Urgent surgical repair is indicated on diagnosis.
   B. Hypocarbia is a prominent feature.
   C. Most defects are on the right.
   D. The diaphragmatic defect is anteromedial.
   E. Extracorporeal membrane oxygenation is useful.

3. A female newborn is in respiratory distress. A chest radiograph demonstrates a hyperlucent left upper lobe with adjacent lobar compression and mediastinal shift to the right. The treatment of choice for this patient is:

   A. Left upper lobectomy
   B. Left tube thoracostomy
   C. Left pneumonectomy
   D. Positive pressure ventilation until condition resolves
   E. Bronchoscopy

4. Which of the following is true regarding esophageal atresia (EA) and tracheoesophageal fistula (TEF)?

   A. The most common type is the H type.
   B. It is suspected prenatally by oligohydramnios.
   C. In most patients, gastrostomy is required before definitive repair.
   D. Twenty percent of patients have cardiac anomalies.
   E. Upper endoscopy is required to make the diagnosis.

5. A 4-week-old infant presents to the emergency department with increasingly projectile vomiting that is nonbilious and a palpable small right upper quadrant mass. The infant has a severe hypochloremic hypokalemic metabolic alkalosis. Which of the following is true?

   A. This condition is more common in females.
   B. The urine pH will likely be acidic.
   C. Emergency surgery is indicated.
   D. Ultrasonography is necessary to confirm the diagnosis.
   E. Surgery will likely require a gastrointestinal bypass.

6. A premature infant develops formula intolerance with vomiting, abdominal distention, and bloody stool. Indications for surgery include all of the following EXCEPT:

   A. Free intraperitoneal air
   B. Pneumatosis intestinalis
   C. Progressive acidosis
   D. Progressive thrombocytopenia
   E. Diffuse peritonitis

7. Surgery for midgut volvulus should include all of the following EXCEPT:

   A. Untwisting the volvulus counterclockwise
   B. Appendectomy
   C. Fixation of the cecum to the right lower quadrant
   D. Dividing the bands between the duodenum and terminal ileum
   E. Dividing the bands between the cecum and abdominal wall

8. An 11-month-old boy presents with crampy abdominal pain, vomiting, and bloody mucus per rectum. All of the following are true about this condition EXCEPT:

   A. It is usually triggered by an antecedent viral infection.
   B. Hypertrophied Peyer patches are a prominent feature.
   C. Air enemas are diagnostic and therapeutic.
   D. Recurrence rates approach 30%.
   E. Laparotomy is indicated if the patient has peritonitis.

9. A 2-month-old boy presents with constipation and abdominal bloating. He failed to pass meconium on the first day of life. Barium enema demonstrates a markedly dilated colon with a constricted rectum. Which of the following is true about this condition?

   A. The dilated colon is likely to show absence of ganglion cells.
   B. Upper gastrointestinal infection with small bowel follow-through is helpful in the diagnosis.
   C. A temporary colostomy is indicated.
   D. Suction rectal biopsy is often diagnostic.
   E. Barium enema is particularly useful in newborns.

10. Which of the following is true regarding imperforate anus?

   A. Males have a higher chance of having a "low" lesion.
   B. Patients with a "high" lesion have a greater chance of achieving continence.
   C. Plain radiographs are not helpful in the evaluation.
   D. Preoperative cardiac assessment is unnecessary.
   E. Patients with a "high" lesion require a colostomy soon after birth.

11. Which of the following is true regarding neuroblastoma?

   A. The tumor originates most commonly in the kidney.
   B. Cure rates in advanced stages are high with aggressive chemotherapy.
   C. The tumor has been known to spontaneously regress.
   D. It is the most common pediatric malignancy.
   E. Measurement of urinary vanillylmandelic acid is unhelpful in the diagnosis.

12. All of the following are true regarding sacrococcygeal teratoma EXCEPT:

   A. It is the most common teratoma in infancy.
   B. Most are benign.
   C. Most are identified at birth.
   D. Management consists of radiation therapy.
   E. It has a high risk of malignant degeneration if treatment is delayed.

13. A newborn is in severe respiratory distress and has a markedly scaphoid abdomen. Which of the following is true regarding this condition?

   A. A chest tube should be promptly placed.
   B. Respiratory compromise is mostly due to mechanical compression of the lungs.
   C. Pulmonary artery vasoconstriction is common and exacerbates the respiratory compromise.
   D. Ventilation with high-frequency oscillation is ineffective.
   E. Nasogastric tube placement is contraindicated.

14. All of the following are true regarding the pediatric trauma victim EXCEPT:

   A. Lap belt injuries are associated with lumbar spine fractures.
   B. Splenic salvage is more important than in adults.
   C. An appropriate bolus for a hypotensive 25-kg infant is 500 mL.
   D. Hypothermia occurs more rapidly than in adults.
   E. Use of nasogastric tubes should be avoided.

15. Which of the following is true regarding jejunal atresia?

   A. It is due to a fetal mesenteric vascular accident.
   B. Most infants present with nonbilious vomiting.
   C. It is the most common cause of surgical vomiting in infancy.
   D. If the infant was born prematurely, surgery should be delayed until the infant weighs more than 8 lb.
   E. A barium enema is contraindicated in the work-up.

16. Which of the following is true regarding omphalocele?

    A. Initial treatment involves an attempt at gentle reduction.
    B. Mortality is most often the result of persistent sepsis.
    C. It is thought to occur due to an umbilical vein vascular accident.
    D. The defect is usually to the right of the umbilicus.
    E. The majority of patients have associated cardiac and genetic abnormalities.

17. A 2-month-old infant has persistent jaundice. Ultrasonography fails to demonstrate a gallbladder. Technetium-99m iminodiacetic acid scanning with phenobarbital pretreatment reveals uptake in the liver but not in the intestine. α_1-Antitrypsin determination is normal. The next step in the management would be:

    A. Kasai operation (hepatoportoenterostomy)
    B. Liver transplantation
    C. Percutaneous transhepatic liver drainage
    D. Endoscopic biliary stent placement
    E. Choledochojejunostomy

18. The Sistrunk procedure is performed for:

    A. Torticollis
    B. Brachial cleft cysts
    C. Thyroglossal duct cysts
    D. Esophageal atresia
    E. Cystic hygroma

19. The most common indication for extracorporeal life support (ECLS) in neonates is:

    A. CDH
    B. Respiratory distress syndrome
    C. Meconium aspiration
    D. Persistent pulmonary hypertension
    E. Congenital cardiac abnormalities

20. Which of the following is true regarding the surgical approach to TEF?

    A. The lower esophagus should be more extensively mobilized than the upper esophagus.
    B. The fistula can usually be located by dividing the azygos vein.
    C. The fistula is usually repaired with a left thoracotomy.
    D. A transpleural approach is preferred over an extrapleural one.
    E. The extrapleural approach is easier.

21. A newborn has bilious vomiting. Plain films reveal a distended gastric air bubble and a markedly dilated proximal duodenum. All of the following are true regarding this condition EXCEPT:

    A. It is associated with Down syndrome.
    B. Management consists of a gastrojejunostomy.
    C. The obstruction is typically distal to the ampulla of Vater.
    D. Upper gastrointestinal contrast study is unnecessary.
    E. It is associated with maternal polyhydramnios.

22. A 2-year-old child presents with an abdominal mass, "raccoon eyes," and "blueberry muffin" skin lesions. This most likely represents:

    A. Rhabdomyosarcoma
    B. Neuroblastoma
    C. Wilms tumor
    D. Hepatoblastoma
    E. Teratoma

23. The most common anomaly associated with gastroschisis is:

    A. Cardiac
    B. Renal
    C. Limb
    D. Intestinal atresia
    E. Down syndrome

24. The most common abnormality associated with omphalocele is:

    A. Cardiac
    B. Renal
    C. Limb
    D. Intestinal atresia
    E. Beckwith-Wiedemann syndrome

25. The most common pathologic lead point for intussusception in children is:

    A. Appendix
    B. Small bowel polyp
    C. Henoch-Schönlein purpura
    D. Meckel diverticulum
    E. Small bowel cancer

26. Management of uncomplicated meconium ileus is generally achieved by:

    A. Water-soluble contrast enemas
    B. Resection of terminal ileum with stoma
    C. Resection of terminal ileum with primary anastomosis
    D. Barium enema
    E. Small bowel enterotomy with evacuation of meconium

27. Which of the following is true regarding the high imperforate anus?

   A. Meconium, along the median raphe of the perineum, is characteristic.
   B. In males, it is usually associated with a cloacal deformity.
   C. In females, the rectum ends in the membranous urethra.
   D. It is associated with spinal cord abnormalities.
   E. It is a surgical emergency.

28. Multiple diffuse dilatations of the intrahepatic ducts are known as:

   A. Alagille syndrome
   B. Beckwith-Wiedemann syndrome
   C. Eagle-Barrett (prune-belly) syndrome
   D. Caroli disease
   E. "Christmas tree" deformity

29. Prune-belly syndrome (Eagle-Barrett syndrome) is associated with:

   A. Inguinal hernia
   B. Undescended testicles
   C. Patent urachus
   D. Imperforate anus
   E. Vertebral abnormalities

30. An inguinal hernia in a premature infant:

   A. Should be repaired if the hernia persists beyond 3 months of age
   B. Should be repaired using the Bassini technique
   C. Has a low risk of incarceration
   D. Is more common than in infants born at full term
   E. Is equally common in males and females

31. A 30-kg child has an estimated daily fluid requirement of:

   A. 40 mL/hr
   B. 50 mL/hr
   C. 60 mL/hr
   D. 70 mL/hr
   E. 80 mL/hr

32. A 28-week-old fetus is noted to have a large cystic hygroma in the neck on ultrasonography. All of the following are true regarding this lesion EXCEPT:

   A. It is associated with oligohydramnios.
   B. Initial surgical treatment involves conservative excision and unroofing of cysts.
   C. Postexcisional fluid accumulation can be treated by injection of sclerosing agents.
   D. It is associated with abnormal karyotypes.
   E. It may require emergency tracheostomy at delivery with the fetus still attached to the placenta.

33. Goldenhar complex consists of biliary atresia, congenital cardiac abnormalities, and:

   A. Brachial cleft abnormalities
   B. Thyroglossal duct remnants
   C. Torticollis
   D. Lipoblastoma
   E. Vascular malformations

34. A useful method of prenatal prediction of survival for fetuses with CDH can be achieved by:

   A. Estimation of the defect size
   B. Presence of associated abnormalities
   C. Gestational age at time of detection
   D. Lung-to-head ratio (LHR)
   E. Karyotyping by amniocentesis

35. All of the following are true regarding hypertrophic pyloric stenosis EXCEPT:

   A. It is linked with early administration of erythromycin.
   B. It has a familial link in some cases.
   C. It is readily diagnosed with ultrasonography.
   D. Repair can be achieved laparoscopically.
   E. Surgery requires a full-thickness division of the pylorus into the mucosa.

36. A 4-week-old infant presents with bilious vomiting, irritability, abdominal wall edema, and erythema. Plain films reveal proximal dilated bowel, with a paucity of distal bowel gas. Which of the following is true regarding this condition?

   A. An urgent upper gastrointestinal series is indicated.
   B. A nonoperative trial of nasogastric tube decompression is often helpful.
   C. Endoscopic decompression is often beneficial.
   D. The condition is caused by bands of tissue between the sigmoid colon and the lateral abdominal wall.
   E. Delay in management may lead to a need for intestinal transplantation.

37. The pathogenesis of necrotizing enterocolitis (NEC) is thought to be related to:

   A. A genetic predisposition
   B. An enzyme deficiency
   C. A period of intestinal hypoperfusion
   D. Preexisting intestinal atresia
   E. An antibiotic reaction

38. The Dance sign is associated with:

   A. Meconium ileus
   B. NEC
   C. Intussusception
   D. Duodenal atresia
   E. Hirschsprung disease

39. In addition to needing abdominal wall reconstruction, infants with prune-belly syndrome (Eagle-Barrett syndrome) will likely also require:
    A. Ureterolysis
    B. Nephrostomy tubes
    C. Renal transplantation
    D. Bilateral orchiopexy
    E. Colostomy

40. A neonate is found to have bilateral undescended testes that are not palpable in the inguinal canal. All of the following are true regarding this condition EXCEPT:
    A. A bilateral orchiopexy should be performed by 2 years of age.
    B. Orchiopexy improves fertility potential.
    C. Orchiopexy reduces the risk of malignancy in the testicles.
    D. Chorionic gonadotropin may aid in testicular descent.
    E. Repair may require transection of the testicular arteries.

41. Fetal surgical interventions have demonstrated improved outcome compared with postpartum intervention for all of the following conditions EXCEPT:
    A. CDH
    B. Lower urinary tract obstruction
    C. Myelomeningocele
    D. Large neck teratomas
    E. Congenital tracheal stenosis

42. Optimal management for an 8-month-old girl with biliary atresia in whom a Kasai operation (hepatoportoenterostomy) failed would be:
    A. Repeat Kasai operation
    B. Liver transplantation
    C. Percutaneous transhepatic liver drainage
    D. Endoscopic biliary stent placement
    E. Choledochojejunostomy

Answers

1. D. The patient described has a thyroglossal duct cyst, which is one of the most common lesions of the neck found in the midline. Most are asymptomatic. Thyroglossal remnants produce midline masses extending from the base of the tongue to the pyramidal lobe of the thyroid. Complete failure of thyroid migration results in a lingual thyroid. Ultrasound or radionuclide imaging may be used to identify the presence of a normal thyroid gland within the neck. The indications for surgery include increasing size, infection, and the presence of carcinoma. The most common complication is infection. The treatment of a thyroglossal duct cyst is the Sistrunk procedure, which involves complete excision of the cyst in continuity with its tract, the central portion of the hyoid bone, and the tissue above the hyoid bone extending to the base of the tongue. The mass is generally not detected at birth because it is obscured by fat.

Reference: Brousseau V, Solares C, Xu M, et al: Thyroglossal duct cysts: presentation and management in children versus adults, *Int J Pediatr Otorhinolaryngol* 67:1285–1290, 2003.

2. E. Approximately 90% of CDHs occur on the left side. Rarely, they may be bilateral. The cause of CDHs is unknown, but it is believed that they result from failure of normal closure of the pleuroperitoneal canal in the developing embryo. As a result, the abdominal contents herniate through the defect in the diaphragm and compress the ipsilateral developing lung. A Bochdalek hernia is in the posterolateral location. Extracorporeal membrane oxygenation is useful in managing patients. The most frequent clinical presentation is respiratory distress due to hypoxemia with associated hypercarbia. Most pediatric surgeons wait 24 to 72 hours to allow the infant's condition to stabilize before performing the repair. Bochdalek hernias are distinguished from Morgagni hernias, which are another type of congenital hernia of the anteromedial diaphragm. The Morgagni hernia defect is small and asymptomatic and typically presents as a density on chest radiograph in adulthood.

Reference: Lally K, Paranka M, Roden J, et al: Congenital diaphragmatic hernia: stabilization and repair on ECMO, *Ann Surg* 216:569–573, 1992.

3. A. Congenital lobar emphysema in its most severe form presents as respiratory distress at birth. It is due to excessive hyperexpansion of one or more lobes of the lung from either abnormal cartilage in the bronchus, creating a one-way valve effect, or external compression from a cardiac abnormality such as left atrial enlargement. As the lung overinflates, atelectasis of the adjacent lobes ensues. Eventually mediastinal shifting occurs with compromise of the opposite lung. It is most common in the upper lobes of the lung. In mild forms, the infant may present later with mild respiratory distress. Diagnosis is made by chest radiograph, which shows a hyperlucent affected lobe, adjacent lobar compression and atelectasis, and mediastinal shift to the opposite side. Bronchoscopy is contraindicated because it will exacerbate the overinflation. Treatment involves resection of the affected lobe. The chest radiograph can be confused with a pneumothorax, and inadvertent placement of a chest tube in the distended lung will further worsen an already life-threatening situation. Immediate thoracotomy with resection of the lung lobe may be lifesaving. Recent studies suggest that in asymptomatic or mild symptomatic cases, nonsurgical therapy is acceptable.

Reference: Mei-Zahav M, Konen O, Manson D, et al: Is congenital lobar emphysema a surgical disease? *J Pediatr Surg* 41:1058–1061, 2006.

4. D. EA with TEF is a congenital interruption or discontinuity of the esophagus resulting in esophageal obstruction. Most present at birth with excessive drooling and choking or coughing after an attempted feed. There are five types (A to E). The most common type is type C in which there is EA with a distal TEF. The H type (type E) is a TEF without EA. This is the most difficult one to diagnose because the esophagus is patent. These infants often present later in infancy with recurrent bouts of pneumonia due to aspiration. Half of patients with EA/TEF have a low birth weight, and two thirds have associated anomalies including association with the VACTERL syndrome (vertebral, anorectal, cardiac, tracheal, esophageal, renal, limb). In approximately 20%, congenital heart disease is present. The diagnosis is now often made prenatally by the detection of maternal polyhydramnios because the infant is unable to swallow the amniotic fluid. The immediate care includes decompression of the proximal EA pouch with a sump type of tube placed for continuous suction. Timing of surgery depends on the underlying condition of the infant, most notably, the presence of associated cardiac abnormalities. If the patient is not able to undergo immediate repair, gastrostomy to decompress the stomach and for feeding may be temporarily needed, although studies have shown that the use of a gastrostomy increases the risk of subsequent reflux. The diagnosis is confirmed by an inability to pass a tube into the stomach. Recent studies have shown that the obstructions can be repaired thoracoscopically.

Reference: Rothenberg S: Thoracoscopic repair of tracheoesophageal fistula in newborns, *J Pediatr Surg* 37:869–872, 2002.

5. B. This patient has pyloric stenosis. Pyloric stenosis occurs in 1 in 300 live births. Most often it occurs in an infant who is a first-born male between 3 and 6 weeks of age. There seems to be a familial link as well as a link to early erythromycin administration. Infants with pyloric stenosis present with projectile, nonbilious vomiting. As the disease progresses, an almost complete gastric outlet obstruction develops, and the infant is no longer able to tolerate even clear liquids. The classic electrolyte disorder that results from protracted vomiting is a hypochloremic hypokalemic metabolic alkalosis. The urine pH level is high initially due to the alkalosis, but eventually becomes acidic. The explanation for this is that the renal tubule initially reabsorbs sodium in exchange for potassium. However, gastric juice has a high potassium concentration, and as vomiting continues, serum potassium levels drop.

To conserve potassium as well, the renal tubule switches to reabsorbing sodium in exchange for hydrogen ions in the urine. The diagnosis is made by the palpation of an olive in the upper right quadrant. An uncooperative infant can sometimes make palpation difficult. When the olive cannot be palpated, the diagnosis can be made by ultrasonography, which demonstrates the hypertrophied pyloric muscle. The treatment is pyloromyotomy. Postoperatively, infants are allowed to resume enteral feedings. Vomiting after surgery occurs frequently but is self-limited. Recent studies indicate that the laparoscopic approach is equally effective and has the advantage of a shorter hospital stay, a quicker recovery, and a smaller scar. Although the scar for open pyloromyotomy is small, it tends to become more sizable and grow as the infant grows.

Reference: Fujimoto T, Lane G, Segawa O, et al: Laparoscopic extramucosal pyloromyotomy versus open pyloromyotomy for infantile hypertrophic pyloric stenosis: which is better? *J Pediatr Surg* 34:370–372, 1999.

6. B. In all infants suspected of having NEC, feedings are discontinued, a nasogastric tube is placed, and broad-spectrum parenteral antibiotics are given. Total parenteral nutrition is also started. Bell created a staging system based on severity. Patients with Bell stage I (suspicious for NEC) are closely monitored and kept NPO and on intravenous (IV) antibiotics for 7 to 10 days before enteral nutrition is reinitiated. Patients with Bell stage II (definite NEC) require close observation. Infants with Bell stage III (advanced NEC) either have definite intestinal perforation or have not responded to nonoperative therapy and require surgery. These patients have signs of peritonitis, acidosis, sepsis, and disseminated intravascular coagulation, all of which are associated with a high mortality rate. Answers A, C, D, and E are all part of Bell stage III and are indications for surgery.

Reference: Bell M, Ternberg J, Feigin R, et al: Neonatal necrotizing enterocolitis: therapeutic decisions based upon clinical staging, *Ann Surg* 187:1–7, 1978.

7. C. A midgut volvulus occurs clockwise and therefore treatment includes untwisting in a counterclockwise direction. The diagnosis should be suspected in an infant presenting with bilious vomiting and evidence of a bowel obstruction. Plain radiograph may suggest volvulus with the finding of a distended stomach and a paucity of distal bowel gas beyond it, but because there are no pathognomonic signs on plain radiograph, some authors have recommended ultrasonography to look for a sonographic clockwise whirlpool pattern of the superior mesenteric vein and mesentery around the superior mesenteric artery. When midgut volvulus is suspected, the infant should be urgently taken to the operating room because a delay risks the development of gangrene of the entire small bowel. The Ladd procedure is performed to broaden the narrow mesenteric pedicle to prevent the volvulus from recurring. The bands between the cecum and abdominal wall and between the duodenum and terminal ileum are sharply divided to splay out the superior mesenteric artery and its branches. This brings the duodenum into the right lower quadrant and the cecum into the left lower quadrant. The appendix is removed to avoid diagnostic errors later in life. Rarely, midgut volvulus presents in adulthood. In adults, computed tomography is useful because it can demonstrate the same whirlpool pattern.

Reference: Pracros J, Sann L, Genin G, et al: Ultrasound diagnosis of midgut volvulus: the "whirlpool" sign, *Pediatr Radiol* 22:18–20, 1992.

8. D. Intussusception is the primary cause of intestinal obstruction in the young child. It is more common in boys, with a male-to-female ratio of 3:1 that increases to 6:1 in older children. It is a condition in which the intestine telescopes or invaginates into itself. It most often begins in the terminal ileum and extends distally into the ascending colon. Intussusception is called *idiopathic* when there is no distinct pathologic leading point. This is the case in most infants aged 6 to 24 months in whom the intussusception is usually due to hypertrophy of the Peyer patches in the terminal ileum from a previous viral infection. The symptoms of intussusception include intermittent bouts of crampy abdominal pain, vomiting with passage of bloody mucus, and "currant jelly" stool, although a minority of infants have all three parts of the triad. Between attacks, the infant may act normally. On examination, an elongated mass is detected in the right upper quadrant or in an epigastric location, with an absence of bowel in the right lower quadrant (Dance sign). In the absence of peritonitis, the child should undergo reduction by barium or air enema, which is both diagnostic and curative. If reduction is incomplete, operative intervention is indicated because gangrene and perforation may result. If peritonitis is present on the initial examination or the child is systemically ill, one should forgo enema attempts, and an urgent operation is indicated. At surgery, the intussusception is reduced manually by gentle distal pressure rather than by pulling out the bowel. Recurrence rates after hydrostatic reduction are in the 5% to 10% range and usually occur within the first 24 hours. Intussusception in an older child or an adult is more likely due to an underlying pathology in the bowel (e.g., tumor, polyp, Meckel diverticulum).

Reference: Guo J, Ma X, Zhou Q: Results of air pressure enema reduction of intussusception: 6,396 cases in 13 years, *J Pediatr Surg* 12:1201–1203, 1986.

9. D. Hirschsprung disease is characterized by an absence of ganglion cells in the Auerbach plexus and hypertrophy of associated nerve trunks. The cause is thought to be a defect in the migration of neural crest cells. The rectosigmoid junction is affected in 75% of cases, the splenic flexure or transverse colon in 17%, and the entire colon with variable extension into the small bowel in 8%. The presentation of the disease is characterized as a functional distal intestinal obstruction. In the neonatal period, the most common symptoms are abdominal distention, failure to pass meconium, and bilious emesis. Infants can also present with enterocolitis, which is characterized by abdominal distention and tenderness and is associated with manifestations of systemic toxicity. Enterocolitis is the most common cause of death in uncorrected Hirschsprung disease. The definitive diagnosis is made by rectal biopsy

at least 2 cm above the dentate line to avoid sampling error. The dilated colon is actually the normal colon, so it will demonstrate ganglion. A barium enema is useful because it will often help localize the transition zone between the dilated proximal ganglion containing the colon and the narrowed aganglionic distal segment, but is not as helpful in the immediate neonatal period because the proximal segment may not be as markedly dilated yet. Multiple surgical operations exist for the management of Hirschsprung disease. Recently, primary repair with a pull-through procedure without a temporary colostomy has been performed.

Reference: Carcassonne M, Guys J, Morrison-Lacombe G, Kreitmann B: Management of Hirschsprung's disease: curative surgery before 3 months of age, *J Pediatr Surg* 24:1032–1034, 1989.

10. E. In patients with an imperforate anus, the rectum fails to descend through the external sphincter complex. It is thought to be caused by a failure of the urorectal septum to descend. The rectal pouch ends blindly in the pelvis, above (high) or below (low) the levator ani. Sixty percent of males have high lesions compared with only 30% of females. In most cases, the blind rectal pouch communicates more distally with the genitourinary system or with the perineum through a fistulous tract. In male patients with a high imperforate anus, the rectum usually ends as a fistula in the membranous urethra. In females, a high imperforate anus often occurs in the context of a persistent cloaca. Approximately 60% of patients have an associated malformation; the most common is a urinary tract defect. Skeletal defects are also seen, and the sacrum is most commonly involved. Spinal cord anomalies are common, especially with high lesions. Imperforate anus is also associated with VACTERL syndrome. Evaluation should include plain radiographs of the spine as well as an ultrasound scan of the spinal cord. A plain chest radiograph and careful clinical evaluation of the heart should be conducted. The most common defect is an imperforate anus with a fistula between the distal colon and the urethra in boys or to the vestibule of the vagina in girls. Low lesions can be repaired by a perineal procedure, whereas high lesions typically require a temporary colostomy with a definitive pull-through procedure at 2 months of age.

Reference: Georgeson K, Inge T, Albanese C: Laparoscopically assisted anorectal pull-through for high imperforate anus: a new technique, *J Pediatr Surg* 35:927–931, 2000.

11. C. Neuroblastoma is an embryonal tumor of neural crest origin. It is the third most common pediatric malignancy. It is most commonly found in the adrenal medulla. Measurement of vanillylmandelic acid and homovanillic acid in the serum and urine can assist in the diagnosis. The majority of patients have advanced disease at the time of presentation. The overall survival rate is less than 30%. Two thirds of cases are first found as an asymptomatic abdominal mass. The tumor may cross the midline, and a majority of patients may show signs of metastatic disease. Because these tumors derive from the sympathetic nervous system, catecholamine and their metabolites will be produced at increased levels. Unlike Wilms tumor, the prognosis in advanced stages is poor with a 2-year survival rate of only 20% in stage 4 disease despite aggressive chemotherapy. Spontaneous regression of neuroblastoma has been well described in infants.

Reference: Evans A, Gerson J, Schnaufer L: Spontaneous regression of neuroblastoma, *Natl Cancer Inst Monogr* 44:49–54, 1976.

12. D. A sacrococcygeal teratoma presents as a large mass extending off of the sacrum in the neonatal period. They are the most common teratomas in neonates. Most tumors are identified at birth and are benign. Malignant yolk sac tumor histology occurs in a minority of tumors. The diagnosis may be established by a prenatal ultrasound scan. In fetuses with evidence of hydrops and a large teratoma, the prognosis is poor; thus, prenatal intervention is being advocated in such patients. The mass may be as small as a few centimeters in diameter or as massive as the size of the infant. The tumor has been classified based on the location and degree of intrapelvic extension. Lesions with growth predominantly into the presacral space often present later in childhood. Complete resection of the tumor as early as possible is essential. The rectum and genital structures are often distorted by the tumor, but can be preserved during resection. Very large teratomas detected antenatally can lead to high output failure and placentomegaly (hydrops) and fetal demise. Hydrops is one indication for intrauterine surgery, which has been successful in case series.

Reference: Hecher K, Hackelöer B: Intrauterine endoscopic laser surgery for fetal sacrococcygeal teratomas, *Lancet* 347:470, 1996.

13. C. Normally neonates have a protruberant abdomen, so the presence of a scaphoid abdomen, combined with respiratory distress at birth, should raise the suspicion for CDH because the majority of the peritoneal contents are herniated into the chest. In infants with CDH, both lungs are hypoplastic and there is decreased bronchial and pulmonary artery branching. The infants are prone to the development of pulmonary hypertension. Intrauterine compression of the lungs results in pulmonary hypoplasia with the ipsilateral lung being the most affected. Pulmonary vasculature is distinctly abnormal in that the medial muscular thickness of the arterioles is excessive and extremely sensitive to the multiple local and systemic factors known to trigger vasospasm. Between 80% and 90% occur on the left side, and the defect is posterolateral as opposed to the Morgagni hernia, which is an anteromedial defect. Because of the lung hypoplasia, prompt reduction of the bowel contents does not improve ventilatory function. Ventilation with high-frequency oscillation is effective, as is the use of inhaled nitric oxide. Placement of a nasogastric tube is also important to prevent gastric distention, which may slightly worsen the lung compression, mediastinal shift, and ability to ventilate. Chest tubes are not indicated initially, but the initial chest radiograph can be confused with a tension pneumothorax.

Reference: Lally K, Paranka M, Roden J, et al: Congenital diaphragmatic hernia: stabilization and repair on ECMO, *Ann Surg* 216:569–573, 1992.

14. E. It is important to use uncuffed endotracheal tubes in children younger than 8 years of age to minimize tracheal trauma. It is important to consider that gastric distention from aerophagia can severely compromise respiration.

A nasogastric tube should be placed early. In patients who show signs of volume depletion, a 20-mL/kg bolus of saline or lactated Ringer's solution should be given. If the patient does not respond to two boluses, 10 mL/kg of blood should be transfused. Small intestinal injuries usually occur in the jejunum in the area of fixation by the ligament of Treitz. These injuries are caused by rapid deceleration while the child is restrained by a lap belt. There may be a hematoma on the anterior abdominal wall caused by a lap belt known as the seat belt sign. Postsplenectomy sepsis most often occurs in young children and immunocompromised adults; for this reason, attempts to salvage the spleen are more vigorous in children.

15. A. Obstruction caused by intestinal atresia can occur at any point along the intestinal tract. Most cases are believed to be caused by in utero mesenteric vascular accidents leading to segmental loss of the intestinal lumen. They are classified into four types based on the severity. Infants with jejunal or ileal atresia present soon after birth with bilious vomiting and progressive abdominal distention. The more distal the obstruction, the more distended the abdomen and the greater the number of loops on upright abdominal radiograph. In cases in which the diagnosis of complete intestinal obstruction is ascertained by the clinical picture and the presence of staggered air–fluid levels on plain abdominal films, the child can be brought to the operating room after appropriate resuscitation. In these circumstances, there is little extra information that can be gained by a barium enema. When the diagnosis is uncertain, a barium enema may be used. The initial treatment of jejunal atresia is nasogastric tube decompression and fluid resuscitation. Definitive treatment involves surgical resection of the atretic loop and primary reanastomosis.

Reference: Touloukian T: Diagnosis and treatment of jejunoileal atresia, *World J Surg* 17:310–317, 1993.

16. E. Omphalocele refers to a congenital defect of the abdominal wall in which the bowel and solid viscera are covered by peritoneum and the amniotic membrane. The abdominal wall defect can measure 4 cm or more in diameter. Omphalocoele is less of a surgical emergency than gastroschisis because the bowel is protected by the covering. Conversely, omphalocoele is associated with many other congenital abnormalities that are not seen with gastroschisis. Omphalocele occurs in association with exstrophy of the cloaca, Beckwith-Wiedemann syndrome, Cantrell pentalogy, ectopic cordis, and anterior midline diaphragmatic hernia. The size of the defect may be small or so large that it contains most of the abdominal viscera. There is an increased occurrence of cardiac and chromosomal abnormalities. Omphalocele is associated with premature and intrauterine growth retardation. Immediate treatment of an infant with omphalocele consists of maintaining normal vital signs and body temperature. The omphalocele should be covered with saline-soaked gauze, and the trunk should be wrapped circumferentially. No pressure should be placed in an effort to reduce the abdominal contents because this maneuver may increase the risk of sac rupture or interfere with abdominal venous return. Treatment is surgical. If the entire sac cannot be reduced, a temporary silo is placed.

17. A. Jaundice that persists beyond 2 weeks after birth is considered pathologic. Pathologic jaundice may be caused by biliary obstruction, increased hemoglobin load, or liver dysfunction. One must rule out obstructive disorders, including biliary atresia, choledochal cyst, and inspissated bile syndrome; ABO incompatibility; Rh incompatibility; spherocytosis; metabolic disorders; α_1-antitrypsin deficiency; galactosemia; and congenital infection including syphilis and rubella. The most important surgical cause of jaundice in the newborn is biliary atresia, which is an obliterative process of the extrahepatic bile ducts and is associated with hepatic fibrosis. The infant produces acholic stools and demonstrates a failure to thrive. Left untreated, it will progress to liver failure and portal hypertension. Nuclear scanning after pretreatment with phenobarbital is a useful study. One is specifically looking to see whether the radionuclide appears in the intestine, which would confirm that the extrahepatic bile ducts are patent. This finding excludes biliary atresia. If the radionuclide is normally concentrated in the liver but not excreted and the metabolic screen results are normal, this is highly suggestive of biliary atresia. The presence of a gallbladder does not exclude the diagnosis of biliary atresia. The most effective treatment of biliary atresia is portoenterostomy, as described by Kasai. The procedure involves anastomosing an isolated limb of jejunum to the transected ducts at the liver plate. The likelihood of surgical success is increased if the procedure is performed before the infant reaches the age of 8 weeks. If the patient remains symptomatic after the Kasai operation, he or she will require liver transplantation. Independent risk factors that predict failure of the procedure include bridging liver fibrosis at the time of surgery and postoperative cholangitis episodes.

Reference: Ohhama Y, Shinkai M, Fujita S, et al: Early prediction of long-term survival and the timing of liver transplantation after the Kasai operation, *J Pediatr Surg* 35:1031–1034, 2000.

18. C. The classic treatment of thyroglossal duct cyst is the Sistrunk procedure, which involves complete excision of the cyst in continuity with its tract, the central portion of the hyoid bone, and the tissue above the hyoid bone extending to the base of the tongue.

19. C. In neonates with respiratory distress syndrome, management includes high-frequency ventilation surfactant and inhaled nitric oxide. When those interventions fail, ECLS is used. ECLS can be performed by either venovenous or venoarterial cannulation. The major indications for ECLS include meconium aspiration, respiratory distress syndrome, persistent pulmonary hypertension, sepsis, and CDH. Meconium aspiration is the most common indication for neonatal ECLS. The most dreaded complication of ECLS is intracranial hemorrhage.

Reference: Kugelman A, Gangitano E, Taschuk R, et al: Extracorporeal membrane oxygenation in infants with meconium aspiration syndrome: a decade of experience with venovenous ECMO, *J Pediatr Surg* 40:1082–1089, 2005.

20. B. The surgical treatment for the most common type of TEF involves an extrapleural thoracotomy through the right fourth intercostal space, although more recently it has been performed thoracoscopically. The azygos vein is a key landmark because once it is divided, the TEF is usually underneath. The TEF is dissected circumferentially and ligated with interrupted nonabsorable sutures. The proximal esophageal pouch is then mobilized as high as possible to afford a tension-free esophageal anastomosis. The blood supply to the upper esophageal pouch is based on arteries derived from the thyrocervical trunk. However, the blood supply to the lower esophagus is more tenuous and segmental, originating from the intercostal vessels. As such, significant mobilization of the lower esophagus should not be done to avoid ischemia of the anastomosis. The extrapleural approach is preferred, although the transpleural one is easier to perform.

21. B. The history and radiograph findings are consistent with duodenal atresia. Duodenal atresia occurs because of failure of vacuolization of the duodenum from its solid core state. It is associated with prematurity, Down syndrome, maternal polyhydramnios, malrotation, annular pancreas, and biliary atresia. In most cases, the duodenal obstruction is distal to the ampulla of Vater, and infants present with bilious emesis in the neonatal period. The classic radiographic finding is the "double-bubble sign" (an air-filled stomach, a functioning pylorus, and a distended proximal duodenal bulb). If there is no distal bowel gas, complete atresia is confirmed and no further studies are necessary. Conversely, if distal air is present, an upper gastrointestinal contrast study should be done because other diagnoses are possible. This is important to exclude midgut volvulus. The finding of distal air in association with a double bubble could also indicate a duodenal stenosis or web or an annular pancreas that does not cause a complete obstruction. The treatment of duodenal atresia is surgical bypass of the obstruction as either a side-to-side or proximal transverse-to-distal longitudinal duodenoduodenostomy or a duodenojejunostomy. When the proximal duodenum is markedly dilated, a tapering duodenoplasty may be performed.

22. B. Neuroblastoma is the most common abdominal malignancy in children. The presenting symptoms depend on the site of the primary tumor, the presence of metastatic disease, the age of the patient, and the metabolic activity of the tumor. The most common presentation is a fixed lobular mass extending from the flank toward the midline. The tumor can also extend into the neural foramina and cause symptoms of spinal cord compression. It tends to metastasize to cortical bones, bone marrow, and the liver, and patients may present with localized swelling and tenderness, limp, or refusal to walk. Periorbital metastases account for proptosis and ecchymoses, resulting in "raccoon eyes." In infants, liver metastases may expand, causing hepatomegaly. Metastatic lesions to the skin produce the blueberry muffin appearance. Wilms tumor also presents as an abdominal mass, in association with Beckwith-Wiedemann syndrome (macroglossia, hypoglycemia, gigantism, and visceromegaly), and as part of the WAGR complex (Wilms tumor, aniridia, genitourinary abnormalities, and mental retardation). Rhabdomyosarcoma is a soft-tissue tumor. The most common primary sites are the head and neck. Sacrococcygeal teratoma is the most common type of teratoma. It presents as a large mass extending off of the sacrum in the newborn period.

23. D. Gastroschisis, unlike omphalocele, is not typically associated with systemic or chromosomal abnormalities. There is an abdominal wall defect to the right of the umbilicus, and the bowel herniates through without a peritoneal covering. Because the bowel is eviscerated and exposed, this condition is a surgical emergency. The bowel can be thickened and covered with an exudate. It is most commonly associated with intestinal atresia in as many as 15% of cases. For this reason, it is imperative that the small bowel be carefully explored at the time of reduction and repair of the abdominal wall defect. If the defect cannot be closed, similar to omphalocele, a silo can be used.

24. A. The incidence of other abnormalities in patients with omphalocele is approximately 60% to 70%. Cardiac anomalies are the most common, followed by musculoskeletal, gastrointestinal, and genitourinary anomalies.

25. D. Infants 6 to 24 months of age with intussusception typically have no pathologic lead point on pathologic examination, but instead have hypertrophied Peyer patches. Conversely, older children have a much higher likelihood of having a pathologic lead point. As such, they have a much greater need for operative intervention to resect the segment of bowel that includes the pathologic area. The most common pathologic lead point for intussusception in children is a Meckel diverticulum. Other causes include polyps, appendicitis, intestinal neoplasms such as lymphosarcoma, submucosal hemorrhage, foreign body, ectopic pancreatic or gastric tissue, and intestinal duplication.

26. A. Meconium ileus is a result of cystic fibrosis, in which the meconium becomes thick and viscous due to deficits in pancreatic enzymes. It creates a small bowel obstruction, and as such, the infant may present with bilious vomiting. In the most severe forms, it can lead to intestinal perforation. The radiograph typically demonstrates a "ground-glass" appearance, which represents small pockets of gas trapped inside the thickened meconium. The treatment strategy depends on whether the patient has complicated or uncomplicated meconium ileus. Patients with uncomplicated meconium ileus can be treated nonoperatively. Administering a water-soluble enema such as dilute gastrograffin per rectum allows the meconium to soften as it takes on more water. Optimally, the contrast should be inserted in the dilated portion of the ileum under fluoroscopic control. The enema may be repeated every 12 hours over several days as needed. Surgery is required if nonoperative management fails or if the patient already has evidence of perforation. Complicated cases are usually amenable to bowel resection and primary anastomosis provided there is no evidence of giant cystic meconium peritonitis.

Reference: Rescorla F, Grosfeld J: Contemporary management of meconium ileus, *World J Surg* 17:318–325, 1993.

27. D. In patients with imperforate anus, the rectum fails to descend through the external sphincter complex. Instead,

the rectal pouch ends blindly in the pelvis, above or below the levator ani. In most cases, the blind rectal pouch communicates more distally with the genitourinary system or with the perineum through a fistulous tract. In male patients with a high imperforate anus, the rectum usually ends as a fistula in the membranous urethra. In females, high imperforate anus often occurs in the context of a persistent cloaca. Approximately 60% of patients have an associated malformation. The most common is a urinary tract defect. Skeletal defects are also seen, and the sacrum is most commonly involved. Spinal cord anomalies are common, especially with high lesions. Meconium along the median raphe would be consistent with a low lesion. Although most surgeons would recommend a temporary colostomy in patients with a high lesion, it is not a surgical emergency. The infants do not usually manifest signs of a bowel obstruction at birth; as such, surgical intervention is not emergent. The site of the fistula may not be immediately obvious for 24 hours. Newer techniques of performing an anorectal pull-through procedure laparoscopically are emerging.

Reference: Georgeson K, Inge T, Albanese C: Laparoscopically assisted anorectal pull-through for high imperforate anus: a new technique, *J Pediatr Surg* 35:927–931, 2000.

28. D. Choledochal cysts have been classified into five types. The most common is type I, which is fusiform dilatation of the bile duct. Caroli disease is a type V choledochal cyst that causes multiple bile duct dilatations that are limited to the intrahepatic bile ducts. The cysts lead to recurrent bouts of cholangitis and have a risk of malignancy. If the Caroli disease is limited to one lobe, partial hepatectomy is potentially curative. In patients with diffuse Caroli disease, liver transplantation can provide satisfying long-term results. Eagle-Barrett syndrome is also known as prune-belly syndrome (see description in next question). Beckwith-Wiedemann syndrome consists of macroglossia, hypoglycemia, gigantism, and visceromegaly. Alagille syndrome is a congenital familial syndrome with onset during the first 3 months of life, marked by intrahepatic cholestasis due to hypoplasia of the interlobular biliary duct, neonatal jaundice, and hepatomegaly. The etiology is unclear; however, it is inherited in an autosomal dominant fashion with reduced penetrance and variable expressivity. "Christmas tree" deformity is a type of intestinal atresia in which the bowel distal to the atresia receives its blood in a retrograde fashion from the ileocolic or right colic artery. The bowel wraps around the mesentery in a spiral fashion.

Reference: Kassahun W, Kahn T, Wittekind C, et al: Caroli's disease: liver resection and liver transplantation: experience in 33 patients, *Surgery* 138:888–898, 2005.

29. B. Prune-belly syndrome is associated with a congenital absence or hypoplasia of the abdominal wall musculature. Urinary tract abnormalities are present including a large hypotonic bladder, dilated ureters, dilated prostatic urethra, and bilateral cryptorchidism. The incidence is higher in males. The most significant comorbidity is pulmonary hypoplasia. Skeletal abnormalities include dislocation or dysplasia of the hip and pectus excavatum.

Despite ureteral dilatation, there is no role for ureteral surgery. The testes are intra-abdominal, and bilateral orchipexy can be performed in conjunction with abdominal wall reconstruction at 6 to 12 months of age.

Reference: Guzetta P, Anderson K, Altman P, et al: Pediatric surgery. In Schwartz SI, editor: *Principles of surgery*, ed 8, New York, 1999, McGraw-Hill, pp 715–754.

30. D. The presence of an inguinal hernia in infants is an indication for surgery. Inguinal hernias result from the processus vaginalis failing to close. Inguinal hernias occur more commonly in males and premature infants and are more common on the right side. Infants are at high risk of incarceration because of the narrow inguinal ring. Inguinal hernias in children only require high ligation of the sac. A Bassini repair is used to reinforce a weakened floor of the inguinal canal in adults and involves sewing the conjoined tendon to the inguinal ligament. It has been largely replaced by the mesh repair, but is useful in the setting of strangulated, perforated bowel when one wants to avoid using mesh.

31. D. Daily maintenance fluids for children can be estimated using the 4-2-1 rule (4 mL/kg/hr for the first 10 kg, 2 mL/kg for the second 10 kg, and 1 mL/kg for any additional kilograms). For this child who weighs 30 kg, maintenance fluids calculate to be 4 mL/kg × 10 kg = 40 mL, 2 mL/kg × 10 kg = 20 mL, 1 mL/kg × 10 kg = 10 mL; 40 mL + 20 mL + 10 mL = 70 mL/hr.

32. A. Cystic hygromas result from sequestration or obstruction of developing lymph vessels. The most common sites are the posterior triangle of the neck, axilla, and groin. They are associated with hydrops fetalis and abnormal karyotypes. The cysts are lined with endothelium and are filled with lymph. The mass may be apparent at birth and may enlarge as lymph accumulates, leading to airway compromise. Percutaneous aspiration is a useful technique to relieve respiratory distress. Sometimes they are not apparent until age 2, when baby fat begins to disappear. The cysts can become infected, most often by skin flora such as *Staphylococcus* and *Streptococcus*. Large lesions can cause polyhydramnios by impairing the ability of the baby to swallow the amniotic fluid. This can lead to airway obstruction and distortion at birth. To prevent such a catastrophe, when diagnosed antenatally, a cesarean section is performed and an airway is secured via orotracheal intubation or tracheostomy while the infant remains attached to the placenta. Surgical excision is the treatment of choice. The excision does not need to be radical. A more conservative excision is recommended to avoid damage to adjacent nerves and unroofing of remaining cysts. Repeated partial excisions can be performed later. Fluid may accumulate beneath the surgically created flaps in the area from which the hygroma was excised, requiring multiple aspirations. Injections of sclerosing agents have been used in Japan and the United States in neonates without systemic toxicity, including bleomycin and OK-432, a lyophilized mixture of group A *Streptococcus pyogenes*.

References: Mikhail M, Kennedy R, Cramer B, Smith T: Sclerosing of recurrent lymphangioma using OK-432, *J Pediatr Surg* 30:1159–1160, 1995.

Tanigawa N, Shimomatsuya T, Takahashi K, et al: Treatment of cystic hygroma and lymphangioma with the use of bleomycin fat emulsion, *Cancer* 60:741–749, 1987.

33. A. Brachial cleft anomalies can occur in association with biliary atresia and congenital cardiac anomalies. This triad of congenital abnormalities is called the *Goldenhar complex*.

34. D. An index of severity for patients with left CDH is the LHR, which is the product of the length and the width of the right lung at the level of the cardiac atria divided by the head circumference measured by prenatal ultrasonography. In a study of 15 patients, an LHR less than 1.0 was associated with a poor prognosis, whereas an LHR greater than 1.4 predicted a more favorable prognosis. No patient with an LHR less than 1.0 survived despite extracorporeal membrane oxygenation, whereas all patients with an LHR greater than 1.4 survived, with one requiring extracorporeal membrane oxygenation. LHR values between 1.0 and 1.4 were associated with a 38% survival rate, with 75% of patients requiring extracorporeal membrane oxygenation.

Reference: Lipshutz G, Albanese C, Feldstein V, et al: Prospective analysis of lung-to-head ratio predicts survival for patients with prenatally diagnosed congenital diaphragmatic hernia, *J Pediatr Surg* 32:1634–1636, 1997.

35. E. Administration of erythromycin in early infancy has been linked to the development of hypertrophic pyloric stenosis. Ultrasonography can establish the diagnosis accurately in 95% of cases by detecting pyloric thickness (>4 mm thick for a length of 16 mm). The key element of initial management is the adequate replacement of fluids and electrolytes. Pyloromyotomy is performed by making an incision in the serosa and muscle layers and separating the muscle until the submucosa bulges out. The submucosa and mucosa are not entered.

36. E. The infant is exhibiting signs of malrotation with midgut volvulus. By the time that abdominal wall edema is evident, there is a high likelihood of intestinal gangrene. As such, no further studies are indicated, and the infant requires urgent laparotomy. Ladd bands extend from the cecum to the lateral abdominal wall, crossing the duodenum, which increases the potential for obstruction. Additional clues to the presence of advanced ischemia include erythema of the abdominal wall. Sometimes gangrenous loops of bowel may be seen transabdominally as a discolored mass. If untreated, the infant will progress to shock and death. It must be reemphasized that the index of suspicion for this condition must be high because abdominal signs are minimal in the early states. Abdominal films show a paucity of gas through the intestine with a few scattered air–fluid levels. In early cases, the patient does not appear ill initially, and the plain films may suggest partial duodenal obstruction. Under these conditions, the patient may have malrotation without volvulus. This is best diagnosed by an upper gastrointestinal series that shows incomplete rotation with the duodenojejunal junction displaced to the right. When volvulus is suspected, early surgical intervention is mandatory if the ischemic process is to be avoided or reversed. Volvulus occurs clockwise and should be untwisted counterclockwise.

37. C. The pathogenesis of NEC is thought to be intestinal hypoperfusion. This occurs most frequently in the setting of perinatal stress. The period of hypoperfusion is followed by a period of reperfusion, and the combination of ischemia and reperfusion leads to mucosal injury. The damaged intestinal mucosa barrier becomes susceptible to bacterial translocation that initiates an inflammatory cascade. Various proinflammatory mediators are released, which in turn leads to further epithelial injury and the systemic manifestations of NEC. It is postulated that maintenance of the gut barrier is essential for the protection of the host against NEC.

38. C. Intussusception is the leading cause of intestinal obstruction in the young child. The Dance sign is the finding on physical examination of an elongated mass in the right upper quadrant or the epigastric area, with an absence of bowel in the right lower quadrant, which is a finding associated with intussusception.

Reference: Guzetta P, Anderson K, Altman P, et al: Pediatric surgery. In Schwartz SI, editor: *Principles of surgery*, ed 8, New York, 1999, McGraw-Hill, pp 715–754.

39. D. Prune-belly syndrome refers to a disorder that is characterized by a constellation of symptoms including extremely lax lower abdominal musculature, a dilated urinary tract including the bladder, and bilateral undescended testes. Despite ureteral dilatation, there is no role for ureteral surgery. The testes are intra-abdominal. Bilateral orchiepexy can be performed in conjunction with abdominal wall reconstruction at 6 to 12 months of age.

Reference: Guzetta P, Anderson K, Altman P, et al: Pediatric surgery. In Schwartz SI, editor: *Principles of surgery*, ed 7, New York, 1999, McGraw-Hill, pp 715–754.

40. C. Children born with bilateral undescended testes have a much higher rate of subsequent infertility. When the testicle is not in the scrotum, it is subjected to higher temperatures, resulting in decreased spermatogenesis. Even when the testicles are placed in the scrotum, fertility, although improved, is still not normal. It is recommended that undescended testicles be repositioned by 2 years of age to maximize chances of improving fertility. The use of chorionic gonadotropin sometimes is effective in achieving descent in patients with bilateral undescended testes, suggesting that they may have a hormonal deficiency. If the intra-abdominal testes can be effectively mobilized to reach down into the scrotum, a two-stage Fowler-Stephens procedure is used. In the first stage, the testicular vessels are clipped laparoscopically. In addition to the testicular arteries, the testicles receive collateral blood from the cremasteric artery, a branch of the inferior epigastric artery, and the vasal artery, a branch of the superior vesical artery. Thus, division of the testicular artery is usually well tolerated and does not usually result in testicular necrosis. The orchiopexy is then performed through the groin approximately 6 months later, after which time collateral flow has increased. Undescended testicles are at higher risk of malignant degeneration, which is not altered by orchiopexy; however, their location in the scrotum facilitates earlier detection.

41. A. Despite advances in perinatal management, some congenital disorders continue to have significant morbidity and mortality both in utero and in the early postnatal period. In selected anomalies, fetal surgical intervention can alter the natural history of the disorder, leading to improved survival rates and functional outcomes. Potential indications for fetal surgery include large neck masses that obstruct the airway, CDH, myelomeningocele, lower urinary obstruction, and tracheal stenosis. Fetal tracheal occlusion was developed as a potential intervention for CDH. However, a recent randomized trial that compared fetal tracheal occlusion with standard postnatal care for left-sided CDH showed no improvement in survival for patients treated with tracheal occlusion. The study was stopped prematurely because the survival rate in the nonprenatal intervention arm was unexpectedly high.

References: Harrison M, Keller R, Hawgood S, et al: A randomized trial of fetal endoscopic tracheal occlusion for severe fetal congenital diaphragmatic hernia, *N Engl J Med* 349:1916–1924, 2003.

Walsh D, Adzick N: Fetal surgical intervention, *Am J Perinatol* 17:277–283, 2000.

42. B. The Kasai operation, in which an isolated limb of the jejunum is anastomosed to the transected ducts at the liver plate, is the operation of choice for biliary atresia. However, in a subset of patients, the Kasai operation is unsuccessful, and they eventually require liver transplantation for progressive liver failure and recurrent bouts of cholangitis. Independent risk factors that predict failure of the procedure include bridging liver fibrosis at the time of surgery and postoperative cholangitic episodes. In one study, elevation of the bilirubin level at 3 months predicted long-term survival and the need for future transplantation.

References: Hackam DJ, Grikscheit TC, Wang KS, et al: Pediatric surgery. In Brunicardi FC, Andersen DK, Billiar TR, et al, editors: *Schwartz's principles of surgery*, ed 9, New York, 2010, McGraw-Hill, pp 1409–1457.

Ohhama Y, Shinkai M, Fujita S, et al: Early prediction of long-term survival and the timing of liver transplantation after the Kasai operation, *J Pediatr Surg* 35:1031–1034, 2000.

Warner BW: Pediatric surgery. In Townsend CM Jr, Beauchamp RD, Evers BM, Mattox KL, editors: *Sabiston textbook of surgery: the biological basis of modern surgical practice*, ed 18, Philadelphia, 2008, WB Saunders, pp 2047–2089.

Peripheral Arterial Disease 18

1. Buerger disease is characterized by:
   A. Frequent coronary artery involvement
   B. Frequent involvement of aortoiliac arterial segments
   C. Recurrent superficial thrombophlebitis
   D. Marked improvement with sympathectomy
   E. Rare progression to gangrene

2. All of the following are true regarding noninvasive hemodynamic assessment EXCEPT:
   A. In normal resting subjects in the supine position, the ankle pressure can be 20% higher than that in the arm.
   B. There is a correlation between ankle-brachial index (ABI) and severity of symptoms.
   C. End-stage renal failure can cause a false elevation of the ABI.
   D. In diabetic patients, toe pressures are more useful than the ABI.
   E. In diabetic patients, transcutaneous oximetry is unreliable.

3. Which of the following is true regarding the use of thrombolytic therapy for acute limb ischemia?
   A. It can safely be used in patients within a week of cataract surgery.
   B. Bleeding risk does not correlate with fibrinogen levels.
   C. It is contraindicated in patients with a profound motor deficit in the ischemic limb.
   D. It is ideal in patients with rapid deterioration to advanced ischemia.
   E. It can safely be used for as long as 72 hours.

4. In the upper extremity, the most common site for an embolus to lodge is:
   A. Subclavian artery
   B. Axillary artery
   C. Brachial artery
   D. Radial artery
   E. Ulnar artery

5. Occlusion of a reverse saphenous vein femoral artery–to–popliteal artery bypass 8 months after surgery is most often due to:
   A. Intimal hyperplasia
   B. Progressive atherosclerosis
   C. Hypercoagulable state
   D. Technical error at the anastomosis
   E. Poor choice of target

6. A 65-year-old man presents with a 4-hour history of sudden onset of left leg pain. He has no history of claudication. He has no pulses in his left femoral artery or distally. The calf is markedly tender to palpation. The foot is cool and pale with markedly diminished capillary refill. He has a sensory deficit in his foot. In his right leg, the femoral, popliteal, and distal pulses are normal. Cardiac examination reveals an irregularly irregular rhythm. After administration of heparin, the next step in management would be:
   A. Diagnostic arteriography
   B. Thrombolytic therapy
   C. Transfemoral embolectomy
   D. Embolectomy via the below-knee popliteal artery
   E. Duplex ultrasound scan

7. When comparing in situ saphenous vein bypass with reverse saphenous vein bypass, the in situ technique:
   A. Has a better 5-year patency
   B. Provides better blood flow
   C. Can be performed with a smaller-diameter saphenous vein
   D. Is technically easier to perform
   E. Maintains the vasa vasorum, which improves short-term patency

8. A 35-year-old woman presents with difficult-to-control hypertension that is requiring four medications. Despite this regimen, her blood pressure is 190/90 mm Hg. Arteriography reveals bilateral high-grade stenosis of the main renal arteries with a string-of-beads appearance. Management should consist of:

   A. Bilateral aortorenal bypass with saphenous vein
   B. Transaortic bilateral renal endarterectomy
   C. Bilateral aortorenal bypass with Dacron
   D. Bilateral renal artery percutaneous transluminal angioplasty
   E. Bilateral percutaneous renal artery stenting

9. The conduit of choice for renal artery bypass in a 6-year-old girl would be:

   A. Greater saphenous vein
   B. Dacron
   C. Polytetrafluoroethylene
   D. Internal iliac artery
   E. Cephalic vein

10. A 60-year-old woman presents with sudden onset of acute abdominal pain. On examination, the patient is writhing in pain, yet the abdomen is only mildly tender, without guarding or rebound. The cardiac examination findings are irregularly irregular. The serum lactate level is elevated. Serum amylase is slightly elevated. Troponins are negative. Plain abdominal radiographs are negative. A computed tomography (CT) scan of the abdomen reveals diffuse edema of the small bowel wall. The next step in the management would be:

    A. Magnetic resonance imaging
    B. Arteriography
    C. Upper gastrointestinal series
    D. Exploratory laparotomy
    E. Duplex ultrasound scan

11. In a hypertensive patent with unilateral renal artery stenosis:

    A. Hypertension is primarily caused by angiotensin II–mediated vasoconstriction.
    B. Diuretics are particularly useful.
    C. Angiotensin-converting enzyme inhibitors are contraindicated.
    D. Patients are predisposed to recurrent episodes of congestive heart failure.
    E. Creatinine clearance is usually reduced.

12. A 65-year-old woman undergoes creation of a forearm brachial artery–to–cephalic vein loop arteriovenous (AV) graft for hemodialysis in the left arm using a 6-mm polytetrafluoroethylene graft. Four days postoperatively, the patient reports marked coolness, pallor, and numbness in the hand as well as decreased strength. On examination, there is no palpable pulse at the radial artery and only a monophasic Doppler signal that becomes biphasic on graft compression. Which of the following is the best management option?

    A. Distal revascularization and interval ligation of the brachial artery
    B. Ligation of the AV graft and placing the upper arm graft in same arm
    C. Ligation of the AV graft and placing the new graft in the other arm
    D. Banding of the AV graft adjacent to the arterial anastomosis
    E. Banding of the AV graft adjacent to the venous anastomosis

13. A 45-year-old man presents with a 1-week history of vague, diffuse abdominal pain and distention. On examination, he has mild diffuse tenderness without guarding or rebound. A CT scan reveals thickened loops of small bowel and failure of opacification of the superior mesenteric vein. Management would consist of:

    A. Intra-arterial thrombolytic therapy
    B. Intravenous (IV) thrombolytic therapy
    C. IV heparin alone
    D. Arteriography with papaverine infusion
    E. Immediate operative exploration

14. Claudication symptoms are most improved with the use of:

    A. Pentoxifylline
    B. Aspirin
    C. Cilostazol
    D. Clopidogrel
    E. Coumadin (warfarin)

15. A 17-year-old boy presents with right calf pain that consistently comes on after walking one block and is relieved by rest. The pain has been present for 3 months. He denies a smoking history. He has seen several physicians who diagnosed a persistent calf muscle strain. Femoral, popliteal, and distal pulses in the foot are normal. The ABI is 1.0. However, a repeat ABI after exercise is 0.6. This most likely indicates:

    A. Popliteal cystic adventitial disease
    B. Popliteal aneurysm
    C. Buerger disease
    D. Popliteal entrapment syndrome
    E. Vasculitis

16. Four days after a left femoral-to-popliteal bypass with ipsilateral reverse saphenous vein, the patient reports swelling in the left leg. This most likely indicates:

    A. Deep venous thrombosis
    B. Reperfusion edema
    C. Decreased venous return from saphenous vein harvest
    D. Cellulitis
    E. Lymphatic disruption

17. The most common site for cardiac embolus to lodge is:

    A. Middle cerebral artery
    B. Common femoral artery
    C. Superficial femoral artery
    D. Popliteal artery
    E. Brachial artery

18. A 65-year-old male smoker presents with right calf claudication that limits his walking to one-half block. He denies rest pain in his foot. On physical examination, he has a normal femoral pulse on the right and absent popliteal and distal pulses. Arterial noninvasive studies reveal a 40-mm Hg decrease in segmental pressure from the upper thigh to the knee. The ABI is 0.7 on the right and 0.8 on the left. The next step in the management of this patient would be:

    A. Standard arteriography
    B. Magnetic resonance arteriography
    C. Duplex ultrasound scan
    D. Smoking cessation and exercise
    E. CT angiography

19. Which of the following is true regarding the use of postoperative duplex ultrasound scanning after a saphenous vein, common femoral artery–to–anterior tibial artery bypass:

    A. It should be performed only if the distal pulse disappears.
    B. It should be performed only if the ABI decreases by more than 0.3.
    C. It is unnecessary because thrombosed vein grafts are readily lysed.
    D. Grafts with a focal peak systolic velocity greater than 300 cm/sec are at highest risk of graft thrombosis.
    E. Detecting and correcting a graft stenosis lowers amputation rates.

20. All of the following are true regarding sympathectomy EXCEPT:

    A. Upper dorsal sympathectomy is helpful in patients with hyperhidrosis.
    B. Lumbar sympathectomy is particularly useful in diabetic patients with nonhealing ulcers.
    C. Horner syndrome is a common complication of upper dorsal sympathectomy.
    D. It is useful in relieving the pain from frostbite.
    E. It is useful in treating complex regional pain syndrome.

21. Fifteen years after an aortobifemoral bypass, a 65-year-old man presents with a painless pulsatile mass in his right groin. He has no other symptoms. CT confirms a 3-cm anastomotic femoral pseudoaneurysm, but findings are otherwise unremarkable. Management would consist of:

    A. Right axillary–to–superficial femoral artery (SFA) bypass followed by excision of the right limb of the aortobifemoral graft
    B. Ultrasonic compression of the pseudoaneurysm
    C. Ultrasonography-guided thrombin injection of the pseudoaneurysm
    D. Interposition graft from the old right graft limb to the more distal femoral artery
    E. Observation

22. A 65-year-old man presents with sudden onset of coolness and pain in his left calf and foot. The foot is pale and appears ischemic. Which of the following best correlates with severe ischemia?

    A. An absent distal pulse
    B. Six-hour duration of the ischemia
    C. A motor deficit in the foot
    D. The etiology of the ischemia
    E. An ABI less than 0.3

23. A 65-year-old female smoker presents to the emergency department with mottling of her skin from the umbilicus to her feet. She has a 2-year history of thigh and buttock claudication. She has no femoral or distal pulses. She has marked weakness in both legs. Definitive management is best achieved by:

    A. Aortobifemoral bypass
    B. Axillobifemoral bypass
    C. Bilateral transfemoral embolectomy
    D. Thrombolytic therapy
    E. Aortoiliac stenting

24. Which of the following best predicts healing of a below-knee amputation?

    A. A popliteal systolic pressure greater than 50 mm Hg
    B. Absence of gangrene above the ankle
    C. Transcutaneous oximetry reading of 25 mm Hg at the calf
    D. Presence of a popliteal pulse
    E. Warm skin above the ankle

25. Two hours after cardiac catheterization for evaluation of congenital heart disease, a 1-year-old boy is noted to have an absent right femoral pulse at the site of the arteriography. The right foot is cool and pulseless. He appears to be moving the foot and withdrawing to pain. Pulses in the other leg and foot are normal. Which of the following is the best option?

    A. Heparinization and observation
    B. Arteriography to evaluate injury
    C. Immediate exploration of the right femoral artery with a Fogarty embolectomy
    D. Immediate exploration of the right femoral artery with an interposition saphenous vein graft
    E. Immediate exploration of the right femoral artery with an arteriotomy and tacking of the intimal flap

26. A 65-year-old man with a history of a coronary artery bypass graft 2 years earlier presents with recurrent chest pain. He describes the pain as substernal and radiating to his jaw. He works as a carpenter and also states that his left arm tires out easily with use. Blood pressure in the right arm is 150/90 mm Hg and 100/60 mm Hg in the left arm. Relief of his chest pain is likely best achieved with:

    A. Redo coronary artery bypass graft
    B. Coronary stenting
    C. Increasing the dose of nitrates
    D. Subclavian artery stenting
    E. Increasing beta-blocker dose

27. A 45-year-old male nonsmoker presents with pain in his right calf with walking a half block for 6 months. Popliteal and distal pulses on the right are absent, with an ABI of 0.7, but are normal on the left. The symptoms do not improve despite an exercise program. Magnetic resonance angiography reveals a curvilinear lesion causing a partial obstruction of the popliteal artery (scimitar sign). This most likely represents:

    A. Chronic embolization
    B. Buerger disease
    C. Popliteal entrapment syndrome
    D. Popliteal cystic adventitial disease
    E. Persistent sciatic artery

28. All of the following are indicated in the surgical management of bowel ischemia due to an embolus to the superior mesenteric artery (SMA) EXCEPT:

    A. Mannitol
    B. Planned second-look laparotomy
    C. Fogarty embolectomy of the SMA
    D. Heparin
    E. Resection of bowel with questionable viability

29. The 5-year risk of limb loss in a patient with claudication is estimated to be:

    A. Less than 1%
    B. Less than 5%
    C. 10%
    D. 20%
    E. 30%

30. A 65-year-old man with ischemic rest pain in both feet is about to undergo an aortobifemoral bypass. He is a smoker and is hypertensive. He denies any history of cardiac or cerebrovascular events. However, he has poor exercise tolerance due to claudication and is only able to walk a half block. His serum creatinine level is 1.2 mg/dL. Which of the following would be the optimal strategy before surgery?

    A. Persantine sestamibi scan and, if abnormal, obtain a coronary angiogram
    B. Persantine sestamibi scan and, if abnormal, perform an axillofemoral bypass
    C. Dobutamine echocardiography and, if abnormal, obtain a coronary angiogram
    D. Dobutamine echocardiography and, if abnormal, attempt endovascular repair
    E. Proceed to surgery with beta-blockade and statins

31. At surgery for suspected acute mesenteric ischemia, almost the entire small bowel as well as the right colon appear ischemic. However, the proximal jejunum, duodenum, and left colon appear healthy. The most likely etiology of these findings is:
    A. Thrombosis of the SMA
    B. Embolus to the SMA
    C. Superior mesenteric vein thrombosis
    D. Portal vein thrombosis
    E. Nonocclusive mesenteric ischemia

32. The most common type of fibromuscular dysplasia (FMD) and most common location are:
    A. Medial fibroplasia, renal artery
    B. Medial fibroplasia, internal carotid artery
    C. Intimal fibroplasia, renal artery
    D. Intimal fibroplasia, internal carotid artery
    E. Perimedial dysplasia, renal artery

33. Arterial complications of thoracic outlet syndrome are most often caused by a:
    A. Cervical rib
    B. Hypertrophied anterior scalene muscle
    C. Narrowed costoclavicular space
    D. Hypertrophied subclavius muscle
    E. Anomalous middle scalene muscle

34. Neurogenic thoracic outlet syndrome most commonly affects which nerve?
    A. Radial
    B. Ulnar
    C. Median
    D. Musculocutaneous
    E. Axillary

35. A 65-year-old man with pain at rest in his left leg is about to undergo a common femoral–to–common femoral crossover bypass with polytetrafluoroethylene. Significant arterial steal is most likely to develop if:
    A. The right iliac artery has a stenosis.
    B. The left iliac artery has a stenosis.
    C. The right SFA is occluded.
    D. The left superficial artery is occluded.
    E. The donor leg ABI is less than 0.6.

36. Horner syndrome after upper extremity sympathectomy is best prevented by preserving:
    A. T1 ganglion
    B. T2 ganglion
    C. T3 ganglion
    D. Kuntz nerve
    E. Upper half of the stellate ganglion

37. A 60-year-old diabetic patient presents with gangrene of his right great toe. The patient has normal femoral and popliteal pulses but no distal pulses. Angiography reveals patent iliac, femoral, and popliteal arteries with a long segment occlusion of the trifurcation vessels with reconstitution of the anterior tibialis artery above the ankle and runoff into the dorsalis pedis artery. The greater saphenous veins in both legs were previously harvested for a coronary artery bypass graft. Which of the following is the best option?
    A. Common femoral–to–anterior tibial bypass with cephalic vein spliced from both arms
    B. Popliteal-to-anterior tibial bypass with lesser saphenous vein
    C. Common femoral–to–anterior tibialis bypass with polytetrafluoroethylene graft
    D. Great toe amputation only
    E. Below-knee amputation

38. Which of the following is the most common cause of death at 5 years in patients with claudication?
    A. Stroke
    B. Myocardial infarction
    C. Cancer
    D. Lower extremity gangrene
    E. Ruptured aortic aneurysm

39. The common denominator that is thought to lead to the development of atherosclerosis is:
    A. Endothelial injury
    B. High shear stress
    C. Low shear stress
    D. Cigarette smoking
    E. Hyperlipidemia

40. The earliest identifiable lesion in atherosclerosis is:
    A. Atheroma
    B. Foam cells
    C. Fibrous plaque
    D. Fatty streak
    E. Clustering of monocytes

41. All of the following are true regarding cilostazol EXCEPT:
    A. It is contraindicated in patients with heart failure.
    B. It inhibits platelet aggregation.
    C. It increases vasodilation.
    D. It inhibits smooth muscle proliferation.
    E. It is contraindicated in diabetic patients.

42. A 32-year-old woman notes that her hands become cold and painful when exposed to cold temperatures. The hand changes in color from pale to cyanotic to red. Her medical history is negative, and vascular pulse examination is normal. Arterial noninvasive studies reveal a marked decrease in digital blood pressure with exposure to cold temperatures. Symptoms persist despite wearing gloves and avoidance of cold exposure. The next step in management is:

   A. Upper extremity sympathectomy
   B. Prostaglandins
   C. Fluoxetine
   D. Arteriography
   E. Diltiazem

43. A 25-year-old right-handed baseball pitcher presents with sudden onset of a painful, blue right index finger. He denies smoking. Cardiac examination is unremarkable. Brachial and radial pulses at both wrists are normal. This most likely indicates:

   A. Buerger disease
   B. Cardiac embolus
   C. Embolus from subclavian artery atherosclerosis
   D. Embolus from subclavian artery aneurysm
   E. Giant cell arteritis

44. A 60-year-old man presents with severe claudication of both buttocks and thighs as well as impotence. He is only able to walk one-fourth block before he has to stop and rest. He also reports waking up at night with pain in his feet, requiring him to get out of bed. He has quit smoking. On examination, he has no pulses in either the femoral artery or distally. The ABI is 0.4 on each side. Magnetic resonance angiography reveals an aortic occlusion just below the renal arteries with reconstitution of the common femoral arteries in the groin. Which of the following would be the recommended management?

   A. Aortobifemoral bypass
   B. Axillobifemoral bypass
   C. Stent graft of one iliac artery and femoral-to-femoral crossover bypass
   D. Stent graft of both iliac arteries
   E. Medical management

Answers

1. C. Buerger disease is a progressive nonatherosclerotic segmental inflammatory disease that most often affects small- to medium-sized arteries, veins, and nerves of the upper and lower extremities. The typical age at onset is 20 to 50 years, and the disorder is more common in men who smoke. The disease also affects the veins, and specifically the upper extremities may be affected by a migratory superficial thrombophlebitis. Patients initially present with foot, leg, arm, or hand claudication. Progression of the disease leads to ischemic rest pain and ulcerations of the toes, feet, and fingers. Characteristic angiographic findings may show disease confinement to the distal circulation, usually infrapopliteal and distal to the brachial artery. The occlusions are segmental and show skip lesions with extensive collateralization, the so-called corkscrew collaterals. The diagnosis is difficult to establish because there are no pathognomonic features. As such, the disease can be confused with chronic embolization and other diseases. Several criteria have been established to confirm the diagnosis: age younger than 45 years; current (or recent) smoker; distal extremity ischemia (claudication, pain at rest, ischemic ulcers, gangrene); exclusion of autoimmune diseases, hypercoagulable states, and diabetes mellitus; exclusion of a proximal source of emboli by echocardiography and arteriography; and characteristic arteriographic findings in the involved limbs. The aortoiliac segments are typically spared, as are the coronary arteries. The treatment revolves around smoking cessation. In patients who are able to abstain, disease remission is impressive and amputation avoidance is increased. The role of surgical intervention is minimal because there is usually no acceptable target vessel for bypass. Sympathectomy may result in mild improvement of symptoms.

   Reference: Olin J: Thromboangiitis obliterans (Buerger's disease), *N Engl J Med* 343:864–869, 2000.

2. E. Normally the ABI varies between 1 and 1.2 because the ankle pressure in the supine position can be as much as 20% higher than in the arm. Peripheral arterial disease has been defined as a value less than 0.9 and indicates some degree of an obstruction. Patients with claudication typically have an ABI between 0.5 and 0.7, and those with rest pain have an ABI less than 0.4. Patients with diabetes and end-stage renal disease are at risk of developing calcification of the arterial medial layer, known as medial calcinosis or Mönckeberg arteriosclerosis. This process makes blood vessels rigid and difficult to compress, causing falsely increased pressure readings. The process tends to affect tibial vessels primarily and spares digital vessels in the toes. As such, toe pressures are more reliable, as are other measures of distal perfusion such as transmetatarsal pulse volume recordings and transcutaneous oximetry.

Reference: Belkin M, Owens CD, Whittemore A, et al: Peripheral arterial occlusive disease. In Townsend CM Jr, Beauchamp RD, Evers BM, Mattox KL, editors: *Sabiston textbook of surgery: the biological basis of modern surgical practice,* ed 18, Philadelphia, 2008, WB Saunders, p 1941–1979.

3. C. Absolute contraindications to thrombolytic therapy include recent stroke or transient ischemic attack, active or recent bleeding, and significant coagulopathy. Relative contraindications include patients with recent major surgery, recent trauma, uncontrolled hypertension, intracranial tumors, and pregnancy. The risk of bleeding is increased with long-term therapy and with decreasing fibrinogen levels. In most series, thrombolytic therapy is used for as long as 48 hours, at which point the bleeding risk increases significantly.

The causes of acute limb ischemia can be divided into embolic and thrombotic. The heart is the most common source of emboli leading to acute ischemia, most often in the setting of atrial fibrillation. Other cardiac sources include mural thrombus after an acute myocardial infarction, valvular disease, and atrial myxoma. Other sources of emboli include arterial aneurysms and atherosclerotic plaques. Thrombosis is most often caused by underlying atherosclerosis in the peripheral artery, and these patients typically will have a history of claudication.

The severity of acute limb ischemia is based primarily on the motor and sensory examination. Patients should be placed in four categories: (1) normal motor and sensory function, (2) sensory deficit only, (3) motor and sensory deficit, and (4) complete motor and sensory loss. In addition, consideration should be given to the duration of ischemia. Muscle can usually tolerate as much as 6 hours of ischemia before irreversible damage ensues. As a general rule, patients with category 1 or 2 ischemia can be treated with multiple options, a trial of heparin alone, thrombolytic therapy, or operative embolectomy/bypass. Patients with category 3 ischemia need prompt restoration of blood flow, and because thrombolytic therapy may require more than 24 to 48 hours to restore flow, category 3 ischemia is a relative contraindication to thrombolysis. Such a patient should be taken to the operating room. Category 4 ischemia is considered irreversible and requires amputation. Irreversible ischemia is confirmed by an absence of arterial or venous Doppler signals, duration of ischemia of more than 6 to 8 hours, presence of mottling of the skin, absence of capillary refill, and complete anesthesia and paralysis.

References: Norgren L, Hiatt W, Dormandy J, et al: Inter-Society Consensus for the Management of Peripheral Arterial Disease (TASC II), *J Vasc Surg* 45(Suppl S):S5–S67, 2007.

Semba CP, Murphy TP, Bakal CW, et al: Thrombolytic therapy with use of alteplase (rt-PA) in peripheral arterial occlusive disease: review of the clinical literature. The Advisory Panel, *J Vasc Interv Radiol* 11:149–161, 2000.

The STILE trial: Results of a prospective randomized trial evaluating surgery versus thrombolysis for ischemia of the lower extremity, *Ann Surg* 220:251–268, 1994.

4. C. The upper extremities are affected in approximately 10% of cases of peripheral embolization. The most common site for the embolus to lodge is in the brachial artery. The pulse examination can be most helpful in determining the site of embolus because a patient with a brachial embolus will typically have a palpable pulse in the axillary artery in the armpit, but no pulse in the brachial or radial arteries. These patients most often present in the setting of atrial fibrillation. Management consists of immediate administration of heparin, fluid hydration (provided the patient is not presenting with an acute coronary syndrome), and placing the limb in a dependent position. The most expeditious management is to take the patient to the operating room to perform an embolectomy. This procedure can easily be performed while the patient is under local anesthesia by making an incision at the elbow. The brachial, radial, and ulnar arteries are isolated, and a transverse arteriotomy is made in the brachial artery near the radial and ulnar artery origins. This allows the Fogarty balloon to be guided into the radial and ulnar arteries.

Reference: Green R, Ouriel K. Arterial disease. In Schwartz SI, editor: *Principles of surgery,* ed 8, New York, 1999, McGraw-Hill, p 953.

5. A. Early failure (within 30 days) after surgery generally indicates a technical error. Technical errors include anastomotic stenosis, a kink or twist within the graft, poor choice of proximal or distal target, and inadequate-caliber saphenous vein. Intermediate failures, from 30 days to 2 years after bypass, are generally caused by intimal hyperplasia. Late graft failures (beyond 2 years) are caused by progression of atherosclerotic occlusive disease, either within the inflow or outflow vessels.

6. C. In an acutely ischemic limb, in addition to the motor and sensory examination, one of the most important aspects of the physical examination is the pulse examination of the nonischemic limb. If the nonischemic limb has normal pulses and no other evidence of chronic ischemia (e.g., hair loss, thin dry skin), then the ischemia is most likely embolic in nature. The heart would be the most likely source because the cardiac examination is critical, which in this case indicates that the patient is in atrial fibrillation. With an absent femoral pulse, the thrombus has lodged in the common femoral artery. Native arterial occlusions due to cardiac embolization tend to respond less favorably to thrombolytic therapy. Thus, the patient is best managed with an embolectomy. A transfemoral approach is optimal because this can be done with the patient under local anesthesia, and it allows selective embolectomy down the superficial femoral and profunda femoral arteries. Given the classic presentation and physical examination, as well as the 4-hour duration of ischemia, further diagnostic studies are not necessary and will simply delay definitive care. The below-knee popliteal artery approach to embolectomy is reserved for situations in which the patient has normal femoral and popliteal pulses and the embolus is lodged in the tibial vessels.

Reference: The STILE trial: Results of a prospective randomized trial evaluating surgery versus thrombolysis for ischemia of the lower extremity, *Ann Surg* 220:251–268, 1994.

7. C. Recent reported results with reverse saphenous vein grafting demonstrated 5-year primary and secondary patency rates of 75% and 80%, respectively, and limb salvage rates of 90%. The in situ technique was developed using the concept that minimizing trauma to the vein would prolong patency; however, this has never been demonstrated. There are several theoretical advantages to the in situ technique. The vasa vasorum are maintained, which prevents ischemia to the endothelial layer of the vein graft. The in situ position allows the surgeon to sew the large end of the greater saphenous vein to the larger femoral vessels and to sew the smaller distal saphenous vein to the smaller distal vessels. This size match at the proximal and distal ends facilitates the completion of a precise anastomosis. Given this technical advantage, it is possible to successfully use smaller greater saphenous veins, which may not be suitable for the reverse vein technique. One disadvantage of the in situ technique is that it is more likely to produce technical errors. The valves need to be cut, which can injure the vein, or an inadequate valvulotomy may result in early thrombosis. All tributaries need to be ligated, and if one is left, this may lead to inadequate distal perfusion.

8. D. The classic string-of-beads appearance of the angiogram is characteristic of FMD. FMD is an angiopathy that affects medium-sized arteries. It occurs predominantly in young women, and most commonly affects the renal arteries. The etiology is unclear, but the predilection for women suggests a possible hormonal influence. Following the renal arteries, the internal carotid arteries are the second most common site, followed by the SMA. There is also an association with intracranial aneurysms. The angiopathy also predisposes to arterial dissection, most classically in the internal carotid artery.

Initial management of FMD should be medical. Intervention should be reserved for those in whom medical management fails. Renal artery FMD is more responsive to percutaneous transluminal angioplasty than renal artery atherosclerosis, and stenting is not routinely needed. Percutaneous transluminal angioplasty has technical success rates ranging from 83% to 100%, improvement rates of 21% to 63%, and cure rates of 14% to 59%. Open surgical bypass should be reserved for patients who do not respond to interventional techniques. The best surgical option is bypass, not endarterectomy. Bypass can be done with saphenous vein or synthetic graft. Success rates with open bypass range from 89% to 97%, with cure rates slightly higher than those with percutaneous transluminal angioplasty.

References: Slovut D, Olin J: Fibromuscular dysplasia, *N Engl J Med* 350:1862–1871, 2004.

Surowiec S, Sivamurthy N, Rhodes J, et al: Percutaneous therapy for renal artery fibromuscular dysplasia, *Ann Vasc Surg* 17:650–655, 2003.

9. D. In adults, hypertension is primarily due to essential hypertension, with only 5% considered surgically correctable causes. In children, conversely, in 85%, the hypertension is due to some underlying pathology. This can include underlying kidney disease, obstructive uropathy, pheochromocytoma, neurofibromatosis, and renal artery stenosis. The most common cause of renal artery stenosis in children is FMD. If a bypass were to be needed, the conduit of choice is autogenous artery, such as the internal iliac artery. Studies have shown that the saphenous vein tends to dilate with time in the pediatric age group and become aneurysmal.

Reference: Broekhuisen-de Gast H, Tiel-Van Buul M, Van Beek E: Severe hypertension in children with renovascular disease, *Clin Nucl Med* 26:606–609, 2001.

10. D. This patient's history and CT scan findings are most consistent with acute mesenteric ischemia. Acute mesenteric ischemia can be divided into four major causes. Embolization from a cardiac source is the most common cause (30%–50% of cases), is seen most often in the setting of atrial fibrillation, and is the likely etiology in the patient presented. The most common site of mesenteric embolization is the SMA. Celiac artery embolization is rare given its take-off at a right angle to the aorta. The inferior mesenteric artery orifice is so small that a cardiac thrombus rarely lodges inside. Another cause is mesenteric arterial thrombosis, which is usually due to underlying mesenteric artery atherosclerosis. In this situation, the patient will typically have a long-standing history of pain after eating, fear of eating, and weight loss, and the physical examination will reveal evidence of diffuse atherosclerosis and bruits. Mesenteric venous thrombosis is a third etiology and is most often seen in patients with hypercoagulable states. The acute venous occlusion leads to massive bowel edema with secondary arterial insufficiency from bowel wall distention. Patients with mesenteric venous thrombosis tend to present in a less dramatic fashion, often with days or weeks of abdominal pain. Finally, nonocclusive mesenteric ischemia results from shock that creates hypoperfusion to the bowel, such as with cardiac failure or severe hypovolemia.

The classic findings in acute mesenteric ischemia are sudden onset of severe pain out of proportion to the physical examination findings. Elevated serum lactate levels should raise the suspicion for ischemic bowel, but are not sensitive enough to detect early bowel ischemia. A plain abdominal radiograph is often unremarkable, although it may demonstrate evidence of edema in the small bowel wall. If the patient has peritoneal signs on abdominal examination, this would indicate that the bowel is already infarcted. In the absence of peritonitis and because the differential diagnosis is extensive, CT provides the greatest diagnostic yield initially. However, CT scan may not be diagnostic because it may not necessarily demonstrate opacification in the mesenteric veins or arteries. Surgery offers the best chance of treatment and would involve an SMA embolectomy. Because the patient has a classic presentation and embolization is best treated with embolectomy, delaying further treatment with arteriography is not necessary. Conversely, if the history were suggestive of underlying mesenteric atherosclerosis and thrombosis, arteriography would help in planning an arterial bypass. If the CT scan revealed a thrombus in a mesenteric vein, treatment would be heparin alone, provided there is not peritonitis. For nonocclusive ischemia, correcting the underlying shock is the initial management. There are some case reports in which mesenteric emboli have been successfully managed with lytic therapy, but this is not the standard approach.

11. A. The Goldblatt kidney refers to the ischemic kidney that produces hypertension. Through a series of animal experiments, Goldblatt and colleagues demonstrated that when only one kidney has renal artery occlusive disease and the other kidney is normally perfused, the hypertension that ensues is primarily caused by angiotensin II–mediated vasoconstriction due to increased renin secretion from the affected kidney. The increased aldosterone secretion that initially leads to sodium and water retention is offset by the normal kidney that increases the glomerular filtration rate and excretes the excess volume. Conversely, with bilateral severe renal artery stenosis, there is no ability to compensate, and thus such patients are prone to the development of fluid and sodium overload and recurrent bouts of intractable congestive heart failure. Angiotensin-converting enzyme inhibitors inhibit the angiotensin II–mediated vasoconstriction of the efferent arteriole at the glomerulus. With bilateral renal artery stenosis, angiotensin-converting enzyme inhibitors can therefore lead to a decrease in the glomerular filtration rate in both kidneys and worsening renal function. Thus, answers B, C, D, and E would be appropriate for bilateral stenosis. With unilateral renal artery stenosis, the normal kidney compensates by increasing the glomerular filtration rate. Thus, therapy for treating the hypertension should be targeted toward the renin-angiotensin system and not with diuretics.

Reference: Goldblatt H, Lynch J, Hanzal R, Summerville W: Studies on experimental hypertension I: the production of persistent elevation of systolic blood pressure by means of renal ischemia, *J Exp Med* 59:347–379, 1934.

12. A. This patient is manifesting symptoms of steal syndrome. Ischemic steal syndrome occurs in approximately 1% to 2% of patients with arteriovenous fistulas created for hemodialysis. The more proximal the fistula is, the greater the chance of creating steal, so that wrist fistulas (Cimino fistulas) have a very low risk of the development of steal. AV grafts also have a greater risk of steal compared with native AV fistulas. This is likely due to the fact that the large diameter of the graft creates a low-resistance bed. In addition, steal secondary AV fistulas tend to occur early after the access placement, whereas steal after native AV fistulas has a bimodal distribution, with some presenting early and others late after the native vein has undergone dilation with lowered resistance. Some degree of physiologic steal occurs in every patient with an AV fistula, but only a small minority manifest severe symptoms. The steal syndrome is caused by a diversion of blood flow from the anastomosed artery to the low-resistance vein. In addition, the low-resistance venous anastomosis leads to blood flowing in a retrograde fashion from the distal circulation into the fistula. Mild steal can be managed conservatively with exercise. More severe symptoms require intervention. Although ligation of the AV graft would have a great chance of resolving the steal syndrome, the patient will

require a new access and will again be at risk of developing steal. Several options exist for the management. The most effective treatment that maintains fistula function is distal revascularization and interval ligation. The disadvantage of this procedure is that it requires creating a new bypass, usually with saphenous vein, from the native artery proximal to the AV graft to the artery distal to it, with interval ligation of the native artery just proximal to the distal anastomosis. Banding or plicating of the AV graft, adjacent to the arterial anastomosis, serves to increase the resistance in the graft and reduce steal. The primary disadvantage of this approach is that inadequate banding leads to persistent steal, and excessive banding causes graft thrombosis. Banding or plication is a more attractive option for steal in an autologous AV fistula, such as a brachial artery cephalic vein fistula, because the vein is more resistant to thrombosis. This is not as yet the standard approach, however.

References: Walz P, Ladowski J, Hines A: Distal revascularization and interval ligation (DRIL) procedure for the treatment of ischemic steal syndrome after arm arteriovenous fistula, *Ann Vasc Surg* 21:468–473, 2007.

Yaghoubian A, de Virgilio C: Plication as primary treatment of steal syndrome in arteriovenous fistulas, *Ann Vasc Surg* 23:103–107, 2008.

Yu, P, Cook T, Canty R, et al: Hemodialysis-related steal syndrome: predictive factors and response to treatment with the distal revascularization-interval ligation procedure, *Ann Vasc Surg* 22:210–214, 2008.

13. C. Mesenteric venous thrombosis accounts for approximately 10 to 15 cases of mesenteric ischemia. It tends to have a slow, insidious onset, as in this case. Risk factors for mesenteric venous occlusion include hypercoagulable states such as factor V Leiden, antithrombin III deficiency, and protein C and S deficiency as well as liver disease with portal hypertension, pancreatitis, and any intraperitoneal inflammatory conditions. Venous thrombosis is less dramatic than arterial occlusion. Abdominal pain is vague, and tenderness is mild or equivocal. CT may demonstrate a thickened bowel wall with delayed passage of intravenous contrast agent into the portal system and lack of opacification of the portal or superior mesenteric vein. If the diagnosis is established from the CT scan, further diagnostic tests are unnecessary. Another useful diagnostic modality is duplex ultrasound scanning. Arteriography may demonstrate venous congestion and lack of prompt filling of the portal system. If the patient is manifesting peritoneal signs, operative exploration is indicated. However, in the absence of peritonitis, therapy should consist of fluid hydration, hemodynamic support, anticoagulation with heparin, and serial examination. If peritonitis subsequently develops, exploratory laparotomy is appropriate to assess bowel viability with segmental bowel resection. Surgical thrombectomy of the venous system is not likely to be successful. Fibrinolytic therapy has been used in a few select cases, but is not the standard treatment of choice.

Reference: Kumar S, Sarr M, Kamath P: Mesenteric venous thrombosis, *N Engl J Med* 345:1683–1688, 2001.

14. C. Cilostazol has a number of functions including inhibiting platelet aggregation and smooth muscle proliferation, increasing vasodilation, and lowering high-density lipoprotein and triglyceride levels. Cilostazol has been shown to significantly increase walking distance by 50% to 67% in patients with claudication in several randomized trials and results in improvement in physical functioning and quality of life. This drug is more effective than pentoxifylline in the treatment of claudication. Pentoxifylline is a methylxanthine derivative that has hemorrheologic properties. Two meta-analyses showed that it improves walking distance, but in some more recent randomized studies, it proved to be no better than placebo. Pentoxifylline improves symptoms of claudication by increasing red blood cell flexibility and reducing blood viscosity. Antiplatelet medications such as aspirin are used in the treatment of peripheral vascular disease, but do not appear to improve walking distance per se. Aspirin has been found to reduce the vascular death rate by approximately 25% in patients with any manifestation of atherosclerotic disease (e.g., coronary, peripheral). Clopidogrel is effective in reducing overall acute cardiovascular events, especially in patients with lower extremity occlusive disease, but is much more expensive. It does not seem to directly improve walking distance. Pure vasodilators have not been efficacious in the treatment of peripheral vascular disease because most patients with such occlusive disease already exhibit marked vasodilation. Anticoagulants also have not been shown to alter the course of peripheral atherosclerosis.

Reference: Money S, Herd J, Isaacsohn J, et al: Effect of cilostazol on walking distances in patients with intermittent claudication caused by peripheral vascular disease, *J Vasc Surg* 27:267–274, 1998.

15. B. The patient most likely has popliteal entrapment syndrome. Popliteal entrapment syndrome is rare but is the most common cause of true claudication in a young nonsmoking male (if the patient were a smoker, one would think of Buerger disease). The claudication is caused by compression of the popliteal artery. This can be due to either an aberrant course of the popliteal artery, medial to the medial head of the gastrocnemius muscle, or by abnormal fibrous bands or an enlarged popliteus muscle that compresses the artery. It is a rare disorder predominantly found in men. The typical patient presents with swelling and claudication of isolated calf muscle groups after exercise. Early on, the diagnosis can be elusive because the pulses at rest can be normal. Evocative tests should be performed by checking for disappearance of the distal pulses with active plantarflexion or passive dorsiflexion. Noninvasive studies with ABIs should be performed with the knee extended and the foot in a neutral, forced plantarflexed, and dorsiflexed position. A decrease in pressure of 50% or greater or dampening of the plethysmographic waveforms in plantarflexion or dorsiflexion is a classic finding. Repeating the ABI after exercise will result in compression of the popliteal artery and a decrease in the ABI. As the disease progresses, the repetitive trauma to the popliteal artery leads to injury and occlusion of the artery with thrombus or aneurysmal formation and the risk of embolization and limb loss. The diagnosis can be confirmed with CT angiography or magnetic resonance imaging. The characteristic feature of entrapment, in which the popliteal artery is deviated more medially than normal, is not seen in all types of entrapment. Thus, CT or magnetic resonance imaging is helpful in demonstrating abnormal muscle bundles compressing the artery. If the diagnosis is made early, before irreversible injury to the popliteal artery, then dividing the abnormal muscle bundles may be appropriate. Otherwise, bypass with reverse saphenous vein is required. Endovascular treatment alone is generally not sufficient because it does not address the abnormal muscle.

Buerger disease is a progressive nonatherosclerotic segmental inflammatory disease, seen in young male smokers, that most often affects small- to medium-sized arteries, veins, and nerves of the upper and lower extremities. Patients initially present with foot, leg, arm, or hand claudication. Progression of the disease leads to calf claudication and eventually ischemic rest pain and ulcerations of the toes, feet, and fingers.

Popliteal cystic adventitial disease is a condition that affects men in their fourth to sixth decades of life. Besides claudication as a symptom, the diagnosis should be considered in young patients who have a mass in a nonaxial vessel in proximity to a related joint. These synovium-like, mucin-filled cysts reside in the subadventitial layer of the vessel wall. They have an appearance similar to that of ganglion cysts. Patients presenting at a young age with bilateral lower extremity claudication and minimal risk factors for atheroma formation should be evaluated for adventitial cystic disease. Angiographically, the lesion will give the appearance of a scimitar (a curved blade).

Popliteal aneurysms are the most common peripheral artery aneurysms. These aneurysms present by a process of chronic distal embolization or sudden-onset occlusion of the popliteal artery. The patients may present with foot ischemia or sudden onset of limb-threatening ischemia. Examination may reveal a pulsatile mass. Foot pulses may be diminished if embolization has been occurring. This would most likely present in much older male smokers.

References: Rich N, Collins G, McDonald P, et al: Popliteal vascular entrapment, *Arch Surg* 114:1377–1384, 1989.

Turnipseed W: Popliteal entrapment syndrome, *J Vasc Surg* 35:910–915, 2002.

16. E. Leg edema after femoral-to-popliteal bypass is common. In most instances, it is due to lymphatic disruption. This disruption occurs at both the groin and popliteal incisions as well as from harvesting of the saphenous vein. Deep venous thrombosis can occur after this procedure but is relatively uncommon.

Reference: AbuRahma A, Woodruff B, Lucente F: Edema after femoropopliteal bypass surgery: lymphatic and venous theories of causation, *J Vasc Surg* 11:461–467, 1990.

17. B. Cardiac clot tends to lodge in areas where the arterial diameter suddenly decreases, such as at bifurcations. Where a clot lodges also depends on flow patterns. Because a cardiac clot is usually large, it lodges preferentially in larger vessels. Approximately 70% of clots lodge in the lower extremities, 13% in the upper extremities, 10% in the cerebral circulation, and 5% to 10% in the visceral circulation. The most common location is the common femoral artery in 34%, followed by the common iliac and popliteal arteries at their bifurcations.

Reference: Green R, Ouriel K. Arterial disease. In Schwartz SI, editor: *Principles of surgery*, ed 8, New York, 1999, McGraw-Hill, p 953.

18. D. The normal ABI ranges from 1 to 1.2, and a value less than 0.9 indicates some degree of peripheral vascular disease. Patients with claudication typically have an ABI in the 0.6 to 0.8 range. Calf claudication is usually due to disease in the SFA. The pulse deficit between the femoral and popliteal arteries further confirms disease in the SFA. The segmental pressures also help to localize the site of the obstruction to the SFA as the pressure decrease is between the upper thigh and knee. Because the initial management of claudication should be medical, no further imaging is needed. Claudication is not considered limb threatening in the absence of ischemic rest pain, ulceration, or gangrene. The goal of medical management is to prevent progression of peripheral vascular disease, reduce the risk of major cardiovascular events elsewhere, and improve function in symptomatic patients. Smoking cessation is the most important factor in determining the outcome of patients with claudication. Smoking cessation has been shown to result in a reduction of the 10-year mortality rate from 54% to 18%. In addition to smoking cessation, the patient should be placed on an exercise program and be prescribed a statin and aspirin. Hypertension should be controlled.

Duplex ultrasound scanning is an appropriate arterial noninvasive study that is often used in conjunction with segmental pressures and ABI. However, given that the patient has already undergone an ABI, the next step would be to institute medical management. Magnetic resonance imaging, CT, or standard arteriography should be reserved for patients in whom an intervention is being planned.

19. D. This is a controversial topic. Numerous prospective studies have demonstrated that a program of routine vein graft surveillance results in improved secondary graft patency because stenoses can be detected and corrected before graft occlusion. One should not wait until the pulse disappears or until there is a marked decrease in the ABI, because at that point, the graft is likely already clotted. In addition, vein grafts, once thrombosed, are difficult to reopen with standard thrombolytic techniques. Graft surveillance of synthetic grafts, however, does not seem to be effective because some grafts thrombose without a pre-existing stenosis, and synthetic grafts can be reopened more readily with thrombolytic therapy.

A recent prospective, randomized European study threw a monkey wrench into the surveillance algorithm. The study demonstrated no benefit of using a surveillance plan in terms of secondary patency or limb salvage rates and showed increased costs. Many U.S. surgeons have raised questions about the study design and thus continue to perform surveillance. Grafts at highest risk of thrombosis are those with a peak systolic velocity greater than 300 cm/sec or a velocity ratio greater than 3.5 at the site of the stenosis.

References: Bandyk D, Kaebnick H, Stewart G, Towne J: Durability of the in situ saphenous vein arterial bypass: a comparison of primary and secondary patency, *J Vasc Surg* 5:256–268, 1987.

Davies A, Hawdon A, Sydes M, et al: Is duplex surveillance of value after leg vein bypass grafting? Principal results of the vein graft surveillance randomized trial (VGST), *Circulation* 112:1985–1991, 2005.

20. B. Lumbar sympathectomy was first used for non-healing foot ulcers well before arterial reconstruction was conceived. The initial interest in sympathectomy was that surgeons noted experimentally and clinically increased skin temperature and hyperemia afterward. However, subsequent experimental evidence indicates that lumbar sympathectomy increases skin temperature by augmenting non-nutrient blood flow through cutaneous AV anastomoses without improving skin capillary blood flow. As such, it is not indicated for the treatment of non-healing ulcers. In addition, in the diabetic patient, there is already autosympathectomy as a result of associated autonomic neuropathy; thus, surgical sympathectomy is even less helpful. The best indications for lumbar sympathectomy are complex regional pain syndrome (reflex sympathetic dystrophy, causalgia) and lower extremity Raynaud syndrome that has not adequately responded to medical management. The most common complication is postoperative neuralgia. Complex regional pain syndrome sometimes develops after injury. The affected limb is painful and swollen, with changes in the color, temperature, and texture of the skin. These symptoms are related to prolonged and excessive activity of the sympathetic nervous system. Because sweating is controlled by the sympathetic nervous system, sympathectomy is also effective in treating hyperhidrosis of the palms, armpits, or face. Postoperative Horner syndrome may occur if portions of the stellate ganglion are removed or inadvertently cauterized.

Reference: Welke K, Cronenwett J: Lumbar sympathectomy for lower extremity cutaneous ischemic ulcers. In Ernst C, Stanley J, editors: *Current therapy in vascular surgery*, St. Louis, 2001, Mosby, pp 483–486.

21. D. Anastomotic femoral pseudoaneurysms develop in approximately 3% to 5% of cases after aortobifemoral bypasses. If a pseudoaneurysm develops early after surgery, one has to be concerned about the possibility of a graft infection. In one study, 60% of treated femoral anastomotic pseudoaneurysms had an occult *Staphylococcus epidermidis* infection. Late anastomotic pseudoaneurysms are thought to be due to deterioration of the Dacron material, suture deterioration, or repetitive hip flexion, causing the sutures to pull through the native artery. Elective surgical management is the treatment of choice because these lesions progressively increase in size. Studies on the natural history indicate that the pseudoaneurysm may lead to rupture or thrombus formation and graft occlusion. The operative repair most frequently used is excising the diseased segment of the artery and graft and placing an interposition prosthesis. Proximally, it is sewn in an end-to-end fashion to the previous graft. Distally, the graft has to be tailored to connect around both the SFA and the profunda femoris artery. Ultrasonography-guided thrombin injection or compression would be indicated for pseudoaneurysms that develop after femoral catheterization, but would not be appropriate for a disrupted graft.

References: Mulder E, van Bockel J, Maas J, et al: Morbidity and mortality of reconstructive surgery of noninfected false aneurysms detected long after aortic prosthetic reconstruction, *J Arch Surg* 133:45–49, 1998.

Seabrook G, Schmitt D, Bandyk D et al: Anastomotic femoral pseudoaneurysms: an investigation of occult infection as an etiologic factor, *J Vasc Surg* 11:629–634, 1990.

22. C. The classic presentation of patients with acute ischemia of the extremities is highlighted by the "five Ps": pain, pallor, pulselessness, paresthesias, and paralysis. Pain is the most common symptom in alert patients. The degree of pain depends on the severity of ischemia, which is generally determined by the location of the occlusion and the degree of collateral flow. Ischemic pain can be severe and difficult to relieve, even with large doses of narcotics. The sudden onset of severe ischemic pain in a previously asymptomatic patient is most suggestive of an embolic occlusion. Patients with spontaneous thrombosis often have had chronic symptoms of claudication or various degrees of pain before the acute event. Pallor is a common but relative finding that depends on the degree of ischemia and the underlying skin color. A sudden and complete embolic occlusion may result in a cool, waxy-appearing white extremity with no signs of cutaneous blood flow. Conversely, a partial occlusion may result in only delayed capillary refill with pallor on elevation of the extremity and rubor on dependency. Because the degree of the occlusion and collateral circulation influence the severity of ischemia, the duration of ischemia alone is not a good guide to irreversibility. With a large embolus and poor collateralization, profound ischemia develops rapidly, and irreversibility develops within 4 to 6 hours. Conversely, with less profound ischemia, the patient may tolerate the ischemic insult for 12 hours and longer.

The majority of patients with acute ischemia will have an absent distal pulse. As such, the pulse examination, although helpful in identifying ischemia, is not good for determining ischemia severity. The ABI was developed for chronic ischemia, and the same criteria are not accurate for acute ischemia. However, the presence of an arterial Doppler signal at the foot and an ankle pressure greater than 30 mm Hg is suggestive of less severe ischemia. The presence of even monophasic Doppler signals over the pedal vessels affirms some degree of distal vascular flow and at least short-term viability of the distal tissues. Conversely, a complete absence of arterial flow is most suggestive of profound ischemia and calls for immediate revascularization.

Of the choices listed, the best answer is the presence of a motor deficit. Within the extremities, the peripheral nerve is the tissue that is most sensitive to ischemia. As such, the degree of neurologic dysfunction is a useful barometer of the degree of ischemia. With mild ischemia, the findings may be subjective and subtle. Early paresthesias may be characterized as numbness of the toes or a slight decrease in sensation of the foot compared with the contralateral extremity to light touch or pinprick. With severe ischemia, however, profound sensory loss may lead to complete anesthesia of the foot, indicative of impending tissue loss without early revascularization. Paradoxically, these patients with the most severe ischemia and complete anesthesia report less pain than those with mild ischemia and intact sensation. As the ischemia progresses, the weakness may progress to frank paralysis of the affected extremity.

In patients with severe ischemia characterized by anesthesia and paralysis, it is important to distinguish reversible from irreversible ischemic changes. Patients with prolonged ischemia have palpable firmness of the extremity muscle and stiffness of the extremity, indicative of muscle rigor. Reperfusion of such an extremity does not restore function and can result in severe systemic injury. Primary amputation is the safest form of management in such cases.

Reference: Norgren L, Hiatt W, Dormandy J et al: Inter-Society Consensus for the Management of Peripheral Arterial Disease (TASC II), *J Vasc Surg* 45(Suppl S):S5–S67, 2007.

23. B. Acute aortic occlusion is a rare vascular catastrophe. It may result from an aortic saddle embolus from atrial fibrillation or an acute myocardial infarction, in situ thrombosis of a preexisting atherosclerotic abdominal aorta, sudden thrombosis of an abdominal aortic aneurysm, or total aortic dissection. Because patient prognosis is time dependent, early recognition, administration of IV heparin and fluids, and prompt diagnosis play a role in management. Because patients often develop rapid onset of neurologic lower extremity deficits, the diagnosis can be confused with an acute neurologic event, and the patient may be "mistriaged" to neurology. Once the diagnosis is made, prompt intervention is mandatory. In general, the management of choice is to go directly to the operating room and perform bilateral transfemoral embolectomies, particularly in patients without a history of claudication/peripheral vascular disease because the cause is usually embolic. However, in this patient, who has a history of thigh and buttock claudication, embolectomies are unlikely to be successful. Thus, definitive management would most likely be achieved with an arterial bypass. The choice of whether to perform an aortobifemoral or an axillofemoral bypass is one of timing. Given the severity of the patient's ischemia, an axillofemoral bypass would be the most expeditious solution, albeit one with worse long-term patency. In planning the axillofemoral bypass, it is important to measure arm pressure and base the bypass on the arm with the higher blood pressure. In one study of 18 patients, 9 of 10 patients with acute aortic occlusion from emboli were treated successfully with bilateral transfemoral embolectomy, whereas none of the 8 patients with in situ aortic thrombosis were successfully treated. Acute aortic occlusion is associated with a mortality rate of 75% with nonoperative treatment. With operative intervention, the mortality rate ranges from 25% to 50%. In patients with suspected in situ abdominal aortic thrombosis with clinically unclear renal or mesenteric arterial involvement, a preoperative angiogram would be useful, but with current endovascular technology, this can be obtained intraoperatively if the patient is severely ischemic. Choice D is not optimal because there would be an inordinate delay in a patient who already has a motor deficit and it would not be definitive because having underlying atherosclerosis, she would likely need stenting as well if the lysis were successful. There are some case reports emerging on the use of aortoiliac stenting for this indication, but it is not as yet the procedure of choice.

Reference: Littooy F, Baker W: Acute aortic occlusion: a multifaceted catastrophe, *J Vasc Surg* 4:211–216, 1986.

24. D. There are no absolute markers for predicting healing of an amputation. In general, the presence of a palpable pulse just above the proposed site of amputation is a strong predictor of healing. Thus, a femoral pulse predicts healing of an above-knee amputation, a popliteal pulse predicts healing of a below-knee amputation, and a dorsalis pedis pulse predicts healing of a transmetatarsal amputation. Conversely, the absence of a pulse above the site of amputation does not predict a failure of healing. The presence of gangrene above the ankle is thought to be predictive of nonhealing of a below-knee amputation, but the absence of gangrene is not helpful. Numerous noninvasive studies were performed to try to predict healing. Transcutaneous oximetry readings greater than 40 mm Hg predict healing, and readings less than 20 mm Hg predict nonhealing. The problem is that many patients fall in the 20- to 40-mm Hg range. A popliteal pressure greater than 70 mm Hg, as measured with Doppler ultrasonography and a blood pressure cuff, is a useful modality for predicting healing. It was associated with 97% healing of below-knee amputations in one study. In the same study, a palpable popliteal pulse was likewise associated with a 97% healing rate.

References: Malone J, Anderson G, Lalka S, et al: Prospective comparison of noninvasive techniques for amputation level selection, *Am J Surg* 154:179–184, 1987.

Nicholas G, Myers J, DeMuth W Jr: The role of vascular laboratory criteria in the selection of patients for lower extremity amputation, *Ann Surg* 195:469–473, 1982.

25. A. Acute ischemia in an infant, particularly one with congenital heart disease, presents a difficult management dilemma given the small size of the vessels and the underlying cardiac condition. The majority of these injuries respond well to a combination of heparin, hydration, and rewarming of the extremity. Given the difficulty in vascular repair in infants, surgical intervention should be reserved for those who do not respond to these measures. If repair were needed, the surgeon must be aware that the vessels have a greater tendency to develop vasospasm due to the greater muscular component of the vessel. As such, the vessel should be injected with papaverine before manipulation. Arteriotomies should be closed with vein patch closure to prevent further narrowing. If replacement of the artery is necessary, saphenous vein is used, but because of the propensity of the vein to become aneurysmal, reinforcing it with Dacron or another synthetic material is recommended. Suturing should be done using interrupted sutures to allow growth of the artery. It is also important to bear in mind that chronic femoral occlusion has been reported in as many as one third of infants undergoing transfemoral catheterization and that this can lead to future limb length discrepancy. However, a chronic occlusion, if asymptomatic, is better treated later in childhood if the ABI is persistently decreased.

References: de Virgilio C, Mercado P, Arnell T, et al: Noniatrogenic pediatric vascular trauma: a ten-year experience at a level I trauma center, *Am Surg* 63:781–784, 1997.

Sarkar R: Iatrogenic pediatric vascular injuries. In Ernst C, Stanley J, editors: *Current therapy in vascular surgery*, St. Louis, 2001, Mosby, pp 637–641.

26. D. The patient's history and examination are most consistent with symptoms of coronary-subclavian steal syndrome. Most patients with a coronary artery bypass graft have undergone a left internal mammary artery–to–left anterior descending graft. In the setting of subclavian artery stenosis or occlusion proximal to the take-off of the internal mammary artery, arm exercise leads to vasodilation of the arm vessels and lower resistance. Blood will travel through the path of least resistance and flow in a reverse fashion from the left anterior descending artery into the left internal mammary artery and toward the arm, leading to the development of angina. The differential blood pressure in the arms is the clue, as is the left arm claudication. Treatment involves relieving the subclavian artery obstruction. This can generally be done by subclavian artery stenting, but on occasion requires a carotid artery–to–subclavian bypass.

Reference: Bryan F, Allen R, Lumsden A: Coronary subclavian steal syndrome: report of 5 cases, *Ann Vasc Surg* 9:115–122, 1995.

27. D. When a young patient presents with symptoms and signs of peripheral vascular disease, one must consider rare causes, including all the ones listed. Popliteal cystic adventitial disease is a condition that affects men in their fourth to sixth decades of life. In addition to claudication as a symptom, the diagnosis should be considered in younger patients who have a mass in a nonaxial vessel in proximity to a related joint. These synovium-like, mucin-filled cysts reside in the subadventitial layer of the vessel wall. They have an appearance similar to that of ganglion cysts. Patients presenting at a young age with bilateral lower extremity claudication and minimal risk factors for atheroma formation should be evaluated for adventitial cystic disease. Angiographically, the lesion will give the appearance of a scimitar (a curved blade). Treatment would consist of excising the segment of diseased artery with an interposition graft.

Persistence of the sciatic artery as the major blood supply to the lower extremity in adults is a rare vascular anomaly that may be of surgical significance. The SFA is usually atretic. Failure to appreciate the persistent sciatic artery as the major inflow into the lower extremity may lead to inappropriate bypass of apparent occlusive disease of the SFA. The persistent sciatic artery is also frequently aneurysmal, which may cause critical limb ischemia resulting from thrombosis or embolization of an aneurysm thrombus. It can also present as a pulsatile buttock mass (do not perform a biopsy!).

Reference: Mandell V, Jaques P, Delany D, Oberheu V: Persistent sciatic artery: clinical, embryologic, and angiographic features, *AJR Am J Roentgenol* 144:245–249, 1985.

28. E. Initial management of patients with acute mesenteric ischemia includes fluid resuscitation and systemic anticoagulation with heparin sulfate to prevent further thrombus propagation. Significant metabolic acidosis should be corrected with sodium bicarbonate. A central venous catheter, peripheral arterial catheter, and Foley catheter should be placed for fluid resuscitation and hemodynamic status monitoring. Appropriate antibiotics are given before surgical exploration. The operative management of acute mesenteric ischemia is dictated by the cause of the occlusion. For an SMA embolus, exposure of the SMA is obtained via rotation of the small bowel to the right and sharply dissecting the ligament of Treitz. The SMA will be found at the root of the mesentery. The primary goal in the surgical treatment of embolic mesenteric ischemia is to restore arterial perfusion with removal of the embolus from the vessel. This is done by performing a Fogarty embolectomy using a transverse arteriotomy. It is important to avoid resecting bowel until perfusion has been restored; that way, bowel viability can be better established. After restoration of SMA flow, an assessment of the intestinal viability is made, and nonviable bowel is resected. Because the amount of bowel resected can be extensive and this places the patient at risk of short bowel syndrome, bowel that is of borderline viability should be left in place with a planned second-look procedure performed 24 to 48 hours later to reassess whether additional bowel resection is needed. Mannitol is a free radical scavenger that helps mitigate the ischemia/reperfusion injury that follows restoration of blood flow.

29. B. Major amputation is a relatively rare occurrence in patients who have claudication without ischemic rest pain or ulceration. In two recent reviews, the risk of major amputation at 5 years ranged between 1% and 3.3%. In the Framingham studies, the risk of limb loss was less than 2%. Thus, when evaluating and counseling patients with claudication, it is important to reassure them that they do not have an imminently limb-threatening problem. Likewise, the low risk of limb loss further supports the premise that the initial management of claudication should be medical.

Reference: Norgren L, Hiatt W, Dormandy J, et al: Inter-Society Consensus for the Management of Peripheral Arterial Disease (TASC II), *J Vasc Surg* 45(Suppl S):S5–S67, 2007.

30. E. Patients undergoing vascular surgery are among those with the highest risk of experiencing an adverse perioperative cardiac event. As such, a great deal of focus has been placed on trying to identify patients at highest risk and potentially to correct coronary artery disease before the vascular operation. Cardiac risk stratification underwent major changes in the past decade as a result of several studies, the most important of which is the CARP (Coronary Artery Revascularization Prophylaxis) study, which demonstrated that prophylactic coronary artery revascularization did not improve perioperative or long-term cardiac morbidity in patients requiring vascular surgery. In addition, several prospective studies demonstrated that an abnormal persantine sestamibi/thallium test result does not predict adverse perioperative cardiac events.

Given the lack of benefit to prophylactic coronary artery revascularization and the poor predictive value of persantine sestamibi/thallium testing, greater focus has been placed on using clinical criteria to identify patients at highest risk of adverse cardiac events and on the use of drugs to medically optimize the patient. The Revised Cardiac Index is a validated and easily calculated score to assess cardiac risk. One point each is assigned for (1) history of coronary artery disease, (2) insulin

dependence, (3) history of a cerebrovascular event, (4) creatinine level greater than 2.0 mg/dL, (5) history of congestive heart failure, and (6) high-risk surgery (aortic, thoracic, major abdominal). Based on this index, the predicted major cardiac complication rates are as follows: 0 points, class I, very low risk (0.4% complication rate); 1 point, class II, low risk (0.9% complication rate); 2 points, class III, moderate risk (6.6% complication rate); 3 or more points, class IV, high risk (>11% complication rate). Patients should be divided into low, intermediate, and high clinical risk using this scoring system, and the proposed operations should likewise be divided into low (skin, breast), intermediate, and high risk (aortic, major thoracic) operations.

Using this scoring system, the patient described would have a Revised Cardiac Index of 1 (low-risk patient), undergoing a high-risk surgery, and can thus proceed to surgery without any additional work-up. Patients with a Revised Cardiac Index of 2 or less can proceed safely to surgery. It is as yet unclear what role stress testing should play in patients with a Revised Cardiac Index of 3 or more.

Likewise the role of beta-blockade in noncardiac surgery is controversial. Routine use in all noncardiac surgery patients is not warranted, and a recent meta-analysis suggested that such a policy may actually increase the risk of stroke. Conversely, in a patient undergoing high-risk vascular surgery, there are data to support not only beta-blockade but a targeted heart rate of less than 65 beats per minute. The concern is that overly aggressive beta-blockade may lead to hypotension and adverse events. Likewise, the use of statins has been shown to reduce perioperative cardiac events. Statins have anti-inflammatory effects that lead to stabilization of atherosclerotic plaques.

References: de Virgilio C, Toosie K, Ephraim L, et al: Dipyridamole-thallium/sestamibi before vascular surgery: a prospective blinded study in moderate-risk patients, *J Vasc Surg* 32:77–89, 2000.

Lee T, Marcantonio E, Mangione C, et al: Derivation and prospective validation of a simple index for prediction of cardiac risk of major noncardiac surgery, *Circulation* 100:1043–1049, 1999.

McFalls E, Ward H, Moritz T, et al: Coronary-artery revascularization before elective major vascular surgery, *N Engl J Med* 351:2795–2804, 2004.

Poldermans D, Bax J, Kertai M, et al: Statins are associated with a reduced incidence of perioperative mortality in patients undergoing major noncardiac vascular surgery, *Circulation* 107:1848–1851, 2003.

Poldermans D, Bax J, Schouten O, et al: Should major vascular surgery be delayed because of preoperative cardiac testing in intermediate-risk patients receiving beta-blocker therapy with tight heart rate control? *J Am Coll Cardiol* 48:964–969, 2006.

31. B. The most common cause of mesenteric ischemia is a cardiac embolus to the SMA. The SMA provides blood to the bowel from the ligament of Treitz to the mid transverse colon. Cardiac embolus tends to lodge just past the SMA origin at a point where the artery begins to narrow, which is just beyond the first jejunal branches. As such, the proximal jejunum is typically spared. Thrombosis of the SMA, conversely, is usually caused by underlying atherosclerotic disease that occurs at the SMA origin and would thus not spare the proximal jejunum. Mesenteric venous thrombosis and nonocclusive mesenteric ischemia would more likely cause patchy areas of ischemia.

Reference: Jens Eldrup-Jorgensen J, Hawkins R, Bredenberg C: Abdominal vascular catastrophes, *Surg Clin North Am* 77: 1305–1320, 1997.

32. A. In addition to atherosclerosis, the second most common cause of renal artery stenosis is FMD. FMD most commonly affects the renal arteries, followed by the internal carotid artery. FMD of the renal artery represents a heterogeneous group of lesions that produce specific pathologic lesions in various regions of the vessel wall, including the intima, media, and adventitia. The most common type is medial fibroplasia, in which thickened fibromuscular ridges alternate with attenuated media, producing the string-of-beads appearance. The cause of FMD remains uncertain, but it seems to be associated with modification of arterial smooth muscle cells in response to estrogenic stimuli during the reproductive years, unusual traction forces on affected vessels, and mural ischemia from impairment of vasa vasorum blood flow. FMD usually affects the distal two thirds of the main renal artery, and the right renal artery is affected more frequently than the left. This entity most commonly occurs in young women who are often multiparous.

References: Gloviczki P, Ricotta JJ: Aneurysmal vascular disease. In Townsend CM Jr, Beauchamp RD, Evers BM, Mattox KL, editors: *Sabiston textbook of surgery: the biological basis of modern surgical practice*, ed 18, Philadelphia, 2008, WB Saunders, pp 1907–1940.

Lin P, Kougias P, Bechara C, et al: Arterial disease. In Brunicardi FC, Andersen DK, Billiar TR, et al, editors: *Schwartz's principles of surgery*, ed 9, New York, 2010, McGraw-Hill, pp 701–775.

33. A. The causes of thoracic outlet syndrome are divided into neurogenic, venous, and arterial. Neurogenic is the most common, and arterial is the least common. Arterial compression is most commonly caused by a cervical rib. It can also be caused by a long transverse process of C7, the abdominal first rib, osteoarthritis, scalene muscle hypertrophy, trauma, fibrous bands, or neoplasm. Patients with arterial thoracic outlet syndrome are prone to the development of poststenotic aneurysmal dilation.

34. B. Neurologic symptoms occur in 95% of cases of thoracic outlet syndrome. The lower two nerve roots of the brachial plexus, C8 and T1, are most commonly (90%) involved, producing pain and paresthesias in the ulnar nerve distribution. The second most common anatomic pattern involves the upper three nerve roots of the brachial plexus, C5, C6, and C7, with symptoms referred to the neck, ear, upper chest, upper back, and outer arm in the radial nerve distribution.

35. A. Significant steal after a femoral-to-femoral bypass is uncommon. It is most likely to occur if there is stenosis of the donor iliac artery above the proposed bypass. Thus, it is important to assess the donor femoral pulse pre- and intraoperatively. If there is any question, a pressure measurement should be obtained in the donor femoral artery intraoperatively, after papaverine injection (to reproduce

the vasodilation associated with exercise), and if it is lower than the brachial artery pressure (by $\geq$10 mm Hg), then the donor iliac artery should be stented before performing the femoral-to-femoral bypass.

Reference: Vogt K: The clinical importance and prediction of steal following femoral-femoral cross-over bypass: study of the donor iliac artery by intravascular ultrasound, arteriography, duplex scanning and pressure measurements, *Eur J Vasc Endovasc Surg* 19:178–183, 2000.

36. E. Upper extremity sympathectomy is most effective for palmar hyperhidrosis. It is also used for complex regional pain syndrome. Horner syndrome may occur if portions of the stellate ganglion are removed or inadvertently coagulated. The symptoms include ptosis, meiosis, and anhidrosis.

Reference: Singh B, Moodley J, Allopi L, Cassimjee H: Horner syndrome after sympathectomy in the thoracoscopic era, *Surg Laparosc Endosc Percutan Tech* 16:222–225, 2006.

37. B. The greater saphenous vein is the conduit of choice for lower extremity distal bypass. When the greater saphenous vein is not available, options include the lesser saphenous and cephalic veins. Ectopic veins (i.e., lesser saphenous, arm veins) are generally inferior to a single-segment saphenous vein, although they are still superior to the performance of synthetic grafts. A composite graft, which is a vein graft sewn to a polytetrafluoroethylene graft, has a patency rate similar to that of a prosthetic graft and tends to develop neointimal hyperplasia. Option A is suboptimal because it involves splicing vein, and with the femoral and popliteal arteries patent, there is no need to perform such a long bypass. Amputation of the toe is unlikely to heal in the absence of a palpable pedal pulse.

Reference: Gentile A, Lee R, Moneta G, et al: Results of bypass to the popliteal and tibial arteries with alternative sources of autogenous vein, *J Vasc Surg* 23:272–279, 1996.

38. B. The 5-year survival rate of patients with claudication is only 70%; 40% to 60% of deaths are caused by coronary artery disease. Cerebrovascular disease accounts for an additional 10% to 20% of deaths. Thus, the primary focus of the management of those with claudication is to aggressively treat the underlying risk factors for atherosclerosis, including the use of aspirin and statins, as well as smoking cessation.

Reference: Norgren L, Hiatt W, Dormandy J, et al: Inter-Society Consensus for the Management of Peripheral Arterial Disease (TASC II), *J Vasc Surg* 45(Suppl S):S5–S67, 2007.

39. A. The modified response to injury hypothesis is as follows: (1) endothelial injury results in growth factor secretion; (2) the local hemodynamic environment facilitates local injury and particle transfer; (3) circulating monocytes attach to the damaged endothelium; (4) subendothelial migration of monocytes may lead to fatty streak formation and further release of growth factors such as platelet-derived growth factor; (5) fatty streaks may then be converted to fibrous plaques by release of growth factors from macrophages, endothelial cells, or both; (6) macrophages may stimulate or injure the overlying endothelium; thus, endothelial cell loss leads to platelet deposition; (7) platelet deposition leads to the release of growth factors and mitogenic factors for smooth muscle cells; and (8) some of the smooth muscle cells in the proliferative lesion itself may form and secrete growth factors.

Reference: Lin P, Kougias P, Bechara C, et al: Arterial disease. In Brunicardi FC, Andersen DK, Billiar TR, et al, editors: *Schwartz's principles of surgery*, ed 9, New York, 2010, McGraw-Hill, p 701–775.

40. D. The fatty streak is the earliest identifiable lesion of atherosclerosis. It has been detected in children as young as 10 years of age and consists of lipid-laden macrophages overlying lipid-laden smooth muscle cells. They occur at the same anatomic sites as subsequent fibrous plaques.

Reference: Lin P, Kougias P, Bechara C, et al: Arterial disease. In Brunicardi FC, Andersen DK, Billiar TR, et al, editors: *Schwartz's principles of surgery*, ed 9, New York, 2010, McGraw-Hill, p 701–775.

41. E. Cilostazol inhibits platelet aggregation, increases vasodilation, inhibits smooth muscle proliferation (by inhibition of phosphodiesterase type 3), and lowers high-density lipoprotein cholesterol and triglyceride levels. This drug has been more effective than pentoxifylline in the treatment of claudication at doses of 100 mg twice daily. Cilostazol has been shown to significantly increase walking distance in patients with claudication in several randomized trials and to result in improvement in physical functioning and quality of life. Improvement has ranged from 35% to 100%. It is contraindicated in patients with congestive heart failure because of its effects on phosphodiesterase. It is safe to use in diabetic patients.

42. E. This is Raynaud disease. First described in 1862 by Maurice Raynaud, the term *Raynaud disease* applies to a heterogeneous symptom array associated with peripheral vasospasm, more commonly occurring in the upper extremities. The characteristically intermittent vasospasm classically follows exposure to various stimuli, including cold temperatures, tobacco, or emotional stress. Formerly, a distinction was made between Raynaud disease and Raynaud phenomenon for describing a benign disease occurring in isolation or a more severe disease secondary to another underlying disorder, respectively. However, collagen vascular disorders develop in many patients at some point after the onset of vasospastic symptoms; the rate of progression to a connective tissue disorder ranges from 11% to 65% in reported series. Characteristic color changes occur in response to the arteriolar vasospasm, ranging from intense pallor to cyanosis to redness as the vasospasm occurs. The digital vessels then relax, eventually leading to reactive hyperemia. The majority of patients are women younger than 40 years of age. As many as 70% to 90% of reported patients are women, although many patients with only mild symptoms may never present for treatment. Geographic regions located in cooler, damp climates such as the Pacific Northwest and Scandinavian countries have a higher reported prevalence of the disease. Certain occupational groups, such as those that use vibrating tools, may be more predisposed to Raynaud disease or digital ischemia. The exact pathophysiologic mechanism behind the development of such severe vasospasm remains elusive, and much attention has focused on increased levels of α_2-adrenergic receptors and their hypersensitivity in patients with Raynaud disease, as well as abnormalities in the thermoregulatory response, which is governed by the sympathetic nervous system.

There is no cure for Raynaud disease; thus, all treatments mainly palliate symptoms and decrease the severity and perhaps frequency of attacks. Conservative measures predominate, including the wearing of gloves, use of electric or chemically activated hand warmers, avoiding occupational exposure to vibratory tools, abstinence from tobacco, and relocating to a warmer, dryer climate. The majority (90%) of patients will respond to avoidance of cold and other stimuli. The remaining 10% of patients with more persistent or severe syndromes can be treated with a variety of vasodilatory drugs, albeit with only a 30% to 60% response rate. Calcium channel blocking agents such as diltiazem and nifedipine are the drugs of choice. The selective serotonin reuptake inhibitor fluoxetine has been shown to reduce the frequency and duration of vasospastic episodes but is not the first-line treatment. Intravenous infusions of prostaglandins have been reserved for nonresponders with severe symptoms. Upper extremity sympathectomy may provide relief in 60% to 70% of patients; however, the results are short-lived, with a gradual recurrence of symptoms in 60% within 10 years.

43. D. The patient presents with acute digital ischemia. Unilateral finger ischemia suggests an embolic source such as an atherosclerotic plaque in the innominate or subclavian artery or a subclavian artery aneurysm due to thoracic outlet syndrome compressing the artery and causing poststenotic aneurysm and thrombus formation. Buerger disease can cause digital ischemia, but it occurs in smokers. Giant cell arteritis is predominantly a disease of elderly women and presents with headaches and pain over the superficial temporal artery. A cardiac embolus is a possibility, but the typical clot that dislodges from atrial fibrillation or mural thrombus is large and thus too big to enter the digital artery. The exceptions would be infective endocarditis, rheumatic heart disease, and small valvular tumors (such as cardiac papillary fibroelastomas) that might shower off smaller particles. Bilateral finger ischemia suggests an underlying systemic vascular disorder, such as diabetes mellitus, chronic renal failure, and a connective tissue disorder (scleroderma).

44. A. The patient presented has Leriche syndrome, a chronic occlusion of the aorta caused by progressive aortoiliac atherosclerosis that includes the triad of buttock/thigh claudication, impotence, and absent femoral pulses. In addition, the patient has critical limb ischemia, based on the symptoms of ischemic rest pain in his foot and very low ABIs. Rutherford categorized peripheral arterial disease into seven categories based on symptoms:

0 (asymptomatic), 1 (mild claudication), 2 (moderate claudication), 3 (severe claudication), 4 (ischemic rest pain), 5 (minor tissue loss), and 6 (major tissue loss). Furthermore, the Trans-Atlantic Inter-Society Consensus established an arteriographic classification system for the severity of the arterial occlusive disease ranging from A to D. Type A lesions are short stenoses, whereas type D lesions are long segments of occlusion. The current consensus is that Trans-Atlantic Inter-Society Consensus type A and B lesions are more amenable to endovascular therapy; type D lesions are better treated with open bypass, and type C lesions.

References: Belkin M, Owens CD, Whittemore AD et al: Peripheral arterial occlusive disease. In Townsend CM Jr, Beauchamp RD, Evers BM, Mattox KL, editors: *Sabiston textbook of surgery: the biological basis of modern surgical practice*, ed 18, Philadelphia, 2008, WB Saunders, pp 1941–1979.

Lin P, Kougias P, Bechara C, et al: Arterial disease. In Brunicardi FC, Andersen DK, Billiar TR, et al, editors: *Schwartz's principles of surgery*, ed 9, New York, 2010, McGraw-Hill, pp 701–775.

Pituitary and Adrenal Glands 19

1. The most common cause of primary adrenal insufficiency is:
    A. Autoimmune
    B. Tuberculosis
    C. Metastatic disease
    D. Adrenal hemorrhage
    E. Exogenous steroid use

2. Initial management of syndrome of inappropriate secretion of antidiuretic hormone consists of:
    A. Restriction of free water
    B. Furosemide
    C. Hypertonic saline solution
    D. Isotonic saline solution
    E. Demeclocycline

3. Which of the following is true regarding the renin-angiotensin system?
    A. The juxtaglomerular cells are located within the renal efferent arteriole.
    B. The juxtaglomerular cells secrete aldosterone in response to decreased blood pressure.
    C. The juxtaglomerular cells detect changes in chloride concentration in the renal tubule.
    D. Renin catalyzes the conversion of angiotensinogen to angiotensin.
    E. Angiotensin I directly stimulates the production of aldosterone.

4. Which of the following is true regarding the anatomy/blood supply to the adrenal glands?
    A. The arterial blood supply is more constant than the venous drainage.
    B. Catheter-based venous hormonal sampling is easier to perform on the right adrenal vein.
    C. On the right, the adrenal vein drains into the right renal vein.
    D. Right adrenalectomy is more likely to lead to life-threatening hemorrhage than left adrenalectomy.
    E. The majority of the arterial blood supply arises from the celiac trunk.

5. A 70-year-old man is found to have an incidental mass in his right adrenal gland on computed tomography (CT) scan. He has no history of malignancy and has a normal blood pressure. The findings of the remainder of the history and physical examination are negative. Plasma free metanephrines are negative. The serum potassium level is normal. Urinary free cortisol is normal, and a 1-mg overnight dexamethasone suppression test shows a low cortisol level (1.5 µg/dL) the following morning. The mass is 4.5 cm on CT scan, has smooth borders, and has a low attenuation value. Which of the following is true regarding this condition?
    A. The patient should undergo a CT-guided needle biopsy.
    B. The patient should undergo a laparoscopic adrenalectomy.
    C. The patient should undergo an open adrenalectomy.
    D. A repeat CT scan should be performed in 6 months.
    E. The mass is most likely malignant.

6. Which of the following is true regarding the histology of the adrenal gland?
    A. The zona glomerulosa is the inner layer of the adrenal cortex.
    B. Cells in the zona fasciculata produce cortisol.
    C. Cells in the zona reticularis produce aldosterone.
    D. Medullary cells are chromaffin negative.
    E. The zona reticularis is the middle layer of the adrenal cortex.

7. The most common symptom/sign of pheochromocytoma is:
    A. Hypertension
    B. Excessive sweating
    C. Palpitations
    D. Chest pain
    E. Headache

8. The hallmark of multiple endocrine neoplasia type 2 (MEN 2) is:
   A. Unilateral pheochromocytoma
   B. Bilateral pheochromocytoma
   C. Mutlifocal and bilateral medullary carcinoma of the thyroid
   D. Unifocal medullary carcinoma of the thyroid
   E. Four-gland parathyroid hyperplasia

9. MEN 2B can be distinguished from MEN 2A by the fact that patients with MEN 2B are:
   A. More likely to develop parathyroid hyperplasia
   B. Less likely to have pheochromocytomas
   C. Less likely to develop early and aggressive medullary carcinoma of the thyroid
   D. More likely to have a marfanoid habitus
   E. Less likely to have tongue neuromas

10. The diagnosis of primary hyperaldosteronism would be supported by which of the following?
    A. Low plasma renin
    B. Increased serum potassium
    C. A decrease in serum aldosterone after captopril administration
    D. Low (<10) plasma aldosterone-to-renin ratio
    E. Hyperpigmentation

11. The most common cause of primary hyperaldosteronism is:
    A. Renal artery stenosis
    B. Glucocorticoid-suppressible aldosteronism
    C. Adrenal adenoma
    D. Idiopathic bilateral adrenal hyperplasia
    E. Adrenal carcinoma

12. The most common cause of congenital adrenal hyperplasia is:
    A. 11β-Hydroxylase deficiency
    B. 3-Hydroxydehydrogenase deficiency
    C. 21-Hydroxylase deficiency
    D. 17-Hydroxylase deficiency
    E. Congenital adrenal lipoid hyperplasia

13. The most common cause of Cushing syndrome aside from exogenous corticosteroid administration is:
    A. Adrenal cortical carcinoma
    B. Adrenal adenoma
    C. Corticotropin (ACTH)-producing pituitary adenoma
    D. Ectopic ACTH syndrome
    E. Ectopic corticotropin-releasing hormone syndrome

14. The most useful first test for Cushing syndrome is:
    A. Serum cortisol
    B. 24-hour urinary free cortisol
    C. Plasma ACTH level
    D. High-dose dexamethasone suppression
    E. Low-dose dexamethasone suppression

15. The test with the highest sensitivity for pheochromocytoma is:
    A. Plasma catecholamine
    B. Plasma metanephrine
    C. Urinary catecholamine
    D. Urinary metanephrine
    E. Urinary vanillylmandelic acid

16. The most common extra-adrenal site of pheochromocytoma is the:
    A. Rectum
    B. Bladder
    C. Neck
    D. Organ of Zuckerkandl
    E. Sacrum

17. The most common symptom of Cushing syndrome is:
    A. Progressive truncal obesity
    B. Acne
    C. Hirsutism
    D. Purple striae
    E. Proximal muscle weakness

18. Which of the following is true regarding neuroblastoma?
    A. It is the third most common abdominal malignancy in children.
    B. Prognosis is better for older children than those diagnosed before 1 year of age.
    C. Prognosis is excellent even in high-risk groups.
    D. In the mediastinum, they are most often located anteriorly.
    E. Amplification of the *N-myc* oncogene has an unfavorable prognosis.

19. Neuroblastoma is associated with all of the following EXCEPT:
    A. Aniridia and hemihypertrophy
    B. Blueberry muffin sign
    C. Cerebellar and truncal ataxia
    D. Verner-Morrison type syndrome
    E. Proptosis and periorbital ecchymosis

20. Which of the following is true regarding adrenal cortical carcinoma?

    A. Associated evidence of hormonal excess is common.

    B. The diagnosis is generally made by CT-guided needle biopsy.

    C. Staging is based on tumor histology.

    D. Because of malignant potential, adrenal masses larger than 3 cm should be excised.

    E. Mitotane is highly effective in patients with positive lymph nodes.

21. The first biochemical abnormality detected in the majority of patients with MEN 1 is:

    A. Hypercalcemia

    B. Hypergastrinemia

    C. Hypoglycemia

    D. Polycythemia

    E. Hyperchloremia

22. All of the following are appropriate in the preoperative management of pheochromocytoma EXCEPT:

    A. Phenoxybenzamine

    B. Propranolol

    C. Doxazosin

    D. Furosemide

    E. Nifedipine

23. The most common pituitary neoplasm associated with MEN 1 secretes:

    A. ACTH

    B. Prolactin

    C. Growth hormone

    D. Thyroid-stimulating hormone

    E. Follicle-stimulating hormone

24. A 45-year-old woman presents with truncal obesity and hypertension. A 24-hour urine free cortisol level is markedly elevated and a low-dose dexamethasone suppression test fails to suppress the elevated plasma cortisol levels. Plasma ACTH levels are also markedly elevated. A high-dose dexamethasone suppression test also fails to suppress the urinary free cortisol level. Which of the following would most likely demonstrate the cause of her symptoms?

    A. CT scan of the sella turcica

    B. Petrosal sinus sampling for ACTH

    C. Chest CT

    D. Magnetic resonance imaging of the sella turcica

    E. CT scan of the abdomen

25. All of the following are true regarding pheochromocytoma EXCEPT:

    A. It is associated with the RET proto-oncogene.

    B. Malignancy is determined histologically by the number of mitoses.

    C. It is associated with von Hippel-Lindau disease.

    D. Metaiodobenzylguanidine scanning is useful for localizing extra-adrenal pheochromocytomas.

    E. It is associated with von Recklinghausen disease.

26. Which of the following is true regarding laparoscopic adrenalectomy?

    A. It is the procedure of choice for small functional adenomas.

    B. It is contraindicated for pheochromocytoma.

    C. It is contraindicated for bilateral pheochromocytoma.

    D. It is contraindicated for tumors larger than 5 cm.

    E. It is the procedure of choice for malignant tumors.

Answers

1. A. Adrenal insufficiency has primary and secondary causes. The most common cause of primary adrenal insufficiency is autoimmune adrenal atrophy. Other less common causes include infections (tuberculosis, fungal cytomegalovirus, human immunodeficiency virus), adrenal hemorrhage, metastases, and infiltrative disorders (amyloidosis). The most common cause of secondary adrenal insufficiency is exogenous glucocorticoid therapy, followed by bilateral adrenal resection and pituitary tumors. Symptoms and signs of acute adrenal insufficiency include fever, nausea and vomiting, abdominal pain, hypotension, hyponatremia, and hyperkalemia. As such, it can readily be confused with septic shock. The most specific test for adrenal insufficiency is the ACTH stimulation test. Cortisol levels are measured at 1, 30, and 60 minutes. Blood and urine cortisol levels normally rise with ACTH; failure to rise is indicative of adrenal insufficiency.

    Reference: Arlt W, Allolio B: Adrenal insufficiency, *Lancet* 361:1881–1893, 2003.

2. A. The syndrome of inappropriate secretion of antidiuretic hormone is seen in association with malignancies (most often small cell lung cancer, but also head and neck cancers and non–small cell lung cancer, thymoma, and pancreatic cancer), trauma (head injury), surgery to the central nervous system, pulmonary and brain infections, and drugs (cytotoxic agents, phenothiazine). The criteria for diagnosis include the presence of hyponatremia with a low serum osmolality, high urine osmolality (>200 mOsm/kg), lack of evidence of severe volume depletion, continued urinary excretion of sodium (>30 mEq/L), and normal renal, adrenal, and thyroid function. The ultimate treatment is to correct the underlying trigger. However, in the short term, the initial management is to restrict free water (to <1 L/day). If free water restriction alone is not sufficient or if the patient is severely symptomatic, hypertonic fluids with furosemide to induce free water loss can be added. Care must be taken to avoid too rapid administration of hypertonic saline because this may induce dangerous hypernatremia. In chronic forms of syndrome of inappropriate antidiuretic hormone, additional drugs can be given. One such drug is demeclocycline, a tetracycline derivative that is known to induce diabetes insipidus via impairment of cyclic adenosine monophosphate.

Reference: Sørensen J, Andersen M, Hansen H: Syndrome of inappropriate secretion of antidiuretic hormone (SIADH) in malignant disease, *J Intern Med* 238:97–110, 1995.

3. D. The juxtaglomerular cells are modified smooth muscle cells located in the afferent arteriole of each glomerulus. They synthesize the precursor prorenin, which is cleaved into the active proteolytic enzyme renin. Renal hypoperfusion, decreased plasma sodium, and increased sympathetic activity are the major stimuli for renin secretion. Renin initiates a sequence of steps that begins with cleavage of angiotensinogen (a protein produced in the liver) to form angiotensin I. Angiotensin I is then converted to angiotensin II by angiotensin-converting enzyme, found primarily in the lung. Angiotensin II causes systemic vasoconstriction and stimulates aldosterone synthesis and release by the adrenal gland, leading to sodium and water retention and expansion of the plasma volume. In the glomerulus, it leads to vasoconstriction of the efferent arteriole. This leads to increased glomerular pressure in an attempt to maintain the glomerular filtration rate despite systemic hypoperfusion.

4. D. The arterial blood supply to the adrenal glands is highly variable, whereas the venous drainage is more constant. The adrenal glands are supplied by three primary sources: the inferior phrenic artery, adrenal branches directly off the aorta, and branches from the renal artery. Additional branches may arise from the intercostal and gonadal arteries. A single left adrenal vein empties into the left adrenal vein and is a relatively longer vein than the single right adrenal vein, which is very short and enters the posterior aspect of the inferior vena cava. Adrenalectomy (open and laparoscopic) is more challenging on the right side because of (1) the need to retract the liver (for a laparoscopic approach), (2) the need to mobilize the duodenum, and (3) the short, posteriorly located adrenal vein that drains into the inferior vena cava, posing a risk of inferior vena cava hemorrhage. Likewise, venous sampling of the right adrenal vein is more challenging.

Reference: Corcione F, Esposito C, Cuccurullo D, et al: Vena cava injury: a serious complication during laparoscopic right adrenalectomy, *Surg Endosc* 15:218, 2001.

5. C. Incidentally discovered adrenal masses are quite common and are termed *adrenal incidentalomas*. Most are nonfunctioning cortical adenomas. The differential diagnosis includes a functional tumor (pheochromocytoma, aldosteronoma, cortisol producing), metastatic cancer (from lung, breast, melanoma), and adrenocortical carcinoma. A careful history and physical examination should be performed to detect evidence of hormonal excess (hypertension, virilization, Cushing disease). If the patient has hypertension and a low potassium level, plasma aldosterone and renin levels should be obtained. If there is no evidence of hormonal excess, the following studies should still be obtained to rule out a functional tumor: plasma free metanephrines to rule out a pheochromocytoma and a 1-mg overnight dexamethasone suppression test to rule out a cortisol-producing tumor (in normal patients, this will markedly suppress endogenous cortisol production to a level <1.8 μg/dL). Characteristics on the CT scan should also be determined. A mass with smooth borders, that is, homogeneous, and low attenuation (using Hounsfield units) is very likely benign, whereas an irregular mass with evidence of local invasion, that is, inhomogeneous, and a high attenuation score is of much more concern for malignancy. Fine-needle aspiration biopsy is not helpful in distinguishing a benign adrenal adenoma from a malignant adrenocortical carcinoma because it is even difficult to distinguish the two on histologic examination. Fine-needle aspiration biopsy would only be useful in the patient with a history of malignancy to rule out an adrenal metastasis. Surgery is generally recommended for functional adrenal adenomas, pheochromocytomas, masses that have CT scan features suggestive of malignancy, and masses larger than 5 cm.

Reference: Grumbach M, Biller B, Braunstein G, et al: Management of the clinically inapparent adrenal mass ("incidentaloma"), *Ann Intern Med* 138:424–429, 2003.

6. B. The adrenal gland is divided into the outer cortex and the inner medulla. The cortex is further subdivided into three layers ("GFR": glomerulosa, fasciculata, reticularis). The zona glomerulosa is the outermost layer and is responsible for aldosterone production. The middle layer, the zona fasciculata, produces glucocorticoids. Adrenal androgens are produced by the deepest cortical layer, the zona reticularis. Cells of the adrenal medulla produce epinephrine (80%) and norepinephrine (20%). Medullary cells are chromaffin positive.

7. A. The most common manifestation (symptom or sign) of pheochromocytoma is hypertension. In most patients, the hypertension is sustained rather than episodic. The most common symptom is headache.

8. C. The hallmark of MEN 2 is medullary thyroid carcinoma (MTC). Eventually, nearly 100% of patients with MEN 2 develop MTC, whereas only approximately 40% develop pheochromocytoma and one third have parathyroid hyperplasia. MTC is characteristically multifocal and bilateral and presents at a young age. MTC is associated with C-cell hyperplasia. It is caused by mutations in the RET proto-oncogene.

9. D. MEN 2B is not associated with parathyroid hyperplasia, whereas it is present in approximately one third of patients with MEN 2A. MEN 2B patients have a characteristic facial appearance with thick upper lips, marfanoid habitus, and tongue neuromas. MTC can be detected in asymptomatic patients by measuring calcitonin levels (>1000 pg) along with increased carcinoembryonic antigen. Once clinical manifestations of MTC develop in association with MEN 2B, it is difficult to cure because it is aggressive. It clinically presents as either a mass in the neck or as metastatic disease. If a neck mass is present, it can be confirmed by fine-needle aspiration as well as by an elevated serum calcitonin level and increased carcinoembryonic antigen.

10. A. Primary hyperaldosteronism (Conn syndrome) should be suspected in patients with hypertension and hypokalemia. Primary hyperaldosteronism results from autonomous aldosterone secretion, which, in turn, leads to suppression of renin secretion. The diagnosis is made by demonstrating a combination of inappropriate potassium excretion in the urine (kaliuresis), low plasma renin, and a high aldosterone-to-renin ratio (>20). However, patients must discontinue drugs that may affect these results (spironolactone and angiotensin-converting enzyme inhibitors). The diagnosis is confirmed by demonstrating increased urine aldosterone in the face of a high-sodium diet with potassium supplementation. After the diagnosis is established, the first study of choice is either a CT scan to look for an adrenal mass. It accounts for approximately 1% of cases of hypertension.

11. C. Renal artery stenosis leads to secondary hyperaldosteronism due to stimulation of renin production. Other causes of secondary hyperaldosteronism include congestive heart failure and cirrhosis. The other causes listed previously are causes of primary hyperaldosteronism. Adrenal adenoma accounts for approximately 70% of cases, followed by idiopathic bilateral adrenal hyperplasia. An adrenal adenoma is managed by surgical resection, whereas idiopathic bilateral adrenal hyperplasia is managed medically (spironolactone, thiazide diuretics, amiloride).

12. C. Congenital adrenal hyperplasia results from inherited enzyme deficiencies that can lead to ambiguous genitalia, postnatal virilization, and problems with salt metabolism. The most common enzyme defect is 21-hydroxylase deficiency (>90% of cases). In the complete form, the deficiency leads to a decrease in both cortisol and aldosterone. This leads to ambiguous genitalia in females (due to androgen excess), salt wasting with hypernatremia, and hypokalemia.

13. C. Cushing syndrome is most often due to exogenous corticosteroid administration. The most common pathology associated with Cushing syndrome is an ACTH-producing pituitary adenoma, which is referred to as *Cushing disease*. Causes of Cushing syndrome are divided into ACTH dependent (ACTH-producing pituitary adenoma, ectopic ACTH syndrome, and ectopic corticotropin-releasing hormone syndrome) and ACTH independent (adrenal carcinoma, adrenal adenoma, and adrenal hyperplasia).

14. B. The term *Cushing syndrome* refers to a complex of symptoms and signs resulting from hypersecretion of cortisol, regardless of the etiology. The aims of diagnostic tests in the evaluation of patients suspected of having Cushing syndrome are twofold: to confirm the presence of Cushing syndrome and to determine its etiology. Measurement of elevated 24-hour urinary cortisol levels is a very sensitive (95%–100%) and specific (98%) modality for diagnosing Cushing disease.

15. B. The diagnosis of pheochromocytoma is established by demonstrating an increased level of catecholamines and their metabolites in the plasma and urine. Plasma metanephrine levels have the highest sensitivity for pheochromocytoma (99% sensitivity) and are used by most as the initial screening test. A recent large study showed that combining tests did not add to the diagnostic yield.

References: Goldstein D, Eisenhofer G, Flynn JA, et al: Diagnosis and localization of pheochromocytoma, *Hypertension* 43:907–910, 2004.

Lenders J, Pacak K, Walther M, et al: Biochemical diagnosis of pheochromocytoma: which test is best? *JAMA* 287:1427–1434, 2002.

16. D. Approximately 10% of pheochromocytomas are extra-adrenal pheochromocytomas (the 10% rule: 10% malignant, 10% bilateral, 10% in children, 10% familial). The organ of Zuckerkandl is a para-aortic structure located at the take-off of the inferior mesenteric artery or at the aortic bifurcation. It consists of a small mass of chromaffin cells that are derived from the neural crest. In the fetal circulation, it is important in the regulation of blood pressure via the secretion of catecholamines, but then regresses.

Reference: Disick G, Palese M: Extra-adrenal pheochromocytoma: diagnosis and management, *Curr Urol Rep* 8:83–88, 2007.

17. A. Progressive truncal obesity is the most common symptom but is not specific. Relatively specific findings include proximal muscle weakness, wide purple striae, spontaneous ecchymoses, and hypokalemic metabolic alkalosis.

18. E. Neuroblastoma is the most common abdominal malignancy in children and the third most common overall and is of neural crest origin. It most often presents as an abdominal mass, and most patients have advanced disease at presentation. For stage I disease, surgical resection is the best treatment. The overall survival rate is less than 30%. The tumor may cross the midline, and a majority of patients show signs of metastatic disease at presentation. Because these tumors are derived from the sympathetic nervous system, catecholamines and their metabolites will be produced at increased levels. Prognosis is based on age at presentation (older or younger than 1 year of age), tumor biology, and tumor histology. Amplification of the *N-myc* oncogene has an unfavorable prognosis. High-risk groups have only a 20% long-term survival rate. In infants, spontaneous regression has been well described. In the mediastinum, they most often present in the posterior mediastinum (the most common location for neurogenic mediastinal tumors).

Reference: Meitar D, Crawford S, Rademaker A, Cohn S: Tumor angiogenesis correlates with metastatic disease, N-myc amplification, and poor outcome in human neuroblastoma, *J Clin Oncol* 14:405–414, 1996.

19. A. Neuroblastoma is associated with many different syndromes, including dancing eyes–dancing feet syndrome (cerebellar ataxia, nystagmus, and involuntary movements), catecholamine release, periorbital metastasis leading to proptosis and periorbital ecchymosis, skin metastasis that gives the appearance of a blueberry muffin, and severe diarrhea (due to release of vasoactive intestinal polypeptide). Aniridia and hemihypertrophy, however, are associated with Wilms tumor.

20. A. Adrenocortical carcinomas are rare. They should be suspected in the presence of large tumors (>5–6 cm) or if the CT scan shows evidence of necrosis, hemorrhage, or local invasion. Approximately 60% of patients with adrenocortical carcinoma present with hormonal excess, including Cushing syndrome and virilization. There are no distinctive histologic or cytologic features that distinguish adrenocortical carcinoma from an adenoma. Thus, one must rely on evidence of local invasion, lymph node metastasis, or distant metastasis. The best chance for cure is surgical resection. Mitotane is an adrenal cytotoxic agent but has poor response rates. Adrenal masses that are hormonally active should be excised. In the absence of hormonal activity and in the absence of CT scan features suggestive of malignancy, resection is recommended for asymptomatic masses if they are larger than 5 to 6 cm.

Reference: Ng L, Libertino J: Adrenocortical carcinoma: diagnosis, evaluation and treatment, *J Urol* 169:5–11, 2003.

21. A. MEN 1 is characterized by lesions in the parathyroid, pituitary, and pancreas. The most common (95%) and earliest manifestation is hypercalcemia from parathyroid hyperplasia. Pancreatic lesions are the next most common and may consist of diffuse islet cell hyperplasia or multiple microadenomas. The most common functional pancreatic tumor is gastrinoma. Pituitary lesions are usually adenomas located in the anterior pituitary.

22. D. The medical management of pheochromocytomas consists of initial alpha-blockade, hydration, and beta-blockade if needed. Because of the vasoconstriction present in these patients, they are frequently volume depleted. As such, diuretics should be avoided. An important principle in the management is to avoid beginning with beta-blockade because this will lead to unopposed alpha stimulation, worsening vasoconstriction, hypertension, and possible heart failure. Phenoxybenzamine has been considered the drug of choice as an alpha-blocker. Others have used doxazosin, another alpha-blocker. Alpha-blockers are initiated 1 to 3 weeks before surgery. Continued excessive sweating provides a guide to inadequate alpha-blockade. Calcium channel blockers are also useful. Beta-blockers, such as propranolol, are added preoperatively in patients who have persistent tachycardia. Volume repletion also aids in the

prevention of postoperative hypotension, which results from the loss of vasoconstriction after tumor removal.

23. B. Pituitary tumors are the third most common tumors in MEN 1. The majority are prolactinomas. They may cause visual field defects due to local compression or may lead to amenorrhea and galactorrhea in women or hypogonadism in men.

24. C. The first test used to establish Cushing syndrome is a 24-hour urine free cortisol test. If the level is elevated, a low-dose dexamethasone suppression test should be performed. Suppression rules out Cushing syndrome. Failure to suppress cortisol levels establishes the diagnosis of Cushing syndrome. ACTH levels should then be measured. Low ACTH levels indicate a primary adrenal source of cortisol, and thus the next step would be to obtain an abdominal CT scan. A high ACTH level suggests either a pituitary or ectopic source of ACTH production. A high-dose dexamethasone suppression test should then be performed because a pituitary source of ACTH will result in some ACTH and cortisol suppression. If cortisol production is suppressed, pituitary magnetic resonance imaging should be performed. Failure to suppress cortisol production with high-dose dexamethasone suggests an ectopic ACTH tumor. The most common causes of ectopic ACTH production are bronchial tumors and small cell lung cancer. Thus, the study of choice would be a chest CT scan.

25. B. Pheochromocytomas occur sporadically, as part of MEN 2A and MEN 2B, in association with von Hippel-Lindau disease and with von Recklinghausen disease. The diagnosis of a benign or a malignant pheochromocytoma cannot be accurately determined by the histologic appearance, but rather is based on evidence of local invasion or the presence or absence of metastasis. The risk of malignancy is lower in patients with familial tumors than in patients with sporadic tumors, although familial tumors are more likely to be bilateral.

26. A. Laparoscopic adrenalectomy has become the procedure of choice for small- and medium-sized functional and benign adrenal tumors. Pheochromocytoma is not a contraindication to the laparoscopic approach and may be used successfully for unilateral or bilateral tumors. Tumor size alone is not a contraindication to the laparoscopic approach. For a large tumor that is clearly malignant based on CT scan evidence of local invasion or lymph node metastasis, the laparoscopic approach is contraindicated.

References: Assalia A, Gagner M: Laparoscopic adrenalectomy, *Br J Surg* 91:1259–1274, 2004.

Du Q-Y, Yeh MW: The pituitary and adrenal glands. In Townsend CM Jr, Beauchamp RD, Evers BM, Mattox KL, editors: *Sabiston textbook of surgery: the biological basis of modern surgical practice*, ed 18, Philadelphia, 2008, WB Saunders, pp 997–1030.

Laimore TC, Moley JF: The multiple endocrine neoplasia syndromes. In Townsend CM Jr, Beauchamp RD, Evers BM, Mattox KL, editors: *Sabiston textbook of surgery: the biological basis of modern surgical practice*, ed 18, Philadelphia, 2008, WB Saunders, pp 1031–1046.

Lal G, Clark OH: Thyroid, parathyroid and adrenal. In Brunicardi FC, Andersen DK, Billiar TR, et al, editors: *Schwartz's principles of surgery*, ed 9, New York, 2010, McGraw-Hill, pp 1343–1407.

Retroperitoneum, Omentum, Mesentery 20

1. All of the following are true regarding desmoid tumors EXCEPT:
   A. They are more common in women.
   B. They do not metastasize.
   C. They are associated with familial adenomatous polyposis.
   D. They have a high rate of local recurrence.
   E. Radiation therapy is the treatment of choice.

2. A 35-year-old woman presents with nausea and vomiting. She reports a 100-lb weight loss as a result of dieting and exercise over the course of 1 year and now weighs 120 lb. Upper gastrointestinal endoscopy demonstrates extrinsic compression of the transverse portion of the duodenum. The most likely diagnosis is:
   A. Superior mesenteric artery compression syndrome
   B. Peptic ulcer stricture
   C. Crohn disease
   D. Median arcuate ligament syndrome
   E. Duodenal adenocarcinoma

3. Which of the following is true regarding retroperitoneal fibrosis?
   A. It is infectious in origin.
   B. It is related to methysergide use.
   C. The erythrocyte sedimentation rate is typically normal.
   D. Intravenous (IV) pyelography is the diagnostic study of choice.
   E. Lateral deviation of the ureters is characteristic.

4. Which of the following are true regarding retroperitoneal sarcomas?
   A. They are best managed by enucleation.
   B. Prognosis is best determined by histologic grade.
   C. Lymph node metastasis is common.
   D. Fibrosarcomas are the most common type.
   E. Radiation therapy alone is often curative for small sarcomas.

5. The most common visceral artery aneurysm is:
   A. Celiac
   B. Splenic
   C. Superior mesenteric artery (SMA)
   D. Hepatic
   E. Pancreaticoduodenal

6. Which of the following is NOT true regarding the mesenteric circulation?
   A. The SMA supplies the gastrointestinal tract from the third portion of the duodenum to the mid transverse colon.
   B. When the SMA is occluded, collaterals from the gastroduodenal artery maintain the blood supply to the proximal jejunum.
   C. The meandering mesenteric artery travels along the mesenteric border of the colon.
   D. The internal iliac artery supplies the rectum via the middle and inferior hemorrhoidal arteries.
   E. The left colic artery is the principal branch of the inferior mesenteric artery (IMA).

7. Which of the following is true regarding a rectus sheath hematoma?
   A. If located above the umbilicus, it is more likely to resemble an acute intra-abdominal process.
   B. If located below the umbilicus, it is more likely to cause severe bleeding.
   C. The majority are associated with a history of trauma.
   D. Operative drainage is the treatment of choice in most cases.
   E. If the mass is palpable, it typically disappears on tensing the rectus muscles.

8. Which of the following is true regarding omental torsion?

   A. Secondary torsion is more common than primary.
   B. Treatment is usually nonsurgical.
   C. If surgery is necessary, management consists of detorsion and omentopexy.
   D. The pain is usually in the left lower quadrant of the abdomen.
   E. It typically produces purulent-appearing peritoneal fluid.

9. The intrinsic hemostatic characteristics of the omentum are due to its:

   A. Ability to recruit platelets
   B. Greater concentration of von Willebrand factor
   C. Greater concentration of tissue factor
   D. Ability to induce local vasoconstriction
   E. Ability to activate the intrinsic coagulation pathway

10. Circulating antibodies to ceroid are seen in association with:

   A. Primary retroperitoneal fibrosis
   B. Mesenteric adenitis
   C. Idiopathic thrombocytopenic purpura
   D. Amyloidosis
   E. Sarcoidosis

11. Which of the following has the strongest causal link with retroperitoneal fibrosis?

   A. Entacapone
   B. Methysergide
   C. α-Methyldopa
   D. Beta-blockers
   E. Hydralazine

12. Initial treatment of retroperitoneal fibrosis consists of :

   A. Cyclosporine
   B. Tamoxifen
   C. Ureterolysis
   D. Prednisone
   E. Azathioprine

13. The most common organism isolated from the infected peritoneal fluid of a patient with a peritoneal dialysis catheter is:

   A. β-Hemolytic *Streptococcus*
   B. *Enterococcus*
   C. *Escherichia coli*
   D. *Staphylococcus epidermidis*
   E. *Staphylococcus aureus*

14. A 70-year-old woman presents with progressive abdominal pain and abdominal distention with nonshifting dullness. A CT scan demonstrates loculated collections of fluid and scalloping of the intra-abdominal organs. At surgery, several liters of yellowish gray mucoid material are present on the omentum and peritoneal surfaces. Which of the following is true about this condition?

   A. There is no role for surgical resection.
   B. Long-term antimicrobials are indicated.
   C. This most likely represents a primary peritoneal malignancy.
   D. It is more common in males.
   E. Cytoreductive surgery is indicated.

15. The most common cause of a retroperitoneal abscess is:

   A. Diverticulitis
   B. Appendicitis
   C. Renal disease
   D. Tuberculosis of the spine
   E. Hematogenous spread from a remote location

16. The organism most commonly associated with acute mesenteric lymphadenitis is:

   A. *Campylobacter jejuni*
   B. *E. coli*
   C. *Enterococcus*
   D. *Yersinia enterocolitica*
   E. Pinworms

17. The most likely site of origin of pseudomyxoma peritonei is the:

   A. Ovary
   B. Stomach
   C. Appendix
   D. Gallbladder
   E. Pancreas

18. All of the following are true regarding spontaneous (primary) peritonitis EXCEPT:

   A. Broad-spectrum antibiotics should be started immediately.
   B. In adults, cirrhosis is the most common risk factor.
   C. In children, nephrotic syndrome is the most common risk factor.
   D. In children, *E. coli* is the most common isolate.
   E. Paracentesis is the most useful diagnostic study.

Answers

1. E. Desmoid tumors are unusual soft-tissue neoplasms that arise from fascial or musculoaponeurotic structures. They are proliferations of benign-appearing fibroblastic cells with abundant collagen and few mitoses. They are associated with Gardner syndrome (intestinal polyposis, osteomas, fibromas, and epidermal or sebaceous cysts), familial adenomatous polyposis, and pregnancy. In addition, in sporadic cases, surgical trauma appears to be an important cause. Patients with familial adenomatous polyposis have a 1000-fold increased risk of the development of desmoid tumors. Desmoids are more common in women of childbearing age and may be linked to estrogen. Desmoid tumors may develop within or adjacent to surgical scars. Patients are typically in their third or fourth decade of life and present with pain, a mass, or both. They are classified as extra-abdominal (extremities, shoulder), abdominal wall, and intra-abdominal (mesenteric and pelvic). There are no typical radiographic findings, but magnetic resonance imaging may delineate muscle or soft-tissue infiltration. Core needle biopsy often reveals collagen with diffuse cellularity with spindle cells, which may suggest a low-grade fibrosarcoma; however, the cells lack mitotic activity and are well differentiated. An open incisional biopsy of lesions larger than 3 to 4 cm is often necessary. Desmoid tumors do not metastasize, but they have a very high local recurrence rate that reaches 50%. The primary treatment is wide local excision with negative margins. Numerous noncytotoxic drugs have been investigated in the treatment of desmoid tumors. Although surgical resection remains the treatment of choice, the agents with the most promise are nonsteroidal anti-inflammatory agents and antiestrogens, which have met with objective response rates of 50%. Case reports using radiation have been reported. The high recurrence rate and locally aggressive nature of these tumors lead to significant morbidity and mortality. In fact, desmoid tumors are the second most common cause of death in patients with familial adenomatous polyposis, after colorectal carcinoma.

References: Ballo M, Zagars G, Pollack A, et al: Desmoid tumor: prognostic factors and outcome after surgery, radiation therapy, or combined surgery and radiation therapy, *J Clin Oncol* 17:158–167, 1999.

Hansmann A, Adolph C, Vogel T, et al: High dose tamoxifen and sulindac as first-line treatment for desmoid tumors, *Cancer* 100:612–620, 2004.

2. A. This patient's history is most consistent with SMA compression syndrome. It is caused by compression of the third part of the duodenum between the SMA and the aorta. Although very rare, it has been reported most often in the setting of rapid weight loss, such that there is loss of mesenteric fat, causing the angle between the SMA and the aorta to narrow and compress the duodenum. The syndrome causes symptoms of a proximal intestinal obstruction, including postprandial epigastric pain, eructation, fullness, and voluminous vomiting. Diagnosis

is suggested by contrast-enhanced spiral CT showing extrinsic compression of the duodenum. Treatment is by high-calorie diet to gain weight and increase the SMA angle. If this is unsuccessful, the patient needs a duodenojejunostomy. Medial arcuate ligament syndrome causes symptoms of mesenteric ischemia from extrinsic compression of the celiac artery by the median arcuate ligament. The patient experiences postprandial pain and subsequent weight loss. An abdominal bruit is heard in almost all patients. Diagnosis is made by arteriography. Treatment involves surgical release of the arcuate ligament.

References: Baltazar U, Dunn J, Floresguerra C, et al: Superior mesenteric artery syndrome: an uncommon cause of intestinal obstruction, *South Med J* 93:606–608, 2000.

Lippl F, Hannig C, Weiss W, et al: Superior mesenteric artery syndrome: diagnosis and treatment from the gastroenterologist's view, *J Gastroenterol* 8:640–643, 2002.

3. B. Retroperitoneal fibrosis is characterized by a periaortic and retroperitoneal proliferation of fibrous tissue that surrounds the ureters and leads to ureteral obstruction, flank pain, and, in some cases, acute renal failure. The disorder may be idiopathic (also known as Ormond disease), or a secondary reaction to an inciting inflammatory process, malignancy, or medication. Idiopathic retroperitoneal fibrosis is rare. It occurs twice as often in men. One theory is that it is related to an autoimmune response. There does not seem to be any support for an infectious etiology. The fibrotic process can eventually encase the ureters, inferior vena cava, aorta, mesenteric vessels, and/or sympathetic nerves. On physical examination, patients are often hypertense and an abdominal or flank mass may be palpated. Compression of pelvic veins may lead to lower extremity edema. Laboratory evaluation often demonstrates elevated blood urea nitrogen and creatinine levels as well as an elevated erythrocyte sedimentation rate. CT scan is the diagnostic study of choice. Medial deviation of the ureters is characteristic but not pathognomonic. It tends to have a symmetrical distribution. Malignant tumors conversely tend to deviate the ureters laterally. It is important to note that malignant tumors can induce retroperitoneal fibrosis. As such, CT-guided needle biopsy is essential.

References: Cronin C, Lohan D, Blake M, et al: Retroperitoneal fibrosis: a review of clinical features and imaging findings, *Am J Roentgenol* 191:423–431, 2008.

Gilkeson G, Allen N: Retroperitoneal fibrosis: a true connective tissue disease, *Rheum Dis Clin North Am* 22:23–38, 1996.

4. B. Most retroperitoneal tumors are malignant and comprise approximately half of all soft-tissue sarcomas. The most common sarcomas occurring in the retroperitoneum are liposarcomas, malignant fibrous histiocytomas, and leiomyosarcomas. Local recurrence and intra-abdominal spread are frequent. Retroperitoneal sarcomas present as large masses because they do not typically produce symptoms until their mass effect creates compression or invasion of adjacent structures. Retroperitoneal sarcomas have a worse prognosis than sarcomas. The best chance for long-term survival is achieved with a margin-negative resection. Tumor stage at presentation, high histologic grade, unresectability, and grossly positive resection margins are strongly associated with increased mortality rates. Tumor grade is a significant predictor of outcome. Complete surgical resection is the most effective treatment for primary or recurrent retroperitoneal sarcomas. Even if surgical resection can be performed, the margins are often compromised because of anatomic constraints.

5. B. Aneurysms of the visceral arteries are rare. Splenic artery aneurysms are the most common type and make up as many as 60% of cases. Hepatic artery aneurysms are the second most common, with as many as 20% of cases. Aneurysms of the celiac, superior mesenteric, and pancreaticoduodenal arteries together compose less than 10% of all visceral aneurysms.

References: Seymour NE, Bell RL: Abdominal wall, omentum, mesentery, and retroperitoneum. In Brunicardi FC, Andersen DK, Billiar TR, et al, editors: *Schwartz's principles of surgery*, ed 9, New York, 2010, McGraw-Hill, pp 1267–1281.

Turnage RH, Richardson KA, Li B, et al: Abdominal wall, umbilicus, peritoneum, mesenteries, omentum and retroperitoneum. In Townsend CM Jr, Beauchamp RD, Evers BM, Mattox KL, editors: *Sabiston textbook of surgery: the biological basis of modern surgical practice*, ed 18, Philadelphia, 2008, WB Saunders, pp 1129–1154.

6. C. The territory of the SMA begins at the third portion of the duodenum and ends at the distal portion of the transverse colon. The IMA territory begins in the region of the splenic flexure. Thus, the splenic flexure is a watershed area of circulation and as such is prone to the development of ischemic colitis in elderly patients during periods of decreased perfusion. A large collateral vessel, the marginal artery (not the meandering artery), connects these two circulations and forms a continuous arcade just along the mesenteric border of the colon. The left colic artery is the most proximal branch of the IMA, supplying the distal transverse colon, splenic flexure, and descending colon. The meandering mesenteric artery, also called the Riolan arch, is a collateral artery that directly connects the proximal SMA with the proximal IMA and may serve as a vital conduit when one or the other of these arteries is occluded. It runs parallel and posterior to the middle colic artery in the transverse mesocolon and is highly variable in size. The meandering mesenteric artery should routinely be preserved in all surgical procedures, including resection for cancer, given its critical function in providing collateral mesenteric circulation. The presence of a large meandering mesenteric artery suggests occlusion of either the SMA or IMA. The name *meandering* is derived from the fact that the vessels can become quite tortuous and enlarged. The middle rectal artery is a branch of the internal iliac artery. The inferior rectal artery is a branch of the pudendal artery, which is a more distal branch of the internal iliac artery.

Reference: Gourley EJ, Gering SA: The meandering mesenteric artery: a historic review and surgical implications, *Dis Colon Rectum* 48:996–1000, 2005.

7. B. Rectus sheath hematomas are clinically significant because of the fact that they can easily be mistaken for an intra-abdominal inflammatory process. The etiology is an injury to an epigastric artery within the rectus sheath. In most cases, there is no clear history of trauma. In particular, in the elderly who are taking oral anticoagulants, they typically occur spontaneously. Patients frequently describe a sudden onset of unilateral abdominal pain, sometimes preceded by a coughing fit. In one series, 11 of 12 patients were women, and in another series, all 8 were women, with an average age in the sixth decade. Below the arcuate line, there is no aponeurotic posterior covering to the rectus muscle. As such, hematomas below this line can cross the midline, causing a larger hematoma to form, and cause bilateral lower quadrant pain resembling a perforated viscus. On physical examination, a mass is often palpable. The Fothergill sign is the finding of a palpable abdominal mass that remains unchanged with contraction of the rectus muscles. This helps distinguish it from an intra-abdominal abscess, which would not be palpable with rectus contraction. The diagnosis is best established with a CT scan, which will demonstrate a fluid collection in the rectus muscle. The hematocrit should be closely monitored. Once the diagnosis is established, management is primarily nonoperative and consists of resuscitation, monitoring of serial hemoglobin/hematocrit levels, and reversal of anticoagulation. On rare occasions, angiographic embolization may be necessary. Surgical management, when rarely necessary, would involve ligation of the bleeding vessel and evacuation of the hematoma. One should suspect a rectus sheath hematoma in older women taking anticoagulants who present the clinical triad of acute abdominal pain, an abdominal wall mass, and anemia.

References: Berná J, Zuazu I, Madrigal M, et al: Conservative treatment of large rectus sheath hematoma in patients undergoing anticoagulant therapy, *Abdom Imaging* 25:230–234, 2000.

Zainea G, Jordan F: Rectus sheath hematomas: their pathogenesis, diagnosis, and management, *Am Surg* 54:630–633, 1988.

8. A. It is important to be aware of omental torsion because it readily mimics an intra-abdominal perforation. Because it is typically very difficult to diagnose preoperatively, the diagnosis is most often made at surgery. Torsion of the omentum describes a twisting of the omentum around its vascular pedicle. Primary torsion, in which case there is no underlying pathology, is extremely rare. Secondary torsion is much more common, and the torsion is usually precipitated by a fixed point such as a tumor, an adhesion, a hernia sac, or an area of intra-abdominal inflammation. Omental torsion is much more common in adults. Children with torsion are typically obese, likely contributing to a fatty omentum that predisposes to twisting. Other factors that predispose a patient to torsion include a bifid omentum and a narrowed omentum pedicle. Interestingly, the twisted omentum tends to be localized to a right side; thus, it is most commonly confused with acute appendicitis, acute cholecystitis, and pelvic inflammatory disease. Complicating the diagnosis is the fact that the omentum itself tends to migrate and envelop areas of inflammation. Laparoscopy is ideal for establishing the diagnosis and to exclude other etiologies. Treatment is to resect the twisted omentum, which can often be infarcted at the time of surgery. The finding of purulent fluid would suggest another diagnosis because it is not consistent with omental torsion.

References: Chew D, Holgersen L, Friedman D: Primary omental torsion in children, *J Pediatr Surg* 30:816–817, 1995.

Saber A, LaRaja R: Omental torsion. http://emedicine.medscape.com, 2007.

Sánchez J, Rosado R, Ramírez D, et al: Torsion of the greater omentum: treatment by laparoscopy, *Surg Laparosc Endosc Percutan Tech* 12:443–445, 2002.

Young T, Lee H, Tang H: Primary torsion of the greater omentum, *Int Surg* 89:72–75, 2004.

9. C. The greater omentum has been called the policeman of the abdomen for its ability to wall off infections and stem bleeding. In fact, omental wrapping is used by trauma surgeons to control bleeding around the liver and spleen. An interesting study that may explain the omentum's hemostatic properties demonstrated that the concentration of tissue factor in omentum is more than twice the amount per gram of that found in muscle. This property facilitates the activation of the extrinsic pathway of coagulation in the settings of trauma, infection, and ischemia, leading to the production of fibrin, which facilitates the adherence of the omentum to these areas.

Reference: Logmans A, Schoenmakers C, Haensel S: High tissue factor concentration in the omentum, a possible cause of its hemostatic properties, *Eur J Clin Invest* 26:82–83, 1996.

10. A. Retroperitoneal fibrosis seems to be an autoimmune process. Supporting this theory, circulating antibodies to ceroid are present in more than 90% of patients. Ceroid is an insoluble polymer of oxidized lipid and protein. Ceroid accumulates in macrophages of the heart, liver, gastrointestinal tract, and brain in the elderly and has been termed the "wear-and-tear" pigment. The immune-mediated mechanism of retroperitoneal fibrosis is further supported by its coexistence with primary biliary cirrhosis, fibrosing mediastinitis, systemic lupus erythematosus, and Hashimoto thyroiditis. Methysergide, an ergot alkaloid used for migraines, is the medication with the strongest causal relationship with retroperitoneal fibrosis.

11. B. Retroperitoneal fibrosis has been associated with several medications. The strongest causal relationship is with the use of methysergide, a semisynthetic ergot alkaloid used to treat migraine headaches. Other medications that have been linked to retroperitoneal fibrosis include beta-blockers, hydralazine, lysergic acid diethylamide, α-methyldopa, amphetamines, phenacetin, cocaine, and entacopone. The retroperitoneal fibrosis may regress upon discontinuation of these medications.

Reference: Graham J, Suby H, LeCompte P, Sadowsky N: Fibrotic disorders associated with methysergide therapy for headache, *N Engl J Med* 274:359–368, 1966.

12. D. Steroids are the mainstay of treatment for retroperitoneal fibrosis. It is important to first obtain a tissue diagnosis. In a prospective study over 10 years, the initial dose of prednisolone was 60 mg on alternate days for 2 months and was tapered during the following 2 months to a daily dose of 5 mg. The total duration of prednisolone use was 2 years (although others recommend discontinuing the medication after 2 months). Ureterolysis, ureteral stenting, or nephrostomy tubes are reserved for those who do not respond or those who have massive hydronephrosis with alteration of renal function. Patients are also at risk of the development of thrombosis of the iliac veins or inferior vena cava. As such, they may require oral anticoagulation. For those who do not respond to oral steroids, cyclosporine, tamoxifen, and azathioprine have been successfully used. The overall prognosis is excellent with 5-year survival rates reportedly in the 90% to 100% range.

Reference: Kardar A, Kattan S, Lindstedt E, et al: Steroid therapy for idiopathic retroperitoneal fibrosis: dose and duration, *J Urol* 168:550–555, 2002.

13. D. Coagulase-negative *Staphylococcus* species (*S. epidermidis*) is by far the most common cause of peritoneal catheter-related infections. The diagnosis is made by a combination of abdominal pain, development of cloudy peritoneal fluid, and an elevated peritoneal fluid white blood cell count greater than $100/mm^3$. Initial treatment consists of intraperitoneal antibiotics, which seem to be more effective than IV antibiotics. If the infection fails to clear, based on abdominal examination, clinical picture, or persistent peritoneal fluid leukocytosis, then the catheter needs to be removed. *S. aureus* and gram-negative organism infections are less likely to respond to antibiotic management alone.

14. E. Pseudomyxoma peritonei is a rare process in which the peritoneum becomes covered with semisolid mucus and large loculated cystic masses. For some time, it has been unclear whether it represents a true malignant process. A useful classification derived from a large series uses two categories: disseminated peritoneal adenomucinosis (DPAM) and peritoneal mucinous carcinomatosis (PMCA). DPAM is histologically a benign process and most often due to a ruptured appendiceal mucinous adenoma. The category PMCA is used for cases with pathologic features of adenocarcinoma. The 5-year survival rates in a series of 109 patients were 84% for patients with DPAM, 37.6% for patients with PMCA with intermediate or discordant features, and 6.7% for patients with PMCA. Pseudomyxoma peritonei is most common in women aged 50 to 70 years. It is often asymptomatic until late in its course. Symptoms are often nonspecific. Physical examination may demonstrate a distended abdomen with nonshifting dullness. Management is surgical, with cytoreduction of the primary and secondary implants, including peritonectomy and omentectomy. If there is a clear origin at the appendix, a right colectomy should also be performed. If the origin appears to be the ovary, total abdominal hysterectomy with bilateral salpingo-oophorectomy is recommended. The recurrence rate is very high (76% in one series).

References: Gough D, Donohue J, Schutt AJ, et al: Pseudomyxoma peritonei: long-term patient survival with an aggressive regional approach, *Ann Surg* 219:112–119, 1994.

Hinson F, Ambrose N: Pseudomyxoma peritonei, *Br J Surg* 85:1332–1339, 1998.

Ronnett B, Zahn C, Kurman R, et al: Disseminated peritoneal adenomucinosis and peritoneal mucinous carcinomatosis: a clinicopathologic analysis of 109 cases with emphasis on distinguishing pathologic features, site of origin, prognosis, and relationship to "pseudomyxoma peritonei." *Am J Surg Pathol* 19:1390–1408, 1995.

15. C. The most common sources of retroperitoneal infections are organs within the retroperitoneum or adjacent spread of peritoneal infections. Renal infections account for nearly 50% of retroperitoneal abscesses. Other common causes include retrocecal appendicitis, perforated duodenal ulcers, pancreatitis, and diverticulitis. Patients typically present with back, pelvic, flank, or thigh pain with associated fever and leukocytosis. Flank erythema may be present. Treatment consists of broad-spectrum antibiotics and drainage as well as identification of the source. If the abscess is a simple, unilocular one, then CT-guided drainage is the treatment of choice. Operative drainage may be required for complex abscesses.

16. D. Acute mesenteric adenitis presents most commonly in children and young adults. It is the disease most often confused with acute appendicitis in children. Usually, an upper respiratory infection is present or has recently resolved. The abdominal pain is usually diffuse, but true rigidity is rare. Laboratory values are of little help in establishing the diagnosis. More than 50% have an elevated white blood cell count. *Yersinia* is the organism most commonly associated with mesenteric lymphadenitis in children. If the diagnosis is clear preoperatively (which is usually not the case), treatment is supportive because it is a self-limited disease. The diagnosis can also be made with CT by the demonstration of enlarged, clustered mesenteric lymph nodes in the right lower quadrant in the absence of acute appendicitis. However, with the increasing reluctance to expose children to the radiation associated with CT scanning, the diagnosis is most often made during laparoscopy.

17. C. In one large series, in approximately 60% of patients with DPAM, the origin was an appendiceal mucinous adenoma. In patients classified as PMCA, in the majority, the origin was either a well-differentiated appendiceal or intestinal mucinous adenocarcinoma.

Reference: Ronnett B, Zahn C, Kurman R, et al: Disseminated peritoneal adenomucinosis and peritoneal mucinous carcinomatosis: a clinicopathologic analysis of 109 cases with emphasis on distinguishing pathologic features, site of origin, prognosis, and relationship to "pseudomyxoma peritonei." *Am J Surg Pathol* 19:1390–1408, 1995.

18. D. Spontaneous (primary) bacterial peritonitis is defined as bacterial infection of ascitic fluid in the absence of an intra-abdominal, surgically treatable source of infection. Secondary peritonitis refers to peritonitis in the setting of a bowel perforation. Although spontaneous bacterial peritonitis is most commonly associated with cirrhosis, it also occurs in patients with nephrotic syndrome or congestive heart failure. One of the key features is that the isolate is usually a single organism and usually is not an anaerobe. Finding multiple organisms in the culture would suggest secondary peritonitis. In adults, the most common pathogens in spontaneous bacterial peritonitis are the aerobic enteric flora *E. coli* and *Klebsiella*. In children with nephrogenic or hepatogenic ascites, group A streptococcus, *S. aureus*, and *Streptococcus pneumoniae* are common isolates. The diagnosis is made by paracentesis demonstrating more than 250 neutrophils/mm^3 of ascetic fluid in the presence of a correlating clinical presentation.

References: Seymour NE, Bell RL: Abdominal wall, omentum, mesentery, and retroperitoneum. In Brunicardi FC, Andersen DK, Billiar, et al, editors: *Schwartz's principles of surgery*, ed 9, New York, 2010, McGraw-Hill, pp 1267–1281.

Turnage RH, Richardson KA, Li B, et al: Abdominal wall, umbilicus, peritoneum, mesenteries, omentum and retroperitoneum. In Townsend CM Jr, Beauchamp RD, Evers BM, Mattox KL, editors: *Sabiston textbook of surgery: the biological basis of modern surgical practice*, ed 18, Philadelphia, 2008, WB Saunders, pp 1129–1154.

Small Bowel 21

1. Early postoperative small bowel obstruction:
   A. Is best managed nonoperatively in the majority of patients
   B. Is more frequent with upper intestinal than lower intestinal surgery
   C. Does not seem to occur after open transperitoneal aortic surgery
   D. Has a higher rate of strangulation than delayed small bowel obstruction
   E. Is associated with high morbidity and mortality rates

2. Which of the following has been shown to be the most efficacious means of reducing postoperative ileus?
   A. Early ambulation
   B. Erythromycin
   C. Alvimopan
   D. Ketorolac combined with reduction in opioid use
   E. Cisapride

3. All of the following are true regarding Crohn disease EXCEPT:
   A. It is more common in individuals of low socioeconomic status.
   B. It is the most common primary surgical disease of the small bowel.
   C. It has a bimodal distribution.
   D. It is more prevalent in smokers.
   E. It is associated with the use of Accutane (isotretinoin).

4. The earliest lesion characteristic of Crohn disease is:
   A. Aphthous ulcer
   B. Caseating granuloma
   C. Noncaseating granuloma
   D. Cobblestone mucosa
   E. Serosal thickening

5. An intraoperative finding that is virtually pathognomonic of Crohn disease is:
   A. Extensive stricturing of the small bowel
   B. Multiple interloop small bowel abscesses
   C. Multiple enterocutaneous fistulas
   D. Terminal ileitis
   E. Extensive mesenteric fat wrapping

6. Which of the following is true regarding the principles of the operative management of the small bowel in Crohn disease?
   A. The optimal margin is at least 4 cm beyond grossly visible disease.
   B. Frozen section should be obtained to confirm the absence of active disease in at least one margin.
   C. Duodenal disease is best managed by resection.
   D. A 10-cm strictured segment of jejunum can be managed by a Heineke-Mikulicz strictureplasty rather than by resection.
   E. Strictures longer than 10 cm are best managed by resection.

7. Which of the following is the best therapeutic option for mild active Crohn disease?
   A. Sulfasalazine
   B. Prednisone
   C. Budesonide
   D. Metronidazole
   E. Infliximab

8. Which intestinal cells have been implicated in the formation of gastrointestinal stromal tumors (GISTs):
   A. Goblet cells
   B. Cajal cells
   C. Enteroendocrine cells
   D. Paneth cells
   E. Absorptive enterocytes

9. Which of the following is true regarding duodenal diverticula?

   A. They tend to occur on the antimesenteric side of the bowel.
   B. They are usually true diverticula.
   C. Treatment with endoscopic interventions is contraindicated.
   D. They are most commonly located in the periampullary region.
   E. When discovered incidentally at surgery, they should be left alone.

10. The most common presentation for a Meckel diverticulum in children is:

   A. Intussusception
   B. Gastrointestinal (GI) bleeding
   C. Incarceration into a hernia sac
   D. Diverticulitis
   E. Obstruction caused by volvulus

11. Two weeks after an open aortic aneurysm repair, the patient presents with marked abdominal distention without nausea or vomiting. There is no tenderness on abdominal examination. Plain films are unremarkable. Computed tomography (CT) scan reveals a large amount of ascites but is otherwise unremarkable. Paracentesis reveals turbid fluid that is culture negative. Fluid analysis reveals a triglyceride level of 400 mg/dL. The white blood cell count is 600 cells/μL with a predominance of lymphocytes. Which of the following is true about this condition?

   A. The patient should be placed on total parenteral nutrition (TPN) and NPO.
   B. Octreotide is not useful.
   C. The patient should immediately be re-explored.
   D. Peritoneovenous shunting is highly successful.
   E. Most patients respond to a high-protein, low-fat diet.

12. Which of the following is true regarding short bowel syndrome in adults?

   A. The presence of an intact ileocecal valve reduces malabsorption.
   B. It is defined as less than 300 cm of residual small bowel.
   C. Resection of the ileum is better tolerated than resection of the jejunum.
   D. The presence of an intact colon does not alter the severity.
   E. It is most commonly caused by multiple operations requiring small bowel resection.

13. Management of short bowel syndrome includes all of the following EXCEPT:

   A. Cholestyramine
   B. Omeprazole
   C. Codeine
   D. Avoidance of enteral feeding
   E. H_2-receptor antagonists

14. A 6-year-old boy has short bowel syndrome caused by midgut volvulus that developed during infancy and has since been dependent on TPN, which he has tolerated well. He has approximately 28 cm of small bowel remaining with an intact colon. The small bowel is markedly dilated without evidence of small bowel obstruction. Which of the following is the best option?

   A. Serial transverse enteroplasty procedure
   B. Continue with TPN
   C. Small bowel transplantation
   D. Small bowel tapering procedure
   E. Tapering and lengthening procedure (Bianchi)

15. Small intestinal lymphoma:

   A. Is most often the Hodgkin type
   B. Is associated with acquired immunodeficiency syndrome
   C. Most commonly occurs in the duodenum
   D. Is the most common small bowel malignancy
   E. Is primarily treated by chemotherapy

16. A 68-year-old woman presents with an exacerbation of congestive heart failure and acute abdominal pain. Physical examination of the abdomen is significant for mild diffuse abdominal tenderness but no rebound or guarding. CT arteriography of the abdomen demonstrates diffuse narrowing of the superior mesenteric artery (SMA) and its branches. Which of the following is the best management option?

   A. Intravenous (IV) heparin drip
   B. Exploratory laparotomy
   C. Observation
   D. Intra-arterial papaverine
   E. Thrombolytic therapy

17. Diagnosis of carcinoid syndrome is best established by:

   A. Serum serotonin levels
   B. Serum substance P levels
   C. A 24-hour urinary 5-hydroxyindoleacetic acid (5-HIAA) test
   D. Serum neurotensin levels
   E. Serum neurokinin A levels

18. Which of the following is the best test for prognosis and for monitoring treatment response in carcinoid tumors?
 A. Platelet serotonin levels
 B. A 24-hour urinary 5-HIAA test
 C. Serum chromogranin A levels
 D. Serum serotonin levels
 E. Neuron-specific enolase

19. Which of the following is least likely to be of benefit in a patient with advanced small bowel carcinoid?
 A. Interferon-α
 B. Hepatic artery chemoembolization
 C. Debulking intra-abdominal disease
 D. Systemic cyclophosphamide and 5-fluorouracil
 E. Lanreotide

20. The most common cardiac valvular lesion associated with carcinoid syndrome is:
 A. Tricuspid stenosis
 B. Tricuspid insufficiency
 C. Pulmonary stenosis
 D. Pulmonary insufficiency
 E. Mitral stenosis

21. Which of the following is the principal fuel used by the small intestine?
 A. Arginine
 B. Alanine
 C. Glutamine
 D. Tyrosine
 E. Carnitine

22. All of the following are true regarding stromal tumors of the small bowel EXCEPT:
 A. They can be treated with tyrosine kinase inhibitors.
 B. They stain positive for CD34.
 C. They typically present as large bulky tumors.
 D. Surgical resection is the management procedure of choice.
 E. Malignancy is primarily determined by evidence of local invasion.

23. A hernia sac containing a Meckel diverticulum is known as:
 A. Petit hernia
 B. Littre hernia
 C. Spigelian hernia
 D. Richter hernia
 E. Grynfeltt hernia

24. The SMA (Wilkie) syndrome:
 A. Involves the second portion of the duodenum
 B. Is more common in men
 C. Is best diagnosed with arteriography
 D. Is associated with body casting
 E. Is best managed by gastrojejunostomy

25. A 45-year-old woman with a history of laparotomy and 5000 cGy of abdominal and pelvic irradiation for ovarian cancer 10 years ago presents with symptoms and signs of an acute bowel obstruction. CT scan shows a complete small bowel obstruction at the level of the mid jejunum with no evidence of any masses. Which of the following is true about this condition?
 A. If a stricture is present, it is best managed by strictureplasty.
 B. The patient should undergo a complete lysis of adhesions.
 C. Chronic radiation enteritis is due to an obliterative arteritis.
 D. A trial of corticosteroids is indicated.
 E. The degree of radiation damage is not affected by whether the patient received chemotherapy.

26. Which of the following is the best first-line option for an acute exacerbation of Crohn disease?
 A. Sulfasalazine
 B. Mesalamine
 C. Natalizumab
 D. Prednisone
 E. Infliximab

27. Which of the following is true regarding acute ileitis?
 A. It is usually a manifestation of Crohn disease.
 B. It is best treated with segmental small bowel resection.
 C. If discovered at surgery, the appendix should be removed, even if the cecum is inflamed.
 D. If lymph nodes are enlarged, a biopsy should be performed.
 E. It is associated with *Campylobacter* infections.

28. A 12-year-old boy presents with a large amount of bright red blood per rectum, combined with melena. He is hemodynamically stable. Subsequent work-up includes lower and upper endoscopies, both of which are negative. A technetium-99m pertechnetate nuclear scan is performed, and it lights up in the bowel in the right lower quadrant region. Further management consists of:

    A. Arteriography
    B. Meckel diverticulectomy
    C. Small bowel follow-through
    D. Segmental resection of ileum to include the Meckel diverticulum
    E. CT scan of the abdomen with oral contrast

29. A 5-year-old boy presents with symptoms and signs of acute appendicitis. He undergoes an open appendectomy. At surgery, the appendix is acutely inflamed but not perforated. A Meckel diverticulum is incidentally discovered. In addition to performing an appendectomy, further management consists of:

    A. Observation
    B. Meckel diverticulectomy
    C. Meckel diverticulectomy only if ectopic mucosa is palpated in the diverticulum
    D. Meckel diverticulectomy only if an adhesive band to the umbilicus is present
    E. Meckel diverticulectomy only if previous signs of inflammation are present

30. A 46-year-old woman is about to undergo hepatic resection for a metastatic carcinoid tumor. During anesthesia induction, her blood pressure decreases to 80 mm Hg systolic and her heart rate increases to 110 beats per minute. Her entire body appears flushed. Her temperature is normal as is end-tidal CO_2. Management consists of:

    A. Corticosteroids
    B. Antihistamine
    C. Octreotide
    D. Abort operation
    E. Dantrolene

31. A 70-year-old woman presents with vague abdominal pain, diarrhea, steatorrhea, and anemia with an elevated mean corpuscular volume. Her medical and surgical history is unremarkable. A CT scan of the abdomen and pelvis is negative. An upper GI series and small bowel follow-through is significant only for a large jejunal diverticulum. All of the following are true about this condition EXCEPT:

    A. A D-xylose test helps to establish the diagnosis.
    B. A medium-chain triglyceride diet may be helpful.
    C. The diverticulum should be resected.
    D. Broad-spectrum antibiotics are indicated.
    E. Vitamin B_{12} is indicated.

32. All of the following are true regarding Peutz-Jeghers syndrome EXCEPT:

    A. The typical small bowel lesion is an adenomatous polyp.
    B. It is autosomal dominant.
    C. Bowel obstruction is the most common presentation.
    D. There is an increased risk of small intestine cancer.
    E. There is an increased risk of breast cancer.

33. All of the following are true regarding pneumatosis intestinalis EXCEPT:

    A. In neonates, it is most often associated with necrotizing entercolitis.
    B. It can lead to a nonsurgical pneumoperitoneum.
    C. In adults, it is commonly associated with chronic obstructive pulmonary disease.
    D. Primary pneumatosis usually requires surgical intervention.
    E. The diagnosis is readily made with plain radiography.

34. The most common cause of obscure GI bleeding in adults is:

    A. Small intestine angiodysplasia
    B. Meckel diverticulum
    C. Crohn disease
    D. Infectious enteritis
    E. Vasculitis

35. A 35-year-old man with recent travel to South America presents with fever, bloody diarrhea, and abdominal pain. On plain radiograph, there is free air under the diaphragm. At surgery, a single perforation is found in the terminal ileum with accompanying mesenteric lymphadenopathy and splenomegaly. Management consists of:

    A. Closure of perforation
    B. Segmental resection with primary anastomosis
    C. Ileocecectomy with ileal ascending colostomy
    D. Resection of terminal ileum with ileostomy and mucous fistula
    E. Resection of terminal ileum with right colectomy and ileotransverse colostomy

36. The most important factor in reducing mortality from a small bowel fistula is:

    A. Early operative intervention
    B. Prevention of skin breakdown
    C. Waiting at least 6 weeks before operative intervention
    D. Control of sepsis
    E. Use of TPN

37. The most common presentation in adults with a Meckel diverticulum is:

A. Occult bleeding
B. Massive lower GI bleed
C. Diverticulitis with localized abscess
D. Diverticulitis with diffuse peritonitis
E. Obstruction

Answers

1. A. Mechanical small bowel obstruction is the most frequently encountered surgical disorder of the small intestine and is most commonly due to intra-abdominal adhesions related to previous abdominal surgery. The risk of readmission for adhesions seems to be greatest for patients undergoing lower abdominal surgery and seems to be in the 9% range long term. Early postoperative (within 30 days) small bowel obstruction similarly seems to be more frequent with lower abdominal surgery. The diagnosis can be confused with a postoperative ileus. The majority of patients can be managed nonoperatively with nasogastric decompression and nutritional support. The incidence of strangulation is no greater than with small bowel obstruction that presents later. If nasogastric decompression fails to resolve the obstruction, surgery is indicated. The timing of surgery is debatable. In one large series, surgery was recommended for failure of nasogastric decompression after 6 days and in another study after 10 to 14 days. The morbidity and mortality rates of early small bowel obstruction are very low.

References: Ellozy S, Harris M, Bauer J, et al: Early postoperative small-bowel obstruction: a prospective evaluation in 242 consecutive abdominal operations, *Dis Colon Rectum* 45:1214–1217, 2002.

Matter I, Khalemsky L, Abrahamson J, et al: Does the index operation influence the course and outcome of adhesive intestinal obstruction? *Eur J Surg* 163:767–772, 1997.

Parker M, Ellis H, Moran B, et al: Postoperative adhesions: ten-year follow-up of 12,584 patients undergoing lower abdominal surgery, *Dis Colon Rectum* 44:822–829, 2001.

Stewart R, Page C, Brender J, et al: The incidence and risk of early postoperative small bowel obstruction: a cohort study, *Am J Surg* 154:643–647, 1987.

2. C. Postoperative ileus remains a major source of prolonged hospitalization in patients undergoing abdominal surgery. The use of early ambulation, early postoperative feeding protocols, and routine nasogastric intubation has not been shown to be associated with earlier resolution of postoperative ileus. Reducing opioid use in combination with the use of nonsteroidal anti-inflammatory drugs such as ketorolac has been shown to reduce the duration of ileus in most studies. The mechanism may be a combination of the reduction in opioids and the anti-inflammatory properties of ketorolac. However, ketorolac has been associated with an increased risk of operative site and GI bleeding as well as fluid retention. Another drug that has been investigated is erythromycin, which is useful for gastric paresis because it works by its agonistic effect on the motilin receptor. However, it does not seem to be useful for ileus. Prepulsid (ciapride) is a serotonin agonist and had shown promise for ileus but was withdrawn in the United States due cardiac toxicity and reported deaths. Metoclopramide is a dopaminergic antagonist with antiemetic and prokinetic properties, but has also not been shown to be useful for ileus. Recent randomized studies have shown that Entereg (alvimopan) is useful for postoperative ileus in patients undergoing bowel resection. Alvimopan is an opioid receptor antagonist. It binds μ-opioid receptors in the GI tract and selectively inhibits the opioid effects on GI function and motility while not affecting opioid analgesia. It is the first U.S. Food and Drug Administration–approved drug for postoperative ileus. It is approved for short-term (maximum 15 doses over 5 days) in-hospital use only.

References: Ludwig K, Enker W, Delaney C, et al: Gastrointestinal tract recovery in patients undergoing bowel resection: results of a randomized trial of alvimopan and placebo with a standardized accelerated postoperative care pathway, *Arch Surg* 143:1098–1105, 2008.

Wolff B, Weese J, Ludwig K, et al: Postoperative ileus-related morbidity profile in patients treated with alvimopan after bowel resection, *J Am Coll Surg* 204:609–616, 2007.

3. A. Crohn disease is the most common primary surgical disease of the small bowel. It has a bimodal distribution, with one large peak in the second and third decades of life and a second smaller peak in the sixth decade. Several risk factors for Crohn disease have been identified, including living in northern latitudes, Ashkenazi Jewish descent, smoking, and a familial inheritance. The relative risk among first-degree relatives of patients with Crohn disease is as high as 14 to 15 times greater than in the general population. It is also more common in urban areas and in patients with a high socioeconomic status. Recently, a link between Crohn disease and Accutane (isotretinoin) has been reported, as well as an exacerbation of preexisting Crohn disease in patients taking Accutane (isotretinoin) for severe acne. Most studies suggest that Crohn disease is approximately of equal prevalence in females and males. Breastfeeding may also be protective against the development of Crohn disease.

Reference: Passier J, Srivastava N, van Puijenbroek E: Isotretinoin-induced inflammatory bowel disease, *Neth J Med* 64:52–54, 2006.

4. A. In the early stages of Crohn disease, patients demonstrate small superficial ulcers in the mucosa known as aphthous ulcers. These superficial ulcers are often surrounded by a halo of erythema. The ulcers form as a result of submucosal lymphoid follicle expansion. As the disease progresses, the ulcers coalesce to form larger ulcers, which are stellate shaped, as well as deep linear ulcers. Further coalescence of the ulcers leads to a cobblestone appearance, which is a hallmark of Crohn disease. Other hallmarks of Crohn disease include noncaseating granulomas, transmural inflammation, and "skip lesions," meaning that the areas of intestinal inflammation are discontinuous. The noncaseating granulomas are found in both areas of active disease, and grossly normal-appearing intestine is seen in all layers of the bowel wall and in mesenteric lymph nodes. Because the inflammation is transmural, inflamed loops of bowel become adhered to one another, leading to fibrosis, stricture formation, intra-abdominal abscess, fistulas, and, rarely, free perforation.

5. E. All the features listed are seen in Crohn disease. However, the finding of "creeping fat" or mesenteric fat wrapping is a gross feature of Crohn disease that is considered pathognomonic. It indicates the encroachment of mesenteric fat onto the serosal surface of the bowel. The presence of fat wrapping correlates well with the presence of underlying acute and chronic inflammation. A recent study suggests that adiponectin, an adipocyte-specific protein with anti-inflammatory properties found in mesenteric adipose tissue, may play an important role in the inflammation seen in Crohn disease. Terminal ileitis refers to any acute inflammation of the distal ileum adjacent to the ileocecal valve. It is associated with numerous infectious causes including *Yersinia* (*enterocolitica* and *pseudotuberculosis*), *Mycobacterium*, cytomegalovirus (in acquired immunodeficiency syndrome), *Salmonella*, *Campylobacter*, and *Shigella*, among others. The finding of terminal ileitis does not warrant bowel resection. Overall, a minority of patients (10% in one study) who present with terminal ileitis progress to Crohn disease on long-term follow-up.

Reference: Yamamoto K, Kiyohara T, Murayama Y, et al: Production of adiponectin, an anti-inflammatory protein, in mesenteric adipose tissue in Crohn's disease, *Gut* 54:789–796, 2005.

6. D. Approximately three fourths of patients with Crohn disease will eventually require surgery. Indications for surgery include failure of medical management, intestinal obstruction, fistula, abscess, bleeding, and perforation. In children, growth retardation is another indication. Because patients with Crohn disease will often require repeat operations, it is important to avoid unnecessary resection of small bowel because this puts the patient at risk of short bowel syndrome. As such, several principles of surgical management should be followed. Surgical resection should be limited to the segment of bowel that is causing the complication. Other areas of active disease should be left alone provided they are not causing obvious complications. Resection margins of 2 cm beyond grossly visible disease are recommended. Resection margins have not been shown to affect recurrence. The presence of microscopic disease in the resection margin also does not adversely affect outcome or recurrence. Thus, frozen section is unnecessary. When the indication for surgery is small bowel obstruction, strictureplasty has been shown to be equally effective as resection for jejunal and ileal disease while sparing bowel length. Two types of strictureplasty are recommended: the Heinecke-Mikulicz pyloroplasty (for strictures <12 cm in length) and the Finney pyloroplasty (for strictures ≤25 cm in length). A potential drawback of these techniques is that they may potentially leave an undetected malignancy behind. Thus, during the course of a strictureplasty, biopsy specimens of any intraluminal ulcerations should be taken. Duodenal Crohn disease is much less common, and thus guidelines are less clear. However, current recommendations are to perform a bypass of duodenal strictures, such as with a gastrojejunostomy and duodenojejunostomy, depending on the location. Duodenal resection is not recommended. Duodenal strictureplasty has been rarely reported. For colon disease, resection is recommended, again limiting resection to the diseased segment causing symptoms. In a meta-analysis, 90% of recurrences occurred at nonstrictureplasty sites.

References: Fazio V, Marchetti F, Church M, et al: Effect of resection margins on the recurrence of Crohn's disease in the small bowel: a randomized controlled trial, *Ann Surg* 224:563–571, 1996.

Tichansky D, Cagir B, Yoo E, et al: Strictureplasty for Crohn's disease: meta-analysis, *Dis Colon Rectum* 43:911–919, 2001.

Yamamoto T, Fazio V, Tekkis P: Safety and efficacy of strictureplasty for Crohn's disease: a systematic review and meta-analysis, *Dis Colon Rectum* 50:1968–1986, 2007.

7. A. Numerous pharmacologic agents are used to treat Crohn disease. Treatment options should be divided into those used for maintenance therapy for mild active disease, those used to treat an acute exacerbation, and drugs for maintaining remission. In patients with mild active disease, the most commonly used drug is Azulfidine (sulfasalazine), an aminosalicylate that acts as an anti-inflammatory agent. This is particularly useful in patients with colitis and ileocolitis. Mesalamine is a newer agent and another anti-inflammatory agent in the same family as sulfasalazine. It seems to have fewer side effects and is a slow-release drug. For acute flare-ups, the treatment of choice remains corticosteroids and, in particular, prednisone. Prednisone is highly effective in inducing remission (in approximately three fourths of patients); however, due to the side effects of long-term use, it is not recommended for long-term prevention of remission. Budesonide, a synthetic glucocorticoid, is another option. It has an advantage over prednisone in that it has a markedly reduced systemic absorption, and thus fewer long-term side effects. Nevertheless, it can also suppress the adrenal gland. If corticosteroids are ineffective in inducing remission, the next step would be to administer Remicade (infliximab), a monoclonal antibody that targets tumor necrosis factor α. Care must be used in administering infliximab. Because it targets tumor necrosis factor α, a cytokine that regulates inflammatory reactions, patients who receive infliximab are at increased risk of acquiring opportunistic infections such as tuberculosis and aspergillosis. It is also associated with activation of latent multiple sclerosis, demyelinating central nervous system disorders, and worsening congestive heart failure. Infliximab has also been shown to be effective in healing complex fistulas associated with Crohn disease. Antibiotics have an adjunctive role in the treatment of infectious complications associated with Crohn disease. They are used to treat patients with perianal disease, enterocutaneous fistulas, and active colon disease and aid in situations in which bacterial overgrowth has occurred. Once remission had been achieved after an acute flare-up, it is important to maintain remission. Although corticosteroids would theoretically be useful, the side effects preclude long-term administration. Infliximab is used to maintain remission, as are azathioprine and 6-mercaptopurine. These latter drugs act by inhibiting DNA synthesis and thus suppressing the function of T cells and natural killer cells. A second-line agent for maintenance of remission is methotrexate.

8. B. There are four main cell types in the small intestine: absorptive enterocytes, which make up 95% of intestinal cells; goblet cells; Paneth cells; and enteroendocrine cells. Goblet cells secrete mucus. Paneth cells secrete several substances including lysozyme, tumor necrosis factor, and cryptidins, which assist in host mucosal defense. There are more than 10 distinct types of enteroendocrine cells that secrete various gut hormones. The interstitial Cajal cell is a specialized cell of mesodermal origin that seems to regulate peristalsis. It is referred to as an intestinal pacemaker cell. The cells normally express KIT, a tyrosine kinase receptor. These cells have been implicated as the cells of origin of GISTs.

References: Miettinen M, Majidi M, Lasota J: Pathology and diagnostic criteria of gastrointestinal stromal tumors (GISTs): a review, *Eur J Cancer* 38(Suppl 5):S39–S51, 2002.

Sircar K, Hewlett B, Huizinga J, et al: Interstitial cells of Cajal as precursors of gastrointestinal stromal tumors, *Am J Surg Pathol* 23:377–389, 1999.

9. E. Duodenal diverticula are most commonly (75%) located adjacent to the ampulla of Vater and as such are referred to as periampullary diverticula. They are false diverticula in that they are made up of mucosa and submucosa and arise on the mesenteric border in areas of weakness in the bowel wall where blood vessels penetrate. These false diverticula are also found in the jejunum and ileum. They are distinguished from a Meckel diverticulum, which is a true diverticulum present at birth. Duodenal diverticula are most often discovered between ages 56 to 76 years during upper endoscopy, endoscopic retrograde cholangiopancreatography, or abdominal imaging in as many as 6% of patients. They are asymptomatic in the majority of patients, and thus surgery is not recommended if they are discovered incidentally. Complications are estimated to occur in 6% to 10% of patients. They may cause symptoms of malabsorption due to bacterial overgrowth within the diverticula. This can be treated with antibiotics. Less commonly, bleeding can arise within the diverticulum

or diverticulitis can develop leading to perforation, which usually occurs into the retroperitoneum. Perforation requires laparotomy, and closure of the duodenal defect can be challenging and may require placing a loop of jejunum over the defect as a serosal patch. Periampullary diverticula are associated with cholangitis, pancreatitis, and sphincter of Oddi dysfunction. Duodenal diverticula are also associated with choledocholithiasis. These latter complications are thought to be due to the location of the periampullary diverticulum, which may lead to obstruction and stasis of the common duct. The majority of patients presenting with biliary complications who are discovered to have a duodenal diverticulum can be safely treated endoscopically. If this is not successful, surgical diverticulectomy is recommended. Care must be taken during diverticulectomy to identify and preserve the sphincter, which may require cannulation of the common bile duct.

References: Kennedy RH, Thompson MH: Are duodenal diverticula associated with choledocholithiasis? *Gut* 29:1003–1006, 1988.

Tham TC, Kelly M: Association of periampullary duodenal diverticula with bile duct stones and with technical success of endoscopic retrograde cholangiopancreatography, *Endoscopy* 36:1050–1053, 2004.

Vaira D, Dowsett JF, Hatfield AR, et al: Is duodenal diverticulum a risk factor for sphincterotomy? *Gut* 30:939–942, 1989.

10. B. Bleeding is the most common presentation of a Meckel diverticulum in children and is in fact the most common cause of lower GI bleeding in children. The bleeding can present as either melena or bright red blood per rectum. The bleeding is due to heterotopic gastric mucosa within the Meckel diverticulum, leading to acid production and an ulcer forming in the ileum adjacent to the diverticulum. A Meckel diverticulum is a true diverticulum that is due to a failure of closure of the vitelline (omphalomesenteric) duct. An adhesive band may remain between the Meckel diverticulum and the umbilicus, leading to adhesive small bowel obstruction or volvulus. In fact, intestinal obstruction is the most common presentation in adults. Bowel obstruction can also occur due to intussusception with the Meckel diverticulum as the lead point or due to incarceration of the diverticulum into a hernia sac (Littre hernia).

11. E. The patient has chylous ascites. In Western countries, chylous ascites is most often due to malignancy and cirrhosis, whereas in Eastern and developing countries, infectious etiologies predominate, such as tuberculosis and filariasis. Other causes include postlaparotomy inflammatory disorders, trauma, radiation therapy, congenital lymphatic abnormalities, and pancreatitis. The operations most associated with this complication include aortic aneurysm repair, retroperitoneal lymph node dissection, inferior vena cava surgery, and liver transplantation because these are operations where retroperitoneal lymphatics are most likely to be interrupted. The mechanisms thought to lead to the development of chylous ascites include exudation of chyle due to obstruction of the cisterna chyli, direct leakage of chyle through a lymphoperitoneal fistula, and exudation through dilated retroperitoneal vessels. The diagnosis of chylous ascites is best established by analysis of the fluid. Chyle typically has a turbid appearance; however, it may be clear in fasting patients. Elevated triglyceride levels in the fluid are considered diagnostic, usually above 200 mg/dL, although some use a threshold above 110 mg/dL. In addition, the white blood cell count is greater than 500, with a predominance of lymphocytes. The total protein level is between 2.5 and 7.0 g/dL. Cultures are negative, except for cases of tuberculosis, in which adenosine deaminase is also positive in the fluid. The initial treatment of chylous ascites is to administer a high-protein, low-fat diet with medium-chain triglycerides. This diet minimizes chyle production and flow. Medium-chain triglycerides are absorbed by the intestinal epithelium and are transported to the liver through the portal vein and do not contribute to chylomicron formation. Conversely, long-chain triglycerides are converted to monoglycerides and free fatty acids, which are then transported to the intestinal lymph vessels as chylomicrons. If this diet regimen fails, placing the patient NPO and on TPN with octreotide has been shown to be useful in patients with postoperative chylous ascites. If these medical approaches fail, then lymphoscintigraphy is often useful to localize lymph leaks and the site of obstruction. Surgical re-exploration with localization and closure of the lymphatic leak should be performed. Peritoneovenous shunting has a poor success rate due to a high rate of occlusion, made worse by the viscous chyle, and a high rate of other complications including sepsis and the induction of disseminated intravascular coagulation. This latter complication may be due to a high plasminogen concentration in the ascitic fluid.

Reference: Cárdenas A, Chopra S: Chylous ascites, *Am J Gastroenterol* 97:1896–1900, 2002.

12. A. The total length of small bowel is approximately 20 feet (each foot is equal to ~30 cm), or approximately 600 cm (6 m). Short bowel syndrome is defined as the presence of less than 180 cm of residual and functional small bowel in adult patients. Thus, resection of less than 50% of the small intestine is generally well tolerated. In approximately 75% of cases, short bowel syndrome results from one massive small bowel resection, as opposed to multiple sequential resections. In adults, the most common etiologies include acute mesenteric ischemia, malignancy, and Crohn disease. In pediatric patients, the most common etiologies include intestinal atresia, midgut volvulus, and necrotizing enterocolitis. Resection of the jejunum is better tolerated than resection of the ileum because the absorption of bile salts and vitamin B_{12} occurs in the ileum. An intact ileocecal valve is thought to reduce malabsorption because it increases the residence time of the chyme in the small intestine. Likewise, an intact colon is important because it has a tremendous water-reabsorbing capacity as well as electrolytes and can also absorb fatty acids. With an intact colon, a shorter small bowel remnant is tolerated. The key to avoiding short bowel syndrome is avoidance of excessive small bowel resection. In Crohn patients, the use of strictureplasty as opposed to resection when possible is recommended, and in acute mesenteric ischemia, one should resect only obviously dead bowel, leaving marginal bowel in situ and performing a second-look procedure.

13. D. In the early phase of short bowel syndrome, treatment is directed at slowing intestinal transit, reducing GI secretions, and maintaining nutrition, fluid, and electrolyte balance. Transit time is slowed by the administration of narcotics such as codeine and diphenoxylate, as well as with the antimotility agents Lomotil (diphenoxylate and atropine) and loperamide. Massive small bowel resection is associated with hypergastrinemia and acid hypersecretion. The increased acidity in the small bowel results in the inhibition of digestive enzymes. This can be controlled with H_2-receptor antagonists or proton pump inhibitors such as omeprazole. Nutrition is achieved with the institution of TPN. In addition, enteral feeding should be instituted as soon as postoperative ileus has resolved. Enteral feeding assists in the process of intestinal adaptation and prevents the development of villous atrophy associated with being NPO for a prolonged period of time. Cholestyramine is also useful in controlling diarrhea due to unabsorbed bile salts. The role of octreotide is controversial. Short-term use leads to a reduction in diarrhea, but long-term use may lead to steatorrhea, gallstones, and an inhibition of intestinal adaptation. More recently, a high-carbohydrate, low-fat enteral diet rich in glutamine combined with growth hormone administration has shown promise in improving intestinal absorptive capacity. Intestinal adaptation occurs over a period of 1 to 2 years in most adults. Thus, the final determination of whether permanent TPN will be necessary is not determined until after this period.

14. A. Many patients with short bowel syndrome can eventually discontinue TPN, particularly if the bowel length is more than 120 cm in adults and more than 60 cm in children. Treatment options for short bowel syndrome depend on the length of small bowel remaining, whether the remnant small bowel is markedly dilated, whether the patient remains TPN dependent, and whether multiple complications of TPN have developed such as catheter-related infections, vena cava thrombosis, and liver damage. A short remnant (<90 cm in adults, <30 cm in children) of small bowel poses a challenging dilemma. If the remnant of small bowel is short and markedly dilated without evidence of obstruction, the best option would be an intestinal lengthening procedure. The dilated bowel lends itself to lengthening by applying a series of transverse linear staples on the mesenteric border and then on the antimesenteric border. The procedure is known as the serial transverse enteroplasty procedure. The Bianchi procedure is another option. However, it is technically much more demanding and associated with a risk of creating ischemia and anastomotic leaks and thus has a higher complication rate and an increased need for reoperation. Tapering of the small bowel alone would be indicated for patients with a longer small bowel remnant (>60 cm in children) who have marked bowel distention with evidence of stasis and bacterial overgrowth. Tapering alone would not be appropriate in someone with such a short segment of small bowel. Small bowel transplantation is also an option but is reserved for the patient with a short segment and who is TPN dependent (such as this patient) in whom, in addition, complications have developed from the TPN, as mentioned. If liver failure has developed in the patient, small bowel transplantation can be combined with liver transplantation.

References: Kim H, Lee P, Garza J, et al: Serial transverse enteroplasty for short bowel syndrome: a case report, *J Pediatr Surg* 38:881–885, 2003.

Sudan D, Thompson J, Botha J, et al: Comparison of intestinal lengthening procedures for patients with short bowel syndrome, *Ann Surg* 246:593–601, 2007.

15. B. Malignant tumors of the small bowel are rare. The most common tumor is carcinoid (50%), followed by adenocarcinoma (30%–40%), lymphoma (~15%), and GISTs (1%–20%). Small bowel lymphomas most commonly involve the ileum (as do carcinoids), whereas adenocarcinomas are most common in the duodenum (periampullary), and GISTs are evenly distributed throughout the small bowel. Small bowel lymphomas are associated with immunodeficient states, and in particular with patients with acquired immunodeficiency syndrome and transplant recipients. They are predominantly the non-Hodgkin type. In children younger than age 10, they are the most common intestinal neoplasm. The propensity for involvement of the ileum is due to its high concentration of lymphoid tissue. Grossly, the majority of small intestine lymphomas are large (>5 cm) at presentation. Symptoms include abdominal pain, weight loss, nausea, vomiting, and change in bowel habits. A CT scan may reveal evidence of intussusception (with a target sign), small bowel obstruction, or perforation. Perforation may occur in as many as 25% of the patients. The primary treatment of small bowel lymphoma (as well as all other small bowel malignancies) is surgical resection including affected mesentery. There is no clear, well-defined role for radiation therapy or chemotherapy for the majority of small bowel malignancies. The exception is the use of Gleevec (imatinib mesylate) for GISTs.

References: Balthazar E, Noordhoorn M, Megibow A, et al: CT of small-bowel lymphoma in immunocompetent patients and patients with AIDS: comparison of findings, *AJR Am J Roentgenol* 168:675–680, 1997.

Cunningham J, Aleali R, Aleali M, et al: Malignant small bowel neoplasms: histopathologic determinants of recurrence and survival, *Ann Surg* 225:300–306, 1997.

16. D. The presentation is most consistent with nonocclusive mesenteric ischemia, which accounts for approximately 20% to 30% of cases of acute mesenteric ischemia. This condition typically affects elderly patients and presents in the setting of a decrease in cardiac output, such as after an acute myocardial infarction, exacerbation of congestive heart failure, or after cardiac surgery. There are no laboratory tests to establish the diagnosis of bowel ischemia with certainty, although the presence of lactic acidosis is considered ominous. The initial diagnostic test of choice for suspected acute mesenteric ischemia is CT angiography. It is helpful in identifying the etiology, which includes an embolus that would be visualized as an occlusion just distal to the origin of the SMA; acute thrombosis of the SMA which would appear as an occlusion in association with diffuse calcifications within the vessel; mesenteric venous thrombosis, which would demonstrate a lack of contrast filling of either the portal or superior mesenteric vein; and

nonocclusive mesenteric ischemia, which would simply show diffuse spasm. The standard treatment for SMA embolus is operative embolectomy, although there are some reports of the use of thrombolytic therapy. The treatment for acute thrombosis is surgical bypass from either the aorta or the iliac artery to the more distal SMA. For mesenteric venous thrombosis, the treatment is heparin alone, provided there is no suggestion of infarcted bowel. For nonocclusive mesenteric ischemia, the treatment is a combination of medical optimization to improve cardiac output and selective intra-arterial infusion of a vasodilator such as papaverine hydrochloride into the SMA. If signs of peritonitis develop or are present, emergent laparotomy should be performed and the infarcted intestine should be resected. The mortality rate for nonocclusive mesenteric ischemia is approximately 50%.

References: Bassiouny HS: Nonocclusive mesenteric ischemia, *Surg Clin North Am* 77:319–326, 1997.

Kozuch P, Brandt L: Review article: diagnosis and management of mesenteric ischemia with an emphasis on pharmacotherapy, *Aliment Pharmacol Ther* 21:201–215, 2005.

Trompeter M, Brazda T, Remy C, et al: Non-occlusive mesenteric ischemia: etiology, diagnosis, and interventional therapy, *Eur Radiol* 12:1179–1187, 2002.

17. C. A 24-hour urinary 5-HIAA test is the best test to establish the diagnosis of carcinoid syndrome in a patient who presents with symptoms and signs suggesting the diagnosis. Chromogranin A is the most sensitive screening test for detecting a carcinoid tumor. The carcinoid syndrome occurs in approximately 20% of patients with midgut carcinoid tumors. Most gut carcinoid tumors do not cause the syndrome because vasoactive substances (serotonin, histamine, dopamine, substance P, prostaglandins) from these tumors enter the portal vein and are metabolized by the liver before reaching the systemic circulation. For carcinoid syndrome to develop, these substances need to be released directly into the systemic circulation. Thus, the syndrome develops in the setting of bronchial carcinoids (which do not drain into the liver), retroperitoneal invasion (where retroperitoneal veins drain directly into the systemic circulation), or in the presence of liver metastasis. The gold standard test for the detection of carcinoid syndrome is the 24-hour urinary 5-HIAA test. Normally, most dietary tryptophan is converted into nicotinic acid (niacin, vitamin B_3). In the presence of carcinoid tumors, there is a shift toward conversion to 5-hydroxytryptophan, which is then converted to serotonin. Serotonin is then metabolized to 5-HIAA. The shift away from conversion to tryptophan to nicotinic acid can result in pellagra (diarrhea, dermatitis, dementia) in carcinoid syndrome. 5-HIAA is thought to be highly sensitive and specific for detecting metastatic carcinoid; thus, it is considered the best test for establishing the diagnosis of carcinoid syndrome. However, it is not as sensitive for detecting nonfunctional carcinoid tumors. Serum serotonin, neurotensin, and neurokinin A levels may be elevated in carcinoid syndrome but are less sensitive. Screening for a carcinoid tumor (as opposed to establishing the diagnosis of carcinoid syndrome) is probably best achieved with serum chromogranin A because it will be elevated in both functioning and nonfunctioning tumors. Chromogranin A is a protein present in the chromaffin granules of neuroendocrine cells. It is more sensitive than 5-HIAA but less specific. It can be elevated with other neuroendocrine tumors as well and is considered to be the best screening test for neuroendocrine tumors.

References: Nobels F, Kwekkeboom D, Coopmans W, et al: Chromogranin A as serum marker for neuroendocrine neoplasia: comparison with neuron-specific enolase and the alpha-subunit of glycoprotein hormones, *J Clin Endocrinol Metab* 82:2622–2628, 1997.

Zuetenhorst JM, Taal B: Metastatic carcinoid tumors: a clinical review, *Oncologist* 10:123–131, 2005.

18. C. Serum chromogranin A is the most sensitive marker for detecting neuroendocrine tumors in general. It has also been shown to be the most useful marker for detecting recurrence and response to treatment. High levels correlate with a worse prognosis. Platelet serotonin levels are also useful in detecting carcinoid tumors. However, the platelet becomes rapidly saturated with serotonin; thus, it is not a useful tool for monitoring treatment response. Because levels of chromogranin A correlate with tumor burden, it is a useful marker for treatment response. 5-HIAA is also thought to be useful; however, several studies indicate that chromogranin A is more sensitive for recurrence and a better prognosticator.

References: Bajetta E, Ferrari L, Martinetti A, et al: Chromogranin A, neuron specific enolase, carcinoembryonic antigen, and hydroxyindole acetic acid evaluation in patients with neuroendocrine tumors, *Cancer* 86:858–865, 1999.

Eriksson B, Oberg K, Stridsberg M: Tumor markers in neuroendocrine tumors, *Digestion* 62(Suppl 1):33–38, 2000.

Janson E, Holmberg L, Stridsberg M, et al: Carcinoid tumors: analysis of prognostic factors and survival in 301 patients from a referral center, *Ann Oncol* 8:685–690, 1997.

Nikou G, Lygidakis N, Toubanakis C, et al: Current diagnosis and treatment of gastrointestinal carcinoids in a series of 101 patients: the significance of serum chromogranin-A, somatostatin receptor scintigraphy and somatostatin analogues, *Hepatogastroenterology* 52:731–741, 2005.

19. D. Because carcinoid tumors are relatively slow growing, patients with advanced metastatic carcinoid may benefit from procedures that debulk the intra-abdominal disease, even though they are not curative because this will lessen the symptoms of carcinoid syndrome and has been shown to provide a survival advantage. Another approach is hepatic artery embolization or chemoembolization. Hepatic artery embolization or chemoembolization seems to be effective because of the fact that metastatic liver tumors primarily receive their blood from the hepatic artery, whereas the majority of the liver receives its blood from the portal vein. Another option is radiofrequency ablation, although the number of patients studied, while undergoing this modality to date is small. Significant palliation of advanced carcinoid has been achieved with medical management. In particular, the somatostatin analogues octreotide and lanreotide, as well as interferon-α, are useful in reducing pain and symptoms of carcinoid syndrome. They also seem to slow tumor growth by the inhibition of angiogenesis. The use of systemic chemotherapy does not seem to offer significant benefit to survival or long-term palliation.

References: Bajetta E, Zilembo N, Di Bartolomeo M, et al: Treatment of metastatic carcinoids and other neuroendocrine tumors with recombinant interferon-alpha-2a: a study by the Italian Trials in Medical Oncology Group, *Cancer* 72:3099–3105, 1993.

Drougas J, Anthony L, Blair T, et al: Hepatic artery chemoembolization for management of patients with advanced metastatic carcinoid tumors, *Am J Surg* 175:408–412, 1998.

O'Toole D, Ducreux M, Bommelaer G, et al: Treatment of carcinoid syndrome: a prospective crossover evaluation of lanreotide versus octreotide in terms of efficacy, patient acceptability, and tolerance, *Cancer* 88:770–776, 2000.

Rougier P, Mitry E: Chemotherapy in the treatment of neuroendocrine malignant tumors, *Digestion* 62(Suppl 1):73–78, 2000.

Wessels FJ, Schell SR: Radiofrequency ablation treatment of refractory carcinoid hepatic metastases, *J Surg Res* 95:8–12, 2001.

20. B. Right-sided valvular disease is a significant source of morbidity and mortality in carcinoid syndrome because it can lead to right heart failure. Vasoactive substances released from liver metastasis are transported to the right heart, where endocardial damage ensues, leading to thickening, retraction, and fixation of the valves. The most common valvular disorder is tricuspid insufficiency. Pulmonary valve lesions are the next most common. Left-sided heart lesions are much less common but do occur.

References: Moyssakis I, Rallidis L, Guida G, Nihoyannopoulos P: Incidence and evolution of carcinoid syndrome in the heart, *J Heart Valve Dis* 6:625–630, 1997.

Pellikka P, Tajik A, Khandheria B, et al: Carcinoid heart disease. Clinical and echocardiographic spectrum in 74 patients, *Circulation* 87:1188–1196, 1993.

Robiolio P, Rigolin V, Wilson J, et al: Carcinoid heart disease. Correlation of high serotonin levels with valvular abnormalities detected by cardiac catheterization and echocardiography, *Circulation* 92:790–795, 1995.

21. C. Glutamine is the principal fuel of the small intestine. The delivery of adequate amounts of glutamine is essential to maintain the integrity of intestinal mucosa and rapidly proliferating cells. Glutamine-enriched nutrition protects against atrophy of the intestinal mucosa.

Reference: O'Dwyer S, Smith R, Hwang T, Wilmore D: Maintenance of small bowel mucosa with glutamine-enriched parenteral nutrition, *J Parenter Enteral Nutr* 13:579–585, 1989.

22. E. GISTs were previously termed *leiomyomas* or *leiomyosarcomas*. It now seems that they are mesenchymal tumors. The cell of origin of these tumors is thought to be the interstitial Cajal cell. GISTs are classified into three types: spindle cell (70%), epithelioid type (20%), and mixed spindle and epithelioid cell type (10%). GISTs stain positive for CD34, the human progenitor cell antigen, as well as for CD177, the c-kit proto-oncogene protein. Determining whether a GIST is benign or malignant is difficult because seemingly benign tumors may behave in a malignant fashion with local recurrence. The risk of recurrence is primarily determined by the mitotic index (>2 suggests malignant behavior) per 50 high-power fields and tumor size. The stomach is the most common site in the GI tract. Small bowel GISTs may be incidental discoveries at surgery for other disorders. However, those that do present with symptoms tend to be very large and bulky at presentation. In one large study, the median size of a symptomatic GIST was 11 cm. They tend to present with evidence of obstruction or GI bleeding. The standard treatment is surgical resection with negative margins. GISTs of the small intestine carry a high mortality rate, likely due to the late presentation. Only 28% of patients were alive at a median follow-up of 20 months in one study. The adjuvant treatment of GISTs includes Gleevec (imatinib), a tyrosine kinase inhibitor. In one study, imatinib controlled tumor growth in as many as 85% of advanced GISTs. Currently, imatinib is recommended for unresectable, metastatic, or recurrent lesions. Adjuvant therapy after successful surgical resection is being used as part of clinical trials. The most useful indicators of survival and the risk of metastasis include the size of the tumor at presentation, the mitotic index, and evidence of tumor invasion into the lamina propria.

References: Blay J, Bonvalot S, Casali P, et al: GIST consensus meeting panelists: consensus meeting for the management of gastrointestinal stromal tumors: report of the GIST Consensus Conference of 20–21 March 2004, under the auspices of ESMO, *Ann Oncol* 16:566–578, 2005.

Crosby J, Catton C, Davis A, et al: Malignant gastrointestinal stromal tumors of the small intestine: a review of 50 cases from a prospective database, *Ann Surg Oncol* 8:50–59, 2001.

23. B. A hernia sac containing a Meckel diverticulum is called a *Littre hernia*. Lumbar hernias can be either congenital or acquired and occur in the lumbar region of the posterior abdominal wall. Hernias through the superior lumbar triangle (Grynfeltt triangle) are more common than those through the inferior lumbar triangle (the Petit triangle). The Petit triangle is bounded by the external oblique muscle, latissimus dorsi muscle, and iliac crest. The Grynfeltt triangle is bounded by the quadratus lumborum muscle, the 12th rib, and the internal oblique muscle. A spigelian hernia occurs through the spigelian fascia, which is composed of the aponeurotic layer between the rectus muscle medially and the semilunar line laterally. Nearly all spigelian hernias occur at or below the arcuate line. The absence of posterior rectus fascia may contribute to an inherent weakness in this area. A Richter hernia occurs when only the antimesenteric border of the bowel herniates through the fascial defect. It involves only a portion of the circumference of the bowel. As such, incarceration and strangulation may occur in the absence of any evidence of bowel obstruction.

24. D. SMA syndrome or Wilkie syndrome is a rare condition characterized by compression of the third portion of the duodenum by the SMA as it passes over this portion of the duodenum. It occurs most often in the setting of profound weight loss. Factors that predispose to the condition include supine immobilization, scoliosis, placement of a body cast, and eating disorders. Symptoms include profound nausea and vomiting, abdominal distention, weight loss, and postprandial epigastric pain, which varies from intermittent to constant depending the severity of the duodenal obstruction. Weight loss usually occurs before the onset of symptoms. It is more common in women. The diagnosis can be made by a CT scan, which demonstrates a decreased aortomesenteric angle and a decreased distance between the aorta and the SMA, as well as evidence of obstruction of the duodenum. It can also be diagnosed by a barium upper GI

series or hypotonic duodenography, demonstrating abrupt or near total cessation of flow of barium from the duodenum to the jejunum. Conservative measures are tried initially that are primarily focused on weight gain. The operative treatment is duodenojejunostomy.

References: Adson D, Mitchell J, Trenkner S: The superior mesenteric artery syndrome and acute gastric dilatation in eating disorders: a report of two cases and a review of the literature, *Int J Eat Disord* 21:103–114, 1997.

Agrawal G, Johnson P, Fishman E: Multidetector row CT of superior mesenteric artery syndrome, *J Clin Gastroenterol* 41:62–65, 2007.

25. C. Small bowel obstruction after radiation therapy presents a daunting challenge because of the risk of radiation enteritis. Chronic radiation enteritis results from an obliterative arteritis in the submucosal vessels. This leads to progressive submucosal fibrosis and stricture formation. The risk of radiation enteritis correlates with the amount of radiation received. It is uncommon if the total radiation dose is less than 4000 cGy. The risk of radiation damage increases if the patient received chemotherapy or has underlying vascular disease or diabetes. Early symptoms of radiation damage include diarrhea, abdominal pain, and malabsorption and are usually self-limited. The treatment of acute radiation enteritis includes antispasmodic agents, analgesic agents, and antidiarrheal agents. Only a small group of patients with chronic radiation enteritis will require surgery for either small bowel obstruction from stricture formation or fistulas. Unlike Crohn disease in which strictureplasty is used, it is not recommended for radiation enteritis because there is a high risk of tissue breakdown. The extent of macroscopic radiation injury is difficult to determine on gross inspection. Extensive lysis of adhesions should be avoided because this creates a risk of an enterotomy and subsequent fistula formation as well. The two main surgical procedures are primary resection with reanastomosis or bypass. If the source of obstruction is a loop of bowel stuck in the pelvis, it is best treated with a bypass rather than an attempt to take down the adhesions and risk injury.

Reference: Galland R, Spencer J: Natural history and surgical management of radiation enteritis, *Br J Surg* 74:742–747, 1987.

26. D. For an acute flare-up of Crohn disease, the gold standard for treatment remains corticosteroids and prednisone in particular. Sulfasalazine and mesalamine are used for mild active disease and are not effective for flare-ups. Infliximab is useful for an acute flare-up, but due to the higher risks of complications and its expense, is not considered the first drug of choice for a flare-up. Natalizumab is a new drug that is a monoclonal antibody directed at α_4 integrin. It inhibits leukocyte adhesion and migration into inflamed tissue. It has been shown to produce only small improvements in Crohn disease. Given its side effects (progressive multifocal leukoencephalopathy), it is not a first-line choice for Crohn disease.

27. E. On occasion, a patient who presents with classic symptoms and signs of acute appendicitis will instead be found to have acute inflammation of the terminal ileum on exploration. This entity is commonly referred to as acute or terminal ileitis. Acute ileitis has numerous causes, including infectious agents such as *Yersinia* (*enterocolitica* and *pseudotuberculosis*), *Mycobacterium*, cytomegalovirus (in acquired immunodeficiency syndrome), *Salmonella*, *Campylobacter*, and *Shigella*. It can also be the first manifestation of Crohn disease, but this is much less common. Because the typical course of acute ileitis is benign, resection of the ileum is not recommended. If it is discovered at surgery for presumed appendicitis, removal of the normal appendix is recommended so that if the same symptoms and signs recur, appendicitis is ruled out. Appendectomy should not be performed if the cecum itself is inflamed because dividing the base of the appendix across an inflamed cecum will increase the risk of a fistula, particularly if the underlying disorder is inflammatory bowel disease. There is no role for lymph node biopsy.

28. D. A Meckel diverticulum is a remnant of the vitelline duct. It occurs within 2 feet of the ileocecal valve on the antimesenteric border of the bowel. It is a true diverticulum found in 2% of the population. It is twice as common in males and frequently presents in the first 2 years of life. The most common cause of lower GI bleeding in children is a Meckel diverticulum. It may contain ectopic gastric or pancreatic mucosa. The gastric mucosa secretes acid, leading to ulcer formation and bleeding, usually in the adjacent ileum, not in the Meckel diverticulum itself. Thus, surgical management consists of segmental resection of the ileum to include the Meckel diverticulum. At surgery, the specimen should be opened to search for the ulceration. The presence of a Meckel diverticulum can be determined with a nuclear scan, which consists of technetium-99m pertechnetate. It will light up if the Meckel diverticulum contains ectopic gastric mucosa.

29. B. The management of an incidentally discovered Meckel diverticulum remains controversial. However, most surgeons would recommend removal in children when it is discovered incidentally at surgery. Guidelines in adults for selective removal include age younger than 50 years, the presence of palpable heterotopic tissue, diverticulum length greater than 2 cm, the presence of a mesodiverticular band, and signs of previous diverticulitis.

References: Cullen JJ, Kelly KA, Moir CR, et al: Surgical management of Meckel's diverticulum: an epidemiologic, population-based study, *Ann Surg* 220:564–568, 1994.

McKay R: High incidence of symptomatic Meckel's diverticulum in patients less than fifty years of age: an indication for resection, *Am Surg* 73:271–275, 2007.

Park JJ, Wolff BG, Tollefson MK, et al: Meckel diverticulum: the Mayo Clinic experience with 1476 patients (1950–2002), *Ann Surg* 241:529–533, 2005.

30. C. The patient has a carcinoid crisis. This has been described after anesthetic induction as well as after other stressful situations such as biopsies or invasive procedures. Carcinoid crisis is characterized by hypotension, bronchospasms, flushing, and tachycardia. The primary treatment is IV octreotide administered as a bolus of 50 to 100 µg. Even more rarely, a carcinoid crisis can manifest with hypertension. Octreotide is effective for a hypertensive

crisis as well. Adjunctive treatment with antihistamines may also be of benefit due to frequent histamine release from carcinoid tumors.

References: Bax N, Woods H, Batchelor A, Jennings M: Octreotide therapy in carcinoid disease, *Anticancer Drugs* 7(Suppl 1): 17–22, 1996.

Warner R, Mani S, Profeta J, Grunstein E: Octreotide treatment of carcinoid hypertensive crisis, *Mt Sinai J Med* 61:349–355, 1994.

31. C. The patient has a blind loop syndrome, which is due to bacterial overgrowth. Symptoms include diarrhea, steatorrhea, megaloblastic anemia, weight loss, abdominal pain, and deficiencies of fat-soluble vitamins. The megaloblastic anemia is due to the utilization of vitamin B_{12} by the bacteria. The underlying cause may be an intestinal abnormality such as a diverticulum, fistula, and intestinal stricture or may follow a Billroth II procedure. In the patient presented, the large jejunal diverticulum is likely the etiology. The diagnosis can be confirmed by various means. A barium study is useful to define the anatomic abnormality. The D-xylose test involves ingesting xylose, which is metabolized by the bacteria. Excessive CO_2 in the breath confirms the diagnosis. Cultures of the small intestine can be obtained; however, passing an intestinal tube distal enough to obtain an adequate culture can be challenging. Another useful study is the Schilling test. Oral radiolabeled vitamin B_{12} is administered along with parenteral unlabeled vitamin B_{12}. The unlabeled vitamin B_{12} saturates liver receptors. Thus, if the oral radiolabeled vitamin B_{12} is properly absorbed and liver receptors are saturated, the radiolabeled vitamin B_{12} will be excreted in high concentrations in the urine. With pernicious anemia and blind loop syndrome, oral absorption will be low and thus urinary excretion of radiolabeled vitamin B_{12} will be low. When the test is repeated after the addition of intrinsic factor, vitamin B_{12} excretion will increase, whereas with blind loop syndrome vitamin B_{12} excretion will remain low. The initial treatment of blind loop syndrome consists of broad-spectrum antibiotics including metronidazole with tetracycline as well as vitamin B_{12} supplementation given parenterally. Prokinetic agents do not seem to help. In addition, dietary modifications are useful, such as a lactose-free diet because patients with blind loop syndrome often become lactose intolerant. Medium-chain triglyceride diets are more readily absorbed than long-chain triglycerides because they do not require digestive enzymes. Resection of the diverticulum is not recommended initially. Surgery should be reserved for patients who fail repeated medical management attempts.

References: Ross B, Richards W, Sharp K, et al: Diverticular disease of the jejunum and its complications, *Am Surg* 56:319–324, 1990.

Woods K, Williams E, Melvin W, Sharp K: Acquired jejunoileal diverticulosis and its complications: a review of the literature, *Am Surg* 74:849–854, 2008.

32. A. Peutz-Jeghers syndrome features mucocutaneous melanotic pigmentation and hamartomatous polyps (not adenomatous) of the small intestine. It is an autosomal dominant inherited syndrome. The skin lesions are found in the circumoral region of the face, buccal mucosa, forearms, palms, soles, digits, and perianal area, whereas the hamartomas are usually in the jejunum and ileum. The most common symptom is recurrent colicky abdominal pain. Symptoms of a bowel obstruction develop in as many as 50% of patients, which is usually due to intussception or obstruction by the polyp itself. Hemorrhage or chronic anemia can also occur as a result of the polyps. The polyps can also undergo adenomatous change. Patients are at significantly increased risk of the development of cancer in the GI tract (esophagus, stomach, small intestine, colon, and pancreas) as well as extraintestinally (testis, breast, uterus, ovary). Over the long term, cancer develops in as many as 90% of patients. Compared with the general population, they are at 500 times increased risk of the development of small intestine cancer.

References: Boardman L, Pittelkow M, Couch F: Association of Peutz-Jeghers-like mucocutaneous pigmentation with breast and gynecologic carcinomas in women, *Medicine (Baltimore)* 79:293–298, 2000.

Giardiello F, Brensinger J, Tersmette AC: Very high risk of cancer in familial Peutz-Jeghers syndrome, *Gastroenterology* 119:1447–1453, 2000.

Wu YK, Tsai CH, Yang JC: Gastroduodenal intussusception due to Peutz-Jeghers syndrome: a case report, *Hepatogastroenterology* 41:134–136, 1994.

33. D. Pneumatosis intestinalis is a radiographic finding and not a disease unto itself. In most cases, it is a benign finding. It has been divided into primary and secondary pneumatosis intestinalis. The primary form is less common and is termed *pneumatosis cystoides intestinalis*. It consists of thin-walled, air-filled cysts within the bowel wall, usually in the colon, but it can occur anywhere in the GI tract. It is an incidental finding on plain radiograph or CT scan. The gas can appear as linear, curvilinear, bubbly, or cystic. There is no specific treatment. Secondary pneumatosis intestinalis occurs when there is an underlying disease process. The exact cause of pneumatosis intestinalis is unclear, but there seem to be several pathways that allow gas to enter the bowel wall. Immunodeficient and inflammatory bowel states lead to a loss of mucosal barrier function that may permit air to enter the bowel wall. Bowel obstruction leads to gas formation under pressure. Alterations in bacteria flora, with invasion of the bowel wall, likewise lead to gas formation. In adults, secondary pneumatosis intestinalis is most often associated with chronic obstructive pulmonary disease. It is also seen with collagen vascular disease, celiac sprue, Crohn disease, and use of steroids and in immunodeficient states. More ominously, it is also associated with ischemic bowel. Thus, it is important to recognize that not all cases of pneumatosis are benign. In neonates, it is most commonly associated with necrotizing enterocolitis. The finding of pneumatosis intestinalis in association with necrotizing enterocolitis does not mandate surgical exploration. It is also seen with pyloric stenosis, Hirschsprung disease, and other causes of bowel obstruction. Pneumoperitoneum can rarely be the result of a benign case of pneumatosis intestinalis because the air-filled cysts are thin walled and can burst.

References: Mularski R, Ciccolo M, Rappaport W: Nonsurgical causes of pneumoperitoneum, *West J Med* 170:41–46, 1999.

Pear BL: Pneumatosis intestinalis: a review, *Radiology* 207:13–19, 1998.

St. Peter S, Abbas M, Kelly K: The spectrum of pneumatosis intestinalis, *Arch Surg* 138:68–75, 2003.

34. A. The majority of lesions responsible for GI bleeding are seen with upper endoscopy or colonoscopy. Obscure GI bleeding refers to persistent or recurrent bleeding for which no source has been identified by these modalities. Obscure bleeding can be either occult (meaning not visible to the eye) or overt (such as melena and hematochezia). In most instances, the source of obscure bleeding is from the small bowel. Small intestine angiodysplasias account for 75% of cases of obscure bleeding in adults. Other causes include Crohn disease, infectious enteritis, neoplasms, and vasculitis. A Meckel diverticulum is the most common cause of obscure GI bleeding in children. Localization of small bowel lesions is difficult with standard studies. Options include push enteroscopy and small bowel barium studies, as well as radiolabeled red blood cell scanning and angiography (although these latter two are only useful in the setting of active bleeding). A more recent modality is capsule endoscopy, which has been shown to be superior to enteroscopy and barium studies.

Reference: Pennazio M, Santucci R, Rondonotti E, et al: Outcome of patients with obscure gastrointestinal bleeding after capsule endoscopy: report of 100 consecutive cases, *Gastroenterology* 126:643–653, 2004.

35. A. The case is most consistent with typhoid enteritis. Diagnosis is confirmed by demonstrating a positive blood or stool culture. The infection is due to *Salmonella typhosa*. The infection leads to hyperplasia of the reticuloendothelial system, including the lymph nodes, liver, and spleen, as well as Peyer patches in the small bowel. Peyer patches may ulcerate, bleed, and perforate, leading to surgical intervention (although this is rare). The perforation is typically solitary and in the terminal ileum and can be managed by simple closure as well as antibiotics. Resection with primary anastomosis is reserved for the rare patient with multiple perforations.

36. D. The primary cause of mortality from a small bowel fistula is sepsis. Thus, control of sepsis is a key element of successful management. A CT scan is essential to ascertain whether the fistula is being adequately captured and to rule out intraperitoneal abscesses. In addition, early management of small bowel fistulas should focus on adequate fluid and electrolyte repletion, early institution of TPN, and protection of the skin. The majority of fistulas will close in 3 to 6 weeks of conservative management. If closure does not occur, then surgery is indicated. Early operative intervention has a high risk of failure and is made more difficult by the density and vascular nature of early adhesions.

37. E. A Meckel diverticulum is found on the antimesenteric border approximately 60 cm (2 ft) from the ileocecal valve. A Meckel diverticulum may be very small or may extend via a fibrous band up to the umbilicus. It is a remnant of the vitelline duct. Because cells from this region are pluripotent during embryologic development, heterotopic tissue may develop within a Meckel diverticulum. Intestinal obstruction is the most common presentation in adults with a Meckel diverticulum. This may be caused by a volvulus of the small bowel around the diverticulum due to a fibrotic band attached to the abdominal wall, intussusception, or, rarely, incarceration of the diverticulum in a hernia. Bleeding is the most common presentation of a Meckel diverticulum in children.

References: Evers BM: Small Intestine. In Townsend CM Jr, Beauchamp RD, Evers BM, Mattox KL, editors: *Sabiston textbook of surgery: the biological basis of modern surgical practice*, ed 18, Philadelphia, 2008, WB Saunders, pp 1278–1332.

Small bowel. In Cameron JL, editor: *Current surgical therapy*, ed 9, Philadelphia, 2008, Mosby, pp 117–160.

Tavakkolizadeh A, Whang EE, Ashley SW, et al: Small intestine. In Brunicardi FC, Andersen DK, Billiar TR, et al, editors: *Schwartz's principles of surgery*, ed 9, New York, 2010, McGraw-Hill, pp 979–1012.

Spleen 22

1. The most common location for an accessory spleen is:

   A. Splenic hilum
   B. Gastrocolic ligament
   C. Greater omentum
   D. Splenorenal ligament
   E. Adjacent to the left testicle

2. The most common cause of spontaneous splenic rupture worldwide is:

   A. Leukemia
   B. Malaria
   C. Sepsis
   D. Hemolytic anemia
   E. Hodgkin lymphoma

3. All of the following are true regarding hyposplenism EXCEPT:

   A. It is associated with ulcerative colitis.
   B. It is associated with sickle cell anemia.
   C. It can occur in the presence of an enlarged spleen.
   D. It is associated with pneumococcal infections.
   E. Howell-Jolly bodies are typically absent on peripheral blood smear.

4. The risk of postsplenectomy sepsis is highest for which of the following?

   A. Trauma
   B. Idiopathic thrombocytopenic purpura (ITP)
   C. Hereditary spherocytosis (HS)
   D. Thalassemia major
   E. Hereditary elliptocytosis

5. After splenectomy for trauma, the optimal timing for administration of the pneumococcal vaccine is on postoperative day:

   A. 1
   B. 4
   C. 7
   D. 10
   E. 14

6. All of the following are true regarding Felty syndrome EXCEPT:

   A. Splenectomy is indicated for intractable leg ulcers.
   B. Patients are prone to recurrent infections.
   C. The neutrophil count markedly improves 24 hours after splenectomy.
   D. Patients have antibodies against neutrophil nuclei.
   E. Corticosteroids are contraindicated.

7. Ectopic or "wandering" spleen:

   A. Is the presence of accessory spleens in unusual locations
   B. Is more common in males
   C. Requires no surgical management even when symptomatic
   D. May result in splenic torsion
   E. Is best diagnosed with mesenteric angiography

8. Which of the following is true regarding HS?

   A. It is transmitted as an autosomal recessive trait.
   B. The spleen is typically smaller than normal.
   C. Associated gallstone formation is rare.
   D. It is associated with leg ulcers.
   E. A positive direct Coombs test result confirms the diagnosis.

9. All of the following are true regarding ITP EXCEPT:

   A. When performing splenectomy, platelets should given just before the skin incision is made.
   B. In children, a splenectomy is less likely needed.
   C. The spleen is typically not palpable on abdominal examination.
   D. Children with platelet counts greater than 30,000 µ/L do not require hospitalization and no medical therapy is needed.
   E. A bone marrow biopsy sample will demonstrate normal or increased megakaryocytes.

10. Which of the following is the best indication for splenectomy?
    A. Sarcoidosis without hypersplenism
    B. Gaucher disease without hypersplenism
    C. Myelofibrosis without hypersplenism
    D. Hairy cell leukemia with neutropenia
    E. Secondary hypersplenism in a cirrhotic patient

11. A 30-year-old woman is found to have a signet ring calcification in the left upper quadrant on a plain abdominal radiograph. A computed tomography (CT) scan confirms a 2-cm splenic artery aneurysm just beyond the take-off of the celiac axis. All of the following are true regarding this condition EXCEPT:
    A. It is more common in women.
    B. It is most likely a true aneurysm.
    C. It is associated with a double-rupture phenomenon.
    D. It is associated with portal hypertension.
    E. It can be safely observed.

12. Two months after a splenectomy for ITP, the patient is noted to have petechiae and a decrease in platelet count. A peripheral blood smear is noteworthy for the absence of Howell-Jolly bodies. Which of the following is the best recommendation for a work-up?
    A. CT scan of the abdomen
    B. Bone marrow biopsy
    C. No work-up needed; administer steroids
    D. Radiolabeled red blood cell (RBC) scan
    E. No work-up needed; administer immunoglobulin

13. Which of the following is true regarding ITP?
    A. It is more common in males.
    B. A chronic form is more likely to develop in adults than in children.
    C. The diagnosis is effectively established by a peripheral blood smear.
    D. Immunoglobulin is ineffective in increasing the platelet count.
    E. In adults, splenectomy should be delayed until after the second relapse.

14. All of the following are true regarding thrombotic thrombocytopenic purpura (TTP) EXCEPT:
    A. It does not lead to hemolysis.
    B. It is associated with renal failure.
    C. Lower extremity petechiae are the most common presentation.
    D. The Coombs test result is negative.
    E. Neurologic complications such as seizures and coma.

15. All of the following are features of the postsplenectomy patient EXCEPT:
    A. Target cells
    B. Schistocytes
    C. Pappenheimer bodies
    D. Howell-Jolly bodies
    E. Leukocytosis that may persist for months

16. The most common source of splenic abscess is:
    A. Hematogenous spread
    B. Secondary infection of a hematoma
    C. Secondary infection of a cyst
    D. Local extension of colonic perforation
    E. Local extension of a pancreatic abscess

17. After splenectomy for a myeloproliferative disorder, a 40-year-old woman presents with anorexia, abdominal pain, and a low-grade fever. Her white blood cell (WBC) count is 14,000 cells/μL and her platelet count is 500,000/μL. A noncontrast CT scan reveals diffuse small bowel edema and mild ascites. The most likely diagnosis is:
    A. Overwhelming postsplenectomy infection
    B. Portal vein thrombosis
    C. Primary peritonitis
    D. Ischemic colitis
    E. Perforated duodenal ulcer

18. In patients with hairy cell leukemia, remission is best achieved with use of:
    A. Leustatin (cladribine)
    B. Radiation therapy
    C. Interferon-alfa
    D. 5-Fluorouracil
    E. Rituxan (rituximab)

19. The most common organism associated with overwhelming postsplenectomy sepsis is:
    A. Group A streptococcus
    B. *Haemophilus influenzae*
    C. *Streptococcus pneumoniae*
    D. *Meningococcus*
    E. *Babesia microti*

20. The most common indication for elective splenectomy is:
    A. Staging for Hodgkin lymphoma
    B. Hereditary spherocytosis
    C. Immune thrombocytopenic purpura
    D. Chronic lymphocytic leukemia
    E. Autoimmune hemolytic anemia

21. In comparing laparoscopic with open splenectomy for hematologic disorders, which of the following is true?

    A. Open splenectomy has better long-term results with respect to response rates.

    B. The length of hospital stay is the same.

    C. The operative mortality rate is lower with laparoscopic splenectomy.

    D. Laparoscopic splenectomy has emerged as the standard of care.

    E. Laparoscopic splenectomy has a lower morbidity rate in cirrhotic patients.

Answers

1. A. More than 80% of accessory spleens are found in the regions of the splenic hilum and vascular pedicle. Other locations for accessory spleens in descending order of frequency are the gastrocolic ligament, the tail of the pancreas, the greater omentum, the greater curvature of the stomach, the splenocolic ligament, the small and large bowel mesenteries, the left broad ligament of the uterus in women, and the left spermatic cord in men. The presence of accessory spleens has clinical implications. In one large series of splenectomy for hematologic disorders, accessory spleens were found in 18%. In patients in whom recurrence of ITP developed, it was eventually found to be due to a missed accessory spleen in a significant number, and reoperation was curative.

    Reference: Rudowski W: Accessory spleens: clinical significance with particular reference to the recurrence of idiopathic thrombocytopenic purpura, *World J Surg* 9:422–430, 1985.

2. B. Spontaneous rupture of the spleen is an uncommon, dramatic abdominal emergency that requires immediate diagnosis and prompt treatment to ensure the patient's survival. Spontaneous rupture rarely occurs in a histologically proven normal spleen and in such cases is called a *true spontaneous rupture*. Spontaneous rupture usually occurs in a diseased spleen and is called *pathologic spontaneous rupture*. Infectious diseases have been cited in most cases involving splenic rupture but are rare in hematologic malignancies despite frequent involvement of the spleen. Malaria is the number one cause worldwide and infectious mononucleosis is the number one cause in the United States. With malaria, changes in splenic structure can result in hematoma formation, rupture, hypersplenism, torsion, or cyst formation. An abnormal immunologic response may result in massive splenic enlargement. Spontaneous rupture of the spleen is an important and life-threatening complication of *Plasmodium vivax* infection, but is rarely seen in *Plasmodium falciparum* malaria.

    Reference: Hamel C, Blum J, Harder F, Kocher T: Nonoperative treatment of splenic rupture in malaria tropica: review of literature and case report, *Acta Trop* 82:1–5, 2002.

3. E. Hyposplenism (reduced splenic function) is associated with sickle cell disease, radiation, celiac disease, malignancy, ulcerative colitis, alcoholism and drug addiction, tropical sprue, systemic lupus erythematosus, Fanconi anemia, human immunodeficiency virus infection, splenic trauma, and amyloidosis. Patients with hyposplenism may be functionally asplenic. Thus, they may display findings associated with the postsplenectomy period including sepsis with encapsulated organisms, mild degrees of thrombocytosis and leukocytosis, Howell-Jolly bodies in RBCs, and an increased number of target cells. Howell-Jolly bodies are nuclear remnants in circulating erythrocytes that appear basophilic (blue). Normally, erythrocytes expel their DNA before exiting the bone marrow.

    References: Fishman D, Isenberg D: Splenic involvement in rheumatic diseases, *Semin Arthritis Rheum* 27:141–155, 1997.

    Piliero P, Furie R: Functional asplenia in systemic lupus erythematosus, *Semin Arthritis Rheum* 20:185–189, 1990.

4. D. The incidence rate and mortality rate for postsplenectomy sepsis are highest for patients with underlying hematologic conditions, in particular, thalassemia major and sickle cell disease. Children have a higher risk than adults. In a large review, the incidence of infection after splenectomy in children (younger than 16 years old) was 4.4% compared with 0.9% in adults. Severe infection after splenectomy for benign disease was very uncommon except in infants and children younger than the age of 5 years. *S. pneumoniae* is the most common infecting organism, accounting for 50% to 90% of cases, followed by *H. influenzae* type B, *Neisseria meningitides*, and group A streptococcus. Patients are also more susceptible to malaria.

    References: Davidson R, Wall R: Prevention and management of infections in patients without a spleen, *Clin Micro Infect* 7:657–660, 2001.

    Holdsworth, R, Irving A, Cuschieri A: Postsplenectomy sepsis and its mortality rate: actual versus perceived risks, *Br J Surg* 78:1031–1038, 1991.

    Leonard A, Giebink G, Baesl T, Krivit W: The overwhelming postsplenectomy sepsis problem, *World J Surg* 4:423–432, 1980.

5. E. In patients who have unanticipated splenectomy (i.e., trauma), administering the pneumococcal vaccine immediately postoperatively will result in a much higher likelihood of the need for revaccination. The optimal timing is 14 days after surgery. Furthermore, in patients undergoing planned splenectomy, those who received the vaccine less than 14 days before surgery were more likely to need revaccination. The timing of immunoprophylaxis for meningococcus and *H. influenzae* type B are less clear, so most would recommend giving it at the same time as pneumococcus. In children, antibiotic prophylaxis with penicillin or amoxicillin is also recommended for at least 2 years after splenectomy. Vaccination against influenza is also recommended because influenza infections predispose to secondary bacterial infection.

References: Shatz D, Romero-Steiner S, Bie C, et al: Antibody responses in postsplenectomy trauma patients receiving the 23-valent pneumococcal polysaccharide vaccine at 14 versus 28 days postoperatively, *J Trauma* 53:1037–1042, 2002.

Shatz D, Schinsky M, Pais L, et al: Immune responses of splenectomized trauma patients to the 23-valent pneumococcal polysaccharide vaccine at 1 versus 7 versus 14 days after splenectomy, *J Trauma* 44:765–766, 1998.

6. E. The triad of rheumatoid arthritis, splenomegaly, and neutropenia is called Felty syndrome. It is present in 3% of patients with rheumatoid arthritis. The pathophysiology involves the coating of the white blood cell surface with immune complexes, leading to their sequestration and clearance in the spleen. An increased risk of infections due to neutropenia ensues. The size of the spleen can vary from nonpalpable to massively enlarged. Initial treatment with corticosteroids typically improves the neutrophil count, but the effects are not always permanent. Hematopoietic growth factors and methotrexate have also been used. There is a tendency for leg ulcers to form in these patients. Other indications for splenectomy include transfusion-dependent anemia and profound thrombocytopenia. Responses to splenectomy are excellent, with more than 80% of patients showing a durable increase in white blood cell count. The neutrophil count typically improves immediately, although the relative number of neutrophils may remain subnormal. However, neutrophil function improves.

7. D. Wandering spleen is rare. It refers to a spleen that lacks its normal peritoneal attachments, thus permitting the spleen to move freely in the peritoneal cavity. It has been postulated to result from failure of the dorsal mesogastrium to fuse to the posterior abdominal wall during embryonic development. The wandering spleen has an unusually long splenic pedicle. Another hypothesis is that an acquired defect in splenic attachment may occur in multiparous women secondary to hormonal changes during pregnancy and associated abdominal laxity. Wandering spleen is most commonly diagnosed in children and in women between 20 and 40 years of age. Most patients with a wandering spleen are asymptomatic. Symptomatic patients often present with recurrent episodes of abdominal pain. This is likely related to tension on the vascular pedicle or intermittent torsion of the splenic vessels. Acute torsion of the splenic vessels may lead to a presentation of severe abdominal pain. The diagnosis of wandering spleen is confirmed by abdominal CT scan. Provided the spleen is not infarcted, treatment is with splenopexy.

References: Hirose R, Kitano S, Bando T, et al: Laparoscopic splenopexy for pediatric wandering spleen, *J Pediatr Surg* 33: 1571–1573, 1998.

Nemcek A Jr, Miller F, Fitzgerald S: Acute torsion of a wandering spleen: diagnosis by CT and duplex Doppler and color flow sonography, *AJR Am J Roentgenol* 157:307–309, 1991.

8. D. Hereditary spherocytosis is a RBC membrane disorder that leads to hemolytic anemia. It is autosomal dominant and the most common hemolytic anemia requiring splenectomy. It is due to an inherited dysfunction or deficiency in one of the RBC membrane proteins (spectrin, ankyrin, band 3 protein, or protein 4.2), which causes the membrane lipid bilayers to destabilize, leading to a lack of membrane deformability. The spleen sequesters and destroys these nondeformable RBCs. Most patients are asymptomatic, although they may have mild jaundice from hemolysis as well as splenomegaly on physical examination. Laboratory features include a mild to moderate anemia, a low mean corpuscular volume, an elevated mean corpuscular hemoglobin concentration, and an elevated red cell distribution width. Laboratory values also reflect the hemolysis and rapid cell turnover, with an elevated reticulocyte count, lactate dehydrogenase, and unconjugated bilirubin. Unlike autoimmune hemolytic anemia, the direct Coombs test result is negative in HS. In HS, RBCs tend to lyse at lower concentrations of salt than normal. Splenectomy is curative for HS and serves as the sole mode of therapy. Due to ongoing red cell lysis, gallstones are common. As such, if gallstones are found, prophylactic cholecystectomy is recommended, particularly in children. Another feature of HS is leg ulceration, which is another indication for early splenectomy. These ulcers heal after splenectomy. The cause of the ulceration is unclear, but may be a result of increased blood viscosity that reduced oxygen levels in the leg tissues. Alternatively, recent studies suggest that hemolysis leads to nitric oxide resistance, endothelial dysfunction, and end-organ vasculopathy, as is seen in sickle cell disease.

Reference: Kato G, McGowan V, Machado R: Lactate dehydrogenase as a biomarker of hemolysis-associated nitric oxide resistance, priapism, leg ulceration, pulmonary hypertension, and death in patients with sickle cell disease, *Blood* 107:2279–2285, 2006.

9. A. ITP is an autoimmune disorder caused by the formation of antiplatelet IgG autoantibodies produced in the spleen. Platelets are opsonized by the antiplatelet antibodies and are then removed prematurely, leading to the low platelet count. In adults, it is two to three times more common in women, whereas it occurs with equal frequency in boys and girls. Patients typically present with ecchymoses or petechiae. Others may exhibit minor bleeding from the gums or nose, excessive menstruation, or blood in the stool or urine. Life-threatening bleeding as an initial presentation is uncommon. In children, the presentation is often preceded by a viral illness. The spleen is usually not enlarged. The diagnosis is one of exclusion and is based on the history, physical examination, complete blood count, and examination of the peripheral smear, which should exclude other causes of thrombocytopenia. The peripheral blood smear frequently shows large, immature platelets. Bone marrow aspiration is not routinely used, but is appropriate in patients older than the age of 60 and in patients considering splenectomy. The bone marrow aspirate shows normal or increased megakaryocytes. The management depends on the age of the patient, the platelet count, and the severity of symptoms. In children, the majority present with mild cases that are self-limited and do not need any medical therapy. In fact, children with platelet counts greater than 30,000 μ/L should not be hospitalized and do not routinely require treatment if they are asymptomatic or have only minor purpura. In adults, that threshold is greater than 20,000 μ/L. The first line of therapy is oral prednisone at a dose of 1 to 1.5 mg/kg/day. Another effective therapy is intravenous (IV) immunoglobulin, which is used if corticosteroids are ineffective. Splenectomy is indicated for failure of medical therapy, for prolonged use of steroids with side effects, and for most cases of a first relapse. Patients with low platelets counts less than 10,000 μ/L should have platelets available for surgery, but should not receive them preoperatively because they will be consumed. Platelets should be given for those who continue to bleed after ligation of the splenic pedicle. Urgent splenectomy plays a role in severe, life-threatening bleeding, in conjunction with medical therapy in both adults and children. Splenectomy provides a permanent response in 75% to 85% of patients.

Reference: George J, Woolf S, Raskob G, et al: Idiopathic thrombocytopenic purpura: a practice guideline developed by explicit methods for the American Society of Hematology, *Blood* 88:3–4, 1996.

10. D. General indications for splenectomy include symptomatic splenomegaly, hypersplenism, hemolytic anemia, thrombocytopenia or other cytopenia, and for diagnostic information for Hodgkin lymphoma. Splenectomy is not indicated for sarcoidosis, Gaucher disease, or myelofibrosis without hypersplenism. Splenectomy is not indicated for patients with portal hypertension. Hairy cell leukemia gets its name from hairlike cytoplasmic projections in lymphocytes that are seen on a peripheral smear. Treatment is with chemotherapy, but splenectomy is useful in increasing cell counts, improving pain, and early satiety. With newer chemotherapeutic agents, the role of splenectomy is decreasing.

11. E. Splenic artery aneurysms are the most common visceral artery aneurysms. Women are four times more likely to be affected than men. The aneurysm usually arises in the middle to distal portion of the splenic artery. The risk of rupture is 3% to 9%; however, once rupture occurs, the mortality rate ranges from 35% to 50%. Splenic artery aneursym is problematic in pregnancy because rupture imparts a risk of mortality to both mother and fetus. Most patients are asymptomatic and seek medical attention based on an incidental radiographic finding (a ringlike calcification on a plain abdominal radiograph located in the left upper quadrant). Indications for treatment include the presence of symptoms, pregnancy, intention to become pregnant, and pseudoaneurysms associated with inflammatory

processes. For asymptomatic patients, size greater than 2 cm is an indication for surgery; however, because this woman is of childbearing age, treatment would be indicated. The majority of splenic artery aneurysms are true aneurysms. Pseudoaneurysms occur most commonly in association with an episode of severe pancreatitis with erosion into the vessel. Splenic artery aneurysms are associated with a double-rupture phenomenon in which there is an initial herald bleed into the lesser sac and then rupture into the peritoneal cavity.

12. D. When a recurrence of a platelet count decrease after splenectomy for ITP develops in a patient, one must consider the possibility of an accessory spleen that was missed. The presence of an accessory spleen is suggested by the absence of Howell-Jolly bodies on a peripheral blood smear and may also be identified by radionuclide imaging. Identification of an accessory spleen in a patient who remains severely thrombocytopenic warrants surgical excision of the accessory spleen.

13. B. Adults are more likely to get a chronic, more insidious form of ITP than children. In adults, women are affected two to three times more often than men, whereas in children, it is equally common in boys and girls. The diagnosis of ITP is one of exclusion. The peripheral blood smear shows a low platelet count as well as large, immature platelets, but does not establish the diagnosis. Intravenous immunoglobulin therapy is effective in both children and adults in increasing the platelet count. In adults, splenectomy is indicated for failure of medical therapy, for prolonged use of steroids beyond 3 to 6 months, and for most cases of a first relapse.

14. A. The surgeon needs to be aware of TTP because it is one of the thrombocytopenic disorders that responds to splenectomy. The first line of treatment is plasma exchange by removing the patient's plasma and exchanging it with fresh-frozen plasma. Splenectomy is reserved for relapses. Features of TTP include thrombocytopenia, microangiopathic hemolytic anemia, and neurologic complications. The pathophysiology involves abnormal platelet clumping, likely due to large multimers of von Willebrand factor, which results in thrombotic episodes in the microvascular circulation. The narrowed lumens in the microvascular circulation lead to increased shear stress on RBCs, causing them to lyse. Symptoms and signs include petechiae; fever; neurologic symptoms such as headaches, seizures, and even coma; and renal failure. The peripheral blood smear shows schistocytes, nucleated RBCs, and basophilic stippling. TTP can be distinguished from autoimmune hemolytic anemia, in that the result of the Coombs test is negative in TTP.

15. B. After splenectomy, target cells, Howell-Jolly bodies, Heinz bodies, and Pappenheimer bodies are seen. These inclusions (bodies) are normally pitted by the spleen. Leukocytosis and increased platelet counts commonly occur after splenectomy as well. The increase in WBC count is primarily mature neutrophils. The WBC count typically increases within 1 day after splenectomy, but may remain elevated for as long as several months. Asplenic patients have been found to have subnormal IgM levels. The spleen is a major site of production for the opsonins properdin and tuftsin, and splenectomy results in decreased serum levels of these proteins. Schistocytes are pathologic and indicate either disseminated intravascular coagulation or traumatic hemolytic anemia (such as TTP)

16. A. Abscesses of the spleen are uncommon. Five distinct mechanisms of splenic abscess formation have been described: (1) hematogenous infection (70%), (2) contiguous infection, (3) hemoglobinopathy, (4) immunosuppression including human immunodeficiency virus and chemotherapy, and (5) trauma. The most common origins for hematogenous spread are infective endocarditis, typhoid fever, malaria, urinary tract infections, and osteomyelitis. Presentation is frequently delayed. Clinical manifestations include fever, left upper quadrant pain, leukocytosis, and splenomegaly. The diagnosis is confirmed by ultrasonography or CT. Upon discovery, broad-spectrum antibiotics should be started, with adjustment to more specific therapy based on culture results and continued for 14 days. If the abscess is unilocular, it can be managed with CT-guided aspiration. If it is multilocular, a splenectomy will usually be required.

Reference: Smyrniotis V, Kehagias D, Voros D, et al: Splenic abscess: an old disease with new interest, *Dig Surg* 17:354–357, 2000.

17. B. This patient most likely has portal vein thrombosis (PVT). It should be suspected in patients with fever and abdominal pain after splenectomy. This patient is predisposed to PVT formation because of her hypercoagulability from a combination of thrombocytosis after splenectomy and the setting of a myeloproliferative disorder. PVT is uncommon (occurrence rate ranging from 2% to 8%) although not rare, and the greatest risk is in cases involving splenomegaly with a myeloproliferative disorder. Postsplenectomy PVT typically presents with anorexia, abdominal pain, leukocytosis, and thrombocytosis, as demonstrated in this patient. A high index of suspicion, early diagnosis with contrast-enhanced CT, and immediate anticoagulation are keys to successful treatment of PVT. Patients undergoing splenectomy should be treated with deep venous thrombosis prophylaxis, including pneumatic compression devices, and with subcutaneous or low-molecular-weight heparin.

References: van't Riet M, Burger J, van Muiswinkel J: Diagnosis and treatment of portal vein thrombosis following splenectomy, *Br J Surg* 87:1229–1233, 2000.

Winslow E, Brunt L, Drebin J, Soper N: Portal vein thrombosis after splenectomy: discussion, *Am J Surg* 184:631–636, 2002.

18. A. Most therapies for hairy cell leukemia begin with Leustatin (cladribine). Nipent (pentostatin) is the next most commonly used. If these are not effective, interferon-alfa and rituximab are used. Splenectomy is used rarely and is more likely used for pain or early satiety or if cell counts fail to increase.

19. C. *S. pneumoniae* accounts for 50% to 90% of cases of postsplenectomy sepsis, followed by *H. influenzae* type B, meningococcus, and group A streptococcus. Splenectomized patients are also more susceptible to protozoan infections that invade the blood cell, in particular, malaria and *B. microti* infections. The risk of overwhelming postsplenectomy sepsis is higher for hematologic indications than for trauma, higher in children than in adults, greater in immunocompromised patients, and highest in the first 2 years after splenectomy.

20. C. The most common indication for splenectomy is trauma to the spleen, whether iatrogenic or accidental. In the past, staging for Hodgkin disease was the most common indication for elective splenectomy. ITP is now the most frequent indication for splenectomy in the elective setting, followed by HS, autoimmune hemolytic anemia, and TTP.

21. D. The laparoscopic approach typically results in longer operative times, shorter hospital stays, and lower morbidity rates. It has similar blood loss and mortality rates compared with open splenectomy. Cost analysis reveals that higher operating room charges are seen with laparoscopic splenectomy. However, several studies have found that the total cost to the patient is less with the laparoscopic procedure due to the shortened hospital stay. The laparoscopic approach has emerged as the standard for nontraumatic, elective splenectomy.

References: Beauchamp RD, Holzman MD, Fabian TC, Weinberg JA: The spleen. In Townsend CM Jr, Beauchamp RD, Evers BM, Mattox KL, editors: *Sabiston textbook of surgery: the biological basis of modern surgical practice*, ed 18, Philadelphia, 2008, WB Saunders, pp 1624–1652.

Parks AE, Godinez CD: Spleen. Brunicardi FC, Andersen DK, Billiar TR, et al, editors: *Schwartz's principles of surgery*, ed 9, New York, 2010, McGraw-Hill, pp 1245–1265.

Stomach 23

1. The most important etiologic factor in peptic ulcer disease is:

   A. Duodenogastric reflux
   B. Acid hypersecretion
   C. Nonsteroidal anti-inflammatory drug ingestion
   D. *Helicobacter pylori* infection
   E. Smoking

2. The most common gastric polyp is:

   A. Adenomatous
   B. Hyperplastic
   C. Hamartomatous
   D. Inflammatory
   E. Heterotopic

3. Bleeding from a Dieulafoy gastric lesion is due to:

   A. Antral vascular ectasia
   B. Abnormal gastric rugal folds
   C. Ingested foreign material
   D. An abnormal submucosal vessel
   E. A premalignant lesion

4. The treatment for low-grade early mucosa-associated lymphoid tissue (MALT) lymphoma is:

   A. Cytotoxic multidrug chemotherapy
   B. Radiation therapy
   C. Gastrectomy
   D. Antibiotics
   E. Combined chemoradiation therapy

5. The most sensitive and specific diagnostic test for gastrinoma is:

   A. Basal and stimulated gastric acid outputs
   B. Octreotide scan
   C. Fasting serum gastrin
   D. Calcium stimulation test
   E. Secretin stimulation test

6. Which of the following is the procedure of choice for an intractable duodenal ulcer that fails to heal despite maximal medical therapy?

   A. Truncal vagotomy and pyloroplasty
   B. Truncal vagotomy and antrectomy with Billroth I reconstruction
   C. Truncal vagotomy and antrectomy with Billroth II reconstruction
   D. Highly selective vagotomy (HSV)
   E. Distal gastrectomy

7. Which of the following is true regarding the types of gastric ulcers?

   A. Type II ulcers are the most common.
   B. Type IV ulcers occur near the gastroesophageal junction.
   C. Type I ulcers usually have increased acid secretion.
   D. Type III ulcers are associated with decreased acid secretion.
   E. Type I gastric ulcers are prepyloric.

8. Which of the following is the procedure of choice for an intractable type I gastric ulcer that fails to heal despite maximal medical therapy?

   A. Truncal vagotomy and antrectomy with Billroth I reconstruction
   B. Truncal vagotomy and antrectomy with Billroth II reconstruction
   C. HSV
   D. Distal gastrectomy with Billroth I reconstruction
   E. Distal gastrectomy with Billroth II reconstruction

9. A 68-year-old woman presents with an upper gastrointestinal (GI) hemorrhage. She has a history of ulcer disease. Upper endoscopy reveals brisk arterial bleeding from a duodenal ulcer located on the posterior wall. Despite numerous attempts to control the bleeding endoscopically, the ulcer continues to bleed. The patient has received four units of blood. Her hematocrit is 25%, her blood pressure is 110/60 mm Hg, and her heart rate is 120 beats per minute. Which of the following is the best management option?

   A. Duodenotomy, oversewing the ulcer, truncal vagotomy, and pyloroplasty
   B. Duodenotomy and oversewing the ulcer
   C. Truncal vagotomy and antrectomy with Billroth I reconstruction
   D. Truncal vagotomy and antrectomy with Billroth II reconstruction
   E. HSV

10. A 60-year-old man presents with a 12-hour history of severe epigastric pain that is now diffuse. He has a history of duodenal ulcer, and the results of a recent biopsy 2 weeks earlier were negative for *H. pylori*. Physical examination reveals an acute abdomen with diffuse tenderness and guarding. Upright chest radiograph demonstrates free air under the diaphragm. The patient is hemodynamically stable. At surgery, a perforated duodenal ulcer is found with mild peritoneal contamination. Which of the following is the best management option?

    A. Graham patch of duodenal ulcer
    B. Graham patch of duodenal ulcer with truncal vagotomy and pyloroplasty
    C. Truncal vagotomy and antrectomy with Billroth I reconstruction
    D. Truncal vagotomy and antrectomy with Billroth II reconstruction
    E. Graham patch of duodenal ulcer with an HSV

11. Which of the following is the most effective treatment for intractable dumping syndrome?

    A. Low-fat, lactose-free diet
    B. Serotonin antagonists
    C. Low-carbohydrate, high-fat diet
    D. Octreotide
    E. Creation of a reversed jejunal segment

12. Which of the following is true regarding postvagotomy diarrhea?

    A. It is effectively treated with octreotide.
    B. It is improved with oral cholestyramine.
    C. It is due to dumping syndrome.
    D. It is best managed by creating a reversed jejunal segment.
    E. It does not respond to dietary interventions.

13. A 45-year-old woman is undergoing an exploratory laparotomy for Zollinger-Ellison syndrome (ZES). Preoperative localization studies failed to demonstrate the location of the tumor. At surgery, no obvious tumor is seen despite an extensive Kocher maneuver and careful inspection and palpation. An intraoperative ultrasound scan is negative. The next step in the management would be:

    A. Closing the abdomen
    B. Distal pancreatectomy and splenectomy
    C. Proximal pancreaticoduodenectomy
    D. Blind proximal duodenotomy
    E. Blind distal duodenotomy

14. The most accurate means of determining T and N staging of gastric adenocarcinoma is:

    A. Triple-phase helical computed tomography (CT) scan
    B. Diagnostic laparoscopy
    C. Endoscopic ultrasonography
    D. Magnetic resonance imaging with gadolinium
    E. Positron emission tomography scan

15. The N staging of gastric adenocarcinoma is based on the:

    A. Number of positive nodes
    B. Anatomic distribution of positive nodes
    C. Proximity of positive nodes to the primary tumor
    D. Immunohistochemical staining of positive nodes
    E. Size of the largest positive node

16. The term that best describes residual postoperative microscopic disease after gastrectomy is:

    A. D1 resection
    B. D2 resection
    C. R0 resection
    D. R1 resection
    E. R2 resection

17. All of the following are risk factors for gastric cancer EXCEPT:

    A. *H. pylori* infection
    B. Blood group O
    C. Achlorhydria
    D. Li-Fraumeni syndrome
    E. Ingestion of nitrates

18. Early gastric cancer is best defined as:

    A. Lymph node negative
    B. Limited to the mucosa
    C. Limited to the mucosa and submucosa with negative nodes
    D. Limited to the mucosa and submucosa regardless of nodes
    E. In the muscularis propria but not the serosa

19. The treatment of choice for high-grade primary gastric lymphoma is:

    A. Radiation therapy
    B. Total gastrectomy
    C. Subtotal gastrectomy
    D. Chemotherapy and radiation
    E. Total gastrectomy followed by chemotherapy

20. A 56-year-old man presents with epigastric pain, diarrhea, and weight loss. Upper endoscopy reveals giant gastric folds in the proximal stomach. A biopsy specimen demonstrates diffuse foveolar hyperplasia with no evidence of malignancy. Twenty-four-hour gastric pH levels are consistent with achlorhydria. All of the following are true about this condition EXCEPT:

    A. It is associated with hypoproteinemia.
    B. It has a familial inheritance.
    C. It is associated with cytomegalovirus infection in children.
    D. It increases the risk of malignancy.
    E. It is associated with *H. pylori* in adults.

21. Which of the following is true regarding postgastrectomy bile reflux?

    A. Most patients with bile reflux into the stomach will develop symptoms.
    B. Symptoms usually correlate with the amount of bile entering the stomach.
    C. In symptomatic patients, medical management is generally effective.
    D. Creation of a Roux-en-Y gastrojejunostomy is an effective surgical option.
    E. It is more likely to occur after a Billroth I than a Billroth II reconstruction.

22. The best test for localization of a gastrinoma is:

    A. Magnetic resonance imaging
    B. CT
    C. Ultrasonography
    D. Octreotide scan
    E. Selective angiography

23. The best test to confirm eradication of *H. pylori* after treatment is:

    A. *H. pylori* serology
    B. Urea breath test
    C. Histologic biopsy
    D. Rapid urease test
    E. Antral mucosal biopsy with culture

24. Which of the following is true regarding an HSV?

    A. The anterior and posterior vagal trunks are divided.
    B. The nerve of Grassi is spared.
    C. The anterior Latarjet nerve is divided.
    D. The crow's feet to the antrum are spared.
    E. The celiac branch is divided.

25. The most common metabolic disorder after gastric resection is a deficiency of:

    A. Iron
    B. Vitamin B_{12}
    C. Folate
    D. Calcium
    E. Vitamin D

26. All of the following are true regarding ZES EXCEPT:

    A. It is associated with a secretory diarrhea.
    B. Ulcers are most often located in the proximal duodenum.
    C. It is most commonly familial.
    D. It is the most common functional neuroendocrine tumor in multiple endocrine neoplasia type 1.
    E. Treatment with proton pump inhibitors can control symptoms in the majority of patients.

27. A 70-year-old man presents with an 8-hour history of acute abdominal pain. On examination, the patient is febrile to 101°F, with a blood pressure of 105/70 mm Hg and a heart rate of 130 beats per minute, and has diffuse abdominal tenderness with rebound and guarding; the rectal examination is guaiac positive. Laboratory values are significant for a white blood cell count of 16,000 μ/L and a hematocrit of 26%. CT demonstrates extravasation of oral contrast in the proximal duodenum. After resuscitation, management consists of:

    A. Closure of the perforation and omental patch plus an HSV
    B. Closure of the perforation and omental patch via the open approach
    C. Closure of the perforation and omental patch, vagotomy, duodenotomy with oversewing of posterior ulcer, and pyloroplasty
    D. Vagotomy and antrectomy with oversewing of the posterior ulcer and omental patch
    E. Closure of the perforation and omental patch via laparoscopic approach

28. A 50-year-old woman presents with symptoms of early satiety, nausea, vomiting, and epigastric pain. Upper endoscopy reveals a large mass of undigested food particles in the stomach that is partially obstructing the pylorus. All of the following are true regarding this condition EXCEPT:

   A. It can be treated with oral administration of meat tenderizer.

   B. It can be treated with oral administration of cellulose.

   C. Psychiatric treatment is critical in long-term management.

   D. It is more common in patients with previous gastric surgery.

   E. Diabetes is a risk factor.

29. Which of the following is true regarding surgical resection for gastric adenocarcinoma?

   A. For cardia cancers, proximal gastric resection is preferable to total gastrectomy.

   B. Splenectomy should be performed to attain adequate lymph node sampling.

   C. Proximal and distal resection margins of 3 cm are considered adequate.

   D. D2 resections provide improved survival with morbidity similar to that with D1 resections.

   E. Total gastrectomy is an acceptable option for palliation in stage IV disease.

30. A 70-year-old man presents to the emergency department with sudden onset of severe epigastric pain associated with retching but with little vomitus. His blood pressure is 140/90 mm Hg and his heart rate is 90 beats per minute. Attempts by the emergency department physician to place a nasogastric tube are unsuccessful. Upright chest radiograph reveals a large gas bubble just above the left diaphragm. All of the following are true regarding this condition EXCEPT:

   A. Mesenteroaxial torsion is more common than organoaxial.

   B. It can lead to gastric necrosis.

   C. It is associated with the Borchardt triad.

   D. It is associated with a wandering spleen.

   E. It can occur without diaphragmatic defects.

31. Which of the following describes the association between Sister Mary Joseph's nodule and gastric cancer?

   A. A metastatic left axillary lymph node

   B. A metastatic left supraclavicular lymph node

   C. An ovarian mass from gastric metastasis

   D. Umbilical metastasis suggesting carcinomatosis

   E. An anterior nodule palpable on rectal examination suggesting drop metastasis

32. All of the following are associated with hypergastrinemia EXCEPT:

   A. Retained gastric antrum

   B. Hypothyroidism

   C. Pernicious anemia

   D. Renal insufficiency

   E. G-cell hyperplasia

33. Which of the following is true regarding gastric stromal tumors?

   A. They rarely present with GI bleeding.

   B. They arise from smooth muscle cells.

   C. Malignant potential is readily determined by histologic features.

   D. They can be managed by laparoscopic wedge resection.

   E. The extent of the tumor is best determined preoperatively by endoscopy.

Answers

1. D. *H. pylori* is considered the most important etiologic factor in peptic ulcer disease. It is reportedly found in 80% to 90% of duodenal ulcers and more than 70% of gastric ulcers. *H. pylori* is a helix-shaped, microaerophilic gram-negative rod with four to six flagella. It is more prevalent in developing countries, where as many as 70% of the population harbor the infection. *H. pylori* also causes acute gastritis. The exact mechanism by which it causes ulceration is unclear, but it may be by the production of local toxic products, induction of a local immune response, or an increase in gastrin levels leading to an increase in acid. In fact, the organism seems to be the cause of hypergastrinemia in duodenal ulcers because the infection reduces the number of antral D cells, thus reducing somatostatin levels, which then disinhibits G (gastrin) cells. *H. pylori* is a potent producer of urease, which splits urea into ammonia and bicarbonate. This allows the bacteria to survive in a microenvironment of relative alkalinity within the stomach. It only lives in gastric epithelium (including heterotopic gastric mucosa) because it expresses specific adherence receptors recognized by the bacteria. After *H. pylori*, ingestion of nonsteroidal anti-inflammatory drugs and smoking are the next most important risk factors. Smoking increases gastric acid secretion and duodenogastric reflux and decreases pancreaticoduodenal bicarbonate production.

Reference: Kurata JH, Nogawa AN: Meta-analysis of risk factors for peptic ulcer. Nonsteroidal anti-inflammatory drugs, *Helicobacter pylori*, and smoking, *J Clin Gastroenterol* 24:2–17, 1997.

2. B. Hyperplastic polyps are by far the most common gastric polyps (70%–90%) Other types include adenomatous, hamartomatous, inflammatory, and heterotopic. Hyperplastic polyps are seen in association with chronic atrophic gastritis, which is due to *H. pylori* infection. Hyperplastic polyps are further classified into polypoid foveolar hyperplasia and typical hyperplastic polyps. Polypoid foveolar hyperplasia does not seem to have malignant potential, whereas the typical hyperplastic polyp has an approximately 2% chance of developing malignancy. Adenomatous polyps have the highest risk of malignancy (10%–20%), and the risk of malignancy seems to be related to size and histology (greater risk for villous than tubular). Hamartomatous, inflammatory, and heterotopic polyps do not seem to have a risk of malignancy. Heterotopic polyps are usually the result of ectopic pancreatic tissue. Treatment for most polyps is simply endoscopic polypectomy. Additional surgical resection is recommended for polyps that are sessile and larger than 2 cm, those with areas of invasive tumor, and those that cause symptoms (bleeding or pain).

Reference: Orlowska J, Jarosz D, Pachlewski J, Butruk E: Malignant transformation of benign epithelial gastric polyps, *Am J Gastroenterol* 90:2152–2159, 1995.

3. D. A Dieulafoy lesion is a congenital malformation in the stomach characterized by a submucosal artery that is abnormally large and tortuous. As a result of its relatively superficial location, it may erode through the mucosa and become exposed to gastric juice, leading to massive upper GI hemorrhage. On endoscopy, the mucosa of the stomach appears normal, and the only finding is a pinpoint area of mucosal defect with brisk arterial bleeding. The lesion may easily be missed if the bleeding is not active. Treatment is endoscopic, via electrocautery, heater probe, or injection with a sclerosing agent. Surgery, which consists of a wedge resection, is reserved for the rare patient that is not controlled endoscopically. Antral vascular ectasia is seen in a condition known as watermelon stomach. Dilated mucosal blood vessels containing thrombus, mucosal fibromuscular dysplasia, and hyalinization are prominent features. It

derives its name from the mucosal vessels that create parallel lines in the mucosal folds. It is seen predominantly in elderly women with autoimmune disease. A Dieulafoy lesion is not premalignant and is not associated with the ingestion of foreign material.

4. D. Low-grade MALT lymphoma develops in association with *H. pylori* infection. The infection induces a lymphoid infiltrate. B cells proliferate as a result of the immunogenic stimulation. The infection also results in the release of toxic oxygen-free radicals by neutrophils. It is thought that these free radicals may trigger a malignant transformation of the B cells. Initial treatment of MALT lymphoma is with antibiotics targeted toward *H. pylori*. Remission was achieved with antibiotics alone in 79% in one study. For patients who do not respond to antibiotics, current recommendations are to proceed to standard lymphoma chemotherapy using CHOP (cyclophosphamide, doxorubicin, vincristine, and prednisone). Factors that predict whether regression will occur with antibiotics include depth of invasion by endoscopic ultrasonography (beyond the mucosa), high-grade lesions, spread beyond the initial location, and the presence of nodal involvement. The overall 5-year survival rate approaches 80%. Antibiotic treatment for *H. pylori* includes a combination of antibiotics (either clarithromycin and amoxicillin, metronidazole and amoxicillin, or metronidazole and tetracycline).

References: Du M, Isaccson P: Gastric MALT lymphoma: from aetiology to treatment, *Lancet Oncol* 3:97–104, 2002.

Nakamura S, Matsumoto T, Suekane H, et al: Predictive value of endoscopic ultrasonography for regression of gastric low grade and high grade MALT lymphomas after eradication of *Helicobacter pylori*, *Gut* 48:454–460, 2001.

Ruskoné-Fourmestraux A, Lavergne A, Aegerter P, et al: Predictive factors for regression of gastric MALT lymphoma after anti-*Helicobacter pylori* treatment, *Gut* 48:297–303, 2001.

5. E. The most sensitive and specific test for gastrinoma (ZES) is the secretin stimulation test. An IV bolus of secretin is administered, and gastrin levels are checked before and after injection. An increase in serum gastrin of 120 pg/mL or greater has the highest sensitivity and specificity for gastrinoma. There are numerous other causes of hypergastrinemia. They can be divided into those associated with an increased acid production and those with a decreased acid production. In the latter situation, the hypergastrinemia is reactive due to hypo- or achlorhydria. In addition to ZES, G-cell hyperplasia, gastric outlet obstruction, and retained antrum after Billroth II reconstruction are associated with increased acid production. Reactive hypergastrinemia is seen with atrophic gastritis, pernicious anemia, and gastric cancer; in patients receiving H_2-receptor antagonists and proton pump inhibitors; and after vagotomy. Hypergastrinemia is also seen in chronic renal failure due to decreased catabolism. Given this broad differential, fasting serum gastrin levels are not sufficiently specific to establish the diagnosis of ZES in the majority of patients unless gastrin levels are extremely high (>1000 pg/mL). The secretin stimulation test has higher sensitivity and specificity than the calcium stimulation test. The calcium stimulation test is used if the secretin test result is negative and there is a high suspicion for ZES in the presence of hypergastrinemia. Once the diagnosis of ZES is established, a nuclear octreotide scan seems to be the most sensitive test to localize the tumor.

Reference: Berna M, Hoffmann K, Long S, et al: Serum gastrin in Zollinger-Ellison syndrome: II. Prospective study of gastrin provocative testing in 293 patients from the National Institutes of Health and comparison with 537 cases from the literature: evaluation of diagnostic criteria, proposal of new criteria, and correlations with clinical and tumoral features, *Medicine (Baltimore)* 85:331–364, 2006.

6. D. An HSV is the procedure of choice for intractable duodenal ulcer in which medical management fails. In the current era of *H. pylori* treatment, surgery for intractable duodenal ulceration is rare. There are three main surgical options: HSV, vagotomy and pyloroplasty, and vagotomy and antrectomy. Vagotomy and antrectomy has the overall lowest rate of ulcer recurrence (<2%). However, because it involves a gastric resection, it has the highest complication rate. The procedure also predisposes the patient to both postvagotomy syndromes and postgastrectomy syndromes. As such, it is the least favored option in this setting. Vagotomy and pyloroplasty has a higher ulcer recurrence rate than vagotomy and antrectomy but less morbidity. An HSV has the highest ulcer recurrence rate (~10%–15%), but the lowest morbidity rate. It requires more time and skill, so it is not an optimal choice in an emergent setting. It also has the advantage that it can be performed laparoscopically. Distal gastrectomy is not an option for duodenal ulcer because it does not reduce acid secretion.

7. B. Gastric ulcers have been categorized into four types. The most common is the type I lesion (~60%), which is located near the angularis incisura at the border between the antrum and the fundus, usually along the lesser curve. These patients usually have normal or decreased acid secretion. Type II gastric ulcers are located in the fundus and are associated with a concomitant duodenal ulcer. Type III gastric ulcers are prepyloric. Both types II and III gastric ulcers are usually associated with increased gastric acid secretion. Type III ulcers are thought to behave like duodenal ulcers. Type IV gastric ulcers are located near the gastroesophageal junction, and acid secretion is normal or below normal. Like type I ulcers, type IV gastric ulcers have normal or low acid production and are associated with impaired mucosal defense.

8. D. With gastric ulcers, one must always be concerned about the risk of malignancy. As such, biopsies should be performed at the time of endoscopy. If they do not heal despite maximal medical therapy, surgical management should include excision of the ulcer. This is achieved via a distal antrectomy. The extent of resection is determined by the ulcer location. Frozen sections should be obtained to rule out malignancy. Because acid hypersecretion is not an issue with type I ulcers, vagotomy is considered unnecessary. Reconstruction can be achieved with a gastroduodenostomy (Billroth I) or a gastrojejunostomy (Billroth II). In general, a Billroth I is preferred because it is more anatomic and thus avoids the complications of a Billroth II

such as a duodenal stump leak, a retained antrum, and afferent loop obstruction. If the duodenal remnant is severely scarred from ulcer disease, a Billroth I may not be feasible. Another option for a type I ulcer would be to excise the gastric ulcer using a wedge excision in combination with an HSV, but an HSV alone would be inadequate. For type II or III ulcers, vagotomy would be added because these ulcers are associated with acid hypersecretion.

9. A. Bleeding from duodenal ulcers can be controlled endoscopically in the majority of patients, and, thus, surgery is rarely indicated. Predictors of failure of endoscopic management include the presence of shock or a large ulcer (<2 cm). When bleeding has been controlled endoscopically and then recurs, endoscopic treatment can again be attempted with a high rate of success, thus avoiding surgery. The bleeding is usually from a posterior ulcer that has eroded into the gastroduodenal artery. Surgical management decisions should be based on the hemodynamic stability of the patient, the patient's overall medical condition, and whether the patient has a history of ulcer disease that has been treated for *H. pylori*. In the patient who is actively bleeding, the duodenum should be opened across the pylorus as is used in a pyloroplasty. The ulcer bed should be oversewn with multiple figure of eight sutures. If the patient has a history of ulcers that have been treated for *H. pylori* and is stable in the operating room, an ulcer operation should be performed. The best option in this type of emergent setting is to perform a truncal vagotomy and to close the longitudinal duodenotomy in a transverse fashion as with a pyloroplasty. If the patient is a high surgical risk and unstable, another option would be to simply perform a smaller duodenotomy, oversew the ulcer, simply close the duodenotomy, and treat postoperatively for *H. pylori*. Although vagotomy and antrectomy is another option, it would seldom be used in the emergent setting due to the higher associated morbidity rate. An HSV would not address the actively bleeding ulcer.

References: Brullet E, Calvet X, Campo R, et al: Factors predicting failure of endoscopic injection therapy in bleeding duodenal ulcer, *Gastrointest Endosc* 43:111–116, 1996.

Lau J, Sung J, Lam Y, et al: Endoscopic retreatment compared with surgery in patients with recurrent bleeding after initial endoscopic control of bleeding ulcers, *N Engl J Med* 340:751–756, 1999.

10. E. In the majority of patients with a perforated duodenal ulcer, simple closure of the ulcer with an omental (Graham) patch is all that is necessary. This is then followed by treatment for *H. pylori*. In addition, a Graham patch alone should be used if the patient is unstable, if there is extensive exudative peritonitis, or if the perforation is long-standing (>24 hours). However, in the setting of a patient with a known ulcer diathesis who has either already been treated for *H. pylori* or is *H. pylori* negative, an ulcer surgery should be added to the operation, provided the patient is a good operative risk, is hemodynamically stable, and does not have extensive peritonitis. The options are either to perform an HSV or a vagotomy and pyloroplasty. An HSV is the preferred approach in the good-risk patient who is stable, provided the surgeon is comfortable with the procedure. The entire procedure can be performed laparoscopically in select patients. Truncal vagotomy and antrectomy is generally not recommended in the setting of perforation because of the high associated morbidity and mortality rates.

References: Cadiere GB, Bruyns J, Himpens J, et al: Laparoscopic highly selective vagotomy, *Hepatogastroenterology* 46:1500–1506, 1999.

Jordan PH Jr, Thornby J: Perforated pyloroduodenal ulcers: long-term results with omental patch closure and parietal cell vagotomy, *Ann Surg* 221:479–486, discussion 486–488, 1995.

Siu WT, Leong HT, Law BK, et al: Laparoscopic repair for perforated peptic ulcer: a randomized controlled trial, *Ann Surg* 235:313–319, 2002.

11. D. Dumping syndrome can occur after any type of gastric surgery and is divided into early and late forms. Early dumping (20–30 minutes after eating) is more common and has both GI (nausea, vomiting, crampy abdominal pain, and explosive diarrhea) and cardiovascular (diaphoresis, dizziness, flushing) symptoms. The symptoms are related to the release of various substances including serotonin, neurotensin, bradykinins, and enteroglucagon. Late dumping (2–3 hours after eating) is the result of a reaction to a large amount of carbohydrates suddenly reaching the small intestine. This leads to a sudden release of large amounts of insulin with subsequent hypoglycemia with resultant diaphoresis, confusion, and tachycardia. The initial therapy for dumping syndrome consists of dietary modification. This includes eating frequent small meals, avoiding large amounts of carbohydrates and instead eating food high in protein and fat, and avoiding large amounts of fluids with meals. Octreotide, a long-acting somatostatin analogue, is the most effective treatment. It is effective against both the GI and cardiovascular symptoms. Long-term use of octreotide is associated with steatorrhea and cholelithiasis. Serotonin antagonists have been used for dumping syndrome but have not been routinely effective.

References: Geer RJ, Richards WO, O'Dorisio TM, et al: Efficacy of octreotide acetate in treatment of severe postgastrectomy dumping syndrome, *Ann Surg* 212:678–687, 1990.

Gray JL, Debas HT, Mulvihill SJ: Control of dumping symptoms by somatostatin analogue in patients after gastric surgery, *Arch Surg* 126:1231–1235, discussion 1235–1236, 1991.

12. B. Postvagotomy syndromes include diarrhea, gastric atony, and incomplete vagotomy (leading to recurrent ulceration). Diarrhea follows truncal vagotomy and may be confused with dumping syndrome. The diarrhea associated with vagotomy is not associated with the other cardiovascular manifestations seen with dumping syndrome. The initial treatment is similar to that for dumping syndrome, with dietary modifications such as frequent small meals with decreased fluid intake and an increase in fiber. A proposed mechanism of the diarrhea is an increase in stool bile salts. Oral cholestyramine is often helpful because it binds bile salts. In the very rare patient who does not respond to medical management, reversal of a segment of jejunum is effective in slowing transit time and improving diarrhea. Octreotide is not effective for postvagotomy diarrhea and may make the situation worse by decreasing pancreatic secretions and thus increasing steatorrhea.

Reference: Duncombe V, Bolin T, Davis A: Double-blind trial of cholestyramine in post-vagotomy diarrhea, *Gut* 18:531–535, 1977.

13. D. More than 80% of gastrinomas are localized preoperatively. For those that cannot be localized, surgical exploration is still indicated because excision of the primary tumor leads to a decreased rate of liver metastasis. When exploring, it is important to be aware that 80% of gastrinomas are found within the gastrinoma triangle, which is an area that includes the first, second, and third portions of the duodenum and the pancreatic head. As many as 60% of gastrinomas are within the wall of the duodenum, primarily in the first and second portions and can be very small. Thus, the next maneuver would be to perform a blind proximal duodenotomy to manually palpate the duodenal wall for tumors. Blind distal pancreatectomy or distal duodenotomy would have very low yields. A pancreaticoduodenectomy (Whipple procedure) would not be indicated in this setting. It is potentially indicated for multiple duodenal or proximal pancreatic head tumors that could not be enucleated.

14. C. Endoscopic ultrasonography is the best modality for assessing tumor depth of invasion and nodal status. It is approximately 80% accurate in determining whether the tumor is transmural (invading serosa, T_3) and 50% accurate in assessing whether pathologically enlarged lymph nodes are present. Endoscopic ultrasonography seems to be more accurate with advanced disease than early disease. CT scanning is the preferred method for determining distant metastases but not as useful for T and N staging. Diagnostic laparoscopy adds additional yield to CT as far as determining distant metastases that preclude curative resection. The routine use of magnetic resonance imaging and positron emission tomography scanning for staging of gastric cancer has not as yet been established.

References: Puli S, Batapati Krishna Reddy J, Bechtold ML, et al: How good is endoscopic ultrasound for TNM staging of gastric cancers? A meta-analysis and systematic review, *World J Gastroenterol* 14:4011–4019, 2008.

Willis S, Truong S, Gribnitz S, et al: Endoscopic ultrasonography in the preoperative staging of gastric cancer: accuracy and impact on surgical therapy, *Surg Endosc* 14:951–954, 2000.

Xi W, Zhao C, Ren G: Endoscopic ultrasonography in preoperative staging of gastric cancer: determination of tumor invasion depth, nodal involvement and surgical respectability, *World J Gastroenterol* 9:254–257, 2003.

15. A. Staging of gastric cancer involves depth of invasion (T1 invades lamina propria; T2, muscularis propria or subserosa; T3, serosa; T4, adjacent structures) and nodes. N1 disease includes 1 to 6 regional nodes; N2, 7 to 15 regional nodes; N3, more than 15 regional nodes.

16. D. R0 resection is resection of all gross and microscopic tumor. R1 indicates removal of all macroscopic disease but microscopic margins are positive for disease. An R2 resection indicates that gross residual disease is left behind. A D1 resection refers to removal of group 1 lymph nodes; D2 refers to resection of lymph nodes in groups 1 and 2. A D3 resection is a D2 resection plus removal of para-aortic lymph nodes.

17. B. Risk factors for gastric cancer include dietary factors such as a large consumption of smoked meats, pickled foods, high nitrates, and high salt, whereas a diet high in fruits and vegetables may be protective. Other risk factors include smoking, *H. pylori* infection, chronic atrophic gastritis, blood type A, previous partial gastrectomy, achlorhydria, pernicious anemia, polyps (adenomatous and hyperplastic), and certain familial syndromes such as hereditary nonpolyposis colorectal cancer, Li-Fraumeni syndrome, familial adenomatous polyposis, and Peutz-Jeghers syndrome. Peutz-Jeghers syndrome is associated with a markedly increased risk of cancer in the esophagus, stomach, small bowel, colon, pancreas, breast, lung, uterus, and ovary, with a cumulative 93% risk of cancer. Gastric cancer has been categorized by Lauren into intestinal and diffuse types based on histology. The intestinal type is thought to be more related to environmental factors, is associated with chronic gastritis, and is well differentiated. The diffuse type is usually poorly differentiated and associated with signet rings, and occurs in younger patients and in association with familial disorders and also with type A blood. The diffuse type has a worse prognosis.

Reference: Giardiello F, Brensinger J, Tersmette A, et al: Very high risk of cancer in familial Peutz-Jeghers syndrome, *Gastroenterology* 119:1447–1453, 2000.

18. D. Early gastric cancers are defined as adenocarcinoma limited to the mucosa and submucosa of the stomach, regardless of lymph node status. In Japan, because of the high prevalence of gastric cancer, aggressive screening programs are used. This has resulted in as many as one half of gastric cancers being detected early, whereas in the United States, less than one fourth are considered early gastric cancer. In one large series of nearly 400 patients with early gastric cancer, 11.9% had positive lymph nodes. Risk factors for lymph node metastasis included large tumor size, lymphatic vessel involvement, and invasion of the submucosa. Lymph node status was the most important determinant of survival.

References: Adachi Y, Shiraishi N, Kitano S: Modern treatment of early gastric cancer: review of the Japanese experience, *Dig Surg* 19:333–339, 2002.

Maehara Y, Orita H, Okuyama T, et al: Predictors of lymph node metastasis in early gastric cancer, *Br J Surg* 79:245–247, 1992.

19. D. Gastric lymphomas were previously treated with surgery because there was concern that chemotherapy would lead to gastric perforation. The risk of perforation now seems to be low (5%), and, therefore, there has been a transition away from surgery. Gastric lymphomas can be divided into low grade and high grade, with or without MALT. Approximately 40% are low grade, and the majority of low-grade lymphomas are of the MALT type, which are treated first by *H. pylori* eradication. Approximately 60% are high grade, with or without MALT. The current recommendation is to treat high-grade lymphomas with chemotherapy and radiation. Surgery is limited to those with residual disease after chemotherapy/radiation (provided the disease is localized) or if a complication develops from these treatments.

Reference: Yoon S, Coit D, Portlock C, Karpeh M: The diminishing role of surgery in the treatment of gastric lymphoma, *Ann Surg* 240:28–37, 2004.

20. B. The patient has Ménétrier disease. Ménétrier disease is an acquired disease with no family predisposition. The etiology is unknown, but it is associated with an increase in transforming growth factor α. Giant rugal folds, particularly in the fundus and body, and a loss of parietal cells develop. Thus, patients have hypo- or achlorhydria. Patients lose a large amount of protein in the stomach due to the hypersecretion of mucus. This results in weight loss and peripheral edema. Giant rugal folds are also seen with ZES; however, the latter can be ruled out by the demonstration of achlorhydria. Mucosal biopsy shows diffuse hyperplasia of the surface mucus-secreting cells as well as loss of parietal cells. There seems to be an increased risk of gastric cancer, although it is not high. It is associated with cytomegalovirus infection in children and with *H. pylori* infection in adults. Most patients with Ménétrier disease are middle-aged men. Symptoms include epigastric pain, weight loss, diarrhea, and hypoproteinemia. Treatment includes a high-protein diet, anticholinergic agents, and *H. pylori* eradication if the patient tests positive. Medical treatment has not been particularly effective, although there are cases of spontaneous resolution. For patients who do not respond to medical therapy, gastric resection may be indicated, particularly for intractable severe hypoproteinemia or if dysplasia or malignancy develops. Recently, Erbitux (cetuximab), which blocks the action of transforming growth factor α, has been used as a potential new treatment.

References: Bayerdörffer E, Ritter M, Hatz R, et al: Healing of protein losing hypertrophic gastropathy by eradication of *Helicobacter pylori*—is *Helicobacter pylori* a pathogenic factor in Ménétrier's disease? *Gut* 35:701–704, 1994.

Burdick J, Chung E, Tanner G, et al: Treatment of Ménétrier's disease with a monoclonal antibody against the epidermal growth factor receptor, *N Engl J Med* 343:1697–1701, 2000.

Hsu CT, Ito M, Kawase Y, et al: Early gastric cancer arising from localized Ménétrier's disease, *Gastroenterol Jpn* 26:213–217, 1991.

21. D. Bile reflux into the stomach can occur without previous surgery, but in most instances follows ablation of the pylorus, such as after gastric resection or pyloroplasty. After such procedures, most patients will have bile in the stomach on endoscopic examination, along with some degree of gross or microscopic gastric inflammation. However, only a small fraction of patients will have a significant degree of symptoms such as nausea, epigastric pain, and bilious vomiting consistent with alkaline (bile) reflux gastritis. Symptoms often develop months or years after the index operation. The differential diagnosis includes afferent or efferent loop obstruction, gastric stasis, and small bowel obstruction. These other diagnoses can be ruled out using a combination of abdominal radiographs, upper endoscopy, an abdominal CT scan. A hepatoiminodiacetic acid scan is particularly helpful for demonstrating bile reflux. Bile reflux and gastritis are more likely to occur after Billroth II reconstruction than after Billroth I and least likely after vagotomy and pyloroplasty. Medical management of symptomatic patients is not particularly effective. The surgical procedure of choice is to convert the Billroth II into a Roux-en-Y gastrojejunostomy with a lengthened jejunal limb (at least 45 cm).

22. D. More than 90% of gastrinomas have receptors for somatostatin. Octreotide scanning (somatostatin receptor scintigraphy) has been shown to be the most sensitive test for localization of gastrinomas. However, successful localization depends on size and location. Somatostatin receptor scintigraphy is poor for very small (<1.1 cm) tumors and for small primary duodenal tumors. Duodenal gastrinomas are best localized by endoscopic ultrasonography. Failure to detect the tumor preoperatively should not preempt surgical exploration because an additional 33% will be found at surgery.

Reference: Alexander H, Fraker D, Norton J, et al: Prospective study of somatostatin receptor scintigraphy and its effect on operative outcome in patients with Zollinger-Ellison syndrome, *Ann Surg* 228:228–238, 1998.

23. B. A urea breath test is the best way to confirm eradication of *H. pylori*. The test relies on the fact that the bacteria hydrolyzes urea. The patient is given radiolabeled urea to ingest orally. If *H. pylori* is present, the urea will be converted to ammonia and radiolabeled bicarbonate, which is then exhaled as carbon dioxide. The amount of exhaled carbon dioxide is quantified. Positive *H. pylori* serology provides evidence of current infection if the patient has never been treated for it, but will remain positive even after successful treatment; thus, it is not useful in this setting. Antral mucosa biopsy with histologic examination for the organism is the gold standard test. It is useful in the initial evaluation of patients with upper GI symptoms because it permits evaluation of the stomach via endoscopy at the time of biopsy. However, given its invasive nature and increased cost, it is not routinely recommended to confirm eradication. Cultures of the gastric mucosa are not routinely available at every laboratory, and a repeat endoscopy is required. The rapid urease test is ideally used if another endoscopy and biopsy are being performed. The study requires placing a sample of gastric mucosa in a urea solution and then using a pH indicator to demonstrate the production of ammonia.

24. D. An HSV is also known as a parietal cell vagotomy or proximal gastric vagotomy. The goal of the operation is to divide the vagal nerves of the proximal two thirds of the stomach where the parietal cells are located and preserve the distal third to maintain antral function and thus not require a drainage procedure (such as a pyloroplasty). This results in fewer complications than the classic truncal vagotomy. The operation spares the main anterior and posterior vagal trunks, but divides the branches of the anterior and posterior Latarjet nerves that directly innervate the proximal stomach. The distal 7 cm (approximately) of nerves, known as the crow's feet, are spared. Likewise, the celiac and hepatic branches are spared. Proximally, it is important to divide the nerve of Grassi, which is a branch off the posterior trunk of the vagus. It is often referred to as the criminal nerve of Grassi because failure to divide this branch leads to a higher ulcer recurrence rate. With the recognition of *H. pylori* as the main etiology of peptic ulcer, the role of surgery has greatly diminished. An HSV is still indicated in certain rare situations, such as patients who do not respond to medical management, patients who are bleeding who do not respond to endoscopic management, or with perforation in patients with a long-standing ulcer diathesis.

25. A. Gastric resection leads to numerous disturbances in metabolism. These include deficiencies of iron, vitamin B_{12}, folate, fat-soluble vitamins, and calcium. Of these, iron deficiency is the most common. Iron is absorbed in the duodenum and is facilitated by an acidic environment. After gastric resection, overall iron intake is decreased, and the reduced acidity impairs absorption. Reduction in the parietal cell mass from gastric resection leads to a decrease in intrinsic factor, which is necessary for the enteric absorption of vitamin B_{12}. This leads to a megaloblastic anemia. Furthermore, an acidic environment facilitates the bioavailability of vitamin B_{12}. Vitamin B_{12} deficiency usually only develops when at least one half of the stomach is resected. Fat malabsorption can occur after gastrectomy (particularly with a Billroth II reconstruction) because of inadequate mixing of food with bile and digestive enzymes. This leads to a decreased absorption of fat-soluble vitamins. Calcium is absorbed in the duodenum and small bowel and is also facilitated by an acid environment. Long-term deficiencies manifest as osteoporosis. Folate deficiency is rare.

26. C. ZES (gastrinoma) is caused by uncontrolled secretion of gastrin by a pancreatic or a duodenal neuroendocrine tumor. Most cases are sporadic, but 20% are inherited. The inherited or familial form of gastrinoma is associated with multiple endocrine neoplasia type 1. Gastrinoma is the most common functional neuroendocrine tumor in multiple endocrine neoplasia type 1. The most common symptoms are epigastric pain, gastroesophageal reflux, and diarrhea. The massive acid hypersecretion leads to a secretory diarrhea that persists even with fasting. The majority will have demonstrable peptic ulceration that is most commonly located in the proximal duodenum. Unlike typical ulcers, those associated with gastrinoma on occasion will be found in the distal duodenum or jejunum. Ulcers in these locations should raise suspicion for gastrinoma, as should recurrent or refractory peptic ulcers, ulcers in association with secretory diarrhea, finding gastric rugal hypertrophy or esophagitis-related stricture on endoscopy, bleeding or perforated ulcer, family history of ulcer, and ulcers in the setting of hypercalcemia or kidney stones. Proton pump inhibitors are highly effective in relieving the symptoms of ZES, although definitive treatment consists of localizing and resecting the tumor.

Reference: Meijer JL, Jansen JB, Lamers CB: Omeprazole in the treatment of Zollinger-Ellison syndrome and histamine H2-antagonist refractory ulcers, *Digestion* 44(Suppl 1):31–39, 1989.

27. C. The presentation of oral contrast extravasation in the proximal duodenum (or free air under the diaphragm) combined with anemia and guaiac-positive stool is highly suggestive of a "kissing" duodenal ulcer. This represents a rare combination of an anterior duodenal ulcer that perforates into the peritoneum and a posterior ulcer that erodes into the gastroduodenal artery and bleeds. The majority of perforated ulcers can be managed by simple ulcer closure with an omental (Graham) patch. This can be achieved via an open or laparoscopic approach. In this patient, one must rule out a bleeding posterior ulcer. This would best be achieved via an anterior duodenotomy across the pylorus. If a posterior ulcer is identified, it should be oversewn. A truncal vagotomy should be performed and the duodenotomy closed as a pyloroplasty.

References: Dasmahapatra KS, Suval W, Machiedo GW: Unsuspected perforation in bleeding duodenal ulcers, *Am Surg* 54:19–21, 1988.

Hunt PS, Clarke G: Perforation in patients with bleeding ulcer, *Aust N Z J Surg* 61:183–185, 1991.

Stabile BE, Hardy HJ, Passaro E Jr: "Kissing" duodenal ulcers, *Arch Surg* 114:1153–1156, 1979.

28. C. Bezoars are accumulations of undigestible material in the stomach. There are two types. Phytobezoars are composed of undigested vegetable matter. Risk factors for phytobezoars include previous gastric surgery and gastroparesis such as from diabetes. Bezoars produce obstructive symptoms, but can also cause ulceration and bleeding. Diagnosis is suggested by an upper GI series and confirmed by endoscopy. Treatment generally consists of a combination of enzymatic degradation, endoscopic disruption, irrigation, and removal. Enzyme therapy can be performed with papain (present in meat tenderizers) or with cellulase. However, the use of papain has been associated with hypernatremia, gastric ulceration, and esophageal perforation, so that cellulase is preferred. More recently, nasogastric Coca-Cola lavage has been successfully used. Trichobezoars are composed of hair. It occurs most commonly in girls and young women who swallow their hair (trichophagy). Interestingly, most have long hair, and many have an underlying psychiatric disorder, so psychiatric care is important in future prevention (unlike phytobezoars). The hair creates a cast of the stomach and strands of hair can extend into the small bowel (the so-called Rapunzel syndrome). Large trichobezoars are likely to require surgical removal because they are less likely to respond to enzymatic degradation.

References: Bonilla F, Mirete J, Cuesta A, et al: Treatment of gastric phytobezoars with cellulose, *Rev Esp Enferm Dig* 91:809–814, 1999.

Ladas S, Triantafyllou K, Tzathas C, et al: Gastric phytobezoars may be treated by nasogastric Coca-Cola lavage, *Eur J Gastroenterol Hepatol* 14:801–803, 2002.

Walker-Renard P: Update on the medicinal management of phytobezoars, *Am J Gastroenterol* 88:1663–1666, 1993.

29. E. Surgical resection is the mainstay of treatment for gastric adenocarcinoma. Survival does not seem to be affected by whether a total or subtotal gastrectomy is performed, provided adequate margins are obtained. However, for patients with a proximal gastric cancer, performing a proximal gastrectomy has been shown to be associated with a higher complication rate than total gastrectomy. Thus, total gastrectomy is preferred for proximal cancers. For distal cancers, there does not seem to be a difference in outcome between a distal gastrectomy and a total gastrectomy, provided margins are adequate. Proximal margins should be at least 6 cm because the tumor tends to spread intramurally. When recurrence rates were compared in one study, those without recurrence had a median proximal margin of 6 cm versus 3.5 cm for those with a recurrence. The extent of lymph node dissection remains controversial. In Japan, a D2 resection (group 1 and 2 nodes as well as splenectomy and distal pancreatectomy) has been shown to improve survival compared with D1 (group 1 nodes only).

In Western countries, D2 resection has not been shown to improve survival and is associated with a higher morbidity rate and perioperative mortality rate. The poorer results with D2 resection in Western countries are likely a reflection of low case volume and the associated morbidity of performing the pancreaticosplenectomy (as such, routine splenectomy is not recommended). For patients with advanced stage IV gastric cancer, total gastrectomy in select patients with symptoms of bleeding or obstruction can provide good palliation with relatively low morbidity and mortality rates.

References: Bozzetti F, Bonfanti G, Bufalino R, et al: Adequacy of margins of resection in gastrectomy for cancer, *Ann Surg* 196:685–690, 1982.

Degiuli M, Sasako M, Ponti A, Calvo F: Survival results of a multicentre phase II study to evaluate D2 gastrectomy for gastric cancer, *Br J Cancer* 90:1727–1732, 2004.

Hartgrink H, van de Velde C, Putter H, et al: Extended lymph node dissection for gastric cancer: who may benefit? Final results of the randomized Dutch gastric cancer group trial, *J Clin Oncol* 22:2069–2077, 2004.

McCulloch P, Niita M, Kazi H, Gama-Rodrigues J: Gastrectomy with extended lymphadenectomy for primary treatment of gastric cancer, *Br J Surg* 92:5–13, 2005.

Monson J, Donohue J, McIlrath D, et al: Total gastrectomy for advanced cancer. A worthwhile palliative procedure, *Cancer* 68:1863–1868, 1991.

Nazli O, Yaman I, Tansug T, et al: Palliative surgery for advanced stage (stage IV) gastric adenocarcinoma, *Hepatogastroenterology* 54:298–303, 2007.

30. A. Gastric volvulus is associated with the Borchardt triad (sudden onset of severe upper abdominal pain, recurrent retching without vomitus, and an inability to pass a nasogastric tube). The volvulus can be either organoaxial (along the long axis of the stomach), which is twice as common, or mesenteroaxial (along the vertical axis). Gastric volvulus most commonly occurs in association with a diaphragmatic defect. The stomach becomes trapped in the defect and twists. In children, the defect is congenital (such as a Bochdalek hernia), whereas in adults, it is more often traumatic or paraesophageal hernias. Gastric volvulus can also occur in the absence of a diaphragmatic defect. In such situations, there is typically a congenital absence of intraperitoneal visceral attachments. It is seen in association with a wandering spleen, a condition in which the spleen also lacks peritoneal attachments and is prone to torsion. Gastric volvulus is a surgical emergency because there is a high risk of gastric necrosis if it is unrecognized. On occasion, there is a delay in diagnosis because the nasogastric tube is successfully passed and subsequent imaging is negative. Management consists of detorsion and repair of the diaphragmatic defect. If a paraesophageal hernia is present, consideration is given to performing a fundoplication. If the stomach is compromised, a gastric resection may be needed. If a volvulus is found without necrosis and without a diaphragmatic defect, then detorsion and gastropexy are performed.

References: Carter R, Brewer L 3rd, Hinshaw D: Acute gastric volvulus. A study of 25 cases, *Am J Surg* 140:99–106, 1980.

Uc A, Kao SC, Sanders KD, Lawrence J: Gastric volvulus and wandering spleen, *Am J Gastroenterol* 93:1146–1148, 1998.

Wasselle JA, Norman J: Acute gastric volvulus: pathogenesis, diagnosis, and treatment, *Am J Gastroenterol* 88:1780–1784, 1993.

31. D. A metastatic left supraclavicular lymph node is called the *Virchow node* (Troisier sign). A metastatic left axillary lymph node from gastric cancer is called an *Irish node*. A Blumer shelf is a palpable nodule on rectal examination suggesting a drop metastasis. An ovarian mass from a gastric metastasis is also known as Krukenberg tumor. An umbilical nodule (Sister Mary Joseph node) suggests carcinomatosis. Although associated with gastric cancer, it may represent any metastatic lesion, most commonly from an intra-abdominal cancer. It was named after Dr. William Mayo's surgical assistant, who made the observation while scrubbing patients for gastric surgery that those with umbilical nodules had widely metastatic and unresectable gastric cancer. Current recommendations are that if such nodules are found on physical examination, the patient should undergo fine-needle aspiration because such umbilical nodules may sometimes represent benign disease.

References: Fleming M, Oertel Y: Eight cases of Sister Mary Joseph's nodule diagnosed by fine-needle aspiration, *Diagn Cytopathol* 9:32–36, 1993.

Giner Galvaň V: [Sister Mary Joseph's nodule. Its clinical significance and management] [in Spanish], *An Med Interna* 16:365–370, 1999.

32. B. When considering gastrinoma, it is important to be aware of the differential diagnosis of an elevated gastrin level. Causes of hypergastrinemia include pernicious anemia, use of acid-suppressive medication, a retained antrum after distal gastrectomy, G-cell hyperplasia, massive small bowel resection, and renal insufficiency. Hypothyroidism is associated with a low gastrin level, whereas hyperthyroidism increases gastrin levels.

Reference: Seino Y, Matsukura S, Inoue Y, et al: Hypogastrinemia in hypothyroidism, *Am J Dig Dis* 23:189–191, 1978.

33. D. GI stromal tumors were previously called *leiomyomas* or *leiomyosarcomas* because they were thought to arise from smooth muscle cells, but they in fact originate from mesenchymal components (from Cajal cells). They stain positive for CD117 (ckit). They are most commonly found in the stomach and, although rare, are the most common mesenchymal tumor of the intestinal tract. Because they are not epithelial tumors and grow in the wall of the stomach, they tend to be large at the time of presentation. They cause mucosal ulceration and frequently present with GI bleeding. Large tumors may also produce symptoms of weight loss, abdominal pain, and fullness and early satiety. An abdominal mass may be palpable. An endoscopic biopsy specimen may be negative in as many as one half of cases due to sampling error because most of the tumor is submucosal. A CT scan provides a better assessment of the extent of the tumor. Determining whether a GI stromal tumor is malignant is not straightforward because there are no discriminating cellular features. The malignant potential is determined by mitotic activity. Treatment is surgical resection to negative margins. Lymph node dissection is not necessary because tumors spread hematogenously and lymph node metastasis is extremely rare. Wedge resection with clear margins is adequate treatment in most cases. This can be performed laparoscopically.

References: Dempsey DT: Stomach. In Brunicardi FC, Andersen DK, Billiar TR, et al, editors: *Schwartz's principles of surgery*, ed 9, New York, 2010, McGraw-Hill, pp 889–948.

Mercer DW, Robinson EK: Stomach. In Townsend CM Jr, Beauchamp RD, Evers BM, Mattox KL, editors: *Sabiston textbook of surgery: the biological basis of modern surgical practice*, ed 18, Philadelphia, 2008, WB Saunders, pp 1223–1277.

Novitsky Y, Kercher K, Sing R, Heniford B: Long-term outcomes of laparoscopic resection of gastric gastrointestinal stromal tumors, *Ann Surg* 243:738–745, 2006.

Sexton J, Pierce R, Halpin V, et al: Laparoscopic gastric resection for gastrointestinal stromal tumors, *Surg Endosc* 22:2583–2587, 2008.

The stomach. In Cameron JL, editor: *Current surgical therapy*, ed 9, Philadelphia, 2008, Mosby, pp 81–115.

Surgical Complications and Nutrition 24

1. The body's response to hypothermia includes all of the following EXCEPT:
   A. Decreased platelet function
   B. Decreased cardiac output
   C. Tachycardia
   D. Cardiac arrhythmias
   E. Increased risk of wound infection

2. All of the following are true regarding malignant hyperthermia EXCEPT:
   A. It is an autosomal dominant disorder.
   B. Creatinine kinase levels are elevated.
   C. It is more common in elderly patients.
   D. It may present as late as 24 hours after anesthesia.
   E. Treatment is with dantrolene.

3. A 65-year-old woman is 3 days status post laparoscopic left colectomy for diverticulitis, and acute shortness of breath develops. On clinical assessment, your suspicion is that the patient has pneumonia, but you have a low to moderate concern for pulmonary embolus. The next test of choice is:
   A. Computed tomography (CT) angiography
   B. Nuclear ventilation/perfusion scan
   C. D-Dimer rapid enzyme-linked immunosorbent assay
   D. Bilateral leg vein duplex ultrasound scan
   E. Pulmonary arteriography

4. A 65-year-old man is 2 days status post gastric bypass procedure. Urine output decreases to 10 mL/hr. All of the following are consistent with prerenal azotemia EXCEPT:
   A. Urine osmolality > 500 mosmol/kg
   B. Urine sodium > 40 mmol/L
   C. BUN/plasma creatinine > 40
   D. BUN/plasma urea > 8
   E. Urine/plasma osmolality < 1.5

5. Abdominal compartment syndrome should be suspected when bladder pressures exceed:
   A. 10 cm H_2O
   B. 25 cm H_2O
   C. 35 cm H_2O
   D. 40 cm H_2O
   E. 45 cm H_2O

6. Five years after a permanent colostomy, a patient develops a bulge adjacent to the stoma. The patient reports no symptoms. Management would consist of:
   A. Observation
   B. Primary repair of fascia defect
   C. Placement of colostomy at new site and primary closure of fascia defect
   D. Mesh repair of fascia defect
   E. Placement of colostomy at new site and closure of fascia defect with mesh

7. Four days after a Whipple procedure, a 65-year-old man presents with fever as well as edema and redness and tenderness over the right cheek. Which of the following is true regarding this condition?
   A. It is usually due to *Streptococcus*.
   B. Massage of the area is beneficial.
   C. It can be prevented with antibiotics.
   D. It is associated with decreased saliva formation.
   E. Tracheostomy is never required.

8. A 69-year-old woman presents with copious diarrhea, fever, dehydration, and abdominal pain. She was hospitalized 4 weeks earlier for pneumonia. The patient demonstrates diffuse abdominal tenderness on examination with guarding and rebound. Plain abdominal radiographs reveal a markedly distended colon without free air. Temperature is 103°F and the white blood cell count is 25,000 µ/L. After fluid hydration, definitive management should consist of:

   A. Oral Flagyl (metronidazole)
   B. Oral vancomycin
   C. Intravenous (IV) Flagyl (metronidazole)
   D. Colonoscopic decompression
   E. Colectomy

9. One day after an emergency Hartmann procedure for perforated diverticulitis, the stoma, which is in the left lower quadrant, appears to be necrotic. Management consists of:

   A. Reexploration resection of ischemic colon and moving the stoma to different site
   B. Reexploration with resection of segment of colon and placement of stoma at same site
   C. Reexploration with on-table bowel prep and then primary colonic anastomosis
   D. Examination of the stoma with a penlight and test tube and, if ischemia is not down to fascia, observe
   E. Reexploration and conversion to ileostomy and mucus fistula

10. Twelve hours after an open cholecystectomy, a high fever to 104°F develops in a 25-year-old woman. On examination, she has foul-smelling "dishwater" pus draining from her wound. A Gram stain reveals gram-positive rods. Which of the following is true regarding this condition?

    A. The causative organism is an aerobe.
    B. Emergency operative débridement of the wound is indicated.
    C. High-dose Flagyl (metronidazole) is the antibiotic of choice.
    D. The organism produces an endotoxin.
    E. Antitoxin therapy is indicated.

11. After an elective low anterior resection for rectal cancer, palpitations develop in a 59-year-old man with a history of congestive heart failure and an ejection fraction of 20% in the intensive care unit. On the electrocardiogram, he is noted to be in a ventricular tachycardia (VT) at a rate of 120 beats per minute. He is currently awake and conversing with the nurse. His blood pressure is 130/75 mm Hg. The best initial treatment of this arrhythmia would be:

    A. Epinephrine 1 mg IV push
    B. Amiodarone 150 mg IV over 10 minutes
    C. Immediate defibrillation with 360 J
    D. Bretylium 5 mg/kg IV
    E. Diltiazem 15 mg IV over 2 minutes

12. A 34-year-old woman undergoes a subtotal thyroidectomy for Graves disease. In the recovery room, she develops anxiety and progressive respiratory distress with stridor. Her neck appears to be full, suggesting a hematoma beneath her collar incision. The most important initial step would be:

    A. Heliox therapy and bronchodilators
    B. Rapid-sequence intubation
    C. Needle aspiration of the neck wound
    D. Ultrasound examination of the neck
    E. Rapidly open the incision at the bedside

13. One day after an emergent left colectomy for perforated diverticulitis, a patient is noted to have an elevation of his serum creatinine. He has a urine output of 30 to 50 mL/hr. A renal ultrasound scan reveals no evidence of hydroureter but significant ascites. Intraventricular pressure demonstrates urine extravasation from the left ureter at the level of the pelvic brim. All of the following about this injury are true EXCEPT:

    A. Placement of ureteral stents would have prevented this complication.
    B. Reoperation with ureteroureterostomy over a stent is usually possible.
    C. Ureteroneocystostomy may be required.
    D. The left ureter crosses the common iliac artery near its bifurcation into the internal and external iliac arteries.
    E. Administration of indigo carmine or methylene blue intravenously often aids in identifying such injuries intraoperatively.

14. Two days after a pedestrian is pinned against a block wall by an automobile with significant crush injury to the lower legs, her urine is noted to be dark brown in color at a rate of 10 to 20 mL/hr. Her serum creatine kinase is 38,000 U/L. Urine dipstick reveals 4+ blood, but only 5 to 10 red blood cells. Treatment of this condition should include all of the following EXCEPT:

   A. Measurement of bilateral lower leg compartment pressures
   B. Cystoscopy and 24-hour urine for creatinine clearance
   C. Aggressive IV fluid hydration
   D. Mannitol 1 g/kg
   E. 5% Dextrose in water with 3 ampules of sodium bicarbonate

15. Five days after a laparoscopic Roux-en-Y gastric bypass, fever with rigors, hypotension, and pain in the left shoulder develops in the patient. This most likely represents:

   A. Gas bloat syndrome
   B. Acalculous cholecystitis
   C. Wound dehiscence
   D. Internal hernia involving the Roux limb
   E. Disruption of the gastric pouch–jejunal anastomosis

16. A 28-year-old woman undergoes a segmental ileal resection during the course of an adhesiolysis for an acute small bowel obstruction. On postoperative day 6, she is noted to have thick bile-colored fluid emanating from the midline wound. After IV hydration, the next step in the management should be:

   A. CT scan of the abdomen
   B. Upper gastrointestinal infection with small bowel follow-through with water-soluble contrast
   C. Fistulogram
   D. Operative re-exploration
   E. Octreotide

17. After excision of multiple subcutaneous lipomas under local anesthesia, a 42-year-old woman seizes violently. The surgeon should be aware that the maximum safe dose of a local anesthetic agent in a 70-kg woman is:

   A. 10 to 20 mL 1% lidocaine
   B. 40 to 50 mL 2% lidocaine with epinephrine
   C. 40 to 50 mL 1% lidocaine with epinephrine
   D. 40 to 50 mL 0.5% lidocaine
   E. 40 to 50 mL 1% lidocaine without epinephrine

18. The most important predictor of colonic ischemia after repair of a ruptured abdominal aortic aneurysm is:

   A. Age
   B. Presence of preoperative shock
   C. Time to operation
   D. Presence of associated cardiac disease
   E. Intraoperative ligation of a patent inferior mesenteric artery

19. A 50-year-old man with end-stage renal failure develops right arm swelling. He has an indwelling internal jugular vein catheter on the right side for hemodialysis and is awaiting permanent access in his left arm. Which of the following is the best management?

   A. Removal of the catheter and IV heparin and Coumadin (warfarin) therapy for 3 to 6 months
   B. Thrombolysis through the catheter
   C. Catheter removal only
   D. IV heparin and Coumadin (warfarin) therapy without catheter removal
   E. Daily low-molecular-weight heparin and continued catheter use

20. Five days after right radical nephrectomy for adenocarcinoma, the patient reports sharp right-sided chest pain and dyspnea. The patient is tachycardic to 110 beats per minute. His Pao_2 is 64 mm Hg on 100% face mask, $Paco_2$ is 32 mm Hg, central venous pressure is 26 mm Hg, and blood pressure is 102/78 mm Hg. There is a high suspicion for pulmonary embolism (PE). The next step in management is:

   A. CT angiography of the chest
   B. Posteroanterior and lateral chest radiographs
   C. Heparin sodium 100 U/kg IV
   D. Immediate duplex scanning of both lower extremities
   E. Ventilation-perfusion lung scan

21. Which of the following is the LEAST likely complication of postpyloric enteral feeding?

   A. Aspiration
   B. Diarrhea
   C. Feeding tube occlusion
   D. Electrolyte abnormalities
   E. Mucosal villi atrophy

22. Red man syndrome is most associated with the use of which of the following antibiotics?

    A. Vancomycin
    B. Clindamycin
    C. Gentamicin
    D. Ciprofloxacin
    E. Levofloxacin

23. The most important amino acid used for gluconeogenesis by the liver is:

    A. Glutamine
    B. Serine
    C. Alanine
    D. Tyrosine
    E. Asparginine

24. Cancer cachexia related to proteolysis-inducing factor is most associated with cancer of the:

    A. Colon
    B. Prostate
    C. Pancreas
    D. Breast
    E. Liver

25. Poor glucose control is a manifestation of deficiency of:

    A. Zinc
    B. Copper
    C. Chromium
    D. Molybdenum
    E. Selenium

26. All of the following are true regarding hepatic dysfunction in infants on long-term total parenteral nutrition (TPN) EXCEPT:

    A. It is more likely to reverse on termination of TPN compared with adults.
    B. It is associated with cholestasis.
    C. It is exacerbated by infection.
    D. It may lead to a need for a combined liver and small bowel transplantation.
    E. It may be improved with carnitine supplementation.

27. A potential for improvement in intestinal absorption efficiency after massive small bowel resection is seen with the administration of:

    A. Glutamine
    B. Serine
    C. Alanine
    D. Tyrosine
    E. Arginine

28. Which of the following is true regarding the use of preoperative TPN to prevent postoperative complications?

    A. It is useful even if used for as little as 3 days.
    B. It is efficacious only if the patient has lost more than 15% of his or her body weight before surgery.
    C. There is no evidence that it lowers the complication rate.
    D. Slightly overfeeding for 7 days with mild to moderate hyperglycemia reduces the risk of septic complications.
    E. Total parenteral nutrition is efficacious even in mild to moderate malnutrition.

29. You are planning an elective umbilical hernia repair in a cirrhotic patient. All of the following are useful in assessing operative mortality in a cirrhotic patient EXCEPT:

    A. Child classification
    B. Child-Pugh classification
    C. MELD (Model for End-Stage Liver Disease) score
    D. American Society of Anesthesiology class
    E. History of diabetes

30. Five days after surgery for perforated appendicitis, liquid stool emanates from the right lower quadrant wound. Which of the following is true about this condition?

    A. Mortality is high for this complication.
    B. The majority will close spontaneously.
    C. The patient should be placed immediately on TPN.
    D. Fluid and electrolyte derangements are common.
    E. The patient should be returned immediately to the operating room for surgical repair.

31. Five days after a Billroth II gastric resection for a bleeding ulcer, high fever, hypotension, and pain in the right shoulder develop in the patient. This most likely represents:

    A. Postoperative pancreatitis
    B. Acalculous cholecystitis
    C. Duodenal stump blow out
    D. Intra-abdominal hemorrhage
    E. Wound dehiscence

32. In patients with acute renal failure, the most immediate threat to the patient is:

    A. Acidosis
    B. Hyperkalemia
    C. Platelet dysfunction
    D. Fluid overload
    E. Malnutrition

33. A 30-year-old woman is involved in a high-speed motor vehicle accident and sustains a femur fracture. Prevention of fat embolism is best accomplished by:
    A. Heparin
    B. Dextran
    C. Steroids
    D. Early fixation of long bone fractures
    E. Prophylactic intubation

34. Two days after an elective right colectomy for colon cancer, a large amount of clear, pink-tinged fluid is noted to suddenly leak from the midline wound between the staples. The abdomen is tensely distended. The management would consist of:
    A. Immediate operative exploration
    B. Removal of all staples to inspect wound
    C. Wound aspiration
    D. IV antibiotics
    E. Ultrasound scan

35. All of the following are true regarding the hepatorenal syndrome EXCEPT:
    A. Type I is rapidly progressive with a poor prognosis.
    B. It is associated with intense renal vasoconstriction.
    C. It is associated with systemic vasodilation.
    D. The urine sodium is typically >40 mEq/L.
    E. Type II is relatively stable.

36. A chest radiograph demonstrating the Westermark sign is indicative of:
    A. Pulmonary embolus
    B. Aspiration pneumonia
    C. Acute respiratory distress syndrome
    D. Acute lung injury
    E. Pulmonary edema

37. Which of the following modalities is LEAST likely to assist in the prevention of postoperative pulmonary complications in a 65-year-old male smoker?
    A. Postoperative use of an incentive spirometer
    B. Postoperative deep breathing exercises
    C. Postoperative use of continuous positive airway pressure
    D. Smoking cessation 1 week before surgery
    E. Placement of a nasogastric tube in a patient who is vomiting

38. Which of the following preoperative studies is most strongly associated with an increased risk of pulmonary-related postoperative complications?
    A. Blood urea nitrogen
    B. Incentive spirometry
    C. Chest radiograph
    D. Serum albumin
    E. Room air arterial blood gas

39. All of the following are known predictors of an increased risk of a perioperative cardiac complication EXCEPT:
    A. History of coronary artery disease
    B. History of congestive heart failure
    C. Smoking
    D. History of stroke
    E. Serum creatinine greater than 2.0 mg/dL

40. The following agent has been shown to clinically reduce the deleterious effects of corticosteroids on wound healing:
    A. Vitamin C
    B. Vitamin A
    C. Zinc
    D. Copper
    E. Transforming growth factor β

Answers

1. C. The body's response to hypothermia includes a decrease in cardiac output, a decrease in heart rate (particularly below 30°C), and, at extremely low temperatures, cardiac arrhythmias. Core temperatures below 35°C (95°F) are defined as hypothermia. Below this temperature, coagulation is affected secondary to decreased platelet function and dysfunction of the clotting cascade. Prolonged operations increase the risk of intraoperative hypothermia, and thus wound infection risk increases due to vasoconstriction and decreased blood flow and oxygen delivery.

Hypothermia also leads to renal dysfunction in association with paradoxical polyuria.

2. C. Malignant hyperthermia is a rare autosomal dominant disorder of skeletal muscle. The condition is characterized by a hypermetabolic state triggered by exposure to certain inhalation anesthetics or succinylcholine. The older anesthetic agents associated with this reaction include halothane and enflurane. Malignant hyperthermia occurs when uncontrolled amounts of intracellular calcium accumulate in skeletal muscle. Symptoms may develop as early as 30 minutes after anesthetic administration and as late as 24 hours postoperatively. The initial clues occur in the operating room after induction. Rather than achieve complete paralysis, the anesthesiologist may notice rigidity in the masseter muscle. Other findings include an increase in end tidal CO_2, tachycardia, and an increase in temperature. It is imperative that all anesthetics are immediately stopped and dantrolene given (2.5 mg/kg every 5 minutes) until resolution of symptoms. Dantrolene stabilizes muscle channels in the sarcoplasmic reticulum. The mortality rate approaches 30%. A functional test on skeletal muscle biopsy, the in vitro contracture test, is used for diagnosis. More than 50% of the families show linkage of the in vitro contracture test phenotype to the gene encoding the skeletal muscle ryanodine receptor. The test requires a muscle biopsy with exposure of the muscle to halothane and caffeine. A positive test will cause significant muscle contraction. The majority of cases occur in children or young adults.

Reference: Jurkat-Rott K, McCarthy T, Lehmann-Horn F: Genetics and pathogenesis of malignant hyperthermia, *Muscle Nerve* 23:4–17, 2000.

3. C. The diagnosis of PE has undergone significant changes in the past 2 decades. The Prospective Investigation of Pulmonary Embolism Diagnosis (PIOPED) study demonstrated that V/Q scanning was not as useful as originally thought for the diagnosis of PE. A high probability scan strongly correlated with PE, but very few patients with a PE had a high-probability scan. Conversely, a low-probability scan did not rule out PE because 12% of patients with a low-probability scan actually had a PE. More recently, the PIOPED II study has permitted the development of a diagnostic pathway. Study investigators recommend beginning with clinical assessment using an objective method followed by testing based on the degree of clinical suspicion. One useful clinical decision scoring system includes (1) evidence on examination of deep venous thrombosis (DVT), (2) likelihood of another diagnosis to explain symptoms, (3) heart rate greater than 100 beats per minute, (4) recent surgery or immobilization, (5) previous PE or DVT, (6) hemoptysis, (7) malignancy. For patients with low or moderate suspicion of PE, the first test recommended by the PIOPED II investigators is the D-dimer rapid enzyme-linked immunosorbent assay. The test relies on the principle that most patients with PE have endogenous fibrinolysis that is not effective enough to prevent PE but breaks down some of the fibrin clot to D-dimers. Elevated D-dimers are highly sensitive for PE but not specific. Particularly in the postoperative period, D-dimers can be elevated in patients for at least 1 week. Sepsis and acute myocardial infarction can also elevate the D-dimers. However, a negative D-dimer in a low- or moderate-risk patient makes the diagnosis very unlikely and thus requires no further testing. If the D-dimer is positive, CT angiography or CT angiography with CT venography is recommended. In patients with high clinical suspicion for PE, the patient should proceed directly to contrast CT.

References: Stein P, Woodard P, Weg J, et al: Diagnostic pathways in acute pulmonary embolism: recommendations of the PIOPED II investigators, *Radiology* 242:15–21, 2007.

Value of the ventilation/perfusion scan in acute pulmonary embolism. Results of the prospective investigation of pulmonary embolism diagnosis (PIOPED): the PIOPED investigators, *JAMA* 263:2753–2759, 1990.

Writing Group for the Christopher Study Investigators: Effectiveness of managing suspected pulmonary embolism using an algorithm combining clinical probability, D-dimer testing, and computed tomography, *JAMA* 295:172–179, 2006.

4. B. The diagnosis of prerenal azotemia is associated with a low urinary sodium of less than 20, an elevated urine osmolarity greater than 500, fractional excretion of sodium less than 1%, a BUN-to-plasma creatinine ratio greater than 40, a BUN-to-plasma urea ratio greater than 8, and a urine-to-plasma osmolality ratio less than 1.5. A high urine sodium (>40) would suggest a renal cause such as acute tubular necrosis.

5. B. Abdominal compartment syndrome occurs in patients who have sustained multiple traumas, severe burns, or retroperitoneal injuries; have undergone an operation for massive intra-abdominal infection; or have undergone a complicated, prolonged abdominal operation. Massive IV fluid resuscitation with resultant third spacing of fluid and marked bowel wall edema places patients at high risk of the development of this complication. The symptoms and signs include progressive abdominal distention, increasing peak airway pressure, decreased cardiac output, and oliguria. These complications are the result of the abdominal pressure decreasing venous return from the inferior vena cava and renal veins and from diaphragm elevation. Renal failure, severe pulmonary compromise, and intracranial hypertension can eventually develop in patients. Pressures transduced from the bladder can be readily measured by instilling 100 mL of saline into the bladder. A pressure of greater than 25 mm Hg with evidence of physiologic compromise as manifested by renal, respiratory, or neurologic compromise is considered diagnostic. Treatment consists of opening the abdomen.

6. A. Management of a peristomal hernia depends on the amount of herniation and the clinical condition of the patient. If the peristomal hernia is small and the patient is asymptomatic, the hernia can be observed. In fact, the majority of these hernias can be managed conservatively. Only 10% to 20% of patients eventually require operative intervention. If the peristomal hernia causes partial obstruction, incarceration, or severe pain, repair of the hernia should be considered. Similarly, a peristomal hernia that becomes very large and cosmetically bothersome should also be repaired. When an operation is indicated, relocating the stoma generally yields better long-term results than does an attempt at local repair of the hernia.

Reference: Rubin M, Schoetz D Jr, Matthews J: Parastomal hernia. Is stoma relocation superior to fascial repair? *Arch Surg* 129:413–418, 1994.

7. D. This patient has postoperative parotitis. Postoperative parotitis most commonly occurs in elderly men with poor oral hygiene, poor oral intake, prolonged nasogastric tube decompression, and dehydration, all leading to a decrease in saliva production. The pathophysiology involves obstruction of the salivary ducts with secondary infection and is more common in the diabetic or immunocompromised patient. Most patients will be diagnosed with parotitis 4 to 12 days postoperatively. Signs and symptoms begin with pain and tenderness over the angle of the jaw that can then progress to high fevers and leukocytosis, as well as significant edema involving the floor of the mouth. If left undiagnosed and untreated, it can lead to life-threatening sepsis. Initial treatment is with high-dose broad-spectrum antibiotics with *Staphylococcus* coverage and warm compresses. If the patient does not improve, surgical incision and drainage is indicated. Rarely, advanced disease may require an emergent tracheostomy. Use of measures to stimulate salivary flow, such as sucking on candy, seems to help prevent this complication.

8. E. The presentation is consistent with toxic megacolon that is most likely secondary to *Clostridium difficile* infection. In the absence of a history of inflammatory bowel disease, a patient presenting with toxic megacolon should be presumed to have *C. difficile* colitis until proven otherwise. The incidence of *C. difficile* colitis is increasing, and patients may not necessarily present with the classic history of diarrhea or previous antibiotic administration. Presumably the patient received antibiotics when hospitalized previously. *C. difficile* makes two toxins, A and B. A particularly virulent strain, known as the NAP1 strain, is more resistant to antibiotics and makes 16 times more toxin A and 23 times more toxin B than other strains. Both oral and IV Flagyl (metronidazole) and oral vancomycin are effective in treating uncomplicated *C. difficile* colitis, but are not the definitive management in this patient with toxic megacolon and peritonitis, whereas IV vancomycin is not effective. The presence of peritonitis mandates exploratory laparotomy. The patient will require colectomy to control her sepsis. Delay in therapy will likely increase the risk of an adverse outcome. In a recent review, the mortality for *C. difficile* colitis with toxic megacolon was 50%.

Reference: Berman L, Carling T, Fitzgerald T, et al: Defining surgical therapy for pseudomembranous colitis with toxic megacolon, *J Clin Gastroenterol* 42:476–480, 2008.

9. D. Ischemia or necrosis of the stoma is a recognized complication of a colostomy creation. It is more likely to occur in situations in which the inferior mesenteric artery was ligated high, near the aorta, such that the stoma is relying on the marginal artery. It is important to determine whether the ischemia extends down to the fascia. If it does, the patient needs re-exploration because otherwise it may progress to necrosis, perforation, and stool spillage into the peritoneum. Conversely, if the ischemia/necrosis is superficial, it can be observed, and a mucosa-cutaneous junction will form by secondary intention. This may lead to recession of the stoma or stricture, but this can be dealt with later when the patient is less critically ill.

10. B. This patient has a rare but well described early postoperative necrotizing soft-tissue infection. The causative organisms are typically *Streptococcus pyogenes* and *Clostridium perfringens*. Clostridia are anaerobic gram-positive rods that produce an exotoxin. There is no effective antitoxin. Effective therapy requires rapid administration of broad-spectrum antibiotics and source control via emergent operative excision of necrotic infected tissue, including fascia. The description of "dishwater pus" is classic for a postoperative clostridial wound infection.

11. B. Patients with underlying cardiac disease are at increased risk of arrhythmias, seeming to be more sensitive to hypoxia, hypercarbia, and electrolyte abnormalities than patients without heart disease. VT is a serious arrhythmia that warrants immediate treatment because it may progress to unstable ventricular rhythms. Management of VT is dependent on the stability of the patient. For those with a pulse palpable at the carotid or femoral artery and normal blood pressure, without dizziness or confusion, pharmacologic treatment is indicated. Amiodarone has become the drug of choice, although lidocaine is also acceptable. If the patient exhibits altered mental status and/or hypotension, immediate cardioversion is indicated, but should begin at 200 J, not 360 J. Cardioversion can be performed on stable patients as well, but the patients must receive premedication given for sedation and pain control, and shocks must be synchronized and started at 100 J. Epinephrine is indicated in pulseless VT and is not first-line management in the stable patient. Diltiazem is useful in atrial tachycardia, but has no place in VT. Most importantly, a search for and correction of any correctable cause should be undertaken.

12. E. Postoperative hematomas after neck surgery (thyroid, parathyroid, carotid artery) can have catastrophic consequences. Physical examination findings can be deceptively benign. Attempts at intubation may be hampered by tracheal compression and deviation. Furthermore, the recent neck dissection, combined with the hematoma, causes venous and lymphatic obstruction, leading to airway edema, further compromising attempts at intubation. Rapidly opening the incision at the bedside is necessary because urgent decompression is the fastest way to restore proper respiratory function. Definitive hemostasis must then be obtained in the operating room. Although ultrasonography is an important diagnostic aid for hematomas, clinical suspicion is sufficient in this emergent situation and the urgency of decompression does not permit waiting for an ultrasound examination. Needle aspiration would not be sufficient. Heliox therapy and bronchodilators are not appropriate in the management of stridor secondary to mechanical upper airway obstruction and are more commonly used for lower airway wheezing.

13. A. The ureters bilaterally pass alongside the transverse processes of the lumbar vertebrae in the retroperitoneum and cross the common iliac arteries near the bifurcation into the internal and external iliac arteries. This anatomic position puts them at high risk during pelvic surgery, and the situation is particularly precarious when inflammation, abscess, and/or phlegmon is present. During mobilization of the left colon and ligation of the inferior mesenteric artery, visualization and protection of the ureter from injury is imperative. Placement of ureteral stents before the operation may help to identify the ureters and identify an injury if made, but does not seem to prevent injury. If unsure whether an injury has occurred, IV injection of indigo carmine and subsequent blue dye seen in the operative field is diagnostic of an injury. If not diagnosed intraoperatively but suspected postoperatively, performance of IV pyelography or retrograde urethrography should reveal the injury. Depending on the location and extent of the injury, ureteroneocystostomy, ureteroureterostomy, or reimplantation along with placement of a ureteral stent is indicated.

Reference: Bothwell W, Bleicher R, Dent T: Prophylactic ureteral catheterization in colon surgery: a five-year review, *Dis Colon Rect* 37:330–334, 1994.

14. B. Crush injury to the extremities causing significant muscle injury is often complicated by rhabdomyolysis, which can cause acute renal failure. Degradation products of both hemoglobin and myoglobin are toxic to the nephron in acidic urine. Further injury results from precipitation of myoglobin in the renal tubules. Elevated serum creatinine phosphokinase, hyperkalemia, and the presence of heme without red blood cells on urine analysis is indicative of rhabdomyolysis. Management consists of aggressive IV hydration to maintain a urine output of more than 100 mL/hr. Myoglobin concentrates in the renal tubules and precipitates readily when it comes in contact with Tamm-Horsfall protein. This precipitation is enhanced under acidic conditions. Alkalinization of the urine increases the solubility of the myoglobin–Tamm-Horsfall protein P complex, thus increasing myoglobin washout; it also prevents lipid peroxidation and renal vasoconstriction. Recommended administration is 1 L of D5W + 2 to 3 ampules of $NaHCO_3$. Mannitol 1 g/kg is also used to force diuresis. It has weak antioxidant properties as well. It may also aid in decreasing muscle swelling and compartment pressures. There is no diagnostic value of cystoscopy or 24-hour creatinine clearance because the pathology occurs on a microscopic level and is usually rapidly reversible.

Reference: Holt S, Moore K: Pathogenesis and treatment of renal dysfunction in rhabdomyolysis, *Intensive Care Med* 27:803–811, 2001.

15. E. Fever, chills, hypotension, and peritoneal irritation occurring together within 1 week of laparoscopic Roux-en-Y gastric bypass should immediately raise suspicion for an anastomotic disruption. Left shoulder pain is often a consequence of left diaphragm irritation and, in this case, correlates with the gastric pouch–jejunal anastomosis. Water-soluble contrast studies can aid in the diagnosis and indicate how large the leak is because contained leaks can often be managed nonoperatively. However, in this patient, hypotension and peritoneal signs indicate operative exploration and repair of the anastomosis.

16. A. This case represents an enterocutaneous fistula, likely resulting from either an anastomotic leak or an unrecognized intraoperative bowel injury away from the anastomosis. Management of enterocutaneous fistulas should begin with stabilizing the patient via aggressive fluid hydration. If the patient is manifesting signs of sepsis, prompt administration of IV antibiotics should be instituted. Sepsis, dehydration, and electrolyte/nutrient losses are

the most devastating early consequences. Prompt return to the operating room is not recommended because the peritoneal cavity will likely have highly vascular adhesions, making re-entry treacherous, and early attempts to reclose fistulas typically fail. Once the patient has been stabilized, the best initial study is a CT scan of the abdomen. This will identify whether any intra-abdominal abscesses are present that might require percutaneous drainage and rule out whether there is a distal obstruction. Fistulas are loosely categorized as high and low output. High output is defined as outputs of more than 500 mL/day and low output as less than 200 mL/day. High-output fistulas are less likely to close and present formidable fluid, electrolyte, and nutritional challenges. Factors that predict whether a fistula will close (mnemonic "FRIEND") include *f*oreign body, *r*adiation to the bowel, *i*nflammation/infection (such as inflammatory bowel disease), *e*pithelialization of the fistula tract, *n*eoplasia at the fistula site, and *d*istal obstruction. The mortality rate of enterocutaneous fistulas remains significant at 10% to 15%. Approximately 50% close spontaneously. Conservative treatment should be continued for at least 6 weeks before any reoperation is performed. Operating before 6 weeks results in higher mortality and fistula recurrence rates. Octreotide has not been shown to aid in fistula closure.

Reference: Sancho J, di Costanzo J, Nubiola P: Randomized double-blind placebo-controlled trial of early octreotide in patients with postoperative enterocutaneous fistula, *Br J Surg* 82:638–641, 1995.

17. C. There are relatively few side effects of local anesthetic agents such as lidocaine, unless they are injected intravenously by mistake or administered in doses higher than recommended. Toxicity begins with light-headedness, facial paresthesias, blurred vision, and tinnitus and can progress to lethargy, tremors, and tonic-clonic seizures. It can rarely progress to cardiac arrest. Maximum doses for local injection of lidocaine are 5 mg/kg without and 7 mg/kg with epinephrine because the vasoconstriction delays the systemic release of lidocaine. Because a 1% solution of lidocaine contains 10 mg/mL, an easy way to remember this is to multiply the patient's weight by either 5 (no epinephrine) or 7 (with epinephrine) and then divide by 10. Therefore, for this patient: 70 kg × 5 mg/kg = 350 mg ÷ 10 mg/mL = 35 mL 1% lidocaine. For lidocaine with epinephrine, 70 kg × 7 mg/kg = 490 mg ÷ 10 = 49 mL of 1% lidocaine. For a 2% lidocaine solution, one would divide by 20 (24.5 mL and 17.5 mL, respectively, with and without epinephrine), and for a 0.5% solution, one would divide by 5 (70 mL and 98 mL, respectively, with and without epinephrine). There have been recent case reports suggesting that "lipid rescue" using an IV intralipid solution, is useful in severe overdose cases.

Reference: Warren J, Thoma R, Georgescu A, Shah S: Intravenous lipid infusion in the successful resuscitation of local anesthetic-induced cardiovascular collapse after supraclavicular brachial plexus block, *Anesth Analg* 106:1578–1580, 2008.

18. B. Colonic ischemia after repair of a ruptured abdominal aortic aneurysm occurs in 1% to 6% of operations, but can occur as much as 25% of the time. The greatest risk factor is the presence of prolonged hypotension preoperatively. In a patient with stable blood pressure, age, time to operation, and the presence of cardiac disease have little effect on the incidence of colonic ischemia after aortic repair. Intraoperative ligation of a patent's inferior mesenteric artery is also not a good predictor of colonic ischemia because many patients will have collateral flow to the rectum via the marginal and internal iliac arteries. Symptoms and signs of ischemia include bloody diarrhea, abdominal pain/distention, and elevated white blood cell count. If the patient has evidence of peritonitis, urgent reoperation is indicated. Otherwise, endoscopy is urgently indicated to view the colonic mucosa. The majority of cases of colonic ischemia can be managed nonoperatively with bowel rest, hydration, and IV antibiotics. If the patient requires colon resection, mortality rates are as high as 75%.

19. A. Until recently, the frequency and significance of upper extremity DVT had been underappreciated. Central venous catheters, thrombophilic states, and a previous leg venous thrombosis were statistically significantly associated with upper extremity DVT in one study. Importantly, objective findings suggestive of a PE were recorded in 36% of the patients with upper extremity DVT. Thus, acute unilateral swelling of the arm without explanation should prompt a Doppler ultrasound examination of the ipsilateral subclavian vein. If thrombosis is present, immediate removal of the catheter is recommended because the clot can continue to extend into the superior vena cava and shower emboli into the heart. IV heparin followed by Coumadin (warfarin) therapy for 3 to 6 months is recommended. Low-molecular-weight heparin is an alternative. Thrombolytics would be relatively contraindicated because the patient has a large catheter puncture site in a deep vein. Both compression ultrasonography and color flow Doppler imaging are accurate methods for diagnosis. Upper extremity DVT may recur and may be followed by postthrombotic sequelae just as in the lower extremity.

Reference: Prandoni P, Polistena F, Bernardi E, et al: Upper-extremity deep vein thrombosis: risk factors, diagnosis, and complications, *Arch Intern Med* 157:57–62, 1997.

20. C. This patient differs from the one in question 3 in that the clinical suspicion is high. Factors of concern include tachycardia, the blood gas findings, lack of another reason to explain hypoxia, recent surgery, and malignancy. Although the study of choice is CT angiography, the clinical picture is worrisome enough that heparin should be immediately instituted. Transesophageal echocardiography has proven effective as well and can be done at the bedside. Chest radiograph should also be obtained to rule out other common etiologies, such as a pneumothorax.

21. E. Aspiration, diarrhea, and feeding tube occlusion are the most common complications associated with enteral feeding. Aspiration has been shown to occur in as many as 80% of cases, regardless of whether the tube is past the pylorus. Elevating the head of the bed can decrease, but not eliminate, the risk. Diarrhea occurs in approximately one third of patients receiving tube feeds and is most commonly a result of hypertonicity of the tube feeds or medicines that contain sorbitol. Eliminating sorbitol and starting tube feeds at half strength and lower rates are usually helpful. Catheter occlusion is of course dependent on the size of the catheter lumen and the particles that are delivered through that lumen. Frequent flushings and avoidance of mixing agents that will precipitate in the catheter will extend the life of the catheter. Electrolyte abnormalities can also occur with enteral feedings, especially in patients with diarrhea or abnormal kidney function. Frequent measurements of blood chemistries while initiating feeds and correction of abnormalities will avoid severe electrolyte problems. Finally, mucosal villi atrophy occurs when enteral feedings are withheld and the intestinal mucosa is deprived of glutamine.

22. A. Rapid infusion of vancomycin is associated with red man syndrome and seems to be due to histamine release. Symptoms and signs include pruritus and erythematous rash of the face, neck, and upper torso. Hypotension and angioedema rarely occur. Patients may become dizzy and agitated, and headache, chills, fever, and paresthesia around the mouth can develop. In the majority of patients, the syndrome is mild. Signs usually commence 4 to 10 minutes after an infusion and seem to occur more often with rapid (<1 hour) infusion of the first dose. This has important implications in the preoperative dosing of prophylactic antibiotics because vancomycin is sometimes used in situations in which a synthetic prosthesis will be implanted. Because the antibiotic needs to be completely infused at least 30 minutes before skin incision, vancomycin infusion should be given over at least 1 hour. The symptoms are relieved by antihistamines. Pretreatment with antihistamines can reduce the symptoms. If the symptoms/signs develop, the vancomycin should be stopped.

Reference: Sivagnanam S, Deleu D: Red man syndrome, *Crit Care* 7:119–120, 2003.

23. C. In humans, the main substrates for gluconeogenesis are lactate, pyruvate, amino acids, and, to a lesser extent, glycerol. Alanine is the most important amino acid precursor in gluconeogenesis. The gut is a major source of alanine release. As such, the gut plays an important role in gluconeogenesis.

24. C. Cachexia is a progressive wasting syndrome characterized by extensive loss of adipose tissue and skeletal muscle. It occurs in approximately one half of all cancer patients and is most prominent in upper gastrointestinal cancers, particularly pancreatic, as well as lung cancer, whereas it is noticeably absent in breast cancer. Patients with cancer often have anorexia, but the energy deficit alone does not explain the pathogenesis of cachexia. Proteolysis-inducing factor has been found in the urine in a large proportion of patients with weight loss due to pancreatic cancer. It is thought that proteolysis-inducing factor induces catabolism in muscle cells and activates the ubiquitin-proteasome pathway in muscle. Eicosapentaenoic acid, found in oily fish, effectively attenuates protein degradation in cachectic muscle by inhibiting the increased proteasome expression and has held initial promise in stabilizing body weight in cachectic cancer patients. However, a recent randomized controlled study failed to observe significant objective or subjective improvement in patients receiving eicosapentaenoic acid compared with placebo.

References: Bruera E, Strasser F, Palmer J, et al: Effect of fish oil on appetite and other symptoms in patients with advanced cancer and anorexia/cachexia: a doubleblind, placebo-controlled study, *J Clin Oncol* 21:129–134, 2003.

Tisdale M: Pathogenesis of cancer cachexia, *J Support Oncol* 1:159–168, 2003.

25. C. Zinc deficiency has numerous manifestations, including alopecia, poor wound healing, immunosuppression, night blindness or photophobia, impaired taste or smell, neuritis, and a variety of skin disorders. Copper deficiency manifests as microcytic anemia, pancytopenia, depigmentation, and osteopenia. It has been observed in patients receiving long-term parenteral nutrition. Chromium is necessary for the adequate utilization of glucose, and deficiency is often manifest as a sudden diabetic state in which blood sugar is difficult to control, along with peripheral neuropathy and encephalopathy. Molybdenum deficiency is characterized by the toxic accumulation of sulfur-containing amino acids and encephalopathy. Selenium deficiency may result in diffuse skeletal myopathy and cardiomyopathy, loss of pigmentation, and erythrocyte macrocytosis.

26. A. Liver dysfunction is commonly observed in patients receiving TPN. It develops in 40% to 60% of infants who require long-term TPN for intestinal failure. The clinical spectrum includes cholestasis, cholelithiasis, hepatic fibrosis with progression to biliary cirrhosis, and the development of portal hypertension and liver failure. Predisposing factors include short gut syndrome, a history of bacterial overgrowth, and recurrent sepsis or a chronic inflammatory state. Lack of enteral feeding contributes by leading to reduced gut hormone secretion, decreased bile flow, and biliary stasis. Deficiencies in particular nutrients such as carnitine, taurine, cysteine, and S-adenosyl methionine are also implicated in TPN-related liver disease. Hepatic steatosis may be improved with carnitine supplementation, but there is no evidence that it will reverse TPN-related liver damage. Hepatic dysfunction is more serious and lethal in infants dependent on TPN compared with adults. Even when enteral feeding is begun and TPN is discontinued, hepatic dysfunction may persist and may progress to cirrhosis and death. The ultimate solution is combined liver and small bowel transplantation.

Reference: Kelly D: Liver complications of pediatric parenteral nutrition: epidemiology, *Nutrition* 14:153–157, 1998.

27. A. Substances such as growth hormone, glutamine, and fiber appear to exert bowel-specific trophic effects and directly or indirectly may influence nutrient absorption. In one randomized study, there were modest improvements in electrolyte absorption and delayed gastric emptying, but no improvements in small bowel morphology, stool losses, or macronutrient absorption.

References: Byrne T, Morrissey T, Nattakom T, et al: Growth hormone, glutamine, and a modified diet enhance nutrient absorption in patients with severe short bowel syndrome, *JPEN J Parenter Enteral Nutr* 19:296–302, 1995.

Scolapio J, Camilleri M, Fleming C: Effect of growth hormone, glutamine, and diet on adaptation in short-bowel syndrome: a randomized, controlled study, *Gastroenterology* 113:1074–1081, 1997.

28. B. Provided nutritional intervention is limited to the group with severe malnutrition and immunologic dysfunction. In the Veterans Affairs multicenter trial, in patients who were judged severely malnourished and who had lost more than 15% of their body weight, preoperative nutritional intervention for 7 to 10 days decreased operative septic complications. However, in the group stratified as having mild to moderate malnutrition, the decrease in surgical complications was more than offset by the increase in catheter-related infectious complications. TPN-induced hyperglycemia is likely a contributor to adverse outcomes. Thus, improperly administered TPN increased the risk of catheter-related and noncatheter-related infection. Buzby proposed the following guidelines: (1) Postoperative TPN should be considered when oral or enteral feeding is not anticipated within 7 to 10 days in previously well-nourished patients or within 5 to 7 days in previously malnourished or critically ill patients. (2) Preoperative TPN should be considered in patients who cannot or should not eat or receive enteral feedings if the operation must be delayed for more than 3 to 5 days. (3) Preoperative TPN should be considered in the most severely malnourished surgical candidates if an operative delay is not contraindicated. In patients with only mild to moderate degrees of malnutrition, preoperative TPN is not indicated.

References: Bozzetti F, Gavazzi C, Miceli R, et al: Perioperative total parenteral nutrition in malnourished, gastrointestinal cancer patients: a randomized, clinical trial, *JPEN J Parenter Enteral Nutr* 24:7–14, 2000.

Buzby G: Overview of randomized clinical trials of total parenteral nutrition for malnourished surgical patients, *World J Surg* 17:173–177, 1993.

29. B. The Child classification system identifies the severity of liver dysfunction from mild to moderate to severe and has been used as a predictor of survival. It was originally designed as a predictor of survival after portosystemic shunting in patients with bleeding varices. The class is determined by five graded factors scored from 1 to 3 based on the presence of hepatic encephalopathy, total serum bilirubin level, presence of ascites, albumin level, and nutritional status. Class A is a score of 5 to 6, Class B is 7 to 9, and Class C is 10 to 15. These criteria were modified by Pugh to create Child-Pugh classes replacing nutritional status, which was deemed too subjective, with prothrombin time. More recently, the MELD score was developed. It was designed to calculate a patient's likelihood of dying within 3 months of their liver disease to better prioritize patients awaiting liver transplantation. The MELD score requires the total serum bilirubin, international normalized ratio (INR), and creatinine and is calculated using the following equation: $3.8 \times \log(e)$ (bilirubin mg/dL) + $11.2 \times \log(e)$ (INR) + $9.6 \log(e)$ (creatinine mg/dL). Seemingly cumbersome to use, the score can easily be calculated on various websites. Scores range from 6 to 40. The MELD score is now being applied to risk stratification in cirrhotics undergoing surgery. In a large Mayo Clinic study, the MELD score, age, and American Society of Anesthesiologists class were found to quantify the risk of mortality postoperatively in patients with cirrhosis, independently of the procedure performed. The 30-day mortality ranged from 5.7% (MELD score, <8) to more than 50% (MELD score, >20) in patients who underwent a wide array of operations.

Reference: Teh S, Nagorney D, Stevens S, et al: Risk factors for mortality after surgery in patients with cirrhosis, *Gastroenterology* 132:1261–1269, 2007.

30. B. This case represents a cecal fistula. The most common causes are slippage of the suture or necrosis of the remaining appendiceal stump, leading to leakage of the enteric contents into the peritoneal cavity. Much less commonly, distal colon obstruction can cause this condition and is usually the result of external compression from an intraperitoneal abscess. Cecal fistulas are low-output fistulas and are not associated with losses of large amounts of fluid, electrolytes, and nutrients. Therefore, TPN is not necessary to maintain adequate nutrition. Spontaneous closure is promoted in as many as 75% of patients maintained on low-residue diets because absorption is mostly complete by the time the contents reach the cecum.

31. C. Duodenal stump blowout occurs after Billroth II operations, where back-pressure on the duodenal stump results in breakdown of the stump closure, leading to abdominal sepsis. Acute pancreatitis is associated postoperatively with Billroth II gastrectomy and jejunostomy, in which increased intraduodenal pressure can cause backflow of activated enzymes into the pancreas. Wound dehiscence is characterized as sudden dramatic drainage of relatively large volumes of a clear, salmon-colored fluid. Acalculous cholecystitis can also occur postoperatively; however, the clinical presentation would mainly consist of right upper quadrant pain. Intra-abdominal hemorrhage would be less likely.

32. B. All are consequences of acute renal failure; however, hyperkalemia is generally the most immediately life-threatening complication and can predispose the patient to VT and fibrillation.

33. D. Fat embolism syndrome is characterized by respiratory distress, altered mental status, and petechiae. Marrow from the fracture site enters the pulmonary vasculature. Early immobilization of fractures reduces the incidence of fat embolism syndrome, and the risk is further reduced by operative fixation rather than conservative management.

Reference: Pinney S, Keating J, Meek R: Fat embolism syndrome in isolated femoral fractures: does timing of nailing influence incidence? *Injury* 29:149–167, 1998.

34. A. Wound dehiscence presents as sudden drainage of relatively large volumes of a clear, salmon-colored fluid. The management depends in part on the timing of the dehiscence and whether the dehiscence appears to be localized or involves a large area of the midline wound.

A minor area of dehiscence that occurs 10 days after surgery can be managed with local wound care and acceptance that an incisional hernia will ensue. Conversely, early dehiscence or large areas of dehiscence are more apt to progress to evisceration, which then becomes a surgical emergency. In this particular patient, the early nature of the dehiscence, coupled with the tense distention would mandate operative re-exploration because the patient is at significant risk of evisceration. If the presentation were more delayed and less dramatic, the choice would be acceptable, provided the wound was probed with a cotton-tip applicator. If probing with the applicator reveals a large segment of the wound that is open all the way to the omentum and intestines, the patient should still be immediately taken back to the operating room.

35. D. Hepatorenal syndrome is a functional renal problem that likely results from relative hypovolemia, systemic vasodilation, and intense vasoconstriction of the renal circulation. The syndrome is probably the final consequence of extreme underfilling of the arterial circulation secondary to arterial vasodilation in the splanchnic vascular bed. It is characterized by azotemia, oliguria, a very low urinary sodium (<10 mEq/day), and a high urine osmolarity. Prognosis is poor. Type 1 is mainly associated with acute liver failure or alcoholic cirrhosis, but it can develop in any other form of liver failure. It is characterized by rapid deterioration of renal function, with a marked increase in serum creatinine and blood urea nitrogen over a short period of time. Optimal treatment is liver transplantation, but the patients may not receive the transplant in time. Hyponatremia and hyperkalemia are typical. Type 2 is a more stable form. The decrease in the glomerular filtration rate and the increase in creatinine are moderate. It occurs mostly in patients with a relatively preserved hepatic function. In one study, a combination of midodrine, an α-agonist, and octreotide improved 30-day survival.

Reference: Ginès P, Guevara M, Arroyo V, Rodés J: Hepatorenal syndrome, *Lancet* 362:1819–1827, 2003.

36. A. The Westermark sign represents a focus of vasoconstriction seen distal to a *pulmonary embolus* (PE). The sign results from a combination of the dilation of the pulmonary arteries proximal to the embolus and the collapse of the distal vasculature, creating the appearance of a sharp cutoff on a chest radiograph. The sign has low sensitivity and high specificity. Although the chest radiograph is abnormal in the majority of PE cases, the Westermark sign is seen in only 2% of patients.

37. D. Smoking is a predictor of postoperative pulmonary complications. However, several studies have reported that current smokers who quit or reduced cigarette consumption within 2 months before surgery were more likely to develop a complication compared with those who did not. The respiratory epithelium is altered in smokers, and poor ciliary activity combined with the production of more viscous mucus leads smokers to be more reliant on coughing to clear secretions from their lungs. Several days after patients have stopped smoking, there may be a transient increase in sputum volume. Postoperative lung expansion modalities such as options A, B, and C each reduce postoperative pulmonary complications, but there is no added benefit from using all three. Routine use of a nasogastric tube may increase aspiration risk because the tube stents open the gastroesophageal junction. However, selective use in patients with nausea, bloating, and/or vomiting is probably protective.

References: Bluman L, Mosca L, Newman N, et al: Preoperative smoking habits and postoperative pulmonary complications, *Chest* 113:883–889, 1998.

Lawrence V, Cornell J, Smetana G: Strategies to reduce postoperative pulmonary complications after noncardiothoracic surgery: systematic review for the American College of Physicians, *Ann Intern Med* 144:596–608, 2006.

38. D. A serum albumin less than 3.5 g/dL is the single most important laboratory predictor of adverse pulmonary events after surgery. Blood urea nitrogen (>21 mg/dL) is also useful, although the correlation is not as strong. Routine spirometry for all operations does not seem to add value beyond a careful history and physical examination. An exception for the use of spirometry would be for lung resection.

References: Lawrence V, Cornell J, Smetana G: Strategies to reduce postoperative pulmonary complications after noncardiothoracic surgery: systematic review for the American College of Physicians, *Ann Intern Med* 144:596–608, 2006.

Qaseem A, Snow V, Fitterman N, et al: Risk assessment for and strategies to reduce perioperative pulmonary complications for patients undergoing noncardiothoracic surgery: a guideline from the American College of Physicians, *Ann Intern Med* 144:575–580, 2006.

39. C. The Revised Cardiac Index is a validated and easily calculated score to assess cardiac risk. One point each is assigned for (1) history of coronary artery disease, (2) insulin dependence, (3) history of a cerebrovascular event,

(4) creatinine more than 2.0 mg/dL, (5) history of congestive heart failure, and (6) high-risk surgery (aortic, thoracic, major abdominal). Based on this index, the predicted major cardiac complication rates are as follows: 0 points, class I, very low risk (0.4% complication rate); 1 point, class II, low risk (0.9% complication rate); 2 points, class III, moderate risk (6.6% complication rate); 3 or more points, class IV, high risk (>11% complication rate). Smoking is not an independent risk factor for adverse cardiac events.

Reference: Lee T, Marcantonio E, Mangione C, et al: Derivation and prospective validation of a simple index for prediction of cardiac risk of major noncardiac surgery, *Circulation* 100:1043–1049, 1999.

40. B. Vitamin A has been shown to counter the deleterious effects of both corticosteroids and radiation and steroids on wound healing in both human and animal studies. The benefit was seen even in patients who were not vitamin deficient. The benefit was seen with both topical application and systemic administration. The mechanism of action of vitamin A is thought to be reversal of the anti-inflammatory effects of steroids. Vitamin A increases lysosomal membrane lability, increases macrophage influx and activation, and stimulates collagen synthesis.

References: Chen CL, Shapiro ML, Angood PB: Patient safety. In Brunicardi FC, Andersen DK, Billiar TR, et al, editors: *Schwartz's principles of surgery*, ed 9, New York, 2010, McGraw-Hill, pp 313–342.

Kulaylat MN, Dayton MT: Surgical complications. In Townsend CM Jr, Beauchamp RD, Evers BM, Mattox KL, editors: *Sabiston textbook of surgery: the biological basis of modern surgical practice*, ed 18, Philadelphia, 2008, WB Saunders, pp 228–370.

Tawa NE, Fischer JE: Metabolism in surgical patients. In Townsend CM Jr, Beauchamp RD, Evers BM, Mattox KL, editors: *Sabiston textbook of surgery: the biological basis of modern surgical practice*, ed 18, 2008, pp 143–190.

Surgical Infection 25

1. The risk of surgical site infection is dependent on all of the following EXCEPT:

   A. American Society of Anesthesiologists physical status
   B. Length of operation
   C. Serum glucose level
   D. Body temperature
   E. Hemoglobin level

2. A 55-year-old man with renal failure secondary to diabetes is scheduled to undergo placement of an arteriovenous polytetrafluoroethylene graft for hemodialysis access. Which of the following best describes the use of prophylactic antibiotics in this patient?

   A. Prophylactic antibiotics are not indicated.
   B. One dose of antibiotics should be given the night before surgery and a second one in the operating room.
   C. One dose of antibiotics should be given 1 hour before surgery.
   D. One dose of antibiotics should be given just before skin incision.
   E. Antibiotics should be given on call to the operating room and continued for 24 hours after surgery.

3. Prophylactic antibiotics are least indicated in which of the following situations?

   A. Duodenal ulcer surgery in a patient receiving H_2 receptor antagonist
   B. Inguinal hernia
   C. Aortobifemoral bypass
   D. Breast surgery
   E. Cholecystectomy for symptomatic cholelithiasis

4. Forty-eight hours after total mastectomy, high fever, diarrhea, vomiting, redness of the skin of the entire body, and hypotension develop in a 30-year-old patient. The mastectomy incision appears unremarkable. The following day diffuse desquamation develops. The most likely etiology is:

   A. *Clostridium perfringens*
   B. *Clostridium difficile*
   C. β-Hemolytic *Streptococcus*
   D. *Staphylococcus aureus*
   E. *Staphylococcus epidermidis*

5. A 60-year-old man presents with gas gangrene of his left leg requiring below-knee amputation. Wound cultures were positive for *Clostridium septicum*. Additional work-up should include:

   A. Head computed tomography scan
   B. Bronchoscopy
   C. Colonoscopy
   D. Human immunodeficiency virus serology
   E. Chest computed tomography scan

6. A 30-year-old government worker opens an envelope and finds a white powdery substance inside. Gram stain of the substance reveals bipolar safety pin–shaped, gram-negative organisms. Postexposure prophylaxis would consist of:

   A. Chloramphenicol
   B. Ciprofloxacin
   C. Amoxicillin
   D. Doxycycline
   E. Gentamicin

7. The leading cause of empyema is:

   A. Pneumonia
   B. Pulmonary infarct
   C. Trauma
   D. Subphrenic abscess
   E. Boerhaave syndrome

8. All of the following are true regarding gentamicin EXCEPT:

   A. It has poor activity against streptococci.
   B. It has a high ratio of therapeutic to toxic levels.
   C. It is toxic to the eighth cranial nerve.
   D. It has some synergism with penicillin against *Enterococcus*.
   E. It has no activity against anaerobes.

9. Peripheral neuropathy with prolonged use is most commonly associated with:

   A. Clindamycin
   B. Metronidazole
   C. Ciprofloxacin
   D. Gentamicin
   E. Vancomycin

10. Vancomycin-resistant *Enterococcus* is treated with:

    A. Azithromycin
    B. Clindamycin
    C. Linezolid
    D. Levofloxacin
    E. Ciprofloxacin

11. All of the following are true regarding tetanus EXCEPT:

    A. The median incubation period is 7 to 8 days.
    B. Wounds should be cleaned extensively and necrotic tissue débrided.
    C. It can develop without any obvious history of injury.
    D. Immunization is indicated even after having survived tetanus.
    E. The diagnosis is established by demonstrating the organisms in a wound.

12. Bacteremia from which of the following organisms is associated with colon cancer?

    A. *Streptococcus bovis*
    B. *C. difficile*
    C. Methicillin-resistant *S. aureus*
    D. *Helicobacter pylori*
    E. *Streptococcus viridans*

13. All of the following antibiotics are useful in the treatment of methicillin-resistant *S. aureus* EXCEPT:

    A. Vancomycin
    B. Linezolid
    C. Rifampin
    D. Amoxicillin
    E. Synercid

14. The most clinically important viral infection in transplant recipients is:

    A. Varicella zoster
    B. Cytomegalovirus (CMV)
    C. Epstein-Barr virus
    D. Hepatitis C virus
    E. Herpes simplex

15. Antibiotics with good bile penetration have higher bile concentrations than serum. Which of the following has *lower* biliary concentrations than serum?

    A. Mezlocillin
    B. Gentamicin
    C. Cefoxitin
    D. Piperacillin
    E. Nafcillin

16. All of the following bacteria are associated with the production of exotoxin EXCEPT:

    A. *Streptococcus pyogenes*
    B. *Bacteroides fragilis*
    C. *Clostridium tetani*
    D. *S. aureus*
    E. *C. perfringens*

17. Which of the following antibiotics is most commonly associated with the development of aplastic anemia?

    A. Amphotericin
    B. Tetracycline
    C. Chloramphenicol
    D. Erythromycin
    E. Clindamycin

18. Which of the following are true regarding hepatitis?

    A. Postexposure hepatitis C immunoglobulin confers protection from infection.
    B. The most common cause of chronic liver disease in the United States is hepatitis B.
    C. The majority of patients with hepatitis B infection progress to a chronic carrier state.
    D. Peginterferon alfa-2b plus ribavirin is ineffective in chronic hepatitis C.
    E. Hepatitis C has a low rate of seroconversion from an accidental solid needle stick.

19. Postexposure prophylaxis for anthrax is best achieved with:

    A. Ciprofloxacin
    B. Second-generation cephalosporin
    C. Rifampin
    D. Trimethoprim-sulfamethoxazole
    E. Clindamycin, rifampin, and ciprofloxacin

20. All of the following are true regarding necrotizing soft tissue except:
    A. Less than half of patients present with hard signs of necrotizing infection.
    B. Laboratory values are helpful in distinguishing these infections from cellulitis.
    C. The majority of these infections are due to *Clostridium* species.
    D. Patients should undergo a planned second-look débridement.
    E. Surgical delays lead to significantly increased mortality.

Answers

1. E. The risk of the development of surgical site infections is related to several factors, including microbial contamination during surgery, length of the operation, and patient factors such as diabetes, nutritional state, obesity, and immunosuppression (cancer, renal failure, immunosuppressive drugs). The National Nosocomial Infection Surveillance risk index is a useful tool to assess the risk of wound infection. This index includes (1) American Society of Anesthesiologists score higher than 2, (2) class III or IV wounds, and (3) duration of an operation greater than the 75th percentile for that particular procedure. Wounds are classified as clean (class I) (e.g., hernia repair, breast biopsy), clean/contaminated (class II) (e.g., cholecystectomy, elective gastrointestinal surgery), contaminated (class III) (e.g., bowel injury from trauma or inadvertent enterotomy), and dirty (class IV) (e.g., perforated appendicitis, diverticulitis, necrotizing soft-tissue infections [NSTIs]). Hemoglobin level has not been shown to increase the risk of wound infection. In a randomized study of patients undergoing colorectal surgery, surgical wound infections were found in 19% who were permitted to become hypothermic but in only 6% who were actively kept normothermic. In a randomized study of clean surgery (breast, varicose vein, hernia), those who were actively warmed 30 minutes before surgery had only a 5% wound infection rate versus 14% in warmed patients. Active control of glucose via continuous infusion was shown to decrease sternal wound infection in diabetic patients undergoing cardiac surgery. The main concern with aggressive glucose control, however, is that it may incite episodes of hypoglycemia. A recent study also highlighted the risk of blood transfusion in wound infection, likely the result of its immunosuppressive effects.

References: Campbell D, Henderson W, Englesbe M, et al: Surgical site infection prevention: the importance of operative duration and blood transfusion—results of the First American College of Surgeons–National Surgical Quality Improvement Program Best Practices Initiative, *J Am Coll Surg* 207:810–820, 2008.

Furnary A, Zerr K, Grunkemeier G, et al: Continuous intravenous insulin infusion reduces the incidence of deep sternal wound infection in diabetic patients after cardiac surgical procedures, *Ann Thorac Surg* 67:352–360, 1999.

Kurz A, Sessler DI, Lenhardt R: Perioperative normothermia to reduce the incidence of surgical-wound infection and shorten hospitalization: Study of Wound Infection and Temperature Group, *N Engl J Med* 334:1209–1215, 1996.

Melling A, Ali B, Scott E, et al: Effects of preoperative warming on the incidence of wound infection after clean surgery: a randomized controlled trial, *Lancet* 358:876–880, 2001.

2. C. Arteriovenous graft construction is considered a clean case. However, prophylactic antibiotics are recommended any time a prosthetic device is inserted due to the potentially catastrophic results of an infected prosthesis. The organisms that pose the greatest risk in clean cases are skin flora (*Staphylococcus* and *Streptococcus*). The timing of antibiotic administration is important. The dose should be given 1 hour before skin incision to achieve the best antibiotic tissue concentration at the time of the incision.

Reference: Classen D, Evans R, Pestotnik S, et al: The timing of prophylactic administration of antibiotics and the risk of surgical-wound infection, *N Engl J Med* 326:281–286, 1992.

3. E. In general, prophylactic systemic antibiotics are not indicated for patients undergoing low-risk, clean operations when no insertion of a graft or foreign material occurs. This is predicated on the fact that the risk of infection is so low (<1%) that antibiotics will not effectively reduce it further, and the liberal use of antibiotics has the potential of introducing resistance or *C. difficile*. The use of H_2 receptor antagonists alters the stomach and duodenal pH, facilitating bacterial growth. Although one would expect a low incidence of wound infection in breast and hernia surgery, in a large randomized study, wound infection occurred in 12.2% of breast surgery patients without antibiotic prophylaxis and in 6.6% with antibiotics. Similarly, the wound infection rate was 4.2% without antibiotics and 2.3% with them.

Furthermore, inguinal hernia involves the use of mesh. Several prospective, randomized studies have been performed for the use of antibiotics in uncomplicated laparoscopic cholecystectomy and have shown no benefit to prophylactic antibiotics.

References: Ilig KA, Schmidt E, Cavanaugh J, et al: Are prophylactic antibiotics required for elective laparoscopic cholecystectomy? *J Am Coll Surg* 184:353–356, 1997.

Platt R, Zaleznik D, Hopkins C, et al: Perioperative antibiotic prophylaxis for herniorrhaphy and breast surgery, *N Engl J Med* 322:153–160, 1990.

4. D. A rare cause of infection in the first 48 hours after an operation is wound toxic shock syndrome. Toxic shock syndrome is an acute onset, multiorgan illness that resembles severe scarlet fever. It was originally described in menstruating women in association with tampon use, but it has been increasingly recognized in postsurgical wounds. In the majority of cases, the illness is caused by *S. aureus* strains that express toxic shock syndrome toxin-1, enterotoxin B, or enterotoxin C. It has rarely been described in association with *S. pyogenes* (group A streptococci). Half of the postsurgical toxic shock syndrome cases present early, within 48 hours of operation. Symptoms include fever, diarrhea, vomiting, diffuse redness of the skin, and hypotension. This is followed a day or two later by diffuse desquamation. Physical examination findings of wound infection are often unremarkable. Wound drainage and antibiotics are recommended. Administration of clindamycin may be helpful because it inhibits exotoxin production.

Reference: Reingold A, Dan B, Shands K, et al: Toxic-shock syndrome not associated with menstruation: a review of 54 cases, *Lancet* 1:1–4, 1982.

5. C. *C. septicum* has been associated with colonic and hematologic malignancies. In a review of the literature involving 162 cases of *C. septicum* infection, 81% had an associated malignancy, including 34% with colon carcinoma and 40% with a hematologic malignancy. In 37%, the malignancy was occult. The survival rate was only 35%.

Reference: Kornbluth A, Danzig J, Bernstein L: *Clostridium septicum* infection and associated malignancy: report of 2 cases and review of the literature, *Medicine (Baltimore)* 68:30–37, 1989.

6. D. Doxycycline is prescribed for postexposure prophylaxis to *Yersinia pestis*. The bacteria are transmitted via aerosolized particles or fleas from rodents. Aerosolized particles cause epidemic pneumonia manifested by blood-tinged sputum, and painful lesions called *buboes* result if fleas are carriers. Patients having a bubo associated with fever and severe malaise should be suspected of having plague. Diagnosis is confirmed with an aspirate of the bubo and a direct antibody stain to detect the bacillus. The typical morphology is that of a bipolar safety pin–shaped, gram-negative organism.

7. A. Bronchopulmonary infection (pneumonia) is the most common cause of empyema. In one large series, it accounted for 73% of cases.

Reference: Alfageme I, Muñoz F, Peña N, et al: Empyema of the thorax in adults: etiology, microbiologic findings, and management, *Chest* 103:839–843, 1993.

8. B. Gentamicin is an aminoglycoside, which is effective against gram-negative rods. It is most active against *Enterococcus* and *Serratia*. It has poor activity against *Streptococcus*. It has some synergism with penicillin or vancomycin against enterococci. It has no activity against anaerobes. It is associated with nephrotoxicity and eighth nerve toxicity. It has a low ratio of therapeutic to toxic levels.

9. B. Metronidazole is effective against anaerobes and protozoa. It is used for perforated bowel, pelvic inflammatory disease, *H. pylori* infections, amebic dysentery, and amebic liver abscesses, among others. It has an Antabuse (disulfiram)-like reaction so it cannot be used in conjunction with alcohol. It is cleared by the liver. Prolonged use has been associated with peripheral neuropathy.

10. C. *Enterococcus* has generally been treated with β-lactams such as ampicillin, aminoglycosides such as gentamicin, or glycopeptides such as vancomycin. With the emergence of vancomycin-resistant *Enterococcus*, there are fewer options for treatment. Options for such situations include Zyvox (linezolid) and Synercid (quinupristin/dalfopristin).

11. E. Tetanus is an acute, often fatal, disease caused by an exotoxin produced by *C. tetani* that enters the body through a wound. It is characterized by generalized rigidity and convulsive spasms of skeletal muscles. It typically involves the jaw muscles (hence the term *lockjaw*) and neck and then becomes generalized. The back spasms can be so intense that they can lead to spontaneous vertebral fractures. Intense facial spasms can lead to a classic appearance known as risus sardonicus (sardonic smile, a smile of contempt or of pain). The causative organism is a gram-positive anaerobic rod. *C. tetani* produces two exotoxins: tetanolysin and tetanospasmin. Tetanospasmin is a neurotoxin and causes the clinical manifestations of tetanus. The toxins act at several sites within the central nervous system, including the peripheral motor end plates, spinal cord, brain, and sympathetic nervous system. The toxin interferes with the release of neurotransmitters, blocking inhibitor impulses, leading to unopposed muscle contraction and spasm. There are no laboratory findings that are characteristic of tetanus. Culture of the wound or blood is not helpful. The diagnosis is clinical. Treatment includes human tetanus immunoglobulin, airway protection by early placement of a tracheostomy, intravenous (IV) magnesium for muscle spasm prevention, high calorie replenishment, and benzodiazepines. Due to the extreme potency of the toxin, contracting tetanus does not result in immunity. Active immunization with tetanus toxoid should begin or continue as soon as the person's condition has stabilized.

12. A. The association between *S. bovis* bacteremia or endocarditis and colonic neoplasia has been appreciated for many years. In several small studies of patients with *S. bovis* bacteremia, colon cancer was noted in 16% to 32% after a diagnostic work-up that was usually initiated because of an *S. bovis* infection. Stool cultures of patients with colon cancer are more likely to grow *S. bovis* compared with stool cultures of patients without colon cancer.

Reference: Klein R, Recco R, Catalano M, et al: Association of *Streptococcus bovis* with carcinoma of the colon, *N Engl J Med* 297:800–802, 1977.

13. D. All are useful in the treatment of methicillin-resistant *S. aureus* except amoxicillin. Another useful drug is Zyvox (linezolid).

14. B. CMV is a member of the herpesvirus family and is the most clinically significant viral infection in transplant recipients. In healthy, nonimmunosuppressed individuals, CMV is clinically silent or mild. In immunosuppressed transplant recipients, CMV is associated with increased mortality and graft loss. In one large study of liver transplant recipients, CMV infection was found to be an independent risk factor for graft failure. In a cardiac transplantation study, CMV-negative recipients of CMV-positive donor hearts had impaired distal epicardial endothelial function and an increased incidence of cardiovascular-related events and death during follow-up.

References: Burak K, Kremers W, Batts K, et al: Impact of cytomegalovirus infection, year of transplantation, and donor age on outcomes after liver transplantation for hepatitis C, *Liver Transpl* 8:362–369, 2002.

Petrakopoulou P, Kübrich M, Pehlivanli S, et al: Cytomegalovirus infection in heart transplant, *Circulation* 110(Suppl 1): II207–II212, 2004.

15. B. All of the antibiotics except gentamicin achieve good bile concentrations. Gentamicin achieves higher levels in the serum than in the biliary system.

16. B. *S. pyogenes* produces streptokinase, which acts as a fibrinolytic. *B. fragilis* does not produce an exotoxin and has defective lipopolysaccharide and lipid A. *C. tetani* produces tetanospasmin, which acts as a neurotoxin. *S. aureus* produces hemolysin and leukocidin, which damage plasma membranes of the host, and exfoliatin, which cleaves desmosomes. *C. perfringens* produces heat-labile enterotoxin causing watery diarrhea.

17. C. Chloramphenicol is a bacteriostatic antimicrobial that inhibits protein synthesis. Because of its mode of action, it is effective against a wide range of bacteria including gram positives (most strains of methicillin-resistant *S. aureus*) and gram negatives. Because it is inexpensive, it is widely used in low-income countries, but in wealthier countries, it is rarely used due to the very rare side effect of aplastic anemia. Aplastic anemia in this setting is often fatal and can occur even weeks after the drug is discontinued.

18. E. Hepatitis C virus is the leading cause of death from liver disease in the United States. Blood products were at one time the leading source of hepatitis C virus transmission. They have become an extremely rare source since 1992, when blood was first effectively tested. In the United States, illicit drug injection is the chief mode of transmission. Postexposure prophylaxis with immunoglobulin has not been effective in preventing infection, nor has the use of antiviral agents for postexposure prophylaxis. A chronic carrier state develops in 75% to 80% of patients with hepatitis C, with chronic liver disease occurring in three fourths of patients with chronic infection. Hepatitis C is not transmitted efficiently during occupational exposures to blood. Seroconversion rates after an accidental needle stick are reported to be 1% to 4% (although this is higher than human immunodeficiency virus and hepatitis B). In one large study, the seroconversion rate was 1.2% for hollow-bore needle sticks and 0% from solid suture needles, sharp object injuries, and mucous membrane contamination. Hepatitis B has chronic carrier rates of 0.1% to 2%. Peginterferon alfa-2b plus ribavirin has been shown to produce a sustained virologic response in chronic hepatitis C. The primary side effects are flulike symptoms and depression.

References: Krawczynski K, Alter MJ, Tankersley D, et al: Effect of immune globulin on the prevention of experimental hepatitis C virus infection, *J Infect Dis* 173:822–828, 1996.

Manns M, McHutchison J, Gordon S, et al: Peg interferon alpha-2b plus ribavirin compared with interferon alpha-2b plus ribavirin for initial treatment of chronic hepatitis C: a randomized trial, *Lancet* 358:958–965, 2001.

Puro V, Petrosillo N, Ippolito G: Risk of hepatitis C seroconversion after occupational exposures in health care workers: Italian Study Group on Occupational Risk of HIV and Other Bloodborne Infections, *Am J Infect Control* 23:273–277, 1995.

Strader DB, Wright T, Thomas DL, Seeff LB: American Association for the Study of Liver Diseases: diagnosis, management, and treatment of hepatitis C, *Hepatology* 39:1147–1171, 2004.

19. A. Postexposure prophylaxis consists of ciprofloxacin or doxycycline. Agents such as cephalosporins and bactrim are not effective against *Bacillus anthracis*. Inhalational anthrax develops after a 1- to 6-day incubation period, with nonspecific symptoms including malaise, myalgia, and fever. Over a short period, these symptoms worsen with the development of respiratory distress, chest pain, and diaphoresis. If symptoms develop in the exposed patient, the mortality rate is very high. Treatment for full-blown anthrax includes combination therapy with ciprofloxacin, clindamycin, and rifampin. Clindamycin is added to block toxin production and rifampin is added for its ability to penetrate the central nervous system and intracellular locations.

20. C. NSTIs is a broad term that encompasses infections limited to skin and subcutaneous tissue (necrotizing cellulitis) and those involving the fascia (necrotizing fasciitis) and muscle (myonecrosis). They can be extremely difficult to accurately diagnose early on because less than half present with obvious hard signs of NSTI, such as bullae, skin necrosis, gas on radiograph, and crepitus. Other signs include tense edema, violaceous skin color, severe pain, and neurologic deficit. Recently, several laboratory values have been shown to be useful in distinguishing NSTI from simple cellulitis. The LRINEC (Laboratory Risk Indicator for Necrotizing Fasciitis) score uses the total white blood cell count, hemoglobin, sodium, glucose, serum creatinine, and C-reactive protein levels. A simpler model uses an admission white blood cell count greater than 15.4×10^9/L and/or a serum sodium level less than 135 mmol/L. This latter model is more useful for its negative predictive value (99%). A low serum sodium is theorized to be the result of either sepsis-induced syndrome of inappropriate antidiuretic hormone or adrenal insufficiency. Risk factors for NSTI include diabetes, illicit IV drug abuse, immunosuppression, and liver disease. Seventy percent to 80% of NSTIs are due to multiorganisms. Of those that are caused by a single organism, *Klebsiella*, *S. pyogenes*, and *C. perfringens* are the most common. Treatment includes rapid administration of broad-spectrum antimicrobial agents, aggressive fluid resuscitation, and aggressive surgical débridement with a planned second-look débridement 12 to 24 hours later. The mortality rate remains at 20% to 40% and is higher with surgical delays, particularly beyond 24 hours. The use of hyperbaric oxygen shows some promise in the management but has not been subject to large randomized studies, which are made more difficult by the lack of widespread availability of such treatment.

References: Anaya DA, Dellinger EP: Surgical infections and choice of antibiotics. In Townsend CM Jr, Beauchamp RD, Evers BM, Mattox KL, editors: *Sabiston textbook of surgery: the biological basis of modern surgical practice*, ed 18, Philadelphia, 2008, WB Saunders, pp 299–327.

Beilman GJ, Dunn DL: Surgical infections. In Brunicardi FC, Andersen DK, Billiar TR, et al, editors: *Schwartz's principles of surgery*, ed 9, New York, 2010, McGraw-Hill, pp 113–133.

Wall D, Klein S, Black S, de Virgilio C: A simple model to help distinguish necrotizing fasciitis from nonnecrotizing soft tissue infection, *J Am Coll Surg* 191:227–231, 2000.

Wong C, Khin L, Heng K, et al: The LRINEC (Laboratory Risk Indicator for Necrotizing Fasciitis) score: a tool for distinguishing necrotizing fasciitis from other soft tissue infections, *Crit Care Med* 32:1535–1541, 2004.

Yaghoubian A, de Virgilio C, Dauphine C, et al: Use of admission serum lactate and sodium levels to predict mortality in necrotizing soft-tissue infections, *Arch Surg* 142:840–846, 2007.

Thoracic Surgery 26

1. A 65-year-old man presents with anorexia, nausea, lethargy, and hyponatremia. A chest radiograph reveals a large right upper lobe nodule. This most likely represents:
   A. Adenocarcinoma
   B. Small cell carcinoma
   C. Large cell carcinoma
   D. Carcinoid
   E. Bronchoalveolar carcinoma

2. All of the following are true regarding Lambert-Eaton myasthenic syndrome EXCEPT:
   A. More than 50% will have a small cell carcinoma of the lung.
   B. 3,4-Diaminopyridine is effective in treating symptoms.
   C. Intravenous (IV) immunoglobulin is effective in treating symptoms.
   D. Thymectomy is effective in patients in whom medical management fails.
   E. Patients present with proximal muscle weakness.

3. The most common mediastinal tumor in adults is:
   A. Neurogenic
   B. Lymphoma
   C. Thymoma
   D. Germ cell tumor
   E. Cyst

4. The most common neoplasm in the anterior mediastinum is:
   A. Lymphoma
   B. Thymoma
   C. Mediastinal cyst
   D. Germ cell tumor
   E. Mesenchymal

5. The most common cause of superior vena cava (SVC) syndrome is:
   A. Radiation therapy
   B. Post–central venous instrumentation
   C. Malignancy
   D. Infectious
   E. Idiopathic

6. Small cell carcinoma of the lung is managed by:
   A. Preoperative chemotherapy followed by surgical resection
   B. Surgical resection
   C. Radiation therapy
   D. Combination chemotherapy and radiation therapy
   E. Preoperative radiation therapy followed by surgical resection

7. The most common cause of lung abscess is:
   A. Aspiration
   B. Bronchial obstruction by tumor
   C. Pneumococcal pneumonia
   D. Pneumocystic pneumonia
   E. Tuberculosis

8. A 17-year-old boy is brought to a physician because of a painful mass in the right side of his chest. History reveals that he bruised his chest while playing football and that he has had malaise and fever. A chest radiograph reveals an expanded lesion with an onion-skin appearance in the boy's right tenth rib. The most likely diagnosis is:
   A. Osteomyelitis
   B. Tuberculosis
   C. Multiple myeloma
   D. Ewing sarcoma
   E. Fibrous dysplasia

9. Which of the following is considered an absolute contraindication to surgical resection of a primary (non–small cell) carcinoma of the lung?

   A. Invasion of the chest wall
   B. A positive ipsilateral mediastinal lymph node
   C. A malignant pleural effusion
   D. Preoperative forced expiratory volume in the first second of expiration (FEV$_1$) of only 1 L
   E. Invasion of parietal pericardium.

10. The most common type of lung cancer in a nonsmoker is:

    A. Squamous cell
    B. Adenocarcinoma
    C. Small cell
    D. Bronchoalveolar
    E. Carcinoid

11. Which of the following is not a factor in TNM staging of lung cancer?

    A. Cell type
    B. Location of tumor
    C. Size of tumor
    D. Spread of tumor to mediastinal lymph nodes
    E. Presence of malignant pleural effusion

12. Which one of the following statements is true regarding thymoma?

    A. The primary treatment modality is chemotherapy.
    B. Malignancy is determined by mitotic activity.
    C. The majority of patients with myasthenia gravis have an associated thymoma.
    D. In patients with myasthenia gravis, thymectomy results are more favorable in those without a thymoma than those with one.
    E. It is not associated with SVC syndrome.

13. A woman who had an osteogenic sarcoma of the femur removed 2 years earlier now presents with two small lesions in the right lung and one small lesion in the left lung. A metastatic work-up reveals no other abnormalities. The treatment of choice is:

    A. Bilateral wedge resections
    B. Chemotherapy
    C. Radiation therapy
    D. Immunotherapy with (bacille Calmette-Guérin) vaccine
    E. Observation

14. A 21-year-old man who was the driver in a head-on collision has a pulse rate of 140 beats per minute, respiratory rate of 36 breaths per minute, and blood pressure of 60 mm Hg palpable. His trachea is deviated to the left, with palpable subcutaneous emphysema and poor breath sounds in the right hemithorax. The most appropriate initial treatment is:

    A. Insertion of two large-bore IV lines for fluid resuscitation
    B. Intubation and ventilation
    C. Tube thoracostomy
    D. Needle thoracostomy
    E. Immediate tracheostomy

15. In the adult, the hypoxemia seen immediately after a flail chest injury is due to:

    A. The underlying pulmonary contusion
    B. Inadequate ventilation of the contralateral lung
    C. Inadequate air exchange from paradoxical movement of the chest wall
    D. Increase in dead space due to movement of air from one lung to another
    E. Pneumothorax secondary to the fractured ribs

16. Four months after prolonged intubation after a motor vehicle accident, a 40-year-old woman presents with dyspnea on exertion and stridor. Endoscopy reveals marked tracheal stenosis 4 cm in length. Management consists of:

    A. Laser ablation
    B. Bronchoscopic dilation
    C. Primary resection of all scarred segments with primary anastomosis
    D. Primary resection of all scarred segments, primary anastomosis, and temporary tracheostomy
    E. Metal stenting

17. Two weeks after a tracheostomy, sudden bright red blood is seen to be oozing from the tracheostomy site. The next step in the management of this patient is:

    A. Arteriography
    B. Immediate sternotomy
    C. Hyperinflation of the tracheostomy cuff
    D. Digital control of the bleeder
    E. Replacing the tracheostomy tube with an endotracheal tube

18. Which of the following is true regarding the trachea?

    A. Blood supply comes predominantly from the superior thyroid arteries.
    B. The rich collateral blood supply allows circumferential mobilization.
    C. As much as 50% of the trachea can be resected with a primary anastomosis.
    D. A tracheostomy tube is ideally placed through the first tracheal ring.
    E. The first complete cartilage ring is the thyroid cartilage.

19. A 45-year-old man presents with 200 mL of hemoptysis. Bleeding persists in the emergency department, although not briskly, and the patient is able to control secretions. His blood pressure is 110/70 mm Hg and his heart rate is 100 beats per minute. A chest radiograph reveals bilateral infiltrates. All of the following are true about this condition and its management EXCEPT:

    A. The patient should be placed in a Trendelenburg position.
    B. IV vasopressin should be administered.
    C. A computed tomography (CT) scan of the chest should be performed.
    D. Pulmonary arteriography with selective embolization will stop the bleeding in the majority of patients.
    E. Flexible bronchoscopy is useful in localizing the source of bleeding.

20. Superior vena cava syndrome most frequently occurs with which lung cancer type?

    A. Small cell
    B. Large cell
    C. Squamous cell
    D. Adenocarcinoma
    E. Bronchoalveolar

21. A 60-year-old male smoker presents with radicular right arm pain. A chest radiograph reveals a bulky tumor in the posterior apex of the chest in the superior sulcus. All of the following are commonly associated with this tumor EXCEPT:

    A. Ptosis
    B. Right eye meiosis
    C. Facial anhidrosis
    D. Right eye exophthalmos
    E. Non–small cell lung cancer

22. In the initial assessment of a patient being considered for lung resection, the most important pulmonary function study is:

    A. Arterial blood gas
    B. FEV_1
    C. Total lung capacity
    D. Minute ventilation
    E. Diffusing capacity of lung for carbon monoxide (D$_{LCO}$)

23. A 65-year-old woman presents with a chronic nonproductive cough of 2 months' duration. A chest radiograph reveals a 2-cm mass in the right upper lobe. A CT scan of the chest confirms the presence of the 2-cm mass corresponding to that found on the chest radiograph, which appears to be malignant, along with 5-mm nodes in the mediastinum. The next step in the management would be:

    A. Positron emission tomography (PET) scan
    B. Abdominal CT
    C. Bone scan
    D. Mediastinoscopy
    E. Brain CT

24. A 50-year-old Central American man presents with a chronic cough and a draining sinus in his left chest wall. Examination of the drainage reveals sulfur granules. Which of the following is true regarding this condition?

    A. Surgical resection is indicated.
    B. The organism involved is likely *Nocardia asteroides*.
    C. The organism involved is an anaerobe.
    D. Optimal treatment consists of trimethoprim-sulfamethoxazole.
    E. Central nervous system involvement is common.

25. Rasmussen aneurysms form in association with:

    A. Aspergillosis
    B. Mucormycoses
    C. Cryptococcosis
    D. Tuberculosis
    E. Small cell lung cancer (SCLC)

26. The most common primary chest wall malignancy is:

    A. Osteochondroma
    B. Chondrosarcoma
    C. Ewing sarcoma
    D. Plasmacytoma
    E. Primitive neuroectodermal tumors

27. A rare but well-recognized complication of bronchial artery embolization performed for massive hemoptysis is:

 A. Esophageal necrosis
 B. Pulmonary infarction
 C. Paraparesis
 D. Vocal cord paralysis
 E. Tracheal necrosis

28. A 24-year-old woman presents with recurrent episodes of right-sided pneumothorax requiring chest tube insertion. A diagnosis of a catamenial pneumothorax as the cause of recurrent pneumothorax in this patient would be supported by the finding of:

 A. *Pneumocystis*
 B. Endometriosis
 C. Cystic fibrosis
 D. Idiopathic pulmonary fibrosis
 E. Apical blebs

Answers

1. B. This patient likely has SCLC with syndrome of inappropriate secretion of antidiuretic hormone (SIADH). This paraneoplastic syndrome develops in as many as 40% of patients with SCLC. The diagnosis is made by a combination of hyponatremia, low serum osmolality, and high urine sodium and osmolality. In mild cases, treatment consists of free water restriction. In more severe cases, treatment consists of hypertonic saline with loop diuretics.

2. D. Lambert-Eaton or Eaton-Lambert myasthenic syndrome is a paraneoplastic syndrome associated with several malignancies, but in particular with small cell carcinoma. It presents with proximal muscle weakness and can be confused with myasthenia gravis. More than 50% have or will be discovered to have SCLC. The syndrome is thought to be caused by antibodies directed against presynaptic calcium channels in the neuromuscular junction that prevent the release of acetylcholine. Treatment is aimed at the underlying malignancy; however, medications shown to improve symptoms include 3,4-diaminopyridine, IV immunoglobulin, and steroids. Unlike in myasthenia gravis, neostigmine is not helpful and thymectomy is not effective.

 References: Illa I: IVIg in myasthenia gravis, Lambert Eaton myasthenic syndrome and inflammatory myopathies: current status, *J Neurol* 252(Suppl 1):I14–I18, 2005.
 Maddison P, Newsom-Davis J: Treatment for Lambert-Eaton myasthenic syndrome, *Cochrane Database Syst Rev* 18(2):CD003279, 2005.

3. A. Neurogenic tumors are the most common, consisting of 20% of all mediastinal tumors. They are most often located in the posterior mediastinum. They arise from the sympathetic ganglia, intercostal nerves, or paraganglia cells. The most common is a neurilemmoma (schwannoma). Other examples include gangliomas, neuroblastomas, and neurofibromas. Most are benign.

4. B. Thymomas are the second most common neoplasm of the mediastinum overall, and the most common anterior mediastinal mass. There is an association between thymoma

and various syndromes, including myasthenia gravis, red cell aplasia, aplastic anemia, Cushing syndrome, and hypogammaglobulinemia.

5. C. More than 80% of cases of SVC syndrome are due to malignancy. The most common malignancy is primary lung cancer, and SCLC is the most common etiology. The presence of SVC syndrome is considered a contraindication to surgical resection of the primary tumor. Relief of symptoms associated with SVC syndrome is best achieved with endovascular stenting of the SVC. The increasing instrumentation of central veins for dialysis access and pacemaker insertion has led to an increase in SVC obstruction from scarring and fibrosis.

6. D. The overall prognosis for SCLC is poor. Patients generally present with advanced bulky disease. The term *limited SCLC* is given to patients with locoregional disease and offers the only hope for cure. In such patients, the recommendation is to administer combination chemotherapy with cisplatin and etoposide with concurrent radiation therapy, with a 5-year survival rate of only 25%. There is generally no role for surgery. The exception is the rare patient who presents with an incidentally discovered small pulmonary nodule in whom the diagnosis is not established preoperatively.

 References: Adjei A: Management of small cell cancer of the lung, *Curr Opin Pulm Med* 6:384–390, 2000.
 Ferraldeschi R, Baka S, Jyoti B, et al: Modern management of small-cell lung cancer, *Drugs* 67:2135–2152, 2007.

7. A. A lung abscess is usually the result of aspiration that results in a suppurative bacterial infection, leading to localized pulmonary parenchymal necrosis. Patients with a history of alcohol abuse, those with poor dentition and gum disease, and patients with seizure disorders are at greatest risk.

8. D. Ewing sarcoma most often presents in the pelvis, humerus, or femur. It is more common in males. Patients report pain and may have systemic symptoms of malaise and fever as well as an increased erythrocyte sedimentation rate and white blood cell count. The classic onion skin appearance on a radiograph is due to periosteal elevation and bony remodeling. The diagnosis can be confirmed by percutaneous needle biopsy. Treatment is with multimodal therapy including chemotherapy, radiation, and surgery.

9. C. Surgery is contraindicated for stages IIIB and IV. Absolute contraindications to surgical resection of primary non-SCLC include the presence of a malignant effusion, distant metastases, a positive contralateral mediastinal lymph node, and bilateral endobronchial tumor. A malignant pleural effusion makes the lesion at least a T4, which makes it at least a stage IIIB. Relative contraindications include recurrent laryngeal nerve involvement, an FEV_1 of less than 0.8 L, Horner syndrome, pericardial involvement, and SVC syndrome. The FEV_1 needs to be assessed in the context of the degree of resection planned and the anticipated postoperative FEV_1. So, for instance, if a lobectomy is planned and the lobe is already completely collapsed, the postoperative FEV_1 will not likely change. Direct extension of tumor to the parietal pericardium or diaphragm makes the lesion at least a T3 lesion and at least a stage IIB, so these findings alone are not a contraindication to surgery because patients with stage IA, IB, IIA, and IIB disease can benefit from surgical resection. Surgery may be indicated for selected patients with stage IIIA disease in combination with neoadjuvant chemotherapy and radiotherapy. A positive ipsilateral mediastinal lymph node is considered N2, which makes it at least a stage IIIA, potentially resectable, whereas a contralateral mediastinal lymph node is at least a stage IIIB. Patients with stage I have only a 50% 5-year survival rate with resection. Stage II patients have a 5-year survival rate after surgery of only 30%, whereas those with stage IIIA have a 17% 5-year survival rate. The stage IIIB survival rate is 5%, and the stage IV survival rate approaches zero.

Reference: Silvestri G, Tanoue L, Margolis M, et al: The noninvasive staging of non-small cell lung cancer: the guidelines, *Chest* 123:147S–156S, 2003.

10. B. Adenocarcinoma is the most common lung cancer in nonsmokers.

11. A. TNM staging of lung cancer assesses each of the factors listed with the exception of cell type.

12. D. Thymoma is the most common neoplasm of the anterosuperior mediastinum, and it is the second most common mediastinal tumor overall. Malignancy is determined based on evidence of local invasion of adjacent structures or capsular invasion, not on cellular or histologic characteristics. Treatment is by surgical resection. Thymomas are radiosensitive, so radiation therapy is used as an adjunct in locally advanced cases. As many as 50% of patients with thymomas have symptoms of myasthenia gravis. Conversely, less than 10% of patients with myasthenia gravis are found to have a thymoma on CT. Nevertheless, thymectomy improves or resolves symptoms of myasthenia gravis in as many as 90% of patients without a thymoma compared with only approximately 25% of patients with thymomas. Due to their location, large thymomas can present with SVC syndrome.

13. A. Prolongation of survival has been achieved with resection of isolated lung metastasis. This is particularly true for osteogenic sarcoma, but has been reported for other malignancies as well. However, several conditions must be met. Ideally, the lung metastasis presents metachronously and the primary tumor has already been controlled, the tumor must be completely resectable, and there should be no evidence of diffuse carcinomatosis. Pulmonary metastasis occurs in as many as 40% to 60% of all primary sarcomas of the limbs within 3 years, and a 30% to 50% 5-year survival rate can be achieved with metastasectomy. In general, solitary metastases have a better prognosis. However, with pulmonary metastasis due to osteogenic sarcoma, similar results have been achieved with multiple and bilateral lesions. Factors associated with survival for metastasectomy of all causes include a disease-free interval from primary tumor to initial evidence of metastasis, resectability, tumor doubling time, and number of metastases.

Reference: Antunes M, Bernardo J, Salete M, et al: Excision of pulmonary metastases of osteogenic sarcoma of the limbs, *Eur J Cardiothorac Surg* 15:592–596, 1999.

14. D. The patient has a tension pneumothorax. Advanced trauma life support protocol states that the initial management is to place a needle in the second intercostal space, midclavicular line, just above the rib using a 4.5-cm (2-inch) catheter (5-cm needle). This should be immediately followed by a tube thoracostomy. Recent studies suggest, however, that the standard recommended needle size may not be long enough to enter the thoracic cavity.

Reference: Zengerink I, Brink P, Laupland K, et al: Needle thoracostomy in the treatment of a tension pneumothorax in trauma patients: what size needle? *J Trauma* 64:111–114, 2008.

15. A. Flail chest occurs when three or more consecutive ribs are fractured in two or more locations. The result is that there is a paradoxical movement of a segment of the chest wall from this free-floating segment. This paradoxical movement, however, is not the major contributor to compromised ventilation. In fact, most patients with flail chest do not need ventilator support. In those patients in whom early respiratory failure develops, it is the result of an underlying pulmonary contusion. Pain control is another important element of management. Most patients do not need fixation of the flail segment.

References: Nason KS, Maddaus MA, Lukeitch JD: Chest wall, lung, mediastinum, and pleura. In Brunicardi FC, Andersen DK, Billiar TR, et al, editors: *Schwartz's principles of surgery*, ed 9, New York, 2010, McGraw-Hill, pp 513–590.

Pettiford B, Luketich J, Landreneau R: The management of flail chest, *Thorac Surg Clin* 17:25–33, 2007.

Varghese TK, Lau CL: The mediastinum. In Townsend CM Jr, Beauchamp RD, Evers BM, Mattox KL, editors: *Sabiston textbook of surgery: the biological basis of modern surgical practice*, ed 18, Philadelphia, 2008, WB Saunders, pp 1677–1697.

16. C. Tracheal stenosis is most commonly due to trauma from prolonged endotracheal intubation or tracheostomy. The risk of stenosis is greater for tracheostomies that are placed too high in the first tracheal ring or for those through the cricothyroid membrane because the trachea is narrowest at this point. Patients with tracheal stenosis present with stridor and dyspnea on exertion, which can be confused with asthma, and usually present within 2 to 12 weeks after decannulation/extubation. The treatment of tracheal stenosis is resection and primary anastomosis. Most patients can be immediately extubated. As much as 6 cm of trachea can be resected using laryngeal release procedures.

Reference: George M, Lang F, Pasche P, Monnier P: Surgical management of laryngotracheal stenosis in adults, *Eur Arch Otorhinolaryngol* 262:609–615, 2005.

17. C. Brisk arterial bleeding from a tracheostomy site, even if it promptly stops, must be considered to be a tracheoinnominate fistula. Patients often have a "herald" bleed before subsequent exsanguination. Factors associated with this complication include pressure necrosis from high cuff pressure, mucosal trauma from a malpositioned cannula tip, a low tracheal incision (ideally it should be placed between the second and fourth tracheal rings), radiation therapy, and prolonged intubation. It typically occurs as early as 3 days and as long as 6 weeks (average 2 weeks) after tracheostomy tube placement, and has been described after percutaneous tracheostomy techniques as well. The initial management is to try to control the bleeding. This is difficult to achieve given the inability to directly compress the innominate artery. The first step is to hyperinflate the tracheostomy cuff to try to tamponade the arterial injury. If this is unsuccessful, the tracheostomy incision should be opened widely, and a finger inserted to compress the artery against the manubrium. If this is successful, the patient should immediately be taken to the operating room. The tracheostomy tube is replaced with an orotracheal tube, and a median sternotomy is performed. The eroded segment of innominate artery is débrided and the ends are ligated.

Reference: Grant CA, Dempsey G, Harrison J, Jones T: Tracheo-innominate artery fistula after percutaneous tracheostomy: three case reports and a clinical review, *Br J Anaesth* 96:127–131, 2006.

18. C. The cricoid cartilage is the first complete cartilage ring of the airway and consists of an anterior arch and a posterior broad-based plate. The tracheal blood supply is segmental via the inferior thyroid and bronchial arteries. Each branch supplies 1 to 2 cm of the trachea. Circumferential mobilization will interrupt that blood supply. The blood supply to the trachea is segmental in nature, meaning that each entering small branch supplies a segment of 1.0 to 2.0 cm, thereby limiting circumferential mobilization to that same distance. The arteries supplying the trachea include the inferior thyroid and the bronchial arteries. The trachea has approximately 18 to 22 rings and is approximately 10 to 13 cm long. As much as about 6 cm can be resected primarily. A tracheostomy is ideally placed between the second and fourth tracheal rings.

19. D. Massive hemoptysis is generally defined as expectoration of 600 mL or more of blood within a 24-hour period. The mortality rate is as high as 30% to 50%. The first step in the management is to stabilize and protect the airway. This is achieved via placing the patient in the Trendelenburg position to assist in the clearance of blood and secretions. Other measures include administering humidified oxygen, bed rest, and giving aerosolized epinephrine and mild sedatives

to prevent excessive reflexive coughing. Desmopressin is also useful in achieving hemostasis. Subsequent studies are geared toward trying to localize the site of bleeding, but depend on the acuity of the bleed. In a patient such as the one presented, in whom bleeding is ongoing but controlled, a chest radiograph is the first study. This should be followed by bronchoscopy to localize the site of bleeding. Bronchoscopy allows determination of the side of the bleeding and helps guide arteriography. This is followed by bronchial, not pulmonary, arteriography because most bleeding arises from the bronchial circulation. If the side of bleeding cannot be determined, then bilateral bronchial arteriography is performed. If that is negative, pulmonary arteriography is recommended. In patients who present with a history of hemoptysis but who are not actively bleeding, CT is useful in helping to localize the site of the bleed. Conversely, patients who present with exsanguinating hemorrhage need to be taken emergently to the operating room, where a double-lumen endotracheal tube is inserted and iced saline lavage is used to try to stop the bleeding. A bronchial blocker can be inflated into the bronchus that is the source of bleeding and left inflated for 24 hours.

References: Hirshberg B, Biran I, Glazer M, Kramer M: Hemoptysis: etiology, evaluation, and outcome in a tertiary referral hospital, *Chest* 112:440–444, 1997.

Osaki S, Nakanishi Y, Wataya H, et al: Prognosis of bronchial artery embolization in the management of hemoptysis, *Respiration* 67:412–416, 2000.

20. A. SVC syndrome is usually of insidious onset, with gradual swelling of the arms, face, head, and neck accompanied by headache. It can less commonly present dramatically, with stridor, massive swelling, and dyspnea on exertion. It is most commonly seen with SCLC.

21. D. This patient has a Pancoast tumor. These tumors are overwhelmingly non-SCLCs (adenocarcinomas and squamous cell) that originate in the posterior apex of the chest in the superior sulcus. Due to the location, the tumor may invade the first rib, chest wall, nerves, and blood vessels, creating symptoms of apical chest wall or shoulder pain, Horner syndrome (unilateral enophthalmos, ptosis, miosis, and facial anhidrosis) from invasion of the stellate sympathetic ganglion, and radicular arm pain (from invasion of T1, and occasionally C8, brachial plexus nerve roots). Treatment is multimodal including a cisplatin-based chemotherapy with etoposide and concurrent radiotherapy as neoadjuvant treatment, followed by surgical resection, provided that there is no evidence of distant metastatic spread. Before intervention, magnetic resonance imaging of the chest is recommended to evaluate the brachial plexus or for vertebral body invasion.

Reference: Pitz C, de la Rivière A, van Swieten H, et al: Surgical treatment of Pancoast tumours, *Eur J Cardiothorac Surg* 26:202–208, 2004.

22. B. Pulmonary function studies are routinely performed when any resection greater than a wedge resection is planned. FEV_1 is regarded as being the best for predicting complications of lung resection in the initial assessment of patients. A general guide states that if the FEV_1 is greater than

2.0 L, the patient can tolerate a pneumonectomy, and if it is greater than 1.0 L, the patient can tolerate lobectomy. One must bear in mind that these rough guidelines do not factor in such things as the patient's age, body size, and predicted post-surgery FEV$_1$. Predictors of increased complications and mortality for pneumonectomy include an FEV$_1$ less than 2.0 L; maximal voluntary ventilation less than 55% of predicted; D$_{LCO}$ less than 50% of predicted; and forced expiratory flow, midexpiratory phase (FEF$_{25\%-75\%}$) less than 1.6 L/sec; and for lobectomy include an FEV$_1$ less than 1.0 L, maximal voluntary ventilation less than 40% of predicted; FEF$_{25\%-75\%}$ less than 0.6 L/sec; and D$_{LCO}$ less than 50% of predicted. If these studies are within accepted limits, no further testing is needed. If they are below these thresholds, however, further testing is recommended including quantitative ventilation-perfusion scanning, differential lung scanning, and/or exercise testing.

Reference: Datta D, Lahiri B: Preoperative evaluation of patients undergoing lung resection surgery, *Chest* 123:2096–2103, 2003.

23. A. The recommended sequential work-up for a potentially resectable lung cancer should begin with a CT scan of the chest, followed by a PET scan. If there are no mediastinal lymph nodes greater than 1 cm, the likelihood of positive lymph nodes is low (<10%), but should be confirmed with a PET scan. If the CT scan shows a mediastinal lymph node less than 1 cm or if a mediastinal lymph node lights up on PET scan, mediastinoscopy is indicated. PET scanning has replaced multiorgan scanning in the search for distant metastases to the liver, adrenal glands, and bones. If PET scanning detects potential metastasis, it is important to obtain a tissue diagnosis before denying a possible resection.

References: Nason KS, Maddaus MA, Lukeitch JD: Chest wall, mediastinum, and pleura. In Brunicardi FC, Andersen DK, Billiar TR, et al, editors: *Schwartz's principles of surgery*, ed 9, New York, 2010, McGraw-Hill, pp 573–590.

Silvestri G, Tanoue L, Margolis M, et al: The noninvasive staging of non-small cell lung cancer: the guidelines, *Chest* 123: 147S–156S, 2003.

24. C. Given the draining sinus and sulfur granules, the patient most likely has actinomycosis, a chronic disease usually caused by *Actinomyces israelii* that occurs most commonly in the head and neck region. Because of its rarity and chronicity, the diagnosis is often delayed and unrecognized. A key to the diagnosis is the finding of chronic sinuses with discharge of purulent material containing yellow-brown sulfur granules. The organisms enter the lungs via the oral cavity. The organisms are often not cultured out because they are anaerobes. Lung involvement can present with progressive pulmonary fibrosis. Prolonged, high-dose penicillin is the treatment of choice. Surgery is generally not indicated; however, pulmonary actinomycosis can easily be confused with a lung cancer, prompting surgical intervention.

Reference: Hsieh M, Liu H, Chang J, Chang C: Thoracic actinomycosis, *Chest* 104:366–370, 1993.

25. D. Active tuberculosis can lead to massive hemoptysis. Most hemoptysis is due to bronchial artery bleeding and is managed via bronchial artery embolization. Rarely, hemoptysis is due to a Rasmussen aneurysm, which is a pulmonary artery aneurysm adjacent to or within a tuberculous cavity. Such an aneurysm would be managed by pulmonary arteriography and selective distal embolization. CT scanning is useful in hemoptysis to help localize the source and guide interventional management.

Reference: Picard C, Parrot A, Boussaud V, et al: Massive hemoptysis due to Rasmussen aneurysm: detection with helicoidal CT angiography and successful steel coil embolization, *Intensive Care Med* 29:1837–1839, 2003.

26. B. Chondrosarcomas are the most common primary malignancy of the chest wall. They usually arise anteriorly. They are a low-grade malignancy and slow growing. Treatment is wide excision. They are not chemo- or radiosensitive.

27. C. Bronchial artery embolization is an effective tool for treating patients with hemoptysis because most cases arise from the bronchial circulation rather than the pulmonary artery circulation. Embolization is highly effective in stopping the hemoptysis; however, recurrent bleeding will develop in as many as 50% of patients. The blood supply to the spine (anterior spinal artery) may have a common origin with a bronchial artery, or the bronchial arteries themselves may contribute to the spinal blood supply. As such, the clinician must be aware of this potential complication.

Reference: Fraser KL, Grosman H, Hyland R, Tullis D: Transverse myelitis: a reversible complication of bronchial artery embolization in cystic fibrosis, *Thorax* 52:99–101, 1997.

28. B. Catemenial pneumothorax is an uncommon cause of pneumothorax in women that occurs around the time of menstruation. The exact etiology is unclear, but in most instances is associated with endometriosis and endometrial deposits on the pleura. The endometrial deposits lead to pleural irritation. Treatment with hormonal therapy has been effective in preventing recurrent attacks. In other instances, however, there is no evidence of endometriosis, and the patient does not respond to hormonal therapy. In such instances, it is postulated that air enters the pleural cavity through diaphragmatic fenestrations. Loss of the cervical mucus plug during the menstrual cycle permits air to enter from the environment into the peritoneal cavity via the fallopian tubes and into the pleural space through these congenital diaphragmatic fenestrations.

References: Nason KS, Maddaus MA, Lukeitch JD: Chest wall, lung, mediastinum, and pleura. In Brunicardi FC, Andersen DK, Billiar TR, et al, editors: *Schwartz's principles of surgery*, ed 9, New York, 2010, McGraw-Hill, pp 513–590.

Peikert T, Gillespie D, Cassivi S: Catamenial pneumothorax, *Mayo Clin Proc* 80:677–680, 2005.

Smythe WR, Reznik SI, Putnam JN: Lung. In Townsend CM Jr, Beauchamp RD, Evers BM, Mattox KL, editors: *Sabiston textbook of surgery: the biological basis of modern surgical practice*, ed 18, Philadelphia, 2008, WB Saunders, pp 1698–1748.

Sugarbaker DJ, Lukanich JM: Chest wall and pleura. In Townsend CM Jr, Beauchamp RD, Evers BM, Mattox KL, editors: *Sabiston textbook of surgery: the biological basis of modern surgical practice*, ed 18, Philadelphia, 2008, WB Saunders, pp 1655–1676.

Varghese TK, Lau CL: The mediastinum. In Townsend CM Jr, Beauchamp RD, Evers BM, Mattox KL, editors: *Sabiston textbook of surgery: the biological basis of modern surgical practice*, ed 18, Philadelphia, 2008, WB Saunders, pp 1677–1697.

Thyroid/Parathyroid 27

1. All of the following are characteristics of medullary thyroid carcinoma (MTC) EXCEPT:
   A. It is more aggressive than papillary thyroid cancer.
   B. It does not take up radioactive iodine.
   C. The majority are multicentric.
   D. The majority of patients with a palpable thyroid mass will have nodal metastasis at presentation.
   E. Chemotherapy is effective for residual disease.

2. The most accurate test for hyperthyroidism is:
   A. Free thyroxine (T_4)
   B. Total T_4
   C. Total triiodothyronine (T_3)
   D. Thyroid-stimulating hormone (TSH)
   E. Thyroid scan

3. All of the following are true regarding the blood supply to the thyroid/parathyroid glands EXCEPT:
   A. The parathyroid glands are usually supplied by the superior thyroid arteries.
   B. The superior thyroid artery is the first branch of the external carotid artery.
   C. The recurrent laryngeal nerves (RLNs) are at risk of injury during ligation of the inferior thyroid arteries.
   D. The external branch of the superior laryngeal nerve is at risk of injury when the superior laryngeal arteries are ligated.
   E. The thyroidea ima artery usually arises from the aorta.

4. All of the following are true regarding the laryngeal nerves EXCEPT:
   A. The internal branch of the superior laryngeal nerve provides sensation to the larynx.
   B. Bilateral injury to the superior laryngeal nerves often results in acute airway obstruction.
   C. The right RLN separates from the vagus after crossing the subclavian artery.
   D. The superior laryngeal nerve is both motor and sensory to the larynx.
   E. The RLNs provide motor function to the intrinsic muscles of the larynx.

5. A non-RLN:
   A. Does not exist
   B. Is more common on the left
   C. Can occur in conjunction with a recurrent nerve on the right
   D. Loops around the aorta on the right side
   E. Is less prone to injury during surgery than a recurrent nerve

6. All of the following are direct effects of parathyroid hormone (PTH) EXCEPT:
   A. Stimulates resorption of calcium and phosphate from the bone
   B. Stimulates reabsorption of calcium by the kidney
   C. Inhibits reabsorption of bicarbonate by the kidney
   D. Stimulates absorption of calcium by the small intestine
   E. Stimulates hydroxylation of 25-hydroxyvitamin D in the kidney

7. Lateral aberrant thyroid in most instances represents:
   A. Metastatic papillary carcinoma
   B. Metastatic follicular carcinoma
   C. Metastatic Hürthle cell carcinoma
   D. A congenital lesion related to thyroid descent
   E. An extension of a thyroglossal duct cyst

8. A 45-year-old woman presents with a 1.5-cm right thyroid nodule. Fine-needle aspiration (FNA) findings are consistent with papillary carcinoma. Her history is significant for radiation therapy for acne as a child. Optimal management of this patient would consist of:

    A. Right hemithyroidectomy
    B. Right hemithyroidectomy plus central lymph node dissection
    C. Total thyroidectomy
    D. Total thyroidectomy with postoperative iodine 131 (^{131}I)
    E. Total thyroidectomy plus right modified radical neck dissection

9. Which of the following is LEAST likely associated with hyperparathyroidism?

    A. Cholelithiasis
    B. Pancreatitis
    C. Osteoclastomas
    D. Diarrhea
    E. Peptic ulcer disease

10. Which of the following laboratory findings are characteristically associated with primary hyperparathyroidism?

    A. Elevated serum phosphate
    B. Increased serum chloride
    C. Decreased urinary calcium
    D. Metabolic alkalosis
    E. Elevated calcium with a decreased PTH

11. Which of the following is true regarding Hürthle cell carcinoma?

    A. It contains an abundance of oncocytic or oxyphilic cells.
    B. Lymph node metastasis is exceedingly rare.
    C. Diagnosis of malignancy is usually made by fine-needle aspiration (FNA).
    D. Residual disease is effectively treated with ^{131}I.
    E. Histologically they demonstrate Orphan Annie cells.

12. A patient presents with fatigue and bone pain. Serum calcium level is 11.1 mg/dL and PTH is elevated. The next step in the diagnostic work-up is:

    A. Operative exploration
    B. Computed tomography scan
    C. Technetium-99m sestamibi imaging
    D. Magnetic resonance imaging
    E. Ultrasound scan

13. Which of the following is true regarding follicular thyroid cancer?

    A. It is the most common thyroid malignancy.
    B. It most commonly spreads via a hematogenous route.
    C. Prophylactic nodal dissection is recommended.
    D. It is best managed by hemithyroidectomy.
    E. Multicentricity is common.

14. A 45-year-old woman presents with symptomatic primary hyperparathyroidism. All of the following would be acceptable surgical management EXCEPT:

    A. Removal of 3½ glands for parathyroid hyperplasia
    B. Removal of all four glands with autotransplantation of half of a gland in the forearm for parathyroid hyperplasia
    C. Removal of one enlarged gland with a biopsy of the other three normal-appearing glands for parathyroid adenoma
    D. Removal of one enlarged gland via mini neck incision under local anesthesia without identification of other glands for single parathyroid adenoma
    E. Removal of two glands for double parathyroid adenoma

15. Treatment of MTC consists of:

    A. Hemithyroidectomy
    B. Hemithyroidectomy with central node dissection
    C. Total thyroidectomy
    D. Total thyroidectomy with central node dissection
    E. Total thyroidectomy with bilateral modified radical dissection

16. A 50-year-old woman presents to the emergency department with nausea, anorexia, irritability, and a serum calcium level of 14.5 mg/dL. Initial management is:

    A. Emergent parathyroidectomy
    B. Furosemide
    C. Intravenous (IV) saline
    D. Mithramycin
    E. Calcitonin

17. A 65-year-old woman with a history of Hashimoto thyroiditis presents with fever, dysphagia, and a painless thyroid mass that has enlarged over a short period of time. This most likely represents:

    A. Lymphoma
    B. Follicular cancer
    C. Anaplastic thyroid cancer
    D. Acute suppurative thyroiditis
    E. MTC

18. Which of the following is true regarding the parathyroid glands?

    A. The inferior glands arise from the fourth branchial pouch and the superior ones from the third pouch.
    B. The superior glands are more likely to be found in an ectopic position.
    C. The superior glands are more likely to be found in the thymus.
    D. Three glands are more common than five glands.
    E. Ectopic superior glands are more likely to be found in the retro- or paraesophageal space.

19. In an asymptomatic patient, surgery for primary hyperparathyroidism would be least indicated for which of the following?

    A. Serum calcium of 11.6 mg/dL
    B. A 40% reduction in creatinine clearance
    C. Age older than 50 years
    D. Bone density at the hip more than 2.5 standard deviations below matched controls
    E. A 24-hour urine calcium excretion greater than 400 mg

20. The most important clinical prognosticator for well-differentiated thyroid cancer is:

    A. Age
    B. Lymph node status
    C. Sex
    D. Tumor size
    E. Local extension

21. Calcified clumps of cells on histology are consistent with:

    A. Papillary cancer
    B. Hürthle cell cancer
    C. Follicular cancer
    D. MTC
    E. Anaplastic cancer

22. Factors related to an increased risk of thyroid cancer include all of the following EXCEPT:

    A. Family history of thyroid cancer
    B. History of low-dose radiation to the head and neck
    C. Low iodine diet
    D. Smoking
    E. Female sex

23. The most common type of thyroid cancer in children is:

    A. Papillary
    B. Follicular
    C. Medullary
    D. Hürthle cell
    E. Anaplastic

24. Which of the following is true regarding secondary hyperparathyroidism?

    A. Serum calcium levels are markedly increased.
    B. It is usually associated with a parathyroid adenoma.
    C. PTH levels are typically normal or high normal.
    D. Cinacalcet is the initial treatment of choice.
    E. Most patients will eventually require parathyroidectomy.

25. Which of the following is true regarding tertiary hyperparathyroidism?

    A. It is usually due to an underlying parathyroid carcinoma.
    B. It is most commonly seen after successful kidney transplantation.
    C. The serum calcium level is usually normal or low.
    D. Distinguishing between secondary and tertiary hyperparathyroidism is essential because the management differs.
    E. It only occurs in patients with chronic renal insufficiency.

26. All of the following are true regarding pseudohypoparathyroidism EXCEPT:

    A. It is the result of a genetic defect.
    B. The serum calcium level is low.
    C. The serum phosphate level is elevated.
    D. Patients have short stubby fingers.
    E. It responds well to exogenously administered PTH extract.

27. A 45-year-old man with episodic severe hypertension is found to have elevated plasma metanephrines and a serum calcium level of 11.5 mg/dL. Which of the following would be indicated in the work-up?

    A. Computed tomography scan of the sella turcica
    B. Calcitonin level
    C. Serum gastrin level
    D. Serum prolactin level
    E. A 24-hour urine cortisol

28. When comparing total thyroidectomy for well-differentiated papillary thyroid cancer with unilateral thyroidectomy and isthmusectomy, all of the following are true EXCEPT:

    A. Total thyroidectomy facilitates detection of metastatic disease via ^{131}I scanning.
    B. Total thyroidectomy facilitates detection of recurrent disease via thyroglobulin levels.
    C. Total thyroidectomy decreases recurrence rates in patients with a history of radiation exposure.
    D. Total thyroidectomy improves overall survival.
    E. Total thyroidectomy increases the risk of postoperative hypocalcemia.

29. A 60-year-old woman presents with a history of kidney stones and a palpable neck mass. Her serum calcium level is 14.1 mg/dL. The most likely diagnosis is:

   A. Parathyroid adenoma
   B. Parathyroid hyperplasia
   C. Parathyroid cancer
   D. Breast cancer with bone metastasis
   E. Secondary hyperparathyroidism

30. During neck exploration for primary hyperparathyroidism, only three parathyroid glands are identified, all of which appear normal in size. Which of the following would be appropriate?

   A. Perform a transcervical thymectomy.
   B. Remove all three glands and reimplant one in the forearm.
   C. Remove two and a half glands and then close.
   D. Perform median sternotomy to look for ectopic parathyroid.
   E. Obtain biopsy samples of all three parathyroid glands and then close.

31. After total thyroidectomy for follicular thyroid cancer, the best test to monitor for recurrent disease is:

   A. Serum TSH
   B. Serum calcitonin
   C. Serum thyroglobulin
   D. ^{131}I scan
   E. Ultrasound scan of the neck

32. The most important test in the work-up of a solitary thyroid nodule is:

   A. FNA
   B. Thyroid function tests
   C. Thyroid scan
   D. Ultrasound scan
   E. CT scan

33. Malignancy within a thyroglossal duct cyst is typically:

   A. Follicular thyroid
   B. Papillary thyroid
   C. Squamous cell
   D. Anaplastic thyroid
   E. Hürthle cells

34. After a total thyroidectomy, the right vocal cord is noted to be fixed in a paramedian position. This most likely represents:

   A. Injury to the RLN
   B. Injury to the external branch of the superior laryngeal nerve
   C. Injury to the internal branch of the superior laryngeal nerve
   D. Trauma from endotracheal intubation
   E. Compression from hematoma

35. The best test to detect hypothyroidism is:

   A. TSH
   B. Free T$_4$
   C. Total T$_4$
   D. Total T$_3$
   E. Anti-TPO antibodies

36. All of the following are true regarding calcitonin EXCEPT:

   A. It does not play an important role in the regulation of calcium levels.
   B. It is produced by thyroid C cells.
   C. It inhibits calcium absorption by osteoclasts.
   D. It is useful for treating hypercalcemic crisis.
   E. It is inhibited by pentagastrin.

37. Factors associated with an elevation of PTH levels include all of the following EXCEPT:

   A. Lithium therapy
   B. Low-dose radiation exposure
   C. Multiple endocrine neoplasia (MEN) type 1
   D. MEN type 2B
   E. Declining renal function

38. The RET oncogene is associated with which of the following malignancies?

   A. Papillary thyroid cancer
   B. MTC
   C. Follicular thyroid carcinoma
   D. Hürthle cell carcinoma
   E. Parathyroid carcinoma

39. Careless division of the superior thyroid arteries during total thyroidectomy would most likely result in which of the following complications?

   A. Voice fatigue
   B. Hoarseness
   C. Loss of airway
   D. Aspiration
   E. Ineffective cough

40. A 45-year-old woman with a history of a goiter presents to the emergency department with a high fever, heart rate of 130 beats per minute, tremors, sweating, and exophthalmos. Treatment may include all of the following EXCEPT:

A. Aspirin

B. Propylthiouracil

C. Beta-blocker

D. Methimazole

E. Steroids

41. Which of the following is true regarding substernal goiter?

A. Surgical resection should be reserved for patients with tracheal deviation.

B. Most are primary mediastinal goiters with a blood supply arising from intrathoracic vessels.

C. Most can be resected by a cervical incision.

D. Most are highly responsive to prolonged thyroid suppression.

E. Because of the risk of tracheomalacia, most patients should have a prophylactic tracheostomy at the time of resection.

Answers

1. E. The characteristics of MTC that affect surgical approach include the following: MTC is more aggressive than other thyroid cancers with higher recurrence and mortality rates. Second, MTC does not take up radioactive iodine, and radiation therapy and chemotherapy are ineffective. Third, MTC is multicentric in 90% of patients. Fourth, in patients with palpable disease, more than 70% have nodal metastases. Last, the ability to measure postoperative stimulated calcitonin levels has allowed assessment of the adequacy of surgical extraction. The two main factors affecting survival are stage and age at diagnosis. A key factor in survival is early detection via calcitonin screening in at-risk patients. In one large study, biochemical cure predicted a survival rate of 97.7% at 10 years.

References: Kebebew E, Ituarte P, Siperstein A, et al: Medullary thyroid carcinoma: clinical characteristics, treatment, prognostic factors, and a comparison of staging systems, *Cancer* 88:1139–1148, 2000.

Modigliani E, Cohen R, Campos J, et al: Prognostic factors for survival and for biochemical cure in medullary thyroid carcinoma: results in 899 patients. The GETC Study Group. Groupe d'étude des tumeurs à calcitonine, *Clin Endocrinol (Oxf)* 48:265–273, 1998.

2. D. TSH is the most accurate test in hyperthyroidism, with significant suppression in hyperthyroid states. In most states of hyperthyroidism, free T_4, total T_4, and total T_3 are elevated.

3. A. The thyroid gland is supplied by paired superior thyroid arteries from the external carotid arteries and the inferior thyroid arteries from the thyrocervical trunk. During thyroidectomy, care must be taken when ligating the superior thyroid arteries to avoid injury to the external branch of the superior laryngeal nerve. To avoid injury, ligating the artery and vein separately and close to the thyroid gland is recommended. In approximately 3% of individuals, a thyroidea ima artery also provides blood to the thyroid gland and arises either from the aorta or the innominate artery. When ligating the inferior thyroid

arteries, care must be taken to avoid injury to the RLNs. The inferior thyroid arteries usually supply the parathyroid glands. Ligation of the main trunk of the inferior thyroid arteries during total thyroidectomy can lead to parathyroid gland ischemia. There are three main pairs of veins draining the thyroid gland: the superior, middle, and inferior thyroid veins. The middle veins are the least constant. The superior and middle veins drain into the internal jugular veins, whereas the inferior veins drain into the brachiocephalic veins.

4. B. The superior laryngeal nerve and RLN arise from the vagus nerve. The superior laryngeal nerve divides into two branches. The internal branch is sensory to the supraglottic larynx, and, although rare, injury during thyroid surgery would lead to aspiration. The external branch innervates the cricothyroid muscle. Injury to the external superior laryngeal nerve causes an inability to tense the ipsilateral vocal cord. This does not cause hoarseness, but rather results in voice fatigue, and in singers creates difficulty in hitting high notes. It has been referred to as the nerve of Amelita Galla Curci or "high note" nerve after the opera singer who underwent thyroid goiter surgery in the 1930s and lost her ability to sing afterward. The left RLN loops around the aorta at the ligamentum arteriosum. The right RLN loops around the right subclavian artery. The RLN innervates the intrinsic muscles of the larynx except the cricothyroid muscle, which is innervated by the external laryngeal nerve. Injury to one RLN leads to paralysis of the ipsilateral vocal cord, which becomes fixed in the paramedian or abducted position. Bilateral RLN injury may lead to airway obstruction and complete loss of the voice.

5. C. A non-RLN is rare and occurs much more commonly on the right. It branches off the vagus nerve in the neck and heads directly to the larynx, as opposed to arising from the vagus after passing the subclavian artery. The anomalous location, as opposed to its normal position in the tracheoesophageal groove, makes it more prone to injury.

On the right, a patient can have both a nonrecurrent nerve and a recurrent nerve. Nonrecurrent left laryngeal nerves have been reported but are extremely rare. The RLN is most vulnerable to injury during the last 2 to 3 cm of its course, but also can be damaged if the surgeon is not alert to the possibility of nerve branches and nonrecurrent nerves, particularly on the right side.

6. D. PTH increases the bone resorption by stimulating osteoclasts and inhibiting osteoblasts, leading to the release of calcium and phosphate into the circulation. At the kidney, PTH limits calcium excretion at the distal convoluted tubule via an active transport mechanism and inhibits phosphate and bicarbonate reabsorption, the latter leading to a mild metabolic acidosis. PTH also enhances hydroxylation of 25-hydroxyvitamin D to 1,25-hydroxyvitamin D in the kidney, which in turn directly increases intestinal calcium absorption (not a direct effect of PTH).

7. A. Lateral aberrant thyroid is a term used to denote what appeared to be ectopic thyroid tissue found within the neck. In most instances, it actually represents metastatic thyroid cancer within a lymph node, most often of the papillary type.

    Reference: De Jong S, Demeter J, Jarosz H, et al: Primary papillary thyroid carcinoma presenting as cervical lymphadenopathy: the operative approach to the "lateral aberrant thyroid," *Am Surg* 59:172–176, 1993.

8. D. The accepted management of low-risk papillary thyroid cancer is either right hemithyroidectomy or total thyroidectomy and postoperative [131]I. There is an increasing trend toward performing a total thyroidectomy. However, in patients with papillary carcinoma with a history of radiation exposure, there is a higher rate of multicentricity. As such, total thyroidectomy is the recommended procedure. Prophylactic neck node dissection is not necessary in patients with papillary thyroid cancers because the overall outcome is excellent using a combination of surgery and radioactive iodine, which seems to effectively ablate micrometastasis in the lymph nodes.

    Reference: Hay I, Thompson G, Grant C, et al: Papillary thyroid carcinoma managed at the Mayo Clinic during six decades (1940–1999): temporal trends in initial therapy and long-term outcome in 2444 consecutively treated patients, *World J Surg* 26:879–885, 2002.

9. D. Hyperparathyroidism is classically associated with "stones (calcium phosphate or oxalate kidney stones), moans (not feeling well), groans (vague abdominal pain, peptic ulcer disease, pancreatitis, gallstones, and constipation), bones (bone pain, osteoporosis, osteitis fibrosa cystica, Brown [osteoclastic] tumors), and psychiatric overtones (depression, fatigue)." Pancreatitis tends to occur in patients with a very high serum calcium level (>12.5 mg/dL). The increased incidence of cholelithiasis is due to increased biliary calcium, leading to formation of calcium bilirubinate stones.

10. B. PTH inhibits phosphate reabsorption at the proximal convoluted tubule, thereby lowering phosphate levels. It also inhibits the Na^+/H^+ antiporter. This leads to an inhibition of bicarbonate excretion in the urine, resulting in a mild metabolic acidosis and corresponding hyperchloremia. This subsequently results in an elevated chloride-to-phosphate ratio (>33). PTH levels are increased.

11. A. Hürthle cell carcinoma accounts for less than 10% of thyroid malignancies and is considered a subtype of follicular cancer. Like follicular cancer, the presence of malignancy is established by the demonstration of vascular or capsular invasion. FNA and frozen section do not reliably establish malignancy. The tumors contain sheets of eosinophilic cells packed with mitochondria, which are derived from oncocytic or oxyphilic cells of the thyroid gland. Hürthle cell carcinomas differ from follicular cell carcinomas in that they are often multifocal and bilateral, usually do not take up radioactive iodine, are more likely to metastasize to local nodes and distant sites, and are associated with a higher mortality rate. Orphan Annie cells are a hallmark of papillary carcinoma. Unlike differentiated thyroid cancer, nodal metastases predict a worse outcome in widely invasive Hürthle cell carcinoma, as does extrathyroidal extension.

    Reference: Stojadinovic A, Ghossein R, Hoos A, et al: Hürthle cell carcinoma: a critical histopathologic appraisal, *J Clin Oncol* 19:2616–2625, 2001.

12. C. Technetium-99m sestamibi imaging is the most widely used and accurate modality, with sensitivity greater than 80% for detection of parathyroid adenomas. High-resolution ultrasonography in particular is complementary. The other imaging techniques are thought to be more useful when sestamibi scanning fails to identify the parathyroid pathology, for the work-up of recurrent hyperparathyroidism, or when surgical exploration fails to identify the parathyroid lesion. Ultrasonography has an overall lower sensitivity, although it may be most useful in identifying intrathyroidal parathyroids. Computed tomography and magnetic resonance imaging are also less sensitive than sestamibi scans, but are helpful in localizing mediastinal glands. Sestamibi combined with single positron-emission computed tomography is particularly useful for localizing ectopic adenomas. False-positive findings with these modalities are most likely to occur in the presence of thyroid nodules or lymphadenopathy. False-negative findings are more likely in patients with hyperplasia or multiple adenomas. More recently, the combination of preoperative technetium-99m sestamibi imaging and the rapid PTH assay has permitted successful directed parathyroidectomy using minimally invasive techniques. An additional modality is intraoperative gamma probe detection, although this approach lengthens the operation and is not routinely used.

    Reference: Dackiw A, Sussman J, Fritsche H Jr, et al: Relative contributions of technetium Tc 99 m sestamibi scintigraphy, intraoperative gamma probe detection, and the rapid parathyroid hormone assay to the surgical management of hyperparathyroidism, *Arch Surg* 135:550–555, 2000.

13. B. Follicular cancer is the second most common thyroid cancer, and it spreads primarily via a hematogenous route. Unlike papillary carcinoma, accurate diagnosis using FNA is not possible because cytologic features cannot distinguish a benign follicular lesion from a follicular carcinoma. To establish malignancy, demonstration of capsular or vascular invasion on histology is necessary. Thus, if FNA demonstrates a follicular neoplasm, the patient should undergo a thyroid lobectomy to determine malignancy. Once histologic confirmation of malignancy is made, total thyroidectomy is recommended with postoperative ^{131}I. Total thyroidectomy also permits the detection of subsequent metastasis using nuclear scanning.

14. C. Surgical management of a solitary parathyroid adenoma consists of resection of the single enlarged gland. On rare occasion, double adenomas are present. For four-gland hyperplasia, resection of all four glands with reimplantation of half of one gland into the brachioradialis muscle in the forearm is recommended. Another option for four-gland hyperplasia is to leave half of a gland in the neck, although this might then require a reoperation in the neck if recurrent hyperparathyroidism develops. On occasion, distinguishing between adenoma and hyperplasia may be difficult if two glands are enlarged and the other two appear normal or slightly enlarged. In this circumstance, removal of the two enlarged glands and biopsy of an additional gland may be performed to rule out four-gland hyperplasia. However, in the presence of one enlarged gland, there is no role for biopsy of the other three glands because this may result in ischemia of the remaining parathyroid glands. Another frequent dilemma occurs when only three glands are found, and all appear normal. If an inferior one is missing, it may be found in the thymus, angle of the mandible, at the skull base, superior to the superior parathyroid glands, or, rarely, within the thyroid gland. If the ectopic gland is not found, transcervical thymectomy is recommended. If the superior gland is missing, it may be found within the thyroid gland, in the paraesophageal or retro-esophageal grooves, or caudal to the inferior glands. Although ectopic glands are found in the mediastinum on rare occasion, median sternotomy is not recommended at initial exploration.

References: Chen H, Sokoll L, Udelsman R: Outpatient minimally invasive parathyroidectomy: a combination of sestamibi-SPECT localization, cervical block anesthesia, and intraoperative parathyroid hormone assay, *Surgery* 126:1016–1021, 1999.

Goldstein R, Billheimer D, Martin WH, Richards K: Sestamibi scanning and minimally invasive radioguided parathyroidectomy without intraoperative parathyroid hormone measurement, *Ann Surg* 237:722–730, 2003.

15. D. Because of the tendency for multicentricity and lymph node metastasis and the lack of response to other treatment modalities, the recommended management of MTC is total thyroidectomy with central lymph node dissection. Most MTCs are sporadic. Sporadic cases are less likely to be multicentric than those associated with MEN type 2. In patients with a family history of MEN or MTC, screening with calcitonin levels is recommended. MTC arises from the parafollicular or C cells of the thyroid, which are concentrated in the superior and lateral aspects of the thyroid lobes. Calcitonin levels are useful for screening in patients with a family history. Familial cases are associated with C-cell hyperplasia, which is considered to be a premalignant lesion. Microscopically, a characteristic

feature of MTC is the finding of abundant collagen and amyloid. Age and TNM stage are the best predictors of outcome.

Reference: Kebebew E, Ituarte P, Siperstein A, et al: Medullary thyroid carcinoma: clinical characteristics, treatment, prognostic factors, and a comparison of staging systems, *Cancer* 88:1139–1148, 2000.

16. C. Severely elevated calcium levels represent a hypercalcemic crisis. Hypercalcemic crisis is a life-threatening emergency. Patients with calcium levels greater than 14 mg/dL or symptomatic patients with calcium levels greater than 12 mg/dL should be immediately and aggressively treated because severe hypercalcemia poses a risk of renal failure as well as severe central nervous system manifestations including coma. In addition, it leads to a shortening of the QT interval, tachycardias, and an increased sensitivity to digitalis. Treatment is divided into fast- and slow-acting modalities. Fast-acting modalities include those that induce a calciuresis (IV fluids), those that prevent bone resorption (bisphosphonates, calcitonin, mithramycin), and those that extract calcium (hemodialysis). Slow-acting measures prevent gastrointestinal absorption of calcium (prednisone, reduced vitamin D and calcium intake). The first-line therapy for hypercalcemic crisis involves rehydration with normal saline. Urine output should be keep at more than 100 mL/hr. Once urine output is established, diuresis with furosemide is instituted. Furosemide works by increasing renal calcium clearance. If these methods are not successful, then additional fast-acting modalities should be used.

Reference: Ziegler R: Hypercalcemic crisis, *J Am Soc Nephrol* 12 (Suppl 17):S3–S9, 2001.

17. A. Hashimoto thyroiditis is an autoimmune disorder that leads to destruction of thyroid follicles by both cell- and antibody-mediated immune processes, including activation of helper lymphocytes and antibody formation against thyroglobulin and thyroid peroxidase. It is the leading cause of hypothyroidism. It results in a lymphocytic infiltration. Treatment of Hashimoto thyroiditis is with thyroid hormone replacement. Hashimoto thyroiditis is associated with primary thyroid lymphoma. The chronic antigenic stimulation coupled with a chronic proliferation of lymphoid tissue in the thyroid is thought to lead to the development of lymphocytic transformation. In a patient with Hashimoto thyroiditis, lymphoma should be suspected in the setting of a rapidly enlarging thyroid mass. Patients additionally may report fever, cervical lymphadenopathy, dysphagia, and hoarseness. Diagnosis is established by FNA. The treatment recommendation is chemotherapy using CHOP (cylophosphamide, doxorubicin, vincristine, and prednisone) and radiation therapy in most cases of thyroid lymphoma.

Reference: Ansell SM, Grant CS, Habermann TM: Primary thyroid lymphoma, *Semin Oncol* 26:316–323, 1999.

18. E. In one large autopsy study, 84% of patients had four parathyroid glands, 13% had more than four glands, and only 3% had 3 glands. The superior parathyroid glands are derived from the fourth branchial pouch, which also gives rise to the thyroid gland. The third branchial pouch gives rise to the inferior parathyroid glands and the thymus. Ectopic inferior glands are more likely to be found within the thymus than the superior glands, whereas the superior glands are more likely to be found in the retro- or paraesophageal position. Given the longer descent of the inferior glands, they are overall much more likely to be in an ectopic position.

19. C. Patients with symptomatic hyperparathyroidism should undergo surgery. Symptoms are defined as having evidence of kidney stones; neuromuscular, neuropsychological, or bone symptoms; hypercalcemic crisis; or a history of pancreatitis or peptic ulcer. Conversely, controversy exists as to whether every patient who is asymptomatic should undergo parathyroidectomy. Natural history studies of patients with asymptomatic hyperparathyroidism indicate that one fourth to one third of patients without symptoms will progress to the development of symptoms over 15 years. Current National Institutes of Health conference guidelines for surgery in asymptomatic patients include at initial evaluation: (1) a serum calcium level more than 1 mg/dL above the upper limit of reference value, (2) reduced creatinine clearance of more than 30% compared with matched controls, (3) an increased urinary calcium excretion of more than 400 mg/day, (4) evidence of bone mass reduction more than 2.5 standard deviations below matched controls, and (5) unwillingness or inability to undergo continued follow-up.

References: Rubin M, Bilezikian J, McMahon D, et al: The natural history of primary hyperparathyroidism with or without parathyroid surgery after 15 years, *J Clin Endocrinol Metab* 93:3462–3470, 2008.

Silverberg S, Shane E, Jacobs T, et al: A 10-year prospective study of primary hyperparathyroidism with or without parathyroid surgery, *N Engl J Med* 341:1249–1255, 1999.

20. A. The TNM system for well-differentiated thyroid cancer takes into account tumor size, the presence of positive lymph nodes, local extension, and the presence of distant metastasis. In addition, however, age is the most critical factor. By definition, patients younger than 45 years of age can only be classified as stage I (no distant metastasis) or II (distant metastasis). For patients younger than age 45, lymph node status and tumor size are not taken into consideration. For patients 45 years or older, the more traditional four stages apply. In general, overall survival is as follows: papillary > follicular > medullary >> anaplastic. The 5-year survival rate for stage I and II papillary and follicular cancers is 100%.

21. A. Psammoma bodies are calcified deposits representing clumps of sloughed cells. It is considered diagnostic of papillary carcinoma. Another histologic characteristic of papillary carcinoma is Orphan Annie nuclei.

22. D. Thyroid cancer is more common in women than men by a ratio of 3:1, and although it can occur at any age, it is seen more often after age 30. It is more aggressive in the elderly. Thyroid cancer occurs more often in people who have been exposed to radiation therapy of the head, neck, and thyroid as children. The risk of thyroid cancer is also increased with a family history of thyroid cancer, and follicular cancer is more common in areas with low iodine in the diet.

23. A. Papillary cancer is the most common thyroid malignancy in adults and children. The rate of malignancy in thyroid nodules is higher in children. In adults, approximately 5% of thyroid nodules are malignant, whereas in children, the rate is approximately 25%. Prognosis in children overall is excellent.

References: Hanks JB, Salomone LJ: Thyroid. In Townsend CM Jr, Beauchamp RD, Evers BM, Mattox KL, editors: *Sabiston textbook of surgery: the biological basis of modern surgical practice*, ed 18, Philadelphia, 2008, WB Saunders, pp 917–954.

Lal G, Clark OH: Thyroid, parathyroid, and adrenal. In Brunicardi FC, Andersen DK, Billiar TR, et al, editors: *Schwartz's principles of surgery*, ed 9, New York, 2010, McGraw-Hill, pp 1303–1407.

Sosa JA, Udelsman R: The parathyroid gland. In Townsend CM Jr, Beauchamp RD, Evers BM, Mattox KL, editors: *Sabiston textbook of surgery: the biological basis of modern surgical practice*, ed 18, Philadelphia, 2008, WB Saunders, pp 955–975.

24. D. Secondary hyperparathyroidism is seen in the majority of cases in association with chronic renal failure. Rarely, it occurs secondary to intestinal malabsorption of calcium and vitamin D. The underlying etiology is a chronic overstimulation of the parathyroid glands. Renal failure leads to a decreased level of calcitriol (vitamin D_3), an elevation in phosphate, and a drop in serum calcium levels. This leads to increased PTH secretion. PTH levels are typically very high, ranging from 500 to 1500 pg/mL (normal is $\leq$ 65 pg/mL). As renal failure progresses, there is a decrease in vitamin D and calcium receptors, leading to parathyroid gland resistance to calcitriol and calcium. This vicious cycle worsens as renal failure worsens. Patients with secondary hyperparathyroidism are generally hypocalcemic or normocalcemic. The typical parathyroid gland pathology is four-gland hyperplasia. Medical management has historically consisted of a low phosphate diet, phosphate binders, and oral supplementation with calcium and vitamin D. More recently, cinacalcet has been approved by the U.S. Food and Drug Administration for the treatment of secondary hyperparathyroidism due to chronic renal failure. Cinacalcet is a calcimimetic agent. It increases the sensitivity of the calcium-sensing receptor to activation by extracellular calcium and thus directly lowers PTH levels. The majority of patients with secondary hyperparathyroidism can be managed medically. The recent introduction of cinacalcet will likely lead to an even further reduction in the need for surgical management. In general, surgery is indicated for failed medical management. Indications include intractable bone pain, severe pruritus, calciphylaxis, and progressive renal osteodystrophy. Surgical treatment consists of removal of all four glands with autoimplantation of parathyroid tissue in the forearm muscle or removal of three and a half glands.

References: Block G, Martin K, de Francisco A, et al: Cinacalcet for secondary hyperparathyroidism in patients receiving hemodialysis, *N Engl J Med* 350:1516–1525, 2004.

Lindberg J, Culleton B, Wong G, et al: Cinacalcet HCl, an oral calcimimetic agent for the treatment of secondary hyperparathyroidism in hemodialysis and peritoneal dialysis: a randomized, double-blind, multicenter study, *J Am Soc Nephrol* 16:800–807, 2005.

Shoback D, Bilezikian J, Turner S, et al: The calcimimetic cinacalcet normalizes serum calcium in subjects with primary hyperparathyroidism, *J Clin Endocrinol Metab* 88:5644–5649, 2003.

Slatopolsky E, Brown A, Dusso A: Pathogenesis of secondary hyperparathyroidism, *Kidney Int Suppl* 73:S14–S19, 1999.

25. B. Tertiary hyperparathyroidism most commonly occurs in the setting of a patient who has had long-standing secondary hyperparathyroidism in whom subsequently autonomously functioning parathyroid glands develop that continue secreting PTH despite high serum calcium levels. The most common clinical scenario in which it develops is the patient who has undergone renal transplantation. Distinguishing between secondary and tertiary hyperparathyroidism is not critical because the initial management is medical, and surgery is indicated for failure of medical management. Surgical treatment consists of removal of 3½ glands rather than all four glands with autoimplantation of parathyroid tissue in the forearm muscle in cases in which all four glands are enlarged.

Reference: Kebebew E, Duh QY, Clark OH: Tertiary hyperparathyroidism: histologic patterns of disease and results of parathyroidectomy, *Arch Surg* 139:974–977, 2004.

26. E. Pseudohypoparathyroidism is a genetic disorder in which there is an insensitivity to PTH. It is characterized by hypocalcemia, hyperphosphatemia, and elevated PTH. Patients are typically of short stature and obese and have a round face and short, stubby fingers with dimpling of the knuckles when the fist is clenched. Because there is an insensitivity to PTH, there is no role for exogenous PTH administration. Treatment is with oral calcium and vitamin D supplementation.

27. B. The elevated plasma metanephrine indicates a high suspicion for pheochromocytoma. Further work-up for this should include a computed tomography or magnetic resonance imaging scan of the abdomen to detect an adrenal mass. The elevated calcium suggests hyperparathyroidism. The patient should have a PTH level measured and, if it is elevated, should undergo a sestamibi scan. Given these findings, the patient most likely has MEN type 2, which is characterized by pheochromocytoma, hyperparathyroidism, and MTC. Screening for MTC involves measuring the serum calcitonin level.

28. D. The role of hemithyroidectomy versus total thyroidectomy for well-differentiated thyroid cancer is somewhat controversial given the overall excellent prognosis. However, the majority of major cancer centers recommend total thyroidectomy with ^{131}I treatment postoperatively. Total thyroidectomy permits the use of radioactive iodine to effectively treat residual disease. It also allows using the thyroglobulin level to detect recurrence. If the thyroglobulin level is elevated, a low-dose radioactive iodine scan can then be performed to detect metastasis in patients who have undergone total thyroidectomy. Total thyroidectomy seems to reduce the rate of local recurrence. Performing hemithyroidectomy is associated with a 5% to 10% recurrence rate in the opposite thyroid lobe, a higher tumor recurrence rate, and a higher incidence of subsequent pulmonary

metastases in some studies. To date, however, the data on the survival rate for well-differentiated papillary thyroid cancer has not shown a survival benefit when comparing total thyroidectomy with hemithyroidectomy in these low-risk patients.

Reference: Mazzaferri E, Kloos R: Current approaches to primary therapy for papillary and follicular thyroid cancer, *J Clin Endocrinol Metab* 86:1447–1463, 2001.

29. C. Parathyroid carcinoma is extremely rare and accounts for less than 1% of cases of primary hyperparathyroidism. It should be suspected in the setting of severe symptoms of hypercalcemia, in association with very high serum calcium and PTH levels and a palpable neck mass. Benign causes of hyperparathyroidism very rarely result in a palpable neck mass. Determination of malignancy is difficult because, similar to other endocrine malignancies, there are not any classic histologic features that reliably distinguish parathyroid malignancy from benign disease. Thus, one must look for evidence of local invasion at the time of surgery as well as enlarged lymph nodes. Treatment is surgical and involves en bloc resection of the parathyroid tumor with the ipsilateral thyroid gland, as well as a modified radical lymph node dissection if nodal metastasis is present. Recently, cinacalcet was approved by the U.S. Food and Drug Administration and is effective in controlling the hypercalcemia associated with parathyroid carcinoma.

Reference: Shane E: Parathyroid carcinoma, *J Clin Endocrinol Metab* 86:485–493, 2001.

30. A. On occasion, despite careful neck exploration, only three parathyroid glands will be encountered. A careful search for the ectopic gland should be conducted. The inferior gland is by far more likely to be ectopic than the superior ones. Most inferior glands are to be found within 2 cm of the inferior thyroid pole. If not found, the next step is to perform a cervical thymectomy and send the tissue for frozen section. If still not found, the carotid sheath should be opened. Intraoperative ultrasonography should then be used to determine whether there is an intrathyroidal parathyroid gland. If ultrasonography is not available, ipsilateral thyroid lobectomy should be considered. Another useful modality in this setting is intraoperative gamma probe detection. Likewise, intraoperative PTH assays can assist in determining whether the pathologic gland has been removed.

31. C. Serum thyroglobulin levels are the most useful modality to monitor patients for recurrence of differentiated thyroid cancer (papillary and follicular) after total thyroidectomy and radioactive iodine ablation. Thyroglobulin is a glycoprotein that is the primary component of colloid matrix within the thyroid follicle. Thyroglobulin levels in patients who have undergone total thyroidectomy should be 3 ng/mL or less when the patient is receiving thyroid hormone replacement therapy and less than 5 ng/mL when thyroid hormone supplementation is withheld. Serum thyroglobulin levels seem to be most predictive of recurrence when patients are hypothyroid as documented by a high TSH level. An increase above these levels is highly suggestive of metastatic disease. The recommendation after thyroidectomy is to check thyroglobulin levels initially at 6-month intervals after surgery. If the thyroglobulin levels are elevated, an ^{131}I scan is recommended. Recurrence of MTC is determined by calcitonin levels.

References: Baudin E, Do Cao C, Cailleux AF, et al: Positive predictive value of serum thyroglobulin levels, measured during the first year of follow-up after thyroid hormone withdrawal, in thyroid cancer patients, *J Clin Endocrinol Metab* 88:1107–1111, 2003.

Duren M, Siperstein A, Shen W, et al: Value of stimulated serum thyroglobulin levels for detecting persistent or recurrent differentiated thyroid cancer in high- and low-risk patients, *Surgery* 126:13–19, 1999.

Lal G, Clark OH: Thyroid, parathyroid, and adrenal. In Brunicardi FC, Andersen DK, Billiar TR, et al, editors: *Schwartz's principles of surgery*, ed 9, New York, 2010, McGraw-Hill, pp 1343–1407.

32. A. The most important test in the evaluation of a solitary thyroid nodule is FNA. This can be performed with ultrasound guidance if the lesion is difficult to palpate. Thyroid scanning to determine whether the lesion is "hot" or "cold" is not recommended as the initial test. Approximately 15% of cold lesions are malignant as opposed to only 1% of hot lesions. However, the scan does not obviate the need for needle biopsy. Four possible results are obtained from FNA: malignant, suspicious, benign, or nondiagnostic. FNA is particularly useful in the diagnosis of papillary cancer, but cannot be used to determine follicular cancer because histologic features of capsular or vascular invasion are needed. Thus, if the FNA suggests a follicular neoplasm, excision of the lesion via lobectomy is recommended, with final pathology needed to determine malignancy. The diagnosis of medullary and anaplastic cancer can be made with FNA.

33. B. The frequency of thyroid carcinoma among patients with a surgically removed thyroglossal duct cyst in one large series was 0.7%. The majority are papillary cancer and are found incidentally after a Sistrunk procedure (performed for the cyst). If discovered incidentally, the patient should subsequently undergo a total thyroidectomy because additional cancer is found within the thyroid gland as well.

Reference: Heshmati H, Fatourechi V, van Heerden J, et al: Thyroglossal duct carcinoma: report of 12 cases, *Mayo Clin Proc* 72:315–319, 1997.

34. A. The RLN innervates the intrinsic muscles of the larynx, except the cricothyroid muscles, which are innervated by the external branch of the superior laryngeal nerve. Injury to one RLN leads to paralysis of the ipsilateral vocal cord. The cord becomes fixed in either the paramedian position or the abducted position. If the cord becomes fixed in the paramedian position, the patient will have a weak voice, whereas if it becomes fixed in the abducted position, the patient will have a hoarse voice and an ineffective cough. If both RLNs are injured, an airway obstruction may develop acutely in the patient.

35. A. Multiple tests are available to assess thyroid function. Although no single test is sufficient to assess thyroid function in all situations, TSH is the best initial test to rule out primary thyroid insufficiency. It is associated with an increased TSH level and decreased T_4 and T_3.

36. E. Calcitonin is produced by thyroid C or parafollicular cells (located in the superior lateral aspect of the thyroid). In humans, it does not play an important role in regulating serum calcium levels. It is useful in treating hypercalcemic crisis by inhibiting osteoclast-mediated bone resorption. Calcitonin production is stimulated by calcium, pentagastrin, and alcohol as well as by catecholamines, cholecystokinin, and glucagon. In the kidney, calcitonin increases phosphate excretion by inhibiting its reabsorption. It is useful as a marker for MTC.

37. D. A causal relationship has been shown between the use of lithium and hyperparathyroidism as well as with low-dose radiation exposure and declining renal function. Hyperparathyoidism is not seen in patients with MEN type 2B (pheochromocytoma, MTC, mucosal neuromas, marfanoid habitus).

Reference: Bendz H, Sjödin I, Toss G, Berglund K: Hyperparathyroidism and long-term lithium therapy—a cross-sectional study and the effect of lithium withdrawal, *J Intern Med* 240:357–365, 1996.

38. B. Germline mutations in the RET proto-oncogene are known to predispose to MEN type 2A, MEN type 2B, familial MTCs, and pheochromocytomas.

39. A. The external branch of the superior laryngeal nerve lies on the inferior pharyngeal constrictor muscle and descends alongside the superior thyroid artery before innervating the cricothyroid muscle. Injury to the external superior laryngeal nerve results in an inability to tense the ipsilateral vocal cord and difficulty hitting high notes, projecting the voice, and voice fatigue during a prolonged speech.

References: Hanks JB, Salomone LJ: Thyroid. In Townsend CM Jr, Beauchamp RD, Evers BM, Mattox KL, editors: *Sabiston textbook of surgery: the biological basis of modern surgical practice*, ed 18, Philadelphia, 2008, WB Saunders, pp 917–954.

Lal G, Clark OH: Thyroid, parathyroid, and adrenal. In Brunicardi FC, Andersen DK, Billiar TR, et al, editors: *Schwartz's principles of surgery*, ed 9, New York, 2010, McGraw-Hill, pp 1343–1407.

Sosa JA, Udelsman R: The parathyroid gland. In Townsend CM Jr, Beauchamp RD, Evers BM, Mattox KL, editors: *Sabiston textbook of surgery: the biological basis of modern surgical practice*, ed 18, Philadelphia, 2008, WB Saunders, pp 955–975.

40. A. In the follicular cell, inorganic iodide is trapped and transported across the basement membrane. Iodide is oxidized to iodine. It is then coupled with tyrosine moieties. This leads to the formation of mono- or di-iodotyrosine, catalyzed by thyroid peroxidase. Two di-iodotyrosine molecules couple to form T_4, and one mono-iodotyrosine and one di-iodotyrosine combine to form T_3, both of which are bound to thyroglobulin. In the periphery, approximately 70% to 75% of T_3 and T_4 is bound to thyroid-binding globulins (not to be confused with thyroglobulin), and most of the remainder is bound to thyroid-binding prealbumin and albumin, leaving only a small amount of unbound or active thyroid hormone. T_4 is relatively inactive but is present in larger amounts. T_4 is converted to the more active form of T_3 in the liver, kidneys, pituitary, and other tissues. Thus, treatment of thyroid storm involves inhibiting several steps: (1) addressing the ABCs by determining whether an airway is needed, administering 100% oxygen, and starting aggressive fluid hydration, (2) decreasing new hormone synthesis, (3) inhibiting the release of thyroid hormone, and (4) blocking the peripheral effects of thyroid hormone. Propylthiouracil and methimazole both inhibit oxidation of iodide to iodine and inhibit the thyroid peroxidase–mediated coupling of iodotyrosines. Propylthiouracil also inhibits the conversion of T_4 to T_3. Catecholamines such as propranolol are useful in controlling the adrenergic response to thyroid storm. Propranolol also inhibits peripheral conversion of T_4 to T_3. Steroids also inhibit the conversion of T_4 to T_3 in the periphery. Aspirin is contraindicated in thyroid storm because it is thought to decrease protein binding of thyroid hormones. Thus, it may increase the levels of unbound T_3 and T_4.

Reference: Nayak B, Burman K: Thyrotoxicosis and thyroid storm, *Endocrinol Metab Clin North Am* 35:663–686, 2006.

41. C. Substernal goiter is divided into primary and secondary forms. Primary forms, defined as ones that originate in the mediastinum with blood supply from intrathoracic vessels, are very rare. Most substernal goiters are extensions from cervical goiters. Most surgeons recommend resection for the mere presence of a substernal goiter because most are symptomatic, and those that are not can cause progressive compression of the trachea. In addition, they may harbor an unsuspected malignancy. The majority can be successfully removed with a cervical collar incision. Sternotomy is very rarely needed nor is tracheostomy because most can be intubated, even in the face of tracheal compression, with a pediatric endotracheal tube.

References: Hanks JB, Salomone LJ: Thyroid. In Townsend CM Jr, Beauchamp RD, Evers BM, Mattox KL, editors: *Sabiston textbook of surgery: the biological basis of modern surgical practice*, ed 18, Philadelphia, 2008, WB Saunders, pp 917–954.

Hedayati N, McHenry CR: The clinical presentation and operative management of nodular and diffuse substernal thyroid disease, *Am Surg* 68:245–251, 2002, discussion 251–252.

Lal G, Clark OH: Thyroid, Parathyroid, and Adrenal. In Brunicardi FC, Andersen DK, Billiar TR, et al, editors: *Schwartz's principles of surgery*, ed 9, New York, 2010, McGraw-Hill, pp 1343–1407.

Sosa JA, Udelsman R: The parathyroid gland. In Townsend CM Jr, Beauchamp RD, Evers BM, Mattox KL, editors: *Sabiston textbook of surgery: the biological basis of modern surgical practice*, ed 18, Philadelphia, 2008, WB Saunders, pp 955–975.

Trauma and Shock 28

1. A 25-year-old man presents with a gunshot wound to the buttocks. Abdominal examination is unremarkable, and the patient is hemodynamically stable. Computed tomography (CT) scan of the abdomen and pelvis is unremarkable. Proctoscopy reveals blood and stool in the distal rectal vault, but an injury cannot be identified. Which of the following is the best management option?

   A. Intravenous (IV) antibiotics with close observation
   B. A proximal diverting colostomy for a distal extraperitoneal rectal injury
   C. Primary closure of the proximal extraperitoneal rectal injury, diverting colostomy, distal rectal irrigation, and presacral drainage
   D. Presacral drainage and IV antibiotics
   E. Abdominal perineal resection

2. A 25-year-old man presents to the emergency department after a high-speed motor vehicle accident (MVA); he is unconscious and has a blown right pupil. Emergent CT scan shows a large right epidural hematoma, multiple rib fractures, a pulmonary contusion, and nonopacification of a normal-size right kidney. There is no free fluid in the abdomen. The left kidney opacifies. The patient is taken emergently to the operating room for a craniotomy. Management of the kidney consists of:

   A. Repair of the renal artery using saphenous vein interposition graft
   B. Repair of the renal artery using a synthetic graft
   C. Endovascular stenting
   D. Nephrectomy
   E. Observation

3. A 30-year-old man sustains a gunshot wound to the abdomen and presents to the emergency department with a systolic blood pressure of 60 mm Hg. Emergent laparotomy reveals a 2-L hemoperitoneum with an injury to the inferior vena cava (IVC) and right iliac vein. Both injuries are successfully repaired. Further exploration demonstrates a distal right ureteral injury below the level of the iliac vessels with a 2-cm defect. After 10 units of blood products, the patient's blood pressure is 80/60 mm Hg, his heart rate is 110 beats per minute, and his temperature is 96°F. Which of the following is the best management option?

   A. Proximal and distal ligation of the ureter
   B. Ureteroureterostomy
   C. Transureteroureterostomy
   D. Psoas hitch
   E. Ureteroneocystostomy

4. Which of the following is true regarding the pregnant trauma patient?

   A. Blood volume increases proportionally less than red blood cell volume.
   B. A pregnant patient tends to have a mild respiratory acidosis.
   C. Use of radiographs is unsafe for the fetus in the third trimester.
   D. The 2,3-diphosphoglycerate level is increased.
   E. The glomerular filtration rate decreases.

5. A 55-year-old man is brought in to the emergency department after a high-speed MVA. The patient is hemodynamically stable. Gross hematuria is present. CT cystography reveals air in the bladder and an accumulation of contrast in the right paracolic gutter. Management consists of:

   A. Foley catheter drainage
   B. Suprapubic cystostomy
   C. Open repair of the intraperitoneal bladder injury with chromic catgut sutures and suprapubic cystostomy
   D. Obtaining a formal cystogram
   E. Open repair of the intraperitoneal bladder injury with silk sutures

6. A 30-year-old man is brought into the emergency department after a 20-foot fall. He is noted to speak using inappropriate words. He withdraws and opens his eyes to pain only. This patient's Glasgow Coma Scale score is:

   A. 10
   B. 9
   C. 8
   D. 7
   E. 6

7. All of the following are true regarding head injury EXCEPT:

   A. Epidural hematomas are associated with a lucid interval.
   B. Subdural hematomas are due to lacerations of bridging veins.
   C. Epidural hematomas are usually associated with a skull fracture.
   D. Some small subdural hematomas can be managed nonoperatively.
   E. Epidural hematomas generally have a worse prognosis than subdural hematomas.

8. In the setting of trauma, ligation is best tolerated for which of the following vessels?

   A. Superior vena cava
   B. Subclavian artery
   C. Brachial artery
   D. Portal vein
   E. Suprarenal IVC

9. Which of the following is true regarding myocardial contusion?

   A. The serial creatine kinase, myocardial bound enzyme determination lacks sensitivity.
   B. It commonly results in serious ventricular arrhythmias.
   C. It is usually the result of traumatic thrombosis of a coronary artery branch.
   D. It commonly results in cardiac pump failure.
   E. It should be suspected in patients with transient sinus tachycardia.

10. A 28-year-old man sustains a gunshot wound just above the right clavicle with no exit wound. On arrival, his systolic blood pressure is 60 mm Hg and he appears agitated. Which of the following is indicated as the next step in the management?

    A. Endotracheal intubation
    B. Right tube thoracostomy
    C. Normal saline hydration
    D. Emergency department thoracotomy
    E. Median sternotomy

11. An 11-month-old boy presents to the emergency department with hypotension after being involved in an MVA. He has obvious deformities of both legs below his knees. Numerous attempts are made to establish venous access at the antecubital fossae without success. The best option for establishing access for fluid administration would be:

    A. Internal jugular central line
    B. Distal saphenous vein cutdown
    C. Femoral vein central line
    D. Interosseous cannulation of the proximal tibia
    E. Interosseous cannulation of the distal femur

12. Exposure is most difficult for which of the following vessels?

    A. Innominate artery
    B. Proximal right subclavian artery
    C. Proximal left subclavian artery
    D. Proximal left common carotid artery
    E. Proximal vertebral artery

13. Exposure of various vascular injuries after trauma may be particularly challenging for the surgeon. Specific maneuvers have been developed to allow adequate exposure of such injuries. Which one of the following injury and maneuver combinations is not correct or not appropriate?

    A. Cattell maneuver for the mid IVC
    B. Transection of the neck of the pancreas for the superior mesenteric vein, splenic vein, portal vein confluence
    C. Mattox maneuver for the suprarenal aorta
    D. Kocher maneuver for the celiac axis
    E. Division of the right common iliac artery for the distal vena cava and common iliac vein bifurcation

14. A 23-year-old man sustains blunt chest trauma after a high-speed MVA. He is hemodynamically stable. Which of the following conditions is an indication for a thoracotomy?

    A. Undrained hemothorax despite a tube thoracostomy
    B. Continuous chest tube drainage of more than 200 mL/hr of blood for 4 hours
    C. Initial chest tube output of 1100 mL
    D. Wide mediastinum
    E. Flail chest

15. A 30-year-old man sustains a gunshot wound to the right chest. His blood pressure in the emergency department is 70/40 mm Hg. A chest tube is placed in the right chest with 500 mL of initial output. A follow-up chest radiograph reveals a complete whiteout of the right lung. The patient is taken to the operating room and a right thoracotomy is performed. On evaluation of the right lung, there is a through-and-through injury to the right lower lobe that appears to have an active air leak and ongoing bleeding: Surgical management should consist of:

    A. Formal right lower lobectomy
    B. Pneumonectomy
    C. Closure of both the anterior and posterior parenchymal defects with interrupted sutures
    D. Pulmonary tractotomy
    E. Ligation of the right lower lobe pulmonary artery

16. A 17-year-old boy is brought to the emergency department after being involved in a high-speed motorcycle accident. He is hypotensive with a systolic pressure of 60 mm Hg. A focused abdominal sonography for trauma (FAST) scan is positive. At laparotomy, he is found to have a large amount of bleeding from behind the liver. Temporary application of a Pringle maneuver does not control the bleeding. However, laparotomy packs are placed, and the bleeding appears to stop. The systolic blood pressure increases to 110 mm Hg after aggressive resuscitation. The patient's pH is 7.06 and his temperature is 34°C. The next step in the management is:

    A. Obtaining control of the IVC above and below the liver
    B. Performing a median sternotomy for placement of a Schrock shunt
    C. Leaving the packs in place and doing a "damage control" closure
    D. Sequentially removing packs and beginning to take down the hepatic ligaments
    E. Dissecting the aorta at the diaphragmatic hiatus

17. After an MVA, a 17-year-old girl with blunt abdominal trauma is found to have free fluid on abdominal CT without evidence of liver or spleen injury. She is hemodynamically stable. She is taken to the operating room. At surgery, she is found to have a 75% luminal circumference injury to the first portion of the duodenum. Surgical management consists of:

    A. Pyloric exclusion
    B. Duodenal diverticulization
    C. Primary duodenal repair
    D. Whipple resection
    E. Resection with duodenoduodenostomy

18. A 19-year-old man presents to the emergency department after an MVA. The patient is alert and oriented but is unable to move his arms and legs. Results of a FAST scan, chest radiographs, and pelvic radiographs are all negative. On physical examination, the patient has a blood pressure of 80/60 mm Hg and a heart rate of 70 beats per minute. His feet are warm and pink, and he is noted to have priapism. Despite aggressive fluid resuscitation, he remains hypotensive. Which of the following is indicated?

    A. Phenylephrine
    B. Dopamine
    C. Dobutamine
    D. Epinephrine
    E. Norepinephrine

19. A 78-year-old woman presents to the emergency department after falling down a flight of stairs. Physical examination is significant for diminished motor function and pain and temperature sensation in the upper extremities. The results of a lower extremity neurologic examination are normal. This spinal cord injury is most likely consistent with:

    A. Brown-Séquard syndrome
    B. Anterior cord syndrome
    C. Middle cerebral artery cerebrovascular accident
    D. Spinal cord injury without radiographic abnormality (SCIWORA)
    E. Central cord syndrome

20. Which of the following is considered a positive diagnostic peritoneal lavage (DPL) in a blunt trauma victim?

    A. Red blood cell count of 85,000/mm^3
    B. White blood cell count of 300/mm^3
    C. Amylase of 145 IU/dL
    D. 5 mL of gross blood
    E. Presence of bile

21. A 46-year-old woman presents to the emergency department hemodynamically stable after a high-speed MVA. A CT scan of the abdomen and pelvis reveals a right perinephric hematoma with a deep laceration in the inferior aspect of the renal parenchyma without involvement of the collecting system. Management consists of:

    A. Observation
    B. Right nephrectomy
    C. Attempt at partial nephrectomy
    D. Attempt at renal salvage with suture repair of the parenchyma
    E. Attempt at renal salvage with omental packing of the laceration

22. All of the following are acceptable in the management of elevated intracranial pressure (ICP) in a patient with severe head injury EXCEPT:

    A. Decompressive craniotomy
    B. Saline 3%
    C. Hyperventilation to keep Paco$_2$ < 30 mm Hg
    D. Mannitol
    E. Barbiturates

23. A 20-year-old morbidly obese man sustains a gunshot wound to the abdomen. His blood pressure is 110/70 mm Hg and his heart rate is 100 beats per minute. At surgery, he is found to have a blast injury to the sigmoid colon involving 75% of the circumference of the bowel, with a moderate amount of fecal contamination. Which of the following is the best option?

    A. Sigmoid colectomy with primary anastomosis with a diverting ileostomy
    B. Primary repair of the sigmoid colon
    C. Sigmoid colectomy with primary anastomosis
    D. Primary repair of the sigmoid colon with exteriorization of the repair
    E. Sigmoid colectomy with a proximal colostomy and oversewing of the rectal stump

24. In a blunt trauma victim, persistent hypotension despite vigorous fluid resuscitation may be indicative of all of the following EXCEPT:

    A. Tension pneumothorax
    B. Air embolism
    C. Pericardial tamponade
    D. Ongoing intracranial hemorrhage
    E. Myocardial infarction

25. A 55-year-old man is brought into the emergency department after a high-speed MVA. He is hypotensive with a systolic pressure of 70 mm Hg despite fluid resuscitation. Chest radiograph demonstrates a wide mediastinum with multiple rib fractures, a left clavicular fracture, a depressed left mainstem bronchus, and a slight shift of the trachea to the right. Pelvic radiograph shows an unstable pelvic fracture. A FAST scan is positive for free fluid in the peritoneum. The Glasgow Coma Scale score is 14. Which of the following is the next step in management?

    A. Left anterolateral thoracotomy
    B. External fixation of the pelvic fracture
    C. Pelvic arterial embolization
    D. Exploratory laparotomy
    E. CT scan of the chest and abdomen

26. Which of the following cord syndromes is thought to have the worst prognosis?

    A. Brown-Séquard syndrome
    B. Anterior cord syndrome
    C. Posterior cord syndrome
    D. SCIWORA
    E. Central cord syndrome

27. Primary amputation should be strongly considered in the mangled lower extremity when popliteal artery transection and tibia and fibula fractures are combined with:
    A. Popliteal vein transection
    B. Tibial nerve transection
    C. Deep peroneal nerve transection
    D. Extensive skin loss
    E. Inability to dorsiflex the foot

28. A 10-year-old boy presents to the emergency department with repeated episodes of vomiting 6 hours after an MVA. Abdominal CT scan with oral and IV contrast is negative for free fluid. However, the wall of the second portion of the duodenum appears to be thickened with a slight amount of adjacent retroperitoneal stranding. There is no extraluminal air and no contrast extravasation. Which of the following is true about this condition?
    A. The patient should undergo exploratory laparotomy.
    B. This type of injury is more common in adults than children.
    C. The surgical procedure of choice is an intestinal bypass.
    D. It can develop in the absence of trauma in patients with hemophilia.
    E. Total parenteral nutrition is rarely needed.

29. All of the following are indications for the damage control approach in a trauma patient EXCEPT:
    A. Diffuse bleeding that cannot be controlled due to coagulopathy
    B. Inaccessible major venous injury
    C. Need to perform time-consuming bowel reanastomosis in a patient who is cold and has not responded appropriately to resuscitation
    D. Inaccessible suprarenal aortic injury
    E. Inability to close the abdominal fascia due to bowel edema

30. A 29-year-old man presents with a gunshot wound to the right upper quadrant. On physical examination, the patient has a tender abdomen. At surgery, the patient is found to have a 500-mL hemoperitoneum with a through-and-through injury to the right lobe of the liver that is no longer actively bleeding. Further management would consist of:
    A. Closing the injury with a liver suture
    B. Packing the injury with omentum
    C. Application of a fibrin sealant
    D. No further management
    E. Drainage with a Penrose drain

31. A 30-year-old man sustains a gunshot wound to the left mid neck. On arrival at the emergency department, the patient appears to be comatose. An airway is immediately established and IV fluids are given. His blood pressure is 70 mm Hg systolic and his heart rate is 120 beats per minute. There is no hematoma in the neck, no active bleeding, and no bruit. The next most appropriate step in management is:
    A. Head CT scan
    B. CT angiography of the neck
    C. Standard four-vessel arteriography
    D. Surgical neck exploration
    E. Triple endoscopy

32. Which of the following is true regarding flail chest?
    A. The initial chest radiograph provides a useful predictor of subsequent pulmonary insufficiency.
    B. Respiratory failure is primarily caused by the paradoxical motion of the chest wall.
    C. Operative chest wall stabilization in patients without pulmonary contusion can shorten the length of intubation.
    D. Aggressive fluid resuscitation is an important management adjunct.
    E. Once the diagnosis is established, the patient should be intubated.

33. A 30-year-old woman presents to the emergency department with a raccoon eye and right hemotympanum after an MVA. The next day marked swelling of the right eye, edema of the conjunctiva, double vision, and pulsatile exophthalmos develop. Management consists of:
    A. Surgical exploration of the eye itself
    B. Medical management to reduce intraocular pressure
    C. Repair of the presumed orbital fracture and muscle entrapment
    D. Close observation
    E. Endovascular embolization

34. Which of the following is true regarding compartment syndrome?
    A. The soleus muscle must be detached from the tibia to decompress the deep posterior compartment of the lower leg.
    B. A compartment pressure greater than 45 mm Hg is necessary to establish the diagnosis.
    C. The lateral compartment is the most commonly affected lower leg compartment.
    D. An early sign of anterior compartment involvement of the lower leg is numbness on the plantar aspect of the foot.
    E. It does not occur in the buttocks.

35. Which of the following is true regarding traumatic peripheral nerve injuries?

   A. Axonotmesis is the most severe grade of nerve injury.

   B. Posterior knee dislocation is the most common cause of traumatic peripheral nerve injury.

   C. Neurotmesis requires surgical repair.

   D. In the upper extremity, the median nerve is the most commonly injured nerve.

   E. Nerve regeneration occurs at a rate of 0.5 mm/week.

36. A 36-year-old woman sustains a gunshot wound to the right upper quadrant and has marked abdominal tenderness. At surgery, she is found to have a blast injury with nearly complete transection of the second portion of the duodenum and a deep laceration to the head of the pancreas. On exploration of the pancreatic wound, the main pancreatic duct and the intrapancreatic portion of the common bile duct are both transected. Management consists of:

   A. Primary repair of duodenum and Roux-en-Y pancreaticojejunostomy and choledochojejunostomy

   B. Pancreaticoduodenectomy (Whipple procedure)

   C. Roux-en-Y duodenojejunostomy and primary repair of the pancreatic and common bile ducts

   D. Primary repair of the duodenum and drainage

   E. Pyloric exclusion

37. A 55-year-old man presents to the emergency department with a stab wound to the left chest just below the nipple. His blood pressure is 100/60 mm Hg, his heart rate is 120 beats per minute, and his respiratory rate is 14. He has distended neck veins, and his heart sounds are muffled. The next step in the management would be:

   A. Endotracheal intubation

   B. Left tube thoracostomy

   C. Pericardiocentesis

   D. IV fluids

   E. Median sternotomy

Answers

1. B. The management of a rectal injury depends on whether it is intra- or extraperitoneal, whether it is from a high-velocity (military type) weapon leading to extensive tissue destruction or a low-velocity civilian weapon, and whether there is associated blood loss from other injuries. As a general rule, intraperitoneal injuries can be repaired primarily (they are treated like a colon injury). If the patient has severe associated injuries with a blood loss of more than six units, then resection with a colostomy is preferred. If it is an extraperitoneal injury, there are two basic options: primary repair of the injury or a diverting colostomy. The decision of whether to do primary repair relates to its accessibility. Proximal extraperitoneal injuries can be repaired primarily. In general, when primary repair of the extraperitoneal injury is performed, diversion via a colostomy is not necessary (thus, choice C is incorrect). In addition, by exposing the extraperitoneal injury to the peritoneal cavity, it effectively renders it an intraperitoneal injury; thus, presacral drainage would not be indicated (again, choice C is incorrect). The goal of presacral drainage is to allow evacuation of an enclosed space. If the extraperitoneal injury cannot be identified and repaired, a proximal diverting colostomy has been shown to be effective in allowing the injury to heal itself. Although still controversial, recent studies indicate that distal irrigation of the rectum and routine drainage of the presacral space are not necessary. In particular, if the injury is to the anterior rectum, the drainage will be ineffective. Abdominoperineal resection would not be indicated. A CT scan is not reliable enough to rule out a distal rectal injury. As such, the finding of blood on proctoscopy is enough of an indication of an injury to proceed with stool diversion.

References: Navsaria P, Edu S, Nicol A: Civilian extraperitoneal rectal gunshot wounds: surgical management made simpler, *World J Surg* 31:1345–1351, 2007.

Velmahos G, Gomez H, Falabella A, Demetriades D: Operative management of civilian rectal gunshot wounds: simpler is better, *World J Surg* 24:114–118, 2000.

2. E. Blunt injury to the renal artery is rare and results from intimal disruption and thrombosis. The likelihood of renal salvage with revascularization is very low, given that the renal artery is an end artery and is immediately subjected to warm ischemia. In most situations, the best management option is observation of the injury, particularly in the patient with multiple other injuries or when there is a delay in recognition. Even in the rare setting where there is an isolated blunt injury to the renal artery with no other injuries and the injury is promptly recognized, the likelihood of restoring significant renal function is so low that most authors recommend leaving the kidney alone (again, provided there is normal renal function in the other kidney). Repair is recommended for bilateral injury or injury in a solitary kidney. Rarely, leaving the kidney in situ leads to hypertension, in which case, a subsequent nephrectomy can be performed.

References: Bruce L, Croce M, Santaniello J, et al: Blunt renal artery injury: incidence, diagnosis, and management, *Am Surg* 67:550–554, 2001.

Sangthong B, Demetriades D, Martin M, et al: Management and hospital outcomes of blunt renal artery injuries: analysis of 517 patients from the National Trauma Data Bank, *J Am Coll Surg* 203:612–617, 2006.

3. A. Injury to the ureter occurs most often after penetrating trauma. The optimal treatment is to débride devitalized tissue, spatulate the two ends, and perform an end-to-end anastomosis over a double J stent (ureteroureterostomy) using an absorbable monofilament. Some mobilization of the ureter is feasible, but mobilization risks interrupting the blood supply that runs just adjacent to the ureter. As such, the dissection should be maintained approximately 1 cm away from the ureter so as not to disrupt its blood supply. A good guide to the viability of the two ends of the ureter is whether the cut edges are bleeding. Lower ureteral injuries may require reimplanting the ureter into the bladder (ureteroneocystostomy) if there is not enough distal ureter for a primary anastomosis. When a large segment of ureter has been injured and primary reanastomosis is not possible, several options are available. A psoas hitch involves mobilization of the bladder, which is then sutured to the iliopsoas fascia above the iliac vessels, to perform a tension-free reimplantation of the ureter. Another option is to anastomose the ureter to the contralateral ureter (transureteroureterostomy). Finally, the kidney itself can be mobilized and brought into the pelvis. In this patient, however, with massive blood loss and hemodynamic instability, a damage control approach should be used. There are two options. The first is to simply ligate the ureter proximally and distally. This will require a percutaneous nephrostomy; however, there is no need to perform the nephrostomy in the operating room because this will further delay rewarming and resuscitating the patient. Rather, the nephrostomy should be performed once the patient is stabilized. The patient can later be taken back for a more elective repair of the ureter. The other option is to perform a temporary cutaneous ureterostomy over a single J stent, placing a tie around the ureter and stent and then bringing the stent up to the skin. Given the location of the injury and the length of injured ureter, the patient would eventually likely need a psoas hitch or other more complex repairs.

4. D. Both blood volume and red cell volume increase in the pregnant patient, but blood volume increases more than red cell volume. Blood volume increases by approximately 50% as term approaches, whereas red cell volume increases by approximately 30%, resulting in a functional hemodilution and manifested by physiologic anemia. The increased blood volume and red cell volume are designed for the anticipated blood loss of delivery. Thus, pregnant patients are less likely to manifest signs of blood loss such as tachycardia and hypotension, and if such signs are present, they are indicative of an even more severe blood loss than in the nonpregnant patient (on the order of 1500–2000 mL of blood loss). The pregnant patient has an increased tidal volume and minute ventilation, designed to increase oxygen release to the fetus. This results in a mild respiratory alkalosis, with a P_{CO_2} in the 27 to 32 range. Oxygen consumption is increased, and functional residual capacity is decreased. In addition, the 2,3-diphosphoglycerate level is increased to enhance release of oxygen to the fetus. However, these physiologic changes result in less pulmonary reserve in an acutely ill pregnant patient. Use of radiographs is thought to be safe for the fetus after the 20th week of gestation. The glomerular filtration rate increases, resulting in a decrease in serum creatinine. Other important aspects to be aware of are that the gravid uterus can compress the IVC, resulting in decreased venous return. Therefore, the pregnant patient should be placed in the left lateral position at approximately 15 degrees. Pregnant patients are more prone to aspiration, so early nasogastric tube decompression is important. Finally, the progressive stretching of the peritoneum leads to desensitization, so that a pregnant patient is less likely to demonstrate peritoneal signs.

Reference: Shah AJ, Kilcline B: Trauma in pregnancy, *Emerg Med Clin North Am* 21:615–629, 2003.

5. C. The majority of bladder injuries occur because of blunt trauma. Bladder rupture may be extraperitoneal, intraperitoneal, or both. Extraperitoneal injuries are the most common (as many as 70%). The majority occur in association with pelvic fractures. Extraperitoneal ruptures often result from perforation due to adjacent bony fragments. Intraperitoneal rupture of the bladder results from dome injuries and is more likely to occur when a full bladder sustains a direct blow (thus, there is an increased risk in patients who have been drinking alcohol). Hematuria in the presence of a pelvic fracture should increase the suspicion for bladder injury. If blood is visible at the urethral meatus, then a Foley catheter should not be inserted until retrograde urethrography is first performed to rule out a urethral injury. Otherwise, in the presence of hematuria, the diagnosis of a bladder injury can usually be made by CT scan performed with contrast inserted into the Foley catheter. If bladder contrast is not given, extraperitoneal injuries may be missed and intraperitoneal injuries may show a large volume of free intraperitoneal fluid combined with air in the bladder and an absence of solid organ injury.

When extravasation is seen, it is important to determine whether it is intraperitoneal, extraperitoneal, or both. Contrast above the peritoneal reflection is intraperitoneal (the paracolic gutter would be intraperitoneal). The management of an extraperitoneal rupture of the bladder is nonsurgical in most instances and consists of placing a Foley catheter for 7 to 10 days and then obtaining a cystogram. Intraperitoneal injuries are repaired via a transabdominal approach, including a three-layer closure using absorbable sutures. Silk suture is not appropriate because permanent sutures in the bladder will increase the risk of ongoing bladder mucosal irritation and bladder stone formation. A suprapubic cystotomy is often placed, in particular for large wounds or those with devitalized tissue. If CT cystography is equivocal, a formal cystogram should be obtained; it is otherwise unnecessary.

Reference: Vaccaro J, Brody J: CT cystography in the evaluation of major bladder trauma, *Radiographics* 20:1373–1381, 2000.

6. B. The Glasgow Coma Scale is based on eye opening, motor response, and verbal response. Motor response has the greatest point total (up to 6 points). A score of 8 or less is considered a severe head injury and is an indication to establish an airway. The scoring is as follows:

Eye opening: 1, does not open eyes; 2, opens to painful stimulus; 3, opens to voice; 4, opens spontaneously

Motor response: 1, no movement; 2, decerebrate posture; 3, decorticate posture; 4, withdraws from pain; 5, localized painful stimulus; 6, obeys commands

Verbal response: 1, no sounds; 2, incomprehensible sounds; 3, inappropriate words; 4, confused; 5, appropriate and oriented

7. E. Epidural hematomas are most typically due to a fracture of the temporal bone and a tear of the middle meningeal artery. Associated parenchymal brain injury is less frequent than with subdural hematomas. Thus, the prognosis in general is better than that for subdural hematomas. Epidural hematomas classically present with loss of consciousness followed by awakening and a lucid interval, with unconsciousness again, but this is not always the case. A CT scan shows a convex or lens-shaped hematoma. Subdural hematomas occur between the dura and cortex and are caused by disruption of bridging veins. Generally, a greater force is required to create this type of disruption, and as such, it is associated with a higher rate of parenchymal brain injury, rendering a worse prognosis. Patients who present with a Glasgow Coma Scale score of 8 or less should be treated with the presumption of a severe head injury. They should be intubated, given mannitol, and mildly hyperventilated to reduce ICP. Small subdurals (<5-mm thickness), without midline shift, and with minimal neurologic symptoms can be treated nonoperatively. Similarly, epidural hematomas that cause alterations in consciousness or in neurologic function should be surgically drained.

8. B. Most veins can be safely ligated in the setting of traumatic injury. However, certain veins are less likely to tolerate ligation well. These include the superior vena cava (as it may result in an acute superior vena cava syndrome), the renal veins close to the renal parenchyma (as there is then inadequate outflow for the kidney; ligation of the left renal vein close to the IVC is well tolerated as drainage can occur via the adrenal, gonadal, and iliolumbar veins), the IVC above the renal veins (as it will impair outflow to both kidneys), or just at the diaphragm (as this will cause an acute Budd-Chiari syndrome), and the portal vein (as it supplies 75% of the blood to the liver). The portal vein has been ligated successfully, provided adequate fluid is administered to compensate for the dramatic but transient edema that occurs in the bowel, but ligation seems to be associated with a higher mortality rate than repair. Ligation of the IVC below the renal veins is better tolerated than the suprarenal IVC; however, marked leg swelling may develop and may require fasciotomies. Ligation of the superior mesenteric vein is also fairly well tolerated and better tolerated than portal vein ligation, although again it is preferable to repair the superior mesenteric vein if the patient is stable and it is technically feasible, as there is similarly marked bowel edema and risk of bowel infarction as with portal vein repair. Arteries for which repair should always be attempted include the carotid, innominate, brachial, superior mesenteric, proper hepatic, iliac, femoral, and popliteal arteries and the aorta. In the forearm, either the radial or ulnar artery can be ligated, provided the other vessel is palpable. Similarly, in the lower leg, at least one of the two palpable vessels (anterior or posterior tibial artery) should be salvaged. Because of the excellent collateralization around the shoulder, ligation of the subclavian artery is well tolerated. In fact, the artery is often occluded during stent-grafting of thoracic aneurysms or aortic transection.

9. A. Myocardial contusion should be suspected in anyone with severe blunt chest trauma. Although the term *myocardial contusion* has been used for many years, an accurate diagnosis of a myocardial contusion remains elusive. This is largely due to the fact that a precise definition of what constitutes a myocardial contusion is not clear. Technically speaking, a myocardial contusion can only be confirmed by either visual inspection of the heart at surgery or at autopsy. Attempts to identify a contusion and stratify severity via creatine kinase, myocardial bound enzymes, electrocardiograms (ECGs), nuclear scans, and echocardiography have not been successful because these modalities lack sensitivity. Most patients with a diagnosis of myocardial contusion have a benign course, with very few developing arrhythmias or pump failure. Given these issues, a proposal has been made to replace the term *cardiac contusion* with the term *blunt cardiac injury* and to be used in the setting of blunt chest trauma with clinically evident cardiac injury. Criteria for blunt cardiac injury include the presence of shock in the absence of hemorrhage or spinal shock, the presence of arrhythmias on ECG requiring treatment, a decreased cardiac index (<2.5 L/min/m^2), and structural abnormalities on echocardiography. Cardiac troponin levels have been shown to be highly sensitive and specific for myocardial injury, but the degree of elevation has not been shown to be a useful tool for stratification of severity. In patients with suspected blunt cardiac injury, a negative cardiac troponin level, combined with a normal ECG, makes significant blunt cardiac injury exceedingly unlikely. If negative, a repeat troponin and ECG should be performed 8 hours later. Two consecutive readings effectively rule out the diagnosis. If the cardiac troponin level and/or ECG are abnormal in a stable patient, the patient should be admitted for observation to a monitored bed. If the patient is unstable, an emergent echocardiogram should be performed. If a tamponade is seen, emergent sternotomy should be performed for suspected cardiac rupture. Very rarely, blunt cardiac injury can lead to coronary artery thrombosis, valvular disruption, or septal disruption. In an unstable patient with blunt cardiac injury without an anatomic abnormality on echocardiography, invasive monitoring with pressor support should be instituted.

References: Kaye P, O'Sullivan I: Myocardial contusion: emergency investigation and diagnosis, *Emerg Med J* 19:8–10, 2002.

Velmahos G, Karaiskakis M, Salim A, et al: Normal electrocardiography and serum troponin I levels preclude the presence of clinically significant blunt cardiac injury, *J Trauma* 54:45–50, 2003.

10. A. In any trauma resuscitation, the ABCs should be addressed first. The first crucial step is to secure the patient's airway via endotracheal intubation because he is agitated and has severe hypotension. Once the airway is secure, adequacy of breath sounds should be determined, and a right chest tube inserted if breath sounds are decreased or diminished. This should be followed by insertion of two large-bore IV catheters into the antecubital fossa and aggressive resuscitation with normal saline or lactated Ringer's solution. Given the location of the injury (if it is zone I of the neck, one should have a high suspicion for a right subclavian artery or innominate artery injury). After instituting the ABCs, the next step would be to take the patient directly to the operating room, given the hemodynamic instability. Proximal control of such an injury on the right is best achieved by a median sternotomy. If the same injury were present on the left, proximal control of the left subclavian artery is best achieved via a left anterolateral thoracotomy. If blood is exsanguinating through the bullet hole, manual compression in this area is ineffective. Temporary tamponade can be achieved via insertion and inflation of a Foley balloon directly into the wound, permitting rapid transportation to the operating room.

Reference Advanced Trauma Life Support, ed 7, Chicago, 2004, American College of Surgeons.

11. E. The preferred access for infants in the trauma setting is the antecubital fossa, as in adults. If this is unsuccessful, the next preferred access is a percutaneous approach to the distal saphenous vein. If neither of these is successful, in a trauma patient younger than 6 years of age, interosseous cannulation of the proximal tibia provides a good short-term access for resuscitation, placed 2 to 3 cm below the tibial tuberosity, using a bone marrow aspiration needle (18 gauge), and angling away from the growth plate. Once the patient has been resuscitated, a follow-up attempt at peripheral access should be made. If a patient has obvious deformities in the tibiae (as in this patient), the next location for interosseous cannulation would be the distal femur just above the femoral condyles. A distal saphenous vein cutdown is another option in children ages 1 to 6 years,

but in a child younger than 1 year of age, it would be challenging and not appropriate in the setting of obvious leg deformity. In hypovolemic pediatric patients younger than 6 years of age, percutaneous femoral vein cannulation is another alternative, but is associated with an increased risk of venous thrombosis and would be much more challenging in a child younger than 1 year. Subclavian and internal jugular central lines would be too difficult to perform in the trauma setting in such a small child and would be associated with an increased risk of iatrogenic injury. The interosseous cannula should be removed expeditiously because of the potential risk of osteomyelitis.

References: Smith R, Davis N, Bouamra O, Lecky F: The utilization of intraosseous infusion in the resuscitation of pediatric major trauma patients, *Injury* 36:1034–1038, 2005.

Vavilala M, Nathens A, Jurkovich G, et al: Risk factors for venous thromboembolism in pediatric trauma, *J Trauma* 52:922–927, 2002.

12. C. Exposure of the innominate, proximal right subclavian, and proximal right and left common carotid arteries is fairly straightforward and is achieved with a median sternotomy. Likewise, exposure of the proximal vertebral artery, just at its take-off from the subclavian artery, is readily achieved with a supraclavicular incision. This will require division of the anterior scalene muscle and clavicular head of the sternocleidomastoid muscle and protection of the phrenic nerve that overlies it and on the left side avoidance of the thoracic duct. Conversely, exposure of the mid portion of the vertebral artery is not readily feasible because it travels through a bony foramina adjacent to the vertebral body. Exposure of the proximal left subclavian artery presents a difficult challenge. The left subclavian artery arises from the aortic arch posteriorly, and thus, it is not readily approached with a median sternotomy. The best exposure of the proximal left subclavian artery is with an anterolateral thoracotomy at the third intercostal space. Distal control can then be achieved via a supraclavicular approach. On occasion, resection of the medial head of the clavicle as well as a partial median sternotomy is needed to connect the two horizontal incisions and raise a chest wall flap. The ribs can also be cut laterally for additional exposure, creating a so-called trapdoor thoracotomy.

13. D. The Cattell maneuver involves a medial visceral rotation of the cecum and ascending colon. It is achieved by incising the peritoneal reflection at the white line of Toldt. It is useful for exposing right retroperitoneal structures, such as the IVC and the right ureter. Further cephalad, mobilization and medial rotation of the duodenum (Kocher maneuver) additionally assist in exposing the suprarenal IVC below the liver. The Kocher maneuver is not useful for exposing the celiac axis. This is best done by combining a Mattox maneuver with division of the left crus of the diaphragm and dividing the celiac plexus. The Mattox maneuver consists of a medial rotation of the left colon (again at the line of Toldt), kidney, and spleen toward the midline. Exposure of injuries to the distal IVC and iliac vein bifurcations can be exceedingly difficult. On occasion, division of the right common iliac artery is needed to expose and repair an injury of this area. A primary repair of the iliac artery can then be performed. On rare occasion, with massive bleeding, the junction of the SMA, splenic, and portal veins may need to be exposed by division of the neck of the pancreas.

References: Cothren CC, Biffl WL, Moore EE: Trauma. Brunicardi FC, Andersen DK, Billiar TR, et al, editors: *Schwartz's principles of surgery*, ed 9, New York, 2010, McGraw-Hill, pp 135–195.

Hoyt D, Coimbra R, Acosta J: Management of trauma. In Townsend CM Jr, Beauchamp RD, Evers BM, Mattox KL, editors: *Sabiston textbook of surgery: the biological basis of modern surgical practice*, ed 18, Philadelphia, 2008, WB Saunders, pp 477–520.

Mullins RJ: Shock, electrolytes, and fluid. In Townsend CM Jr, Beauchamp RD, Evers BM, Mattox KL, editors: *Sabiston textbook of surgery: the biological basis of modern surgical practice*, ed 18, Philadelphia, 2008, WB Saunders, pp 69–112.

14. B. Indications for operative treatment of penetrating thoracic injuries include a caked hemothorax, large air leak with inadequate ventilation or persistent collapse of the lung, drainage of more than 1500 mL of blood when the chest tube is first inserted, continuous hemorrhage of more than 200 mL for more than 3 hours, esophageal perforation, and pericardial tamponade. Thus, for option A, a second chest tube would be inserted. If after the second chest tube, a large hemothorax persists, this is termed a *caked hemothorax*, and a thoracotomy is indicated. For a wide mediastinum, a CT scan of the chest would be obtained to rule out an aortic transection. Flail chest is not typically an indication for a thoracotomy, although there are some recent studies that indicate that early internal fixation may improve pulmonary function and hasten recovery.

15. D. In the past, the injury described would have been dealt with by performing a formal lobectomy. However, pulmonary tractotomy was introduced approximately 15 years ago as a less aggressive alternative. The technique involves using a linear stapling device to insert directly into the injured bullet tract. Two hemostatic staple lines are created, and the lung is divided in between. This allows direct access to the bleeding vessels within the parenchyma as well as any leaking bronchi. Bleeding vessels can then be oversewn with a polypropylene monofilament. Lobectomy is a better choice for a completely devascularized or destroyed lobe. A pneumonectomy is rarely indicated and in the trauma setting is associated with an 80% mortality rate.

References: Asensio J, Demetriades D, Berne J et al: Stapled pulmonary tractotomy: a rapid way to control hemorrhage in penetrating pulmonary injuries, *J Am Coll Surg* 185:486–487, 1997.

Cothren C, Moore E, Biffl W, et al: Lung-sparing techniques are associated with improved outcome compared with anatomic resection for severe lung injuries, *J Trauma* 53:483–487, 2002.

16. C. The management of liver injuries has undergone a major evolution in the past 15 years, from routine laparotomy in the past to the current use of selective nonsurgical management in hemodynamically stable patients, a more liberal use of angiographic embolization, and operative management with selective packing and damage control when the patient is cold and coagulopathic. In a patient who has sustained blunt trauma and is hemodynamically stable, a CT scan with IV contrast should be performed. If a contrast blush is seen in the liver, the patient should be

taken to angiography for embolization, provided there are no other injuries that require operative intervention. Conversely, if the patient is hemodynamically unstable (as in this patient), the patient should be taken to the operating room, and all four quadrants packed. Most liver bleeding can be controlled with a combination of packing and manual compression, topical hemostatic agents, and argon beam coagulator. The Pringle maneuver is another useful adjunct to temporarily control bleeding. Continued bleeding despite the Pringle maneuver (compression of the portal vein and hepatic artery through the foramen of Winslow) suggests bleeding from the retrohepatic IVC or hepatic veins (as in this patient). A juxtahepatic IVC or a central major hepatic vein injury is considered a grade V injury (on the Liver Injury Scale from I to VI) and is associated with a high mortality rate. If the bleeding is controlled with packing, and in addition, the patient is cold (temperature <34°C), coagulopathic, and with a refractory acidosis (as in this patient), the best option would be to proceed to a damage control mode. If, conversely, the bleeding is not controlled, the next step would be to rapidly take down the hepatic ligaments including the ligamentum teres, falciform ligament, triangular ligament, and the right coronary ligament, and perform a Kocher maneuver. This allows better direct compression with packing in the retrohepatic space. A decision must then be made as to whether to attempt repair of a retrohepatic IVC injury. This decision depends on the experience of the surgeon, the clinical status of the patient, and whether bleeding is controlled. If bleeding has now stopped with packing, one option is to take the patient back to the intensive care unit to resuscitate and rewarm. If bleeding persists, total vascular exclusion of the liver is now possible as control of the IVC just below the diaphragm and just inferior to the liver can be performed, combined with the Pringle maneuver.

References: Asensio J, Demetriades D, Chahwan S, et al: Approach to the management of complex hepatic injuries, *J Trauma* 48:66–69, 2000.

Sriussadaporn S, Pak-art R, Tharavej C, et al: A multidisciplinary approach in the management of hepatic injuries, *Injury* 33:309–315, 2002.

17. E. Management of duodenal injuries depends on location, extent of injury, associated pancreatic injury, and clinical status of the patient. Duodenal injuries are graded from I to V, with grade I being a hematoma or partial-thickness injury and grade V being a massive disruption of the pancreaticoduodenal complex or complete duodenal devascularization. If a simple duodenal hematoma is recognized preoperatively, it can be managed without surgery, with nasogastric decompression and parenteral nutrition. If it is found intraoperatively, it is left alone if small. If it is a large hematoma (involving >50% of the lumen), it is recommended to incise the serosa, drain the hematoma, and then reclose the serosa. The majority of full-thickness lacerations of the duodenum can be repaired primarily in a transverse fashion to avoid narrowing the lumen, with placement of an overlying omental patch. Conversely, if the injury involves more than 50% of the luminal circumference, more extensive surgical treatment is required. If such an injury is in the first or fourth portion of the duodenum, then resection with duodenoduodenostomy can be performed (as in this patient). If the injury is in the second or third portion of the duodenum and the ampulla is not injured, then a Roux-en-Y duodenojejunostomy is a better option. The second portion is tethered to the head of the pancreas by its blood supply and the ducts of Wirsung and Santorini, so the length of duodenum that can be mobilized from the pancreas is very limited. Attempts to suture repair the second portion when tissue is lost often result in an unacceptably narrow lumen, and end-to-end anastomosis is not possible. If the injury is distal to the ampulla of Vater, the distal portion of the duodenum is oversewn, the jejunum is anastomosed end to end to the proximal duodenum, and the defunctionalized distal duodenum and proximal jejunum are drained into the jejunum. Pyloric exclusion is rarely needed and involves either stapling or oversewing the pylorus and creating a gastrojejunostomy. Duodenal diverticularization requires repairing the duodenal injury, antrectomy, vagotomy, gastrojejunostomy, duodenostomy, choledochostomy, and feeding jejunostomy. It is not generally recommended. When there is a combined duodenal and pancreatic injury, it is recommended to treat each one separately. In other words, perform duodenal repair for a less than 50% circumference injury and pancreatic drainage for a pancreatic injury without ductal disruption, or distal pancreatectomy for a distal pancreatic injury with ductal disruption. A Whipple procedure is rarely needed in the situation of a combined massive disruption of the pancreatic head and duodenum.

18. A. The presentation is consistent with neurogenic shock. Findings suggestive of neurogenic shock include hypotension with relative bradycardia, warm, well-perfused extremities reflecting loss of sympathetic tone, evidence of a high spinal cord injury, and priapism (sustained erection due to unopposed parasympathetic stimulation). In a patient with a high cervical spine injury, the first step is to secure an airway. The phrenic nerve is supplied by the C3 to C5 nerve roots. Thus, patients with an injury above C5 will routinely require ventilatory support. After the airway is secured and ventilation is adequate, fluid resuscitation and restoration of intravascular volume will often improve perfusion in neurogenic shock. Most patients with neurogenic shock will respond to restoration of intravascular volume alone, with satisfactory improvement in perfusion and resolution of hypotension. It is always important to rule out hypovolemia in the trauma setting. In addition, one must always be aware that in the presence of spinal cord injury, one cannot rely on the abdominal examination. Thus, an abdominal and pelvic CT scan would be indicated to rule out visceral injury. If the patient does not respond to fluids, administration of vasoconstrictors will improve peripheral vascular tone, decrease vascular capacitance, and increase venous return, but should only be considered once hypovolemia is excluded as the cause of the hypotension, and the diagnosis of neurogenic shock is established. If the patient's blood pressure has not responded to what is thought to be adequate volume resuscitation, a pure α-agonist such as phenylephrine may be used. The need for vasoconstrictor support is typically brief and lasts 24 to 48 hours. Restoration of blood pressure and circulatory perfusion is also important to improve perfusion to the spinal cord, prevent progressive spinal cord ischemia, and minimize secondary cord injury.

19. E. Central cord syndrome usually occurs in older persons who suffer hyperextension injuries such as those resulting from an MVA or fall. It is more frequent in someone who has a chronic preexisting cervical spondylolysis. The central part of the spinal cord is preferentially injured. There is a disproportionate deficit in motor function in the upper extremities compared with the lower extremities. Motor function and pain and temperature sensation are diminished in the upper extremities but preserved in the lower extremities. Central cord syndrome generally has a good prognosis for neurologic and functional improvement with rehabilitation, although not usually a complete recovery. Anterior cord syndrome results from ischemia to the anterior two thirds of the spinal cord caused by compression of the anterior spinal artery. It is characterized by diminished motor function and pain and temperature sensation below the level of the injury, with preservation of position, vibratory sense, and crude touch. It is thought to have the worst prognosis of all the cord syndromes. Brown-Séquard syndrome due to a hemisection of the spinal cord. It can be caused by blunt or penetrating trauma or by a spinal cord tumor. It is characterized by ipsilateral hemiplegia with contralateral pain and temperature sensation deficits because of the crossing of the fibers of the spinothalamic tract. SCIWORA occurs more commonly in children. It has been termed an *occult instability of the spinal column*. However, with the increasing use of magnetic resonance imaging, it is now apparent that the instability is not as occult as originally described. Rather, the injuries are just not readily apparent on plain radiograph because they are due to injuries to nonbony supporting tissues of the vertebral column such as the anterior and posterior longitudinal ligaments, the intervertebral disc, and the muscular and interspinal ligaments. Magnetic resonance imaging provides a better assessment of the extent of spinal cord injuries in SCIWORA, which have been classified into five categories that are predictive of outcome: complete transection, major hemorrhage, minor hemorrhage, edema only, and normal. Complete transection and major hemorrhage are associated with a poor outcome; 40% of patients with minor hemorrhage show significant improvement; 75% with edema only show significant improvement and the remainder return to normal; and all patients with normal cord signals make a complete recovery.

References: Pang D: Spinal cord injury without radiographic abnormality in children, 2 decades later, *Neurosurgery* 55:1325–1342, 2004.

Roth E, Lawler M, Yarkony G: Traumatic central cord syndrome: clinical features and functional outcomes, *Arch Phys Med Rehabil* 71:18–23, 1990.

20. E. The role of DPL has diminished considerably over the past two decades with the increasing availability of the FAST scan and the ability to rapidly perform a CT scan. However, DPL is still useful in the setting of a hemodynamically unstable patient for whom a bedside ultrasound scan is unavailable or when results of FAST scanning are equivocal. Another situation in which DPL is useful is when a patient is in the operating room for neurosurgical trauma, and unexplained hemodynamic instability develops. The results of DPL are considered grossly positive if more than 10 mL of free blood can be aspirated after insertion of the catheter. In this situation, it is not necessary to insert fluid into the peritoneal cavity, and an exploratory laparotomy should be performed. If less than 10 mL is withdrawn, a liter of normal saline is instilled. Positive DPL findings include a red blood cell count greater than $100,000/mm^3$ for blunt trauma or greater than $5000/mm^3$ for penetrating trauma, the detection of bile or amylase or vegetable or fecal material, and a white blood cell count greater than $500/mm^3$. For the DPL to be reliable, at least 250 mL of fluid should be aspirated back. It should be kept in mind, however, that if the patient is hemodynamically unstable and there is no gross blood, it is unlikely that the abdomen is the source of hypotension even if the DPL aspirate is positive. In addition, once fluid is infused into the peritoneum, if the patient later stabilizes and a CT scan is performed, the DPL makes subsequent interpretation of the CT scan more difficult because there will be fluid and air within the peritoneal cavity.

21. A. Kidney injuries are graded from I to V, with grade I being a contusion or subcapsular, nonexpanding hematoma and grade V a completely shattered kidney or an avulsion of the renal hilum. Grade I and II injuries are considered minor, grade III injuries are deep lacerations that do not involve the collecting system, whereas grade IV injuries are lacerations extending into the collecting system or an injury to the main renal artery. The vast majority of blunt renal trauma (approximately 98%) can be managed nonoperatively. The injury described in this patient would be a grade III and, in a stable patient, can be managed nonoperatively. Even a grade IV injury from blunt trauma can be managed nonoperatively provided the patient is hemodynamically stable. If there is urinary extravasation, this usually resolves, and if it does not, it can be treated later by percutaneous drainage or by placing a urinary stent. Although penetrating traumas should theoretically be managed the same based on injury grade, they are much more frequently explored because of the high incidence of associated penetrating injury to the bowel. Absolute indications for operative exploration include a renal injury in the setting of hemodynamic instability and if the patient is already being explored and a retroperitoneal hematoma overlying the kidney is rapidly expanding or pulsatile. If during exploration a nonexpanding, nonpulsatile hematoma is found in the retroperitoneum, it can be safely observed in a stable patient. Surgery is indicated for vascular or renal pedicle injury or in a completely shattered kidney. A recent study confirmed that the injury grade correlates with both the need for surgery (grade I = 0%, grade II = 15%, grade III = 76%, grade IV = 78%, and grade V = 93%) and the need for nephrectomy (grade I = 0%, grade II = 0%, grade III = 3%, grade IV = 9%, and grade V = 86%).

Reference: Santucci R, McAninch J, Safir M, et al: Validation of the American Association for the Surgery of Trauma organ injury severity scale for the kidney, *J Trauma* 50:195–200, 2001.

22. C. Intracranial pressure (ICP) monitoring is recommended for patients with severe head injury (Glasgow Coma Scale score ≤8) and in patients with moderate head injury (Glasgow Coma Scale score 9–12) who are undergoing anesthesia and thus cannot be clinically monitored. Treatment is instituted if the ICP increases to more than 20 to 25 mm Hg. It is important to remember this formula: Cerebral perfusion pressure = Mean arterial pressure − ICP. Normal cerebral perfusion pressure is approximately 80 mm Hg. Cerebral ischemia ensues when the cerebral perfusion pressure decreases to less than 50 mm Hg, but an adverse neurologic outcome is seen even with a cerebral perfusion pressure less than 70 mm Hg if it is sustained for long periods of time. Not only is it important to keep the ICP low, but it is also vital to maintain the mean arterial pressure at normal levels. Several methods are used to lower the ICP. Although hyperventilation has been used for more than two decades, its use has recently fallen out of favor. Overly aggressive hyperventilation has been shown to worsen intracranial injury because the severe vasoconstriction leads to a reduction in cerebral blood flow, thus counteracting any potential benefit of lowering the ICP. Early mild to moderate hyperventilation (>30 mm Hg) is still used and seems to be safe. Mannitol induces an osmotic diuresis that leads to a decreased ICP. Hypertonic saline, using either a 7.5% solution in small boluses or a 3% solution as a maintenance fluid, is also effective. The target is to increase the serum sodium level to between 155 and 160 mEq/L. Drainage of cerebrospinal fluid via a ventriculostomy is another option to lower the ICP, although placement of a ventriculostomy is not always feasible in the trauma patient because of ventricular space compression. Finally, a barbiturate coma, targeted to induce burst suppression on the electroencephalogram, is another useful treatment because it lowers cerebral metabolism and ICP. Mannitol and barbiturates should only be instituted when the patient is adequately hydrated and has an adequate blood pressure because they will otherwise lead to counterproductive decreases in blood pressure. Decompressive craniotomy to lower the ICP is controversial. However, anecdotal reports and a small randomized study in children seem to indicate that it is effective in lowering the ICP, particularly when instituted early.

References: Cormio M, Gopinath SP, Valadka A, Robertson C: Cerebral hemodynamic effects of pentobarbital coma in head-injured patients, *J Neurotrauma* 16:927–936, 1999.

Diringer M, Yundt K, Videen T, et al: No reduction in cerebral metabolism as a result of early moderate hyperventilation following severe traumatic brain injury, *J Neurosurg* 92:7–13, 2000.

Taylor A, Butt W, Rosenfeld J, et al: A randomized trial of very early decompressive craniectomy in children with traumatic brain injury and sustained intracranial hypertension, *Childs Nerv Syst* 17:154–162, 2001.

23. C. Increasingly, colon injuries are being treated with either primary repair, if feasible, or resection with a primary anastomosis. This approach is being applied to both right- and left-sided colon injuries. Primary repair is used when less than 50% of the circumference of the bowel is involved, whereas resection is recommended for larger wounds. Once a resection is performed, a decision must be made as to whether to perform a primary reanastomosis or a colostomy. The primary contraindication to attempting a primary reanastomosis is the clinical condition of the patient. A colostomy should be strongly considered in a patient who has a destructive colon injury that requires a resection and is in shock, has received more than five units of blood transfusion, or has other major comorbidities (cardiac, pulmonary, renal). Ischemia at the anastomosis with subsequent breakdown and leakage in such patients is more likely to develop. Using this approach, in a recent large series, only 7% of patients required an ostomy. Certainly the presence of fecal contamination (as in this patient) will increase the risk of complications. However, the increased complication rate does not seem to be related to whether a primary reanastomosis or colostomy is performed. Another important consideration is obesity. Morbid obesity makes the creation of a stoma difficult, predisposes the stoma to the development of ischemia, and, if this occurs, increases the risk of the development of a necrotizing soft tissue infection. It also makes the subsequent colostomy takedown more challenging. As such, strong consideration should be given in obese patients to a primary reanastomosis.

Reference: Murray J, Demetriades D, Colson M, et al: Colonic resection in trauma: colostomy versus anastomosis, *J Trauma* 46:250–254, 1999.

24. D. In the absence of a clear source of ongoing hemorrhage, when a patient manifests persistent hypotension despite vigorous fluid resuscitation after trauma, cardiogenic sources need to be considered. These include a tension pneumothorax, pericardial tamponade, myocardial infarction from coronary artery thrombosis, air embolism, and other blunt cardiac injuries. A closed head injury, conversely, should not generally be considered the source of hypotension. Because it is a limited space, one generally cannot bleed a sufficient volume to create hypotension. Furthermore, traumatic intracranial bleeding often manifests with the Cushing reflex (hypertension and bradycardia). The work-up of a persistently hypotensive patient should include an echocardiogram to look for blunt cardiac injury, a repeat FAST scan to confirm the absence of blood in the peritoneal cavity, and a repeat chest radiograph. Retroperitoneal bleeding is another potential source of major blood loss and is usually due to pelvic fractures. These can be readily diagnosed with a pelvic radiograph.

25. D. The patient presents a difficult challenge because there are three potential sources of bleeding: the abdomen, the chest, and the retroperitoneum. As a general rule, bleeding into the peritoneal cavity takes precedence over other potential sites of bleeding. Thus, this patient should first undergo an exploratory laparotomy. The chest radiograph is highly suspicious for a partial aortic transection (widened mediastinum, depressed left main stem bronchus, shift of the trachea). However, there is no evidence of a massive hemothorax on the chest radiograph. Thus, if there is an aortic injury, it is likely a partial tear. Recent studies indicate that thoracic aortic injuries can be addressed in a delayed fashion, particularly if the patient is hemodynamically stable. Granted this patient is not stable, but the source of instability points toward the abdomen given the positive

FAST scan findings. A recent study of patients with pelvic fractures and positive FAST scan results confirmed that the finding of intraperitoneal fluid strongly correlated with significant intra-abdominal lesions requiring surgical intervention. During laparotomy, after control of bleeding, if a large retroperitoneal hematoma is encountered, packing can be placed and the patient then transported to the angiography suite for embolization. With regard to the definitive management of thoracic aortic injuries, recent studies indicate that endovascular stent grafting is associated with lower mortality and morbidity rates and lower rates of paraplegia than open thoracic repair.

Reference: Ruchholtz S, Waydhas C, Lewan U, et al: Free abdominal fluid on ultrasound in unstable pelvic ring fracture: is laparotomy always necessary? *J Trauma* 57:278–285, 2004.

26. B. Brown-Séquard syndrome is rare and is thought to have the best prognosis, likely due to the fact that there is not a complete cord transection but a hemitransection at most. Anterior cord syndrome is the second most common spinal cord syndrome and is thought to have the worst prognosis. This is likely due to the fact that it is caused by interruption of the anterior spinal artery, which leads to infarction of the anterior two thirds of the spinal cord. Central cord syndrome is the most common spinal cord syndrome and carries a fair prognosis. Posterior cord syndrome is very rare. It is due to a loss of dorsal column function (deep pressure and proprioception). Motor function is preserved. Because patients lose vibration and position sense, walking is difficult because of the persistent impairment of proprioception. Pain and temperature sensation is intact. The Romberg sign is positive. The prognosis of SCIWORA depends on the extent of spinal cord damage, which is best determined by magnetic resonance imaging. Patients with SCIWORA with edema only or with a normal spinal cord on magnetic resonance imaging have an excellent prognosis.

27. B. The decision to perform a primary amputation or attempt reconstruction in a mangled extremity is a complex one. Factors that need to be taken into consideration include (1) the degree of soft tissue and bony defects, (2) the hemodynamic stability of the patient, (3) the severity of ischemia in the extremity, (4) the duration of ischemia, and (5) the mechanism of injury. Numerous scoring systems have been developed in an attempt to predict which patients require amputation. One of the more commonly cited is the Mangled Extremity Severity Score. The scoring is based on four factors: the degree of energy of the injury, degree of limb ischemia, presence and degree of shock, and patient age. Attempts at prospective validation of this and other scoring systems have been met with mixed results. Good scores generally predict limb salvage, but high scores do not necessarily rule out the ability to save the limb. Although attempting limb salvage and reconstruction intuitively seems appropriate for all mangled extremities, this must be tempered by the fact that such attempts may lead to literally dozens of operations for nonunion and osteomyelitis and yet may still result in an anesthetic, nonfunctional limb that will be prone to ulceration. Thus, the trauma surgeon in conjunction with the orthopedic surgeon must use their best clinician judgment. Interestingly, a recent prospective multi-institutional study observed that patients with a mangled extremity reported a quality of life that was similar whether they underwent primary amputation or limb salvage.

Primary amputation should generally be considered for patients with a mangled lower extremity who are hemodynamically unstable and those with profound ischemia of more than 6 hours' duration, a complete amputation of the limb, and a Gustilo grade IIIC tibia/fibula fracture (>10 cm of soft-tissue defect that will require coverage and with arterial injury) with a transection of the tibial nerve. Tibial nerve transection is critical because this injury leads to paralysis of the muscles in the superficial and deep posterior compartments as well as complete anesthesia of the plantar surface of the foot. The Gustilo classification was created for open tibia fractures and is based on the degree of soft-tissue defect and on the vascular status (types I, II, IIIA, IIIB, and IIIC). Injury to the deep peroneal nerve would lead to loss of function of muscles in the anterior compartment with a subsequent footdrop due to an inability to dorsiflex the foot as well as numbness in the first web space. Such a deficit could be managed with an ankle-foot orthotic.

References: Bosse M, MacKenzie E, Kellam J, et al: A prospective evaluation of the clinical utility of the lower-extremity injury-severity scores, *J Bone Joint Surg Am* 83A:3–14, 2001.

Bosse M, McCarthy M, Jones A, et al, The Lower Extremity Assessment Project (LEAP) Study Group: the insensate foot following severe lower extremity trauma: an indication for amputation? *J Bone Joint Surg Am* 87A:2601–2608, 2005.

Quirke T, Sharma P, Boss W Jr, et al: Are type IIIC lower extremity injuries an indication for primary amputation? *J Trauma* 40:992–996, 1996.

28. D. Duodenal hematomas are caused by a direct blow to the abdomen and occur more often in children than adults. Blood accumulates between the seromuscular and submucosal layers, eventually causing obstruction. The diagnosis is suspected by the onset of vomiting after blunt abdominal trauma. A CT scan is the best diagnostic modality and helps differentiate a duodenal hematoma from a free perforation. The presence of contrast extravasation or free air indicates a free perforation and mandates exploratory laparotomy. In the absence of these findings, a presumptive diagnosis of a duodenal hematoma is made. If there is any question about perforation, a water-soluble upper gastrointestinal study can be performed. The classic finding on a contrast study is a coiled-spring appearance of the duodenal wall. The majority of such injuries in children are effectively managed nonoperatively by nasogastric tube decompression and parenteral nutrition because the hematoma impinges on the bowel lumen and leads to obstructive symptoms. Resolution of the obstruction in most patients occurs at an average of 14 days. If surgical intervention becomes necessary, evacuation of the hematoma by a partial-thickness incision in the duodenal wall, followed by closure, is associated with equal success but fewer complications than with a bypass.

References: Kunin J, Korobkin M, Ellis J, et al: Duodenal injuries caused by blunt abdominal trauma: value of CT in differentiating perforation from hematoma, *AJR Am J Roentgenol* 160:1221–1223, 1993.

Shilyansky J, Pearl R, Kreller M, et al: Diagnosis and management of duodenal injuries in children, *J Pediatr Surg* 32:880–886, 1997.

29. D. Damage control surgery consists of three phases. The first phase is abbreviated resuscitative surgery in which hemorrhage and bowel contamination are controlled. Definitive repairs that are not imminently life threatening, such as a reanastomosis of stapled small bowel, are delayed. The peritoneal cavity is packed, and temporary abdominal closure is quickly achieved. The second phase consists of rewarming, resuscitation, and correction of coagulopathy in the intensive care unit while performing a careful examination for additional injuries that may have been missed. The third phase involves re-exploration after normal physiology has been restored to remove packs and complete any additional procedures. All of the choices listed are indications for damage control except for choice D. Arterial injuries generally do not respond well to intra-abdominal packing and damage control. Proper exposure of such an injury would require a medial rotation of the left colon, kidney, and spleen.

Reference: Shapiro M, Jenkins D, Schwab C, Rotondo M: Damage control: collective review, *J Trauma* 49:969–978, 2000.

30. D. Various methods are used for liver bleeding. The simplest are topical hemostatic approaches using electrocautery, an argon beam coagulator, microcrystalline collagen, and fibrin glue, which is now available in a human recombinant form. If these are unsuccessful, liver stitches can be placed, using a chromic suture with a blunt-tipped needle. This is best used for relatively superficial lacerations. Another option is to perform a hepatotomy via a finger fracture technique to access the bleeding site to directly suture it. However, profuse bleeding from a small hole in the liver presents a more difficult dilemma because bleeding may be emanating from the center of the liver, and a hepatotomy may not be feasible. In this circumstance, one novel approach that has been well described is to fashion a balloon tamponade catheter. A catheter with side holes is placed through a Penrose drain, and a tie is placed on either end of the Penrose drain. The catheter is advanced into the bullet wound, and air is insufflated into the catheter, effectively inflating the Penrose drain and creating a tamponade effect. In this case, however, because the bleeding has stopped, there is no role for any additional treatment. Placing liver stitches is unnecessary and does increase the risk of causing liver necrosis. Packing the injury with omentum is useful in large stellate lesions, but hemostasis is better achieved in that setting with packing. Use of fibrin sealant has been associated with anaphylaxis, particularly when bovine sources are used; thus, its application in a nonbleeding liver is not recommended. Finally, the use of drains is controversial. For smaller wounds, drains are not recommended. For larger injuries, closed suction drainage is used by some surgeons. However, an open drain, such as a Penrose drain, is not recommended, because it seems to increase the risk of liver abscess.

31. D. The first step in the management algorithm of a penetrating neck trauma is establishing the airway, particularly in the presence of an expanding hematoma (which may rapidly compress the trachea), shock, or altered mental status. Next, it must be determined whether the patient has a "hard sign" of a vascular injury. In the presence of a rapidly expanding hematoma or visible exsanguination, the patient should be directly taken to the operating room for a neck exploration. The decision to go directly to the operating room is sometimes more difficult to make in the absence of these two signs. However, in the presence of hemodynamic instability, the presumption should be that the patient exsanguinated in the field. Thus, shock is another indication for immediate surgical exploration. In the absence of these findings in the hemodynamically stable patient, the next step would be to perform arteriography of the neck vessels. This historically has been achieved with formal arteriography, but is becoming replaced by CT angiography given the ease and rapidity of its use. In addition, an assessment for injuries to the aerodigestive tract (triple endoscopy and/or esophagography) and cervical spine needs to be performed. The treatment of penetrating carotid artery injuries remains controversial, particularly in the setting of a comatose patient. As a general guide, repairing a carotid artery injury in a patient with a neurologic deficit is recommended because it may result in improved neurologic function, whereas carotid ligation typically does not. If at surgery, the carotid artery is thrombosed, most vascular and trauma surgeons would recommend repair in the face of a neurologic deficit, provided back-bleeding from the internal carotid artery is obtained after resecting the injured segment. Repair can be achieved by arteriorrhaphy, resection with a primary reanastomosis, or interposition graft placement (saphenous vein or polytetrafluoroethylene). If a graft is needed, saphenous vein is preferred, provided the patient has now been stabilized in the operating room. While harvesting the vein, a temporary shunt should be inserted in the proximal and distal ends of the artery. If the patient does not adequately stabilize, the shunt can be placed inside the polytetrafluoroethylene graft. This allows the distal anastomosis and part of the proximal anastomosis to be performed while maintaining cerebral perfusion. The shunt can then be removed just before completing the second anastomosis. As soon as the repair is complete and provided the patient is stable, it is important not to forget to search for the bullet via radiograph of the head, neck, and chest.

32. C. Flail chest occurs when three or more ribs are fractured in at least two locations. Paradoxical movement of this free-floating segment of chest wall is typically not sufficient alone to compromise ventilation. Rather chest flail is due to the severe force that leads to an underlying pulmonary contusion. Most patients can be managed without intubation. Respiratory failure often does not occur immediately, and frequent re-evaluation is warranted. The initial chest radiograph usually underestimates the degree of pulmonary contusion, and the lesion tends to evolve with time and with fluid resuscitation. Intravenous fluid administration should be limited. The most important aspect of treatment of flail chest is pain control. Standard approaches include the use of patient-controlled analgesia and oral pain medications and the placement of continuous epidural catheters. Although the treatment of flail chest has historically been nonoperative, recent literature indicates that internal fixation of the chest wall in select patients without pulmonary contusion decreases intubation time, decreases complications, and improves cosmetic and functional results. In the presence of a pulmonary contusion, however, internal fixation does not seem to be as beneficial. Situations in which internal fixation should be considered include flail chest in patients who are already undergoing thoracotomy for an intrathoracic injury, flail chest without pulmonary contusion, noticeable paradoxical movement of a chest wall segment while a patient is being weaned from the respirator, and severe deformity of the chest wall.

References: Ahmed Z, Mohyuddin Z: Management of flail chest injury: internal fixation versus endotracheal intubation and ventilation, *J Thorac Cardiovasc Surg* 110:1676–1680, 1995.

Lardinois D, Krueger T, Dusmet M, et al: Pulmonary function testing after operative stabilization of the chest wall for flail chest, *Eur J Cardiothorac Surg* 20:496–501, 2001.

Voggenreiter G, Neudeck F, Aufmkolk M, et al: Operative chest wall stabilization in flail chest—outcomes of patients with or without pulmonary contusion, *J Am Coll Surg* 187:130–138, 1998.

33. E. A fistula between the internal carotid artery and the cavernous sinus is rare. It has been reported after basilar skull fractures as well as with penetrating trauma. It has also been reported to be caused by overaggressive inflation of a Fogarty catheter distally into the intracranial carotid artery. In one large study of 312 inpatients with basilar skull fractures, the overall incidence of a carotid cavernous fistula was 3.8% and was most common with a middle fossa fracture (8.3%). Basilar skull fractures should be suspected in the presence of hemotympanum and/or raccoon eyes, as in this patient. Symptoms and signs of a carotid cavernous fistula include eyelid edema, pulsatile exophthalmos, and auscultation of a bruit over the eye. Failure to recognize and treat this complication can lead to permanent vision loss. Treatment options include an open neurosurgical approach and endovascular embolization. This latter technique is emerging as the procedure of choice.

Reference: Liang W, Xiaofeng Y, Weiguo L, et al: Traumatic carotid cavernous fistula accompanying basilar skull fracture: a study on the incidence of traumatic carotid cavernous fistula in the patients with basilar skull fracture and the prognostic analysis about traumatic carotid cavernous fistula, *J Trauma* 63:1014–1020, 2007.

34. A. Compartment syndrome can occur anywhere in the extremities, including the thighs, buttocks, arms, and hands. The mechanisms of compartment syndrome are numerous and can be divided into extrinsic and intrinsic causes. Extrinsic causes include constriction by a cast, pneumatic garment, or tight circumferential dressings or eschar from a burn. Intrinsic causes are divided into bleeding, edema, and exogenous fluid. Bleeding is usually due to trauma, but can also be seen after relatively minor injuries in patients with an underlying coagulopathy or those receiving anticoagulants. Edema of the compartment is the largest and broadest category. It is most often seen after reperfusion of an ischemic limb, from either an arterial embolus or thrombosis or trauma. Ischemia/reperfusion is also seen in a person with a drug overdose or an alcoholic who falls asleep on the limb, in patients with profound shock in whom diffuse muscle ischemia with subsequent reperfusion develops, and after massive iliofemoral deep venous thrombosis. Finally, inadvertent infusion of IV fluid into the subcutaneous tissue can lead to compartment syndrome. Diagnosis of compartment syndrome begins by having a high clinical index of suspicion and knowing the clinical scenarios in which it occurs. The most common features are severe pain in the limb typically out of proportion to the injury, pain on passive motion of the limb, and tense edema with tenderness on palpation of the compartment. Distal arterial pulses typically remain palpable with compartment syndrome. The anterior compartment of the leg is usually the first compartment to be involved in the lower extremity. The deep peroneal nerve runs within it, so that numbness in the first web space of the toe is one of the early findings. Once the diagnosis is suspected, confirmation is sought by doing direct pressure measurements of the individual compartments. If the pressures are increased more than 30 mm Hg in any of the compartments, then strong consideration should be given to performing a four-compartment fasciotomy. It is also important to remember that there is no absolute pressure level that rules compartment syndrome in or out. The measurements should be used in conjunction with the patient's clinical examination. The deep posterior compartment is the one that is most commonly inadequately decompressed. Because this compartment contains the tibial nerve, missing this compartment can have devastating consequences. The soleus muscle must be detached from the tibia to decompress the deep posterior compartment.

35. C. Traumatic peripheral nerve injuries are divided into three grades based on severity. Neurapraxia is the mildest and is due to focal demyelination, as from a mild stretch or compression. The axon is left intact. Nerve conduction proximal and distal to the lesion is preserved. Axonotmesis is more severe than neurapraxia. The axon is damaged but the neural connective tissue sheath, epineurium, and Schwann cell tubes are preserved. Because these latter components are intact, axonal regeneration can occur. Axonotmesis is associated with distal wallerian degeneration. Neurotmesis is the most severe form and is seen with complete transection, damage, or disruption of the nerve. Regeneration cannot occur, and, thus, surgical repair is indicated. Traumatic peripheral nerve injury is much more common in the upper extremity. The most common injury is the radial nerve, associated with a humerus fracture. In the lower extremity, the peroneal nerve is the most commonly injured nerve. Posterior knee dislocation is associated with popliteal artery injury and rarely with tibial nerve injury. Regeneration of a peripheral nerve occurs at approximately 1 mm per day.

Reference: Noble J, Munro CA, Prasad VS, Midha R: Analysis of upper and lower extremity peripheral nerve injuries in a population of patients with multiple injuries, *J Trauma* 45:116–122, 1998.

36. B. Pancreatic injuries are graded from I to V. Grade I is a minor contusion or laceration without a duct injury, whereas grade V is a massive disruption of the pancreatic head. Most pancreatic injuries can be managed by closed suction drainage. The key issue is whether the main pancreatic duct is injured and whether such an injury is to the left of the superior mesenteric vessels. Determining whether the main pancreatic duct is injured can be done by intraoperative pancreatography, which can be performed by a needle injection of contrast into the gallbladder. A disruption of the pancreatic duct to the left of the superior mesenteric vessels can be managed by a distal pancreatectomy. Injury to the main duct to the right of the superior mesenteric vessels in the absence of major pancreatic head disruption is best managed by drainage with subsequent pancreaticoenteric anastomosis if an ensuing fistula fails to heal. Performing such an anastomosis in the emergent trauma setting poses a high risk of anastomotic breakdown. If there is massive destruction of the pancreatic head, as in the present case, a pancreatoduodenectomy will be necessary. It is important to note that such an operation does not have to be performed immediately. Undoubtedly, most of these patients will often have associated extensive bleeding. Therefore, a damage control procedure can be performed and a definitive procedure delayed until after resuscitation. Another indication for a Whipple procedure would be massive devascularization of the duodenum.

37. D. The patient's presentation is highly suggestive of a cardiac injury and pericardial tamponade. However, there is no immediate indication for endotracheal intubation, tube thoracostomy, pericardiocentesis, or thoracotomy/sternotomy. Tamponade is associated with the classic findings of the Beck triad (hypotension, distended neck, and muffled heart sounds) and pulsus paradoxus, but these are not reliably present. Pericardial tamponade impairs right heart filling, reducing right ventricular preload while increasing central venous pressure. It also leads to a decreased myocardial blood flow, subendocardial ischemia, and further reduction in cardiac output. Thus, the first step is to give the patient IV fluids. Early in tamponade, fluid administration will overcome the tamponade and lead to an improvement in hemodynamics. It is important for the trauma surgeon not to be lulled by this temporary improvement. Provided the patient remains hemodynamically stable, the next step would be to perform an emergent FAST scan to look for pericardial and intra-abdominal fluid. If the FAST scan findings are positive for pericardial fluid, the diagnosis of tamponade is confirmed, and the patient should be rapidly transported to the operating room. The incision of choice is a median sternotomy. If the patient were to suddenly decompensate before transport or before the FAST scan, a left anterolateral thoracotomy should be performed in the emergency department. The pericardium should first be opened longitudinally with care to avoid the phrenic nerve. The clot should be removed, and the cardiac injury temporarily controlled with a finger. In general, the insertion of Foley balloon catheters into the cardiac wound should be avoided because this tends to enlarge the wound. It is also important to be aware that positive-pressure ventilation can have a deleterious hemodynamic effect on patients with tamponade. Several authors have suggested a higher threshold for intubation in such patients. As such, if tamponade is suspected and a patient needs emergent intubation, rapid decompression of the pericardium needs to follow.

References: Cothren CC, Biffl WL, Moore EE: Trauma. In Brunicardi FC, Andersen DK, Billiar TR, et al, editors: *Schwartz's principles of surgery*, ed 9, New York, 2010, McGraw-Hill, pp 135–195.

Ho A, Graham C, Ng C, et al: Timing of tracheal intubation in traumatic cardiac tamponade: a word of caution, *Resuscitation* 80:272–274, 2009.

Hoyt DB, Coimbra R, Acosta J: Management of acute trauma. In Townsend CM Jr, Beauchamp RD, Evers BM, Mattox KL, editors: *Sabiston textbook of surgery: the biological basis of modern surgical practice*, ed 18, Philadelphia, 2008, WB Saunders, pp 477–520.

Möller C, Schoonbee C, Rosendorff C. Hemodynamics of cardiac tamponade during various modes of ventilation, *Br J Anaesth* 51:409–415, 1979.

Trauma and emergency care. In Cameron JL, *Current surgical therapy*, ed 9, Philadelphia, 2008, Mosby, pp 921–1083.

Venous and Lymphatic Disease 29

1. All of the following are true regarding venous circulation EXCEPT:

   A. The perforating veins in the leg direct blood flow from deep to the superficial system.
   B. The inferior vena cava (IVC) has no valves.
   C. In a healthy person, venous pressure decreases with walking.
   D. In patients with obstructed deep veins, venous pressure increases with walking.
   E. During ambulation, the calf muscle acts as a pump to overcome hydrostatic forces.

2. A 45-year-old woman presents with a nonhealing ulcer at the medial malleolus associated with leg edema and hyperpigmentation. Management consists of:

   A. Wet-to-dry dressings
   B. Split-thickness skin grafting
   C. Subfascial perforator ligation
   D. Linton procedure
   E. Compression dressings

3. Which of the following is the most common risk factor for spontaneous venous thromboembolism?

   A. Antithrombin III deficiency
   B. Factor V Leiden
   C. Protein C deficiency
   D. Protein S deficiency
   E. Antiphospholipid syndrome

4. All of the following are true regarding deep venous thrombosis (DVT) EXCEPT:

   A. Iliofemoral DVT can lead to gangrene.
   B. Iliac vein DVT is more common on the right than the left.
   C. Duplex ultrasonography is the diagnostic test of choice.
   D. Varicose veins are a risk factor for DVT.
   E. Smoking is a risk factor for DVT.

5. A 40-year-old woman presents with pain and tenderness at the site of a long-standing varicose vein in her calf. There is a palpable cord with surrounding erythema. Management consists of:

   A. Intavenous (IV) heparin sodium
   B. Subcutaneous low-molecular-weight heparin
   C. Warm compresses and nonsteroidal anti-inflammatory drugs
   D. Ligation of saphenofemoral junction
   E. IV antibiotics

6. All of the following are known complications of heparin EXCEPT:

   A. Teratogenesis
   B. Thrombocytopenia
   C. Arterial thrombosis
   D. Osteoporosis
   E. Skin necrosis

7. Which of the following is the best indication for placement of an IVC filter?

   A. For planned gastric surgery in someone with a recent DVT
   B. In a patient with severe pelvic fractures
   C. For a patient with a large free-floating vena cava thrombus
   D. For a recurrent DVT in a patient already taking Coumadin (warfarin)
   E. Before planned thrombolysis of a new DVT

8. A 25-year-old male college swimmer presents with sudden onset of right arm swelling and pain. A duplex ultrasound scan demonstrates thrombosis of the axillary-subclavian vein. The patient is started on IV heparin. Further management of this condition consists of:

   A. First rib resection
   B. Catheter-guided thrombolysis, stenting, and first rib resection
   C. Six months of Coumadin (warfarin)
   D. Catheter-guided thrombolysis and stenting
   E. Catheter-guided thrombolysis followed by first rib resection

9. The most common electrocardiographic change after pulmonary embolism (PE) is:

   A. Atrial fibrillation
   B. Right bundle branch block
   C. Nonspecific ST and T wave changes
   D. S1, Q3, T3 pattern
   E. Sinus tachycardia

10. A 25-year-old woman presents with a 1-day history of left leg pain, swelling, and a sense that the leg is going to burst. Physical examination is significant for massive diffuse swelling of the entire leg and thigh. Her medical history is negative. She does not use oral contraceptives and has had no recent plane flights. A duplex ultrasound scan shows an iliofemoral DVT. The recommended management approach would be:

    A. IV heparin, then 6 months of Coumadin (warfarin)
    B. Low-molecular-weight heparin, then 6 months of Coumadin (warfarin)
    C. Thrombolytic therapy and stenting of the left iliac vein if stenosis is found
    D. Thrombolytic therapy and angioplasty of the left iliac vein if stenosis is found
    E. Operative iliofemoral vein embolectomy

11. A reddish blue nodule develops in the left arm of a 70-year-old woman. The arm has been chronically swollen for 20 years after a modified radical mastectomy for breast cancer. The nodule most likely represents:

    A. Lymphangiosarcoma
    B. Kaposi sarcoma
    C. Capillary hemangioma
    D. Port-wine stain
    E. Strawberry hemangioma

12. The most common cause of primary lymphedema is:

    A. Congenital lymphedema
    B. Lymphedema praecox
    C. Lymphedema tarda
    D. Filariasis
    E. Malignancy

13. Primary management of lymphedema consists of:

    A. Complete decongestive physiotherapy
    B. Benzopyrone (coumarin)
    C. Prophylactic long-term antibiotics
    D. Graded compression stockings
    E. Diuretics

14. All of the following are characteristics of lymphedema EXCEPT:

    A. Predisposition to recurrent cellulitis
    B. "Buffalo hump" appearance of the dorsum of the foot
    C. Hyperpigmentation of the skin
    D. Peau d'orange appearance of the skin
    E. Thickening and squaring of toes

15. The test of choice for suspected lymphedema is:

    A. Lymphoscintigraphy
    B. Lymphangiography
    C. Computed tomography scan
    D. Magnetic resonance imaging
    E. Positron emission tomography scan

16. The following are true regarding hypercoagulable states EXCEPT:

    A. Prothrombin 20210 defect is the second most common inherited condition.
    B. Screening for antithrombin III deficiency cannot be done when a patient is taking heparin.
    C. Warfarin-induced skin necrosis is more common in patients with protein C deficiency.
    D. Lupus anticoagulant should be suspected if a patient has a prolonged activated partial thromboplastin time.
    E. Factor V Leiden is not a risk factor for arterial thromboembolic events.

17. All of the following are true regarding elevated serum homocysteine levels EXCEPT:

 A. It is associated with an increased risk of venous thrombosis.

 B. It is associated with an increased risk of coronary and cerebrovascular events.

 C. Elevated levels can be lowered by folic acid and vitamin B_{12} supplementation.

 D. Medically lowering levels reduces the risk of stroke and cardiovascular death.

 E. Aspirin supplementation is ineffective in lowering levels.

18. Warfarin inhibits the action of all of the following EXCEPT:

 A. Protein C

 B. Protein S

 C. Factor II

 D. Factor V

 E. Factor VII

19. Trauma patients sustaining what type of injury are at highest risk of venous thromboembolism?

 A. Head trauma

 B. Femur fracture

 C. Pelvic fracture

 D. Splenectomy

 E. Spinal cord injury

20. Argatroban:

 A. Activates antithrombin

 B. Is cleared by the kidneys

 C. Is reversed with fresh-frozen plasma

 D. Can be monitored by the activated partial thromboplastin time

 E. Has a 3-hour half-life

21. A 55-year-old man presents with erythema, warmth, and tenderness in the mid thigh along the course of the greater saphenous vein (GSV). On examination, a firm, tender cord is palpated along the medial thigh. The next step in the management consists of:

 A. Duplex ultrasound scan of the saphenous vein

 B. Duplex ultrasound scan of the saphenous and deep veins

 C. Oral antibiotics

 D. Oral nonsteroidal anti-inflammatory drugs

 E. IV heparin

22. A 45-year-old woman presents with a nonhealing ulcer along the medial malleolus for 1 year. She has associated hyperpigmentation of the adjacent skin and varicose veins. Findings of a distal pulse examination are normal. A duplex ultrasound scan reveals incompetence of the superficial veins. A trial of compression therapy was unsuccessful in achieving healing. Which of the following is the preferred surgical approach?

 A. Subfascial endoscopic perforator ligation

 B. Vein valve transplantation to the popliteal vein

 C. GSV vein stripping

 D. GSV vein high ligation

 E. Stab avulsion of varicose veins

23. Lepirudin:

 A. Is a direct thrombin inhibitor

 B. Is cleared by the liver

 C. Is reversed with cryoprecipitate

 D. Is monitored by the international normalized ratio

 E. Binds to platelet factor 4

Answers

1. A. The lower extremity veins are divided into superficial, perforating, and deep veins. The superficial venous system consists of the greater saphenous and lesser saphenous veins. The deep veins follow the course of major arteries. Paired veins parallel the anterior and posterior tibial and peroneal arteries and join to form the popliteal vein. The popliteal vein becomes the superficial femoral vein as it passes through the adductor hiatus. In the proximal thigh, the superficial femoral vein joins with the deep femoral vein to form the common femoral vein. Multiple perforating veins traverse the deep fascia to connect the superficial and deep venous systems. The most important perforators are the Cockett and Boyd perforators. The Cockett perforators drain the lower part of the leg medially, whereas the Boyd perforators connect the GSV to the deep vein higher up in the medial lower leg, approximately 10 cm below the knee. Blood flows from the superficial to the deep venous system. Incompetence of these perforators is a major contributor to the development of venous stasis and ulceration. There are no valves in the portal vein, superior vena cava or IVC, or common iliac vein. The calf muscles serve an important function in augmenting venous return by acting as a pump to return blood to the heart. For this reason, patients who are bedridden are prone to venous stasis.

Venous pressure drops dramatically with walking due to the action of the calf muscles, but increases in patients with venous obstruction.

2. E. This patient has classic signs of chronic venous insufficiency. Venous stasis ulcers are classically located at the medial malleolus. The precise cause of venous stasis ulcers is unclear, but seems to be multifactorial. The increased venous pressure from incompetent valves results in an impedance of capillary flow, which leads to leukocyte trapping. These leukocytes release oxygen free radicals and proteolytic enzymes that lead to local inflammation. The increased venous pressure also leads to the leakage of protein. The first-line therapy for treatment of venous stasis ulcers is compression therapy. The work-up for this patient should include a duplex ultrasound scan of the venous system, specifically looking for valvular incompetence of the deep, superficial, and perforating veins. A popular and effective compression bandage is the Unna boot, which contains zinc oxide, glycerin, gelatin, and calamine lotion. The boot should be wrapped starting at the foot, up to just below the knee. It can remain in place for as long as a week. It should not be used in the setting of an active infection of the ulcer.

3. B. The primary risk factors for spontaneous venous thromboembolism (VTE), as described by Virchow, include stasis of blood flow, endothelial injury, and hypercoagulability. In cases of spontaneous VTE, hypercoagulability is most important. Factors that contribute to hypercoagulability include factor V Leiden, prothrombin gene mutation, protein C and S deficiency, antithrombin III deficiency, elevated homocysteine levels, and antiphospholipid syndrome. In addition, smoking, obesity, pregnancy, malignancy, and use of oral contraceptives are also known to induce hypercoagulability. In surgical patients, the cause of VTE is multifactorial because postoperative stasis from prolonged bed rest and endothelial injury from trauma or recent surgery are significant factors. In trauma patients, spinal cord injury has the highest risk for VTE. Other risk factors for VTE include history of VTE, advanced age, obesity, varicose veins, cardiac disease, oral contraceptive use, smoking, and pregnancy. Factor V Leiden is the most common genetic defect associated with thrombophilia. Factor V Leiden is a single-point mutation in the gene that codes for coagulation factor V. The mutation is transmitted in an autosomal dominant fashion. It makes factor V resistant to inactivation by activated protein C (which is a natural anticoagulant protein). Factor V Leiden accounts for 92% of cases of anticoagulant protein resistance. Other causes include pregnancy, oral contraceptive use, and cancer. The mutation is present in 4% to 6% of the general population and is associated with a sixfold increased risk of VTE in heterozygotes. In homozygotes, the risk is 80-fold. In patients with their first VTE, factor V Leiden was present in 15% to 20%. Interestingly, in one study, the risk of recurrent VTE was similar among carriers of the factor V Leiden gene compared with those without this mutation, suggesting that they do not need longer anticoagulation than standard recommendation for a first-time event.

Reference: Mazza J: Hypercoagulability and venous thromboembolism: a review, *WMJ* 103:41–49, 2004.

4. B. A massive DVT, particularly one involving the iliac and common femoral veins, results in marked leg swelling due to significantly impaired venous return leading to phlegmasia cerulea and alba dolens. These entities can lead to gangrene of the extremity if not promptly managed. Iliac vein DVT occurs more commonly on the left. This is likely the result of the left iliac vein frequently being compressed by the right iliac artery (known as May-Thurner syndrome). In addition to the commonly known risk factors for DVT, smoking and varicose veins have been shown to be independent risk factors. Ultrasonography is the diagnostic study of choice to assess for the presence of DVT. Diagnostic features include the presence of thrombus and noncompressibility of the vein.

References: Hansson P, Eriksson H, Welin L, et al: Smoking and abdominal obesity: risk factors for venous thromboembolism among middle-aged men: "the study of men born in 1913," *Arch Intern Med* 159:1886–1890, 1999.

Heit J, Silverstein M, Mohr D, et al: Risk factors for deep vein thrombosis and pulmonary embolism: a population-based case-control study, *Arch Intern Med* 160:809–815, 2000.

5. C. The patient has superficial venous thrombosis (SVT) or superficial thrombophlebitis (STP). This entity is essentially a clotted surface vein. A palpable cord is suggestive of the diagnosis, as are the accompanying pain and erythema. There are a few pitfalls in the diagnosis and management of STP. First, patients with STP have a high rate of concomitant DVT (5%–40%); thus, a duplex ultrasound scan of the venous system is essential. Second, STP can easily be misdiagnosed as cellulitis, in which case antibiotics may be inappropriately prescribed and a duplex ultrasound scan not obtained. Third, STPs in the upper thigh, within 1 cm of the saphenofemoral junction, have a significant risk of propagating into the deep system. STPs near the saphenofemoral junction should be treated with systemic anticoagulation or ligation of the saphenous vein at the junction. If it is not close to the femoral vein, a follow-up duplex ultrasound scan should be performed in 5 to 7 days to determine evidence of more proximal propagation. STPs are usually sterile, but if they develop in association with an IV line, with fever and leukocytosis, this may represent suppurative thrombophlebitis. This would mandate removal of the line, IV antibiotics, and, on occasion, surgical removal of the infected vein. Finally, patients in whom STPs develop spontaneously, in the absence of varicose veins or a recent IV line, should have a careful history and physical examination to try to uncover evidence of hypercoagulability. Multiple episodes of migratory STP are associated with malignancy (Trousseau sign). Treatment of an STP consists of compression and administration of anti-inflammatory therapy.

References: Chengelis D, Bendick P, Glover J, et al: Progression of superficial venous thrombosis to deep vein thrombosis, *J Vasc Surg* 24:745–749, 1996.

Jorgensen J, Hanel K, Morgan A, et al: The incidence of deep venous thrombosis in patients with superficial thrombophlebitis of the lower limbs, *J Vasc Surg* 18:70–73, 1993.

6. A. Heparin-induced thrombocytopenia (HIT) is a well-recognized complication of heparin therapy. It is caused by heparin-dependent, platelet-activating IgG antibodies against the heparin–platelet factor 4 complex. The resulting platelet activation is associated with increased thrombin generation. HIT typically presents 5 to 10 days after heparin is instituted. If the patient has had a recent previous exposure, the platelet count drop can occur sooner (within a day) with re-exposure. The condition can lead to thrombotic complications, including stroke, myocardial infarction, PE, and peripheral arterial thrombosis. The 4T scoring system has been established to determine the pretest probability of HIT. The four factors include the degree of thrombocytopenia (>50% decrease, 30%–50% decrease, and <30% decrease), the timing of the heparin drop (typically from 5 to 10 days, although sooner if there has been recent previous heparin exposure), evidence of thrombosis, and whether a definite alternative explanation exists for thrombocytopenia. The scoring system is most useful for its negative predictive value. Testing for HIT involves performing an enzyme-linked immunosorbent assay to detect antibodies against the heparin–platelet factor 4 complex. Because false positives occur, if the results of this test are positive, an additional assay is performed using platelets and serum from the patient (called a serotonin release assay). If the results of this test are positive, the patient is considered to have HIT. Because these tests take time, it is imperative that medical management be instituted without waiting for the test results. Management consists of discontinuing all forms of heparin (including heparin flushes) and administering one of two alternative anticoagulants: argatroban or lepirudin. Both are direct thrombin inhibitors. Both can be monitored by the activated partial thromboplastin time, and both have relatively short half-lives (60–90 minutes for lepirudin and 40–50 minutes for argatroban). Neither can be reversed. Argatroban is cleared by hepatic metabolism, whereas lepirudin is cleared by the kidneys. Lepirudin is made by recombinant DNA, but was first derived from the leech (and called hirudin). Heparin-induced skin necrosis is a well-described complication of either IV or SC injection of unfractionated heparin. It is less common than warfarin-induced skin necrosis. Affected areas are usually fat laden, such as the abdomen, as in warfarin-induced necrosis; however, the distal extremities and the nose can also be involved. The appearance of erythema is followed by purpura and hemorrhage, leading to skin necrosis. Although the lesions appear similar to warfarin-induced skin necrosis, deficiencies of protein C and S are not present. Another complication of prolonged heparin use is osteopenia, which results from impairment of bone formation and enhancement of bone resorption by heparin. This complication has most often been reported in pregnant women receiving long-term heparin for DVT. Heparin is a category C drug and can be used in pregnancy, whereas warfarin is teratogenic.

References: Dahlman T: Osteoporotic fractures and the recurrence of thromboembolism during pregnancy and the puerperium in 184 women undergoing thromboprophylaxis with heparin, *Am J Obstet Gynecol* 168:1265–1270, 1993.

Hirsh J, Heddle N, Kelton J: Treatment of heparin-induced thrombocytopenia: a critical review. *Arch Intern Med* 164:361–369, 2004.

Lo G, Juhl D, Warkentin T, et al: Evaluation of pretest clinical score (4 T's) for the diagnosis of heparin-induced thrombocytopenia in two clinical settings, *J Thromb Haemost* 4:759–765, 2006.

7. D. Enthusiasm for the aggressive use of IVC filters is tempered by the sobering fact that filters left in place for long periods of time, although effective in preventing PE, lead to a significantly increased risk of recurrent DVT in the extremities. In a prospective randomized study of patients with DVT, the routine addition of an IVC filter did not improve mortality compared with heparin and warfarin alone. IVC filters are either permanent or retrievable. Retrievable filters should optimally be removed within 2 weeks. So they are ideally used in a situation in which there is a short-term need for protection against PE. Absolute indications for permanent IVC filter placement include a venous thromboembolic event (VTE [DVT or PE]) in a patient who has a contraindication to anticoagulation (such as active gastrointestinal bleeding), a new VTE that develops in a patient who is already receiving anticoagulation, or a patient with a VTE who is already receiving anticoagulation and in whom a major hemorrhage develops. Relative indications for a retrievable filter placement include before planned thrombolysis of a new DVT (as the thrombus may break off toward the lungs during the lysis process), a recent DVT and planned major surgery, and prophylaxis in severe head, pelvic, or spinal cord trauma. Relative indications for a permanent IVC filter include a patient with a VTE who is poorly compliant with anticoagulant therapy, recurrent episodes of VTE, and the presence of a large free-floating thrombus in the IVC. There are eight different permanent filters and three different retrievable filters available in the United States.

References: Decousus H, Leizorovicz A, Parent F, et al: A clinical trial of vena caval filters in the prevention of pulmonary embolism in patients with proximal deep-vein thrombosis, *N Engl J Med* 338:409–415, 1998.

Millward S, Oliva V, Bell S, et al: Günther tulip retrievable vena cava filter: results from the Registry of the Canadian Interventional Radiology Association, *J Vasc Interv Radiol* 12:1053–1058, 2001.

8. E. The Paget-Schroetter syndrome, also known as effort-induced thrombosis, is a spontaneous thrombosis of the axillary-subclavian vein. It is thought to be, in most instances, a manifestation of thoracic outlet syndrome, whereby a hypertrophied or aberrant muscle compresses the axillary-subclavian vein as it passes between the first rib and the clavicle. It tends to develop in young active patients after vigorous activity, although it can also occur spontaneously. It usually presents in young and otherwise healthy patients and in men more often than women. Diagnosis is best established via duplex ultrasonography. The patient should be promptly started on IV heparin. Numerous studies have shown the benefit of catheter-directed thrombolysis for this condition, currently using tissue plasminogen activator. After completion of thrombolytic therapy, a follow-up venogram is obtained to identify any correctable anatomic abnormalities. Stenting a residual stenosis in this area without decompressing the thoracic outlet is contraindicated because the ongoing compression will invariably crush the stent and cause further venous damage. Residual venous stenoses can be treated with angioplasty, although some authors recommend doing this after the first rib resection. One area of debate is whether routine first rib resection is necessary after successful thrombolysis. The majority of articles favor performing a first rib resection, which is most often done via a transaxillary approach. In an active athlete, and in particular one who performs repetitive movement with the arm overhead (which by itself can compress the vein), first rib resection is the best option. The timing of first rib resection is also controversial. In the past, first rib resection was delayed after lysis, treating the patient with 3 months of Coumadin (warfarin). Recent studies indicate that the first rib resection can be safely and effectively performed at the initial hospitalization after thrombolysis.

References: Angle N, Gelabert H, Farooq M, et al: Safety and efficacy of early surgical decompression of the thoracic outlet for Paget-Schroetter syndrome, *Ann Vasc Surg* 15:37–42, 2001.

Lee W, Bradley B, Harris E, et al: Surgical intervention is not required for all patients with subclavian vein thrombosis, *J Vasc Surg* 35:57–67, 2000.

Machleder HI: Evaluation of a new treatment strategy for Paget-Schroetter syndrome: spontaneous thrombosis of the axillary-subclavian vein, *J Vasc Surg* 17:305–315, 1993.

Urschel H, Razzuk M: Paget-Schroetter syndrome: what is the best management? *Ann Thorac Surg* 69:1663–1668, 2000.

9. E. The most common finding on electrocardiography after a PE is sinus tachycardia (present in almost one half of patients). A heart rate greater than 100 beats per minute in the setting of suspected PE should further raise concern. The classic finding on an electrocardiogram is the S1, Q3, T3 pattern, which consists of a prominent S wave in lead I and a Q wave and inverted T wave in lead III. This electrocardiographic finding indicates right ventricular strain from a large PE, but it is not commonly present. A large PE will lead to an enlargement of the right ventricle causing the interventricular septum to deviate to the left. The right bundle branch stretches, leading to a right bundle branch block.

10. C. This patient has a DVT of the left iliac and femoral veins. There are several issues to be considered in this patient. The first is why the DVT developed. In a young patient with no other risk factors and a left-sided iliofemoral DVT, one must consider May-Thurner syndrome. Because of the markedly reduced venous return, patients with iliofemoral DVT are at particular risk of chronic swelling and manifestations of chronic venous stasis. Given this, several authors have investigated the use of thrombolytic therapy for iliofemoral DVT. Thrombolysis has been shown to decrease the incidence of post-thrombotic symptoms and improve the quality of life in patients with iliofemoral DVT compared with standard heparin and Coumadin (warfarin) therapy. If lysis is successful but a residual stenosis is evident in the iliac vein, long-term patency seems to be improved with the placement of a stent. Operative iliofemoral embolectomy is rarely used today, but might be indicated in the setting of phlegmasia alba dolens that does not respond to catheter-guided thrombolysis.

References: Comerota A, Throm R, Mathias S, et al: Catheter-directed thrombolysis for iliofemoral deep venous thrombosis improves health-related quality of life, *J Vasc Surg* 32:130–137, 2000.

O'Sullivan G, Semba C, Bittner C, et al: Endovascular management of iliac vein compression (May-Thurner) syndrome, *J Vasc Interv Radiol* 11:823–836, 2000.

Patel N, Stookey K, Ketcham D, et al: Endovascular management of acute extensive iliofemoral deep venous thrombosis caused by May-Thurner syndrome, *J Vasc Interv Radiol* 11:1297–1302, 2000.

11. A. Lymphangiosarcoma (Stewart-Treves syndrome) is a rare, highly lethal malignancy that develops in extremities with chronic lymphedema, in particular after axillary lymph node dissection for breast cancer. Lymphangiosarcoma actually arises from blood vessels instead of lymphatic vessels (and thus is more appropriately named angiosarcoma) and may manifest as soon as 1 year or as late as 30 years after the onset of lymphedema. Presenting symptoms and signs include purple-colored patches that then form plaques or nodules, a palpable subcutaneous mass, or a poorly healing eschar with recurrent bleeding and infection. Small satellite areas may develop around the nodules. The tumor does not respond well to chemotherapy or radiation. Surgical therapy is the best option. A comparison of early amputation with wide local excision showed no difference in outcome. Despite surgical management, the prognosis is poor, with a high rate of local recurrence and metastasis. The best chance for a good outcome is to alert the patient with lymphedema for the symptoms and signs and take an early and aggressive surgical approach. Kaposi sarcoma has some clinical and histologic features that are similar to those of Stewart-Treves syndrome and has been reported very rarely to develop in lymphedematous extremities.

Reference: Grobmyer S, Daly J, Glotzbach R, Grobmyer A: Role of surgery in the management of postmastectomy extremity angiosarcoma (Stewart-Treves syndrome), *J Surg Oncol* 73:182–188, 2000.

12. B. Lymphedema is divided into primary (with no cause) and secondary (there is a known cause). Primary lymphedema is subdivided into three types: congenital, praecox, and tarda. Congenital lymphedema is present at birth. A familial version of congenital lymphedema is called Milroy disease. Lymphedema praecox develops during childhood or teenage years and accounts for 80% to 90% of cases of primary lymphedema and is 10 times more common in women. It starts usually in the foot or lower leg. Lymphedema tarda is defined as starting after age 35. Secondary lymphedema is more common than primary lymphedema. Worldwide infestation by *Wuchereria bancrofti* (filariasis) is the most common cause, whereas in the United States, the most common cause is post–axillary node dissection.

13. D. It is important when treating patients with lymphedema that they recognize that there is no curative therapy. Patients with lymphedema are at significantly increased risk of contracting recurrent infections and the development of progressive swelling and disability of the leg. With this in mind, compression stockings have been shown to be useful in reducing edema and are the mainstay of treatment. The stockings should ideally be custom fitted. The amount of compression needed for lymphedema is typically greater than for venous stasis and is as high 60 mm Hg. The effect of benzopyrones (coumarin) on lymphedema has been studied in two prospective randomized trials. In one study, there was benefit, and in the other, there was none. The latter study was limited to women with postsurgical arm lymphedema, whereas the first study included primary lymphedema. Coumarin (which has no anticoagulant effect) is thought to reduce edema through the stimulation of macrophages that enhance proteolysis. Complete decongestive physiotherapy has been shown to be effective and involves manual massage of the extremity. It must be used in combination with compression stockings. Compression pumps have also been shown to be effective. Diuretics may temporarily improve lymphedema, especially with mild cases and early on, but do not have any long-term benefit. Patients with lymphedema are predisposed to the development of cellulitis, and these infections can further damage lymphatics. As such, an aggressive approach to the treatment of infection is warranted. However, prophylactic antibiotics have no role. For advanced cases that do not respond to conservative management, the Charles procedure has been performed, which involves complete and circumferential excision of the skin, subcutaneous tissues, and deep fascia of the leg and dorsum of the foot. The exposed muscle is then grafted with a full- or split-thickness skin graft.

References: Casley-Smith J, Morgan R, Piller N: Treatment of lymphedema of the arms and legs with 5,6-benzo-[alpha]-pyrone, *N Engl J Med* 329:1158–1163, 1993.

Ko D, Lerner R, Klose G, et al: Effective treatment of lymphedema of the extremities, *Arch Surg* 133:452–458, 1998.

Loprinzi C, Kugler J, Sloan J, et al: Lack of effect of coumarin in women with lymphedema after treatment for breast cancer, *N Engl J Med* 340:346–350, 1999.

14. C. Distinguishing between chronic venous stasis and lymphedema on physical examination can be difficult, particularly early in their course. Both patient groups will report heaviness and fatigue in the limb, which tends to worsen at the end of a day of prolonged standing. Venous stasis tends to be more pitting and lymphedema nonpitting. Venous stasis tends to spare the foot and toes, whereas lymphedema involves them. The swollen dorsum of the foot has a buffalo hump appearance, and toes look squared off. Recurrent cellulitis is a common complication of lymphedema. In advanced lymphedema, the skin develops a peau d'orange appearance (similar to inflammatory disease of the breast), lichenification, and hyperkeratosis. Hyperpigmentation of the skin, due to hemosiderin deposition, is seen in venous insufficiency and not usually with lymphedema.

15. A. Although the diagnosis of lymphedema can be fairly obvious in advanced stages, early on it may be difficult to determine based on physical examination alone. If the cause of the lymphedema is obvious, such as post–lymph node dissection, then further work-up is not necessary. Conversely, in situations in which lymphedema is suspected but the diagnosis is unclear, lymphoscintigraphy is the diagnostic test of choice. Once the diagnosis of lymphedema is established, computed tomography and/or magnetic resonance imaging can be useful to rule out other pathology that may be precipitating the lymphedema and to more accurately stage the degree of lymphedema. Lymphangiography is more invasive, involves direct injection of dye into the lymphatic vessels, and can irritate the lymphatic vessels, leading to further damage, so it is only recommended for the rare patient who is to undergo a direct lymphatic reconstruction.

Reference: Cambria R, Gloviczki P, Naessens J, et al: Noninvasive evaluation of the lymphatic system with lymphoscintigraphy: a prospective, semiquantitative analysis in 386 extremities, *J Vasc Surg* 18:773–782, 1993.

16. E. Warfarin acts in the liver by inhibiting vitamin K–dependent procoagulant factors II, VII, IX, and X and anticoagulants (proteins C and S). Warfarin takes several days to achieve its full effect because residual normal coagulation factors have to be cleared. An unusual complication of warfarin is the development of skin necrosis. This complication, which usually occurs on the first days of therapy, is associated with protein C and S and factor VII deficiency and malignancy. When warfarin is instituted, protein C and S levels drop quickly (due to their short half-life) and do so earlier than do the procoagulants. This drop creates an early hypercoagulable effect and is exacerbated in patients with preexisting protein C and S deficiency. This can lead to thrombus formation in venules feeding the skin, resulting in extensive skin and subcutaneous fat necrosis. Heparin acts as an anticoagulant by binding to antithrombin and potentiating antithrombin's inhibition of thrombin and activated factor X. The administration of heparin creates a drop in antithrombin III levels. Patients with factor V Leiden are predisposed to venous and arterial thromboembolic events, although venous events are much more common. Prothrombin 20210 defect (G20210A mutation) is the second most common inherited predisposition to hypercoagulability. Antiphospholipid syndrome includes two main types: the lupus anticoagulants and the anticardiolipin antibodies. Lupus anticoagulants prolong the activated partial thromboplastin time. Anticardiolipin antibodies are detected by enzyme-linked immunosorbent assay. The syndrome is associated with several autoimmune disorders such as systemic lupus erythematosus, Sjögren syndrome, and rheumatoid arthritis and leads to venous or arterial thrombosis.

Reference: Nowak-Göttl U, Koch H, Aschka I, et al: Resistance to activated protein C (APCR) in children with venous or arterial thromboembolism, *Br J Haematol* 92:992–998, 1996.

17. D. Several studies have demonstrated that elevated serum levels of homocysteine are an independent risk factor for both venous thrombosis and peripheral artery disease. Likewise, several studies have shown that vitamin supplementation, in particular with folate and vitamin B_{12}, is effective in lowering serum homocysteine levels. Some newer studies suggest that vitamin B_{12} may be more important than folate. Intuitively, one would expect, therefore, that aggressive lowering of homocysteine levels with vitamin supplementation would be effective in preventing cardiovascular events. In fact, in one study, the rate of coronary restenosis was decreased with vitamin supplementation. However, a recent large trial indicated that moderate reduction of total homocysteine after nondisabling cerebral infarction had no effect on vascular outcomes during the 2 years of follow-up. As such, current guidelines are backpedaling away from an aggressive vitamin regimen for homocysteine lowering.

References: Clarke R, Daly L, Robinson K, et al: Hyperhomocysteinemia: an independent risk factor for vascular disease, *N Engl J Med* 324:1149–1155, 1991.

Hankey G, Eikelboom J: Folic acid-based multivitamin therapy to prevent stroke: the jury is still out, *Stroke* 35:1995–1998, 2004.

Schnyder G, Roffi M, Pin R, et al: Decreased rate of coronary restenosis after lowering of plasma homocysteine levels, *N Engl J Med* 345:1593–1600, 2001.

Toole J, Malinow R, Chambless L, et al: Lowering homocysteine in patients with ischemic stroke to prevent recurrent stroke, myocardial infarction and death: the Vitamin Intervention for Stroke Prevention (VISP) randomized controlled trial, *JAMA* 291:565–575, 2004.

18. D. Warfarin inhibits vitamin K–dependent coagulation factors, including factors II, VII, IX, and X as well as proteins C and S.

19. E. The increased risk of the development of VTE in surgical patients is multifactorial. Patients will have a period of activated coagulation, transient depression of fibrinolysis, and temporary immobilization. In addition, many patients may have a central venous catheter in place and have concomitant cardiac disease, malignancy, or intrinsic hypercoagulable states. Trauma patients, in particular, have a high risk of VTE. In trauma patients, spinal cord injury (odds ratio, 8.33) and fracture of the femur or tibia (odds ratio, 4.82) were the injuries with the greatest risk of VTE. In one large prospective study, other risk factors in trauma patients on multivariate analysis included older age, blood transfusion, and need for surgery.

Reference: Geerts W, Code K, Jay R, et al: A prospective study of venous thromboembolism after major trauma, *N Engl J Med* 331:1601–1606, 1994.

20. D. Argatroban and lepirudin are both direct thrombin inhibitors and used for HIT and thrombosis. Both can be monitored by the activated partial thromboplastin time and both have relatively short half-lives (60–90 minutes for lepirudin and 40–50 minutes for argatroban). Neither can be reversed and neither requires the presence of antithrombin to be effective. Argatroban is cleared by hepatic metabolism, whereas lepirudin is cleared by the kidneys. In addition to being used for HIT, argatroban is approved in patients with or at risk of HIT who are undergoing percutaneous coronary intervention. Argatroban has a short half-life (39–51 minutes) and reaches a steady state with IV infusion at 1 to 3 hours. Because it is cleared by hepatic metabolism, it is the drug of choice for patients with HIT and renal insufficiency.

21. B. As discussed in question 5, this patient has superficial thrombophlebitis of the GSV. This case is more concerning, however, because the superficial clot is closer to his saphenofemoral junction. The patient requires a duplex ultrasound scan to rule out concomitant DVT and to determine how far the clot is from the saphenofemoral junction. Provided the clot is not within a centimeter of the junction, the patient can be managed with nonsteroidal anti-inflammatory drugs. A repeat duplex ultrasound scan should be obtained within 5 to 7 days. If the clot is close to the saphenofemoral junction, then IV heparin and Coumadin (warfarin) would be recommended rather than ligation of the saphenofemoral junction.

References: Chengelis D, Bendick P, Glover J, et al: Progression of superficial venous thrombosis to deep vein thrombosis, *J Vasc Surg* 24:745–749, 1996.

Freischlag JA, Heller JA: Venous disease. In Townsend CM Jr, Beauchamp RD, Evers BM, Mattox KL, editors: *Sabiston textbook of surgery: the biological basis of modern surgical practice*, ed 18, Philadelphia, 2008, WB Saunders, pp 2002–2019.

Jorgensen J, Hanel K, Morgan A, et al: The incidence of deep venous thrombosis in patients with superficial thrombophlebitis of the lower limbs, *J Vasc Surg* 18:70–73, 1993.

Liem TK, Moneta GL: Venous and lymphatic disease. In Brunicardi FC, Andersen DK, Billiar TR, et al, editors: *Schwartz's principles of surgery*, ed 9, New York, 2010, McGraw-Hill, pp 777–801.

Piponos IL, Baxter BT: The lymphatics. In Townsend CM Jr, Beauchamp RD, Evers BM, Mattox KL, editors: *Sabiston textbook of surgery: the biological basis of modern surgical practice*, ed 18, Philadelphia, 2008, WB Saunders, pp 2020–2028.

22. C. As mentioned in the response to question 2, the primary management for venous stasis ulceration is compression therapy. However, the work-up for a newly diagnosed venous stasis ulcer should include a duplex ultrasound scan to look for incompetence of the valvular system. Incompetence can be present in any one or a combination of the superficial, deep, or perforating veins. In patients in whom compression therapy fails, correcting or eliminating valvular incompetence can lead to ulcer healing. Studies comparing results of compression therapy with those of surgery indicate that the percentage of ulcers that heal overall is about the same. However, patients undergoing surgery heal faster and have significantly lower ulcer recurrence rates. Isolated superficial vein (GSV) incompetence is underrecognized as a cause of venous stasis ulcer, yet studies have shown that it is present in as many as 50% of patients with ulcers. As a general rule, if a patient has superficial vein incompetence, that is corrected first because eliminating superficial vein incompetence is relatively straightforward and involves stripping of the GSV and is effective in the majority of patients in achieving healing. Simple high ligation of the GSV is not as effective. More recently, this is being performed with radiofrequency ablation. However, the role of radiofrequency ablation for venous ulceration has yet to be defined. If the patient has perforator incompetence, subfascial endoscopic perforator surgery (SEPS) has been shown to be effective in achieving healing. This technique has largely replaced the Linton procedure, which involved a large open incision to essentially achieve the same effect. The Linton procedure created potential for immense wound healing complications. Subfascial endoscopic perforator surgery involves placing endoscopic trocars subfascially. Carbon dioxide is used to insufflate the subfascial space. The perforators are identified and doubly clipped and divided. This can also be used in combination with GSV stripping if the patient has combined superficial and perforator incompetence. Before performing these procedures, it is important to document the patency of the deep system. If a patient has isolated deep system incompetence, numerous techniques of deep venous valve correction have been reported, such as transplanting a segment of brachial vein containing a valve to the popliteal vein (so-called vein valve transplantation). However, in patients with ulceration, 40% to 50% had persistence or recurrence of ulcers in the long term.

References: Bello M, Scriven M, Hartshorne T, et al: Role of superficial venous surgery in the treatment of venous ulceration, *Br J Surg* 86:755–759, 1999.

Gohel M, Barwell J, Earnshaw J, et al: Randomized clinical trial of compression plus surgery versus compression alone in chronic venous ulceration (ESCHAR study)—hemodynamic and anatomical changes, *Br J Surg* 92:291–297, 2005.

Zamboni P, Cisno C, Marchetti F, et al: Minimally invasive surgical management of primary venous ulcers vs. compression treatment: a randomized clinical trial, *Eur J Vasc Endovasc Surg* 26: 337–338, 2003.

23. A. Lepirudin is made by recombinant DNA, but was first derived from the leech (and called hirudin). The loading dose is 0.4 mg/kg, followed by a continuous infusion of 0.15 mg/kg. Because it is cleared by renal metabolism, it is the drug of choice for patients with HIT and hepatic insufficiency. It does not bind to platelet factor 4.

References: Freischlag JA, Heller JA: Venous disease. In Townsend CM Jr, Beauchamp RD, Evers BM, Mattox KL, editors: *Sabiston textbook of surgery: the biological basis of modern surgical practice*, ed 18, Philadelphia, 2008, WB Saunders, pp 2002–2019.

Liem TK, Moneta GL: Venous and lymphatic disease. In Brunicardi FC, Andersen DK, Billiar TR, et al, editors: *Schwartz's principles of surgery*, ed 9, New York, 2010, McGraw-Hill, pp 777–801.